Radiology Core Review

Edited by

Alexander G Pitman BMedSci MBBS FRANZCR

Director of Radiology, Department of Radiology
Specialist in Nuclear Medicine, Department of Nuclear Medicine
and Centre for Positron Emission Tomography
Peter MacCallum Cancer Institute
Melbourne, Australia
Senior Fellow, Department of Radiology
Senior Fellow, Department of Anatomy
The University of Melbourne
Melbourne, Australia

Nancy M Major MD

Associate Professor of Radiology and Surgery
Division of Orthopaedics
Duke University Medical Center
Durham, NC, USA

Richard Tello BS BSE MS(MIT) MD (Stanford) MPH (Harvard)

Professor of Radiology, Epidemiology and Biostatistics
Boston University School of Medicine
Boston, MA, USA

SAUNDERS

An Imprint of Elsevier Science

Edinburgh   London   New York   Oxford   Philadelphia   St Louis   Sydney   Toronto   2003

WB SAUNDERS
An imprint of Elsevier Science Limited

First published 2003

ISBN 0702026190

British Library Cataloguing in Publication Data
A catalogue record for this book is available from the British Library

Library of Congress Cataloging in Publication Data
A catalog record for this book is available from the Library of Congress

Notice
Medical knowledge is constantly changing. Standard safety precautions must be followed, but as new research and clinical experience broaden our knowledge, changes in treatment and drug therapy may become necessary or appropriate. Readers are advised to check the most current product information provided by the manufacturer of each drug to be administered to verify the recommended dose, the method and duration of administration, and contraindications. It is the responsibility of the practitioner, relying on experience and knowledge of the patient, to determine dosages and the best treatment for each individual patient. Neither the Publisher nor the editors/contributors assume any liability for any injury and/or damage to persons or property arising from this publication.
The Publisher

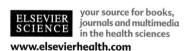

your source for books, journals and multimedia in the health sciences
www.elsevierhealth.com

Printed in the United Kingdom by MPG Books Ltd, Bodmin, Cornwall

Contents

Contributors

J Stephen Fasulakis

BSc MBChB FC Rad D SA FRANZCR

Consultant Radiologist
Department of Medical Imaging
Royal Children's Hospital
Melbourne, Australia

Nicholas J Ferris

MBBS (Hons) MMed FRANZCR

Radiologist, Director of Magnetic
 Resonance Imaging
Department of Radiology
Peter MacCallum Cancer Institute
Melbourne, Australia

Rodney J Hicks

MBBS MD FRACP

Director of Nuclear Medicine and Positron
 Emission Tomography
Department of Nuclear Medicine and Centre
 for Positron Emission Tomography
Peter MacCallum Cancer Institute
Melbourne, Australia
Associate Professor
Department of Medicine
The University of Melbourne
Melbourne, Australia

Caroline L Hollingsworth MD

Clinical Associate
Department of Radiology, Pediatrics Division
Duke University Medical Center
Durham, NC, USA

W F Eddie Lau

BPharm MBBS FRANZCR

Radiologist, Department of Radiology
Specialist in Nuclear Medicine
Department of Nuclear Medicine
 & Centre for Positon Emission Tomography
Peter MacCallum Cancer Institute
Melbourne, Australia

Meng Law   MB BS FRANZCR

Assistant Professor of Radiology
Department of Radiology
New York University Medical Center
New York, USA

Nancy M Major   MD

Associate Professor of Radiology and Surgery
Division of Orthopaedics
Duke University Medical Center
Durham, NC, USA

Alexander G Pitman

BMedSci MBBS FRANZCR

Director of Radiology, Department of
 Radiology
Specialist in Nuclear Medicine, Department
 of Nuclear Medicine and Centre for
 Positron Emission Tomography
Peter MacCallum Cancer Institute
Melbourne, Australia
Senior Fellow, Department of Radiology
Senior Fellow, Department of Anatomy
The University of Melbourne
Melbourne, Australia

John F Seymour

MB BS FRACP

Head of Leukaemia/Lymphoma Service
Division of Haematology and Medical
 Oncology
Peter MacCallum Cancer Institute
Melbourne, Australia

Dinesh A Sivaratnam

BMedSci (Hons) MBBS (Hons) FRACP
Cardiologist
Department of Cardiology
Physician in Nuclear Medicine
Department of Nuclear Medicine
The Royal Melbourne Hospital
Melbourne, Australia

Richard Tello

BS BSE MS(MIT) MD (Stanford) MPH (Harvard)

Professor of Radiology, Epidemiology and
 Biostatistics
Boston University School of Medicine
Boston, MA, USA

Preface

This book was conceived as an overview text for trainees approaching their final exams, and as a review and first line reference for subsequent general radiology practice. It is organised in a way which facilitates study for the US Radiology Boards and British and Australian Radiology Part II examinations.

The chapters are grouped into larger sections organised by organ system: musculoskeletal, abdominal, CNS, head and neck, thoracic, pediatric and female reproductive (obstetrics, gynecology and breast imaging). The last section contains material common to all organ systems: basics of nuclear medicine and PET, general pathology, and examination techniques and study recommendations. There are no separate chapters dedicated to ultrasound or to clinical application of nuclear medicine despite US Boards in these subjects. It is our firm belief that such knowledge is inseparable from other information about the pathology and imaging of particular disease, and properly belongs to the single unified discussion of such diseases. In order to facilitate study for these Boards and also to assist nuclear medicine trainees and practitioners to navigate the book, all the nuclear medicine and ultrasound gamuts in each chapter are grouped together, and nuclear medicine, PET and ultrasound imaging findings for each relevant disease are listed under their specific headings.

In allocation of space and coverage to different diseases we have strived to maintain both a clinical and an exam oriented perspective. Common conditions which comprise the 'bread and butter' of clinical imaging and of exams have been given the most space and detail. We have also deliberately attempted to present those diseases which merit inclusion because of their importance even if they are rare. The extent of the 'knowledge base' material presented in the book reflects what a competent general radiologist should be aware of. We have deliberately avoided sub-specialist knowledge, and have erred on the generalist end of the specialist-generalist spectrum. To this end the book should serve as a concise but complete first line reference long after a candidate has passed his or her boards.

Acknowledgements

This book would not have been possible without the support and help of many persons over the years of its gestation and birth. I would like to thank Dr Norm Eizenberg and Dr Jo Kavanagh, who were the first to enthuse me with teaching anatomy and radiology. My sincere thanks go to Professor Emeritus Bill Hare and Professor Brian Tress, both of the Radiology Department of the University of Melbourne and the Royal Melbourne Hospital, who have patiently taught and encouraged my peers and myself towards excellence in academic radiology.

Several persons in my life bore the brunt of the inevitable daily sacrifices of writing a book, in particular Anna and Greg Sapozhnikov and Lana Zylan, and I truly appreciate the support they gave me during that time.

I would like to acknowledge Dr Allan McKenzie, Director of Diagnostic Imaging at the Peter MacCallum Cancer Institute and my immediate predecessor, without whose practical support this book would not have been written. Michael Houston, Publishing Manager at Elsevier Science, was a key individual in converting this book from a concept and draft to reality. He would not let the dream die even when the outlook was bleak, and to his effort and vision I am eternally grateful.

I would like to acknowledge and thank my two co-authors, Dr Nancy Major and Dr Richard Tello, who shared the long haul with me, and provided me with perspective and guidance.

I would also like to thank and acknowledge our chapter co-authors and contributors for their selfless effort, time and expertise: Dr Stephen Fasulakis, Dr Nick Ferris, Dr Caroline Hollingsworth, Dr Rod Hicks, Dr Eddie Lau, Dr Meng Law, Dr John Seymour and Dr Dinesh Sivaratnam. Finally, the inspiration for this book has been my peers and my successors in radiology and nuclear medicine: those trainees who have studied and sat the exams with me, and all those who are coming after me to undertake the same voyage of learning and trial.

AGP

Abbreviations

2D: two dimensional
3D: three dimensional
A/B ratio: umbilical artery peak systolic velocity (A) to minimal diastolic velocity (B) ratio
A: atomic mass (number of protons and neutrons)
a1AT: alpha 1 antitrypsin
AA: arteries
ABC: aneurysmal bone cyst
Abdo: abdomen/abdominal
ABPA: allergic bronchopulmonary aspergillosis
AC: abdominal circumference; acromioclavicular
ACA: anterior cerebral artery
ACE: angiotensin converting enzyme
ACL: anterior cruciate ligament
ACommA: anterior communicating artery
ACTH: adrenocorticotrophic hormone
AD: Alzheimer's disease; autosomal dominant
ADEM: acute disseminated encephalomyelitis
AFB: acid fast bacilli
AFH: angiofollicular (lymph node) hyperplasia
AFI: amniotic fluid index
AFP: alphafetoprotein (see also alphaFP)
AFS: anterior fibromuscular stroma
AICA: anterior inferior cerebellar artery
AIDS: acquired immune deficiency syndrome
AJCC: American Joint Committee on Cancer staging
Al: aluminium
ALD: adrenoleukodystrophy
ALL: acute lymphoblastic leukemia; anterior longitudinal ligament:
alphaFP: alphafetoprotein
ALPSA: anterior labrum periosteal sleeve avulsion
AMI: acute myocardial infarction
AML: acute myeloid leukemia
ANA: antinuclear antibody
Angio: angiography
AoV: aortic valve
AP: anteroposterior
APCKD: adult polycystic kidney disease
APO: acute pulmonary oedema (edema)
APP: amyloid precursor protein

APTT: activated partial thromboplastin time
APUD: amine precursor uptake and decarboxylation
AR: autosomal recessive
ARC: architectural distortion
ARDS: adult respiratory distress syndrome
ARF: acute renal failure
AS: ankylosing spondylitis
ASA: anterior spinal artery
ASD: atrial septal defect
AT: antitrypsin
ATN: acute tubular necrosis
ATP: adenosine triphosphate
AV: arteriovenous; atrioventricular
AVF: arteriovenous fistula
AVM: arteriovenous malformation
AVN: avascular necrosis
AVSD: atrioventricular septal defect
AXR: abdominal X-ray

Ba: barium
BBB: blood–brain barrier
BCG: bacille Calmette–Guérrin
Be: beryllium
beta hCG: beta human chorionic gonadotrophin
BFCD: benign fibrous cortical defect
BFH: benign fibrous histiocytoma
BM: bone marrow
BMD: bone mineral density
BOOP: bronchiolitis obliterans organizing pneumonia
BP: blood pressure
BPD: biparietal diameter; bronchopulmonary dysplasia
BPH: benign prostatic hyperplasia
bpm: beats per minute
BPP: biophysical profile
BrIDA: bromotriethyl IDA, mebrofenin
BTS: Blalock–Taussig shunt
Ca: calcium, cancer
CADASIL: Cerebral Autosomal Dominant Arteriopathy, Subcortical Infarcts, Leukoencephalopathy
CAL: calcification
CAM: cystic adenomatoid malformation
CBD: common bile duct
CC fistula: caroticocavernous fistula
CC: craniocaudal
CCA: common carotid artery
CCF: chronic cardiac failure

CCK: cholecystokinin
CF: cystic fibrosis
CHAD: calcium hydroxyapatite deposition disease
CHD: congenital heart disease
CIN: cervical intraepithelial neoplasia
CIRC: circumscribed mass
CK: creatine kinase
CK-MB: creatine kinase-myocardial band
Cl: chlorine
CLL: chronic lymphocytic leukemia
CMI: cell mediated immunity
CML: chronic myeloid (myelogenous) leukemia
CMV: cytomegalovirus
CN: cranial nerve or nerves
CNS: central nervous system
CO: carbon monoxide
COAD/
COPD: chronic obstructive airways (pulmonary) disease
CPPD: calcium pyrophosphate dihydrate deposition disease
CPS: complex partial seizures
CREST: Calcinosis, Raynaud's phenomenon, Esophageal dysmotility, Scleroderma and Telangiectasia syndrome
CRF: chronic renal failure
CRL: crown–rump length
CS: chondrosarcoma
CSF: cerebrospinal fluid
CT: computed tomography
CTA: computed tomographic angiography
CTAP: computed tomography arterial portography
CTG: cardiotocography
CTIVC: computed tomography intravenous cholangiogram
CVS: chorionic villus sampling
CXR: chest X-ray
CZ: central zone

DA: dopamine
DAD: diffuse alveolar damage
DBP: diastolic blood pressure
DCIS: ductal carcinoma in situ
DDH: developmentally dysplastic hip
DDx: differential diagnosis
DEXA: dual energy X-ray absorptiometry
DIC: disseminated intravascular coagulation

DiDi (twins): dichorionic diamniotic twins

DiMono (twins): monochorionic diamniotic twins

DIP: desquamative interstitial pneumonia/pneumonitis; distal interphalangeal (joint)

DIS: discrete mass

DISH: diffuse idiopathic skeletal hyperostosis

DISI: dorsal intercalated segment instability

DISIDA: disopropyl IDA, disofenin

DJD: degenerative joint disease

DKA: diabetic ketoacidosis

DMSA: dimercaptosuccinic acid

DNA: deoxyribose nucleic acid

DNET: dysembryoplastic neuroepithelial tumor

DNT: dysembryoplastic neuroepithelial tumor

DORV: double outlet right ventricle

D-TGA: dextro-transposition of great arteries

D-TGV: dextro-transposition of great vessels

DTH: delayed type hypersensitivity

DTPA: diethylenetriamine pentaacetic acid

DU: duodenal ulcer

DVT: deep venous thrombosis

EAA: extrinsic allergic alveolitis

EBCT: electron beam computed tomography

EBV: Epstein–Barr virus

ECA: external carotid artery

ECD: ethylcysteinate dimer (NeuroliteTM)

ECG: electrocardiogram

ECMO: extracorporeal membrane oxygenation

EDD: estimated date of delivery

EDTA: edetate; edetic acid

EDV: end diastolic volume

EF: ejection fraction

EFW: estimated fetal weight

EG: eosinophilic granuloma

ENT: ear, nose and throat

ERCP: endoscopic retrograde cholangiography

ERPF: estimated renal plasma flow

ESR: erythrocyte sedimentation rate

ESV: end systolic volume

fat sat: fat saturated/fat saturation

FB: foreign body

FCC: fibrocystic change

FD: fibrous dysplasia

FDA: Food and Drug Administration

FDG: fluorodeoxyglucose

FDI: International Dental Federation

Fe: iron

FESS: functional endoscopic sinus surgery

FET: fluoroethyltyrosine

FIGO: Federation Internationale de Gynecologie et d'Obstetrique

FIRP: first international reference preparation

FL: femur length

FLAIR: fluid-attenuated inversion-recovery

fluoro: fluoroscopy

FMH: fibromuscular hyperplasia

FMISO: fluoromisonidazole

FMT: fluoromethyltyrosine

FNA: fine needle aspiration

FSE: fast spin echo

FSPGR: fast spoiled gradient recalled acquisition in steady state

Ga: gallium

GA: gestational age

GBM: glomerular basement membrane; glioblastoma multiforme

GCT: giant cell tumor

GCTTS: giant cell tumor of tendon sheath

Gd: gadolinium

GFR: glomerular filtration rate

GH: growth hormone

GI: gastrointestinal

GIT: gastrointestinal tract

glx/glu: glutamine/glutamate

GN: glomerulonephritis

GpA Strep: group A Streptococcus

GRE: gradient echo

GS: gestational sac

GU: gastric ulcer

Gy: Gray (mGy: milliGray)

H+E: hematoxylin and eosin

HAV: hepatitis A virus

Hb: hemoglobin

HBV: hepatitis B virus

HC: head circumference

HCC: hepatocellular carcinoma

HCV: hepatitis C virus

HD: Hodgkin's disease

HDP: hydroxymethyl diphosphonate (oxidronate)

HDV: hepatitis D virus

HELLP: Hemolysis, Elevated LFTs, Low Platelets

HEV: hepatitis E virus

HH: hiatus hernia

HHT: hereditary hemorrhagic telangiectasia

HIDA: 'hepatic' IDA (dimethyl IDA, lidofenin)

HIV: human immunodeficiency virus

HLA: human leukocyte antigen

HMA: homovanillic acid

HMD: hyaline membrane disease

HMPAO: hexamethyl propyleneamine oxime (CeretecTM)

HOA: hypertrophic osteoarthropathy

HOCM: primary hypertrophic obstructive cardiomyopathy

HONK: hyperosmolar non ketosis

HP: Helicobacter pylori

HPTH: hyperparathyroidism

HPV: human papilloma virus

HR: heart rate

HRCT: high resolution computed tomography

HRT: hormone replacement therapy

HSC triad: Hand–Schuller–Christian triad

HSV: herpes simplex virus

HT: hypertension

HTLV: human T lymphotrophic virus

HU: Hounsfield units

HUS: hemolytic uraemic syndrome

HZV: herpes zoster virus

I: iodine

IAC: internal auditory canal

IAM: internal auditory meatus

IBD: inflammatory bowel disease

ICA: internal carotid artery

ICRP: International Commission on Radiation Protection

ICU: intensive care unit

IDA: imino-diacetic acid

IDDM: insulin dependent diabetes mellitus

IF: intrinsic factor

IGA: interstitial gone airspace

IHD: ischemic heart disease

IJV: internal jugular vein

IL: interleukin

IM: intramuscular

IMA: inferior mesenteric artery

In: indium

INR: international normalized ratio

iso: isointense, isodense, isoechoic (i.e. of same signal intensity, density, echogenicity)

ITP: idiopathic thrombocytopenic purpura

IUGR: intrauterine growth retardation

IV: intravenous

IVC: inferior vena cava; intravenous cholangiogram

IVDU: intravenous drug use

IVF: in vitro fertilization

IVP: intravenous pyelogram

IVU: intravenous urogram

JCA: juvenile chronic arthritis

K: potassium

keV: kiloelectron volt

KS: Kaposi's sarcoma

KUB: kidney–ureter–bladder film (abdominal X-ray)

kVp: kilovolt peak

LA: left atrium

LAB: laboratory

LAO: left anterior oblique

LAT/lat: lateral

LB: large bowel

LBO: large bowel obstruction

LCA: left circumflex artery

LCIS: lobular carcinoma in situ

LCL: lateral collateral ligament

LH: luteinizing hormone

LL: lower lobe

LLL: left lower lobe

LMP: date of last menstrual period

L-TGA: levo-transposition of great arteries

L-TGV: levo-transposition of great vessels

LUL: left upper lobe

LUS: lower uterine segment

LV: left ventricle

LVEDP: left ventricular end diastolic pressure

LVEF: left ventricular ejection fraction

LVF: left ventricular failure

LVOT: left ventricle outflow tract

MAA: macroaggregated albumin

MAC: Mycobacterium avium complex

MAG3: mercaptoacetyltriglycine

MALT: mucosa associated lymphoid tissue

mammo: mammography

mAs: milliAmpere-second

MBq: MegaBecquerel

MC: metacarpal

MCA: middle cerebral artery

MCHC: mean corpuscular hemoglobin concentration

mCi: millicurie

MCL: medial collateral ligament

MCP: metacarpophalangeal

MCQ: multiple choice question

MCTD: mixed connective tissue disease

MCU: micturating cystourethrogram

MCV: mean corpuscular volume

MDP: methylenediphosphonate

MELAS: Myopathy, Encephalopathy, Lactic Acidosis, Stroke like episodes

MEN: multiple endocrine neoplasia

MERRF: Myoclonic Epilepsy, Ragged Red Fibers

meV: mega (million) electron volt

MFH: malignant fibrous histiocytoma

MI: myocardial infarction; myo-inositol

MIBG: I-123 or I-131 metaiodobenzylguanidine

MIBI: methoxy isobutyl isonitrile

MID: multiinfarct dementia

MLO: mediolateral oblique

MM: multiple myeloma

MNG: multinodular goitre

MonoMono (twins): monochorionic monoamniotic twins

MPS: mucopolysaccharidoses

MR: magnetic resonance

MRA: magnetic resonance angiography

MRCP: magnetic resonance cholangiopancreatography

MRPA: magnetic resonance projection angiography

MRS: magnetic resonance spectroscopy

MRV: magnetic resonance venography

MS: multiple sclerosis

MSH: melanocyte stimulating hormone

MSK: medullary sponge kidney

MTP: metatarsophalangeal

MV: mitral valve

Na: sodium

NAA: N-acetyl aspartate

NF1: neurofibromatosis 1

NF2: neurofibromatosis 2

NHL: non Hodgkin's lymphoma

NIDDM: non insulin dependent diabetes mellitus

NOF: non ossifying fibroma

NON: non specific density

NOS: not otherwise specified

NPC: nasopharyngeal carcinoma

NPV: negative predictive value

NSAIDs: non steroidal antiinflammatory drugs

NSCLC: non small cell lung carcinoma

NUC MED: nuclear medicine

OA: osteoarthritis (osteoarthrosis)

OCD: osteochondritis dissecans

OCL: osteochondral lesion

OCP: oral contraceptive pill

OFD: occipitofrontal diameter

OM: osteomyelitis

OPG: orthopantomogram (radiographs)

OS: osteosarcoma

PA: pulmonary artery

PAN: polyarteritis nodosa

P-ANCA: P-antineutrophil cytoplasmic antibody

PAS: paraaminosalicylic acid

PBC SHOST: Prostate, Breast, Carcinoid, Stomach, Hodgkin's lymphoma, Osteosarcoma, Small cell lung carcinoma, Transitional cell (urothelial) carcinoma (see bone gamuts)

PC: Pneumocystis carinii

PCA: posterior cerebral artery

PCKD: polycystic kidney disease

PCL: posterior cruciate ligament

PCommA: posterior communicating artery

PCP: Pneumocystis carinii pneumonia

PCV: packed cell volume

PD: Parkinson's disease; proton density

PDA: patent ductus arteriosus

PE: pulmonary embolism

PET: positron emission tomography

PFC: persistent fetal circulation

PFO: patent foramen ovale

pheo: pheochromocytoma

PICA: posterior inferior cerebellar artery

PID: pelvic inflammatory disease

PIE: pulmonary interstitial emphysema

PIOPED: progressive investigation of pulmonary embolism diagnosis

PIP: proximal interphalangeal

PKU: phenylketonuria

PLL: posterior longitudinal ligament

plt: platelet(s)

PMF: progressive massive fibrosis

PML: progressive multifocal leukoencephalopathy

PN: pyelonephritis

PNET: primitive neuroectodermal tumor

POEMS: Polyneuropathy, Organomegaly, Endocrinopathy, Myeloma, Skin lesions

ppm: parts per million

PPV: positive predictive value

PRESS: point resolved spectroscopy

PRL: prolactin

PROM: premature rupture of membranes

PSA: posterior spinal artery; prostate specific antigen

PSV: peak systolic velocity

PTC: percutaneous transhepatic cholangiography

PTH: parathyroid hormone

PTT: parenchymal transit time

PUJ: pelviureteric junction

PV: per vagina; portal vein; pulmonary (pulmonic) valve

PVNS: pigmented villonodular synovitis

PZ: peripheral zone

QCT: quantitative computed tomography

RA: rheumatoid arthritis; right atrium

RAO: right anterior oblique

RB: retinoblastoma

RBC: red blood cell

RCA:	right coronary artery	STEAM:	stimulated echo acquisition mode	UBC:	unicameral bone cyst
rem:	roentgen equivalent man	STEL:	stellate lesion	UBO:	unidentified bright object
RF:	risk factor	STEMI:	ST elevation myocardial injury	UC:	ulcerative colitis
RI:	resistive index	STIR:	short tau inversion recovery	UGT:	urogenital tract
RLL:	right lower lobe	SUV:	standardized uptake value	UICC:	Union Internacional Contra la Cancrum
RLN:	recurrent laryngeal nerve	Sv:	Sievert (mSv: milliSievert)		
RML:	right middle lobe	SVC:	superior vena cava	UIP:	usual interstitial pneumonitis
RNA:	ribonucleic acid			UL:	upper lobe
ROI:	region of interest	T 1/2:	half-life (in units of time)	US:	ultrasound
RS:	Reed–Sternberg (cell)	TAPVR:	total anomalous pulmonary venous return	UTI:	urinary tract infection
RUL:	right upper lobe			UV:	ultraviolet
RUQ:	right upper quadrant	TB:	tuberculosis		
RV:	right ventricle	TCC:	transitional cell carcinoma	V/Q:	ventilation/perfusion
RVEF:	right ventricular ejection fraction	TcO4:	Tc-99m pertechnetate	VA:	vertebral artery
RVOT:	right ventricle outflow tract	TDLU:	terminal ductal lobular unit	VACTERL:	Vertebral, Anal, Cardiac, Tracheal, Esophageal, Renal, Limb (malformation)
		tds:	three times a day		
S/D ratio:	systolic/diastolic (velocity) ratio	TE:	echo time		
SAA:	serum amyloid A	TEF:	tracheoesophageal fistula	VATER:	Vertebral, Anal, Tracheo-Esophageal, Renal and Radial (malformation)
SAH:	subarachnoid hemorrhage	TFT:	thyroid function test		
SAM:	systolic anterior motion	Tg:	thyroglobulin		
SASD:	subacromial subdeltoid bursa	TGV:	transposition of great vessels	VCUG:	voiding/micturating cystourethrogram
SB:	small bowel	TIMI:	thrombolysis in myocardial infarction		
SBC:	solitary bone cyst			vHL:	von Hippel–Lindau syndrome
SBO:	small bowel obstruction	TIN:	tubulointerstitial nephritis	VIP:	vasoactive intestinal polypeptide
SBP:	systolic blood pressure	TIPS:	transjugular intrahepatic portosystemic shunt		
SC:	subcutaneous			VISI:	volar intercalated segment instability
SCA:	subclavian artery; superior cerebellar artery	Tl:	thallium		
		TMJ:	temporomandibular joint	VMA:	vanillylmandelic acid
SCC:	squamous cell carcinoma	TNM:	tumor, nodes, metastases	VofG:	vein of Galen
SCLC:	small cell lung carcinoma	TORCH:	Toxoplasmosis, Other (listeria, syphilis), Rubella, Cytomegalovirus, Herpes simplex virus, Human immunodeficiency virus	VSD:	ventricular septal defect
SD:	sectorial duct; standard deviation			VT:	ventricular tachycardia
SE:	spin echo (sequence)			VUJ:	vesicoureteric junction
SH:	Salter–Harris			VUR:	vesicoureteric reflux
SI:	sacroiliac			VV:	veins
SIJ:	sacroiliac joint	TR:	repetition time (MR sequence parameter)	VZV:	varicella zoster virus
SLAP:	superior labrum anterior to posterior				
		TRUS:	transrectal ultrasound	WAGR:	Wilms' tumor, Aniridia, Genital abnormalities, Retardation
SLE:	systemic lupus erythematosus	TS:	tuberous sclerosis		
SLL:	small lymphocytic leukemia	TSH:	thyroid stimulating hormone	WBC:	white blood cell
SMA:	superior mesenteric artery	TTN:	transient tachypnea of newborn	WM:	white matter
SMV:	superior mesenteric vein	TTP:	thrombotic thrombocytopenic purpura		
SOL:	space occupying lesion			Xe:	xenon
SONK:	spontaneous osteonecrosis of the knee	TURP:	transurethral resection of prostate	XGP:	xanthogranulomatous pyelonephritis
		TV:	tricuspid valve		
SPECT:	single photon emission computed tomography	TZ:	transitional zone	XR:	X-ray
				Z:	atomic number (number of protons)
SPN:	solitary pulmonary nodule	UA:	umbilical artery		
ST:	soft tissue			Zr:	zirconium

Musculoskeletal

1 Musculoskeletal normal and gamuts

1. NORMAL

1.1 ARTICULAR CARTILAGE ON MR

T1W: intermediate
T2W: intermediate
GRE (cartilage targeted): high
T2W fat saturated: intermediate (gray)
STIR: intermediate

1.2 ARTICULAR STRUCTURES ON US

JOINT CAPSULE: hyperechoic
LABRUM: triangular hyperechoic uniform
ARTICULAR CARTILAGE: smooth
    hypoechoic
SUBCHONDRAL ARTICULAR BONE: smooth
    echogenic shadowing

1.3 BONE MARROW

Red bone marrow
40% fat, 40% water, 20% protein
intermediate on T1W, intermediate on T2W,
    intermediate on STIR

Yellow bone marrow
80% fat, 15% water, 5% protein
high on T1W, low on T2W, low on STIR
    (follows fat)

Distribution

ADULT DISTRIBUTION
red marrow in vertebral bodies, pelvis,
    proximal femora and humeri (slowly
    recedes); diploic bone marrow mixed,
    clivus yellow

CHILD DISTRIBUTION:
    EPIPHYSES ARE YELLOW
begins with extensive red marrow in
    diametaphyseal areas of long bones
normal epiphyses contain yellow marrow
slowly shrinks to adult pattern

Normal skull diploe on MR

MATURATIONAL PATTERN
diploic bone marrow prominently red
    <1 year old
diploic bone marrow predominantly yellow
    (adult signal) >10 years

PROMINENT RED CONVERSION OF
SKULL DIPLOIC MARROW IN
ADULTS
smokers, diabetics

1.4 CERVICAL SPINAL ALIGNMENT LINES

Trauma films
lateral (to see C7–T1 junction); AP; open
    mouth
as above and obliques (or pillar views: head
    rotated to contralateral side;
    approximately 15 degrees caudal
    angulation to image facet joints)
FLEXION EXTENSION VIEWS: voluntary
    non forced, in conscious patient;
    abnormal displacement may be masked
    by spasm

Anterior spinal line
lateral view; line along anterior vertebral
    bodies, follows anterior longitudinal
    ligament to odontoid tip

Posterior spinal line
lateral view; line along posterior verterbral
    bodies, follows posterior longitudinal
    ligament to odontoid tip

Spinolaminar line
lateral view; line formed by junction of
    laminae (visible as anterior 'edge of
    spinous process' on the lateral, follows
    ligamenta flava/posterior dura to
    posterior margin of foramen magnum
modified spinolaminar line (C1 to C3 only)
    should have C2 fall on the line (beware of
    hangman's or Jefferson's fractures)

Spinous process line
lateral view; line formed by tips of spinous
    processes, more curved than
    spinolaminar line
excessive separation of two spinous
    processes – ?hyperflexion injury

Soft tissue line
lateral view; interface of air column and
    prevertebral soft tissues
less reliable if endotracheal tube present
below approximately C4, esophagus
    intervenes between air column and spine
in children, palatal adenoids increase soft
    tissue width in front of C1/C2
widening–?traumatic hematoma
see MEASUREMENTS

Craniocervical alignment

NORMAL APPEARANCE
C1 anterior arch moves with dens in
    extension and flexion (see
    MEASUREMENTS)
posterior arch often lies on smooth line:
    spinolaminar line C2–posterior margin
    foramen magnum (opisthion)
odontoid process aligned with anterior
    margin of foramen magnum (basion, tip
    of clivus) in flexion and extension;
    equidistant from lateral masses on open
    mouth view

Other lines of alignment
articular pillars on AP, lateral, obliques
end-on laminae shingle
end-on pedicles align
spinous processes on AP view align and are
    equidistant

Alignment at each segment
disk spaces regular, symmetrical anterior to
    posterior
no single space opens excessively on flexion
    or extension
facet joints align (both columns)
no single facet joint angulates or slides
    excessively on flexion or extension

1.5 ELBOW OSSIFICATION TIMES AND ALIGNMENT

see Ch 17

1.6 NORMAL MEASUREMENTS

Achilles tendon
5–6 mm thick

Adult acromioclavicular joint
normal separation <4 mm

Cervical spine measurements

SWISCHUK'S C1 C2 C3 (pediatric)
line drawn from posterior arch of atlas to
    spinolaminar line C3
C2 spinolaminar line within 1 mm (neutral)
    of the C1–C3 line, up to 3 mm anterior in
    flexion, up to 3 mm posterior in
    extension

PREVERTEBRAL SOFT TISSUE

convenient upper limit of normal is 3 mm at C2 in adults, and 7 mm for children (this has both false negatives and false positives)

upper limit at C7 is up to 2 cm

HARRIS'S POSTERIOR AXIAL LINE

basion (anterior margin of foramen magnum, tip of clivus) within 12 mm anterior (or 4 mm posterior) of C2 posterior longitudinal ligament line AND basion to odontoid interval <12 mm

CERVICAL CANAL DIAMETER

lateral view, as little magnification as possible; posterior spinal line to spinolaminar line

if canal diameter <14 mm, space available for cord is too narrow

in acute trauma reduced canal diameter is usually produced by fracture or at C1 a rupture of transverse and alar ligaments

Distal radioulnar angle

RADIOULNAR ANGLE approx 12 degrees in both projections

1.7 ROTATOR CUFF US LAYERS

SUBCUTANEOUS FAT: hyperechoic reference

DELTOID: hypoechoic, multipennate; echogenicity increases with age

SASD (subacromial subdeltoid bursa): thin hypoechoic line (<2 mm) between two thin echogenic fat layers (peribursal fat)

ROTATOR CUFF TENDON: hyperechoic, fibrillary, anisotropic; 5–10 mm thick; within 2 mm of other side; 'critical zone' is 1–1.5 cm from tip of distal tendon insertion, postulated to be most avascular zone and (in supraspinatus) subject to impingement

ARTICULAR CARTILAGE: hypoechoic smooth

SUBCHONDRAL ARTICULAR BONE: echogenic shadowing smooth

1.8 TENDON ON MR

Normal

normal size tendon

low signal (black) on T1W, T2W

(collagen I has short T2 constant and is black on all sequences; loosely bound water in degenerating collagen I has progressively increasing T2 constant – it is detected progressively first on GRE, then short TE, then long TE sequences)

minimal/no fluid in tendon sheath or around tendon

increasing signal does not equal clinical significance (common age related change)!

Magic angle

55 degrees to main magnetic field on 1.5 Tesla magnets

increased signal on short TE sequences (T1W, PD, GRE)

not on long TE sequences (T2W)

1.9 TENDON ON US

Normal

uniform diameter or gently tapering with sharp margins

fibrillary pattern in longitudinal view: reflectors parallel to tendon surface producing pattern of alternating thin regular bright and dark lines

ovoid echogenic with homogeneous 'speckled' internal echostructure in transverse view

muscle hypoechoic with intrasubstance echogenic surfaces (internal fibrous septa)

tendon sheaths usually contain no or a sliver of fluid

Anisotropy

anisotropy: different sonic reflectivity and pattern depending on angle of insonation

tendons are anisotropic and most reflective at 90 degrees of insonation

other transducer angles may produce artifactual defects in fibrillary pattern

2. GAMUTS

2.1 GENERIC (all modalities)

2.1.1 AVASCULAR NECROSIS – CAUSES

Idiopathic is the most common

Secondary: mnemonic is GESTALT

G-AUCHERS

E-MBOLISM (fat: trauma, pancreatic; gas)

S-TEROIDS

T-RAUMA

A-LCOHOL

L-UPUS AND OTHER VASCULITIDES

T-HROMBOSIS (esp SICKLE CELL DISEASE)

2.1.2 BACK PAIN IN CHILDREN

see Ch 17

2.1.3 BONY MALIGNANCY (child)

see Ch 17

2.1.4 DISK DISEASE DIFFERENTIALS

see Ch 10

2.1.5 HIP ARTHRITIS WITH EFFUSION

see Ch 17

2.1.6 HYPERTROPHIC OSTEOARTHROPATHY (HOA)

also termed hypertrophic pulmonary osteoarthropathy

MANIFESTATIONS

CLINICAL

reactive periostitis of unclear mechanism

finger clubbing, possibly swelling of wrists and ankles

swelling is occasionally painful (common in cancer)

X-RAY

linear bilateral variably symmetrical periosteal reaction with normal underlying bone

distal radius, ulna, tibia, fibula; metacarpals, metatarsals are less common but do not occur in thyroid acropachy

MDP

markedly increased distal appendicular surface tracer uptake (see Nuc Med gamuts)

CAUSES

LUNG

CARCINOMA, LYMPHOMA,
   BRONCHIECTASIS, CYSTIC FIBROSIS,
   ABSCESS

PLEURA

FIBROMA, MESOTHELIOMA

HEART

CYANOTIC HEART DISEASE (UNCOMMON)

GIT

INFLAMMATORY BOWEL DISEASE, CELIAC
   DISEASE, PRIMARY BILIARY CIRRHOSIS

THYROID

THYROID ACROPACHY
term for HOA occurring in Graves' disease

PACHYDERMOPERIOSTITIS
   (DIFFERENTIAL OF HOA)
rare hereditary disorder of thickened skin
   ('pachydermo'), finger clubbing and
   symmetrical periosteal reaction
   ('periostitis') male < female;
   commoner in blacks
no underlying malignancy or other causative
   disease by definition (unless coincidental
   second pathology)

2.1.7 JOINT LOOSE BODY

FRACTURED OSTEOPHYTE

OSTEOCHONDRAL FRACTURE
   FRAGMENT

OSTEOCHONDRITIS DISSECANS,
   FRAGMENT

SYNOVIAL (OSTEO)
   CHONDROMATOSIS

NEUROPATHIC JOINT

2.1.8 LOCALIZED GIGANTISM

INFECTION

NEUROFIBROMATOSIS

KLIPPEL–TRENAUNAY–WEBER
   SYNDROME

BECKWITH–WIEDEMANN SYNDROME

LOCAL AV MALFORMATION OR
   FISTULA, LOCAL HEMANGIOMA

MACRODYSTROPHIA LIPOMATOSUM

2.1.9 LUMPY BUMPY ARTHRITIS

GOUT

AMYLOID

MULTICENTRIC
   RETICULOHISTIOCYTOSIS

2.1.10 MADELUNG AND REVERSE MADELUNG

Madelung (ulna too long)

POST TRAUMATIC

TURNER'S SYNDROME

KLINEFELTER'S SYNDROME

DYSCHONDROOSTEOSIS (Leri–Weill
   syndrome)
MALE > FEMALE

IDIOPATHIC

Reverse Madelung (ulna too short)

DIAPHYSEAL ACLASIA (HEREDITARY
   MULTIPLE EXOSTOSIS)

2.1.11 POSTERIOR VERTEBRAL (NEURAL ARCH) LESION

TB, INFECTION

METASTASIS

OSTEOBLASTOMA

ABC (ANEURYSMAL BONE CYST)

GCT (GIANT CELL TUMOR) – LESS
   COMMON

2.1.12 PRESACRAL MASS (child)

see Ch 17

2.1.13 PROTRUSIO ACETABULI

MNEMONIC: TRAUMATIC PROOF I

TRAUMA

P-AGET'S

R-HEUMATOID ARTHRITIS

O-STEOMALACIA (and rickets)

O-STEOGENESIS IMPERFECTA

F-IBROUS DYSPLASIA

I-DIOPATHIC (Otto's pelvis)

2.1.14 RECURRENT SYMPTOMS AFTER BACK SURGERY

Acute

EPIDURAL HEMATOMA

EPIDURAL ABSCESS

SEQUESTERED FRAGMENT

Chronic

RECURRENT DISK, PERSISTENT
   DISK, SEQUESTERED FRAGMENT

DISK PROTRUSION ELSEWHERE

EPIDURAL FIBROSIS

DISCITIS, EPIDURAL ABSCESS

ARACHNOIDITIS

DIFFUSE SPINAL DEGENERATIVE
   DISEASE

PAIN FROM NON SPINAL SOURCE

NEURITIS?
persistent intrathecal contrast enhancement
   beyond 6 months of uncertain
   significance

2.1.15 TUMORS WITH GIANT CELLS ON HISTOLOGY

GIANT CELL TUMOR

ANEURYSMAL BONE CYST

BROWN TUMOR

CHONDROBLASTOMA

TELANGIECTATIC OSTEOSARCOMA

2.2 XR (and CT)

2.2.1 ACROOSTEOLYSIS

CREST, SCLERODERMA

HYPERPARATHYROIDISM, RENAL
   OSTEODYSTROPHY

THERMAL INJURY

NEUROPATHIC AND LEPROSY

(PVC POISONING)

(EPIDERMOLYSIS BULLOSA,
   PORPHYRIA)

2.2.2 CALCIFICATION

Metastatic

HYPERCALCEMIA AND RELATIVES

HYPERPARATHYROIDISM

RENAL OSTEODYSTROPHY

TUMORAL CALCINOSIS

HYPERVITAMINOSIS D

HYPERCALCEMIA

SARCOIDOSIS

HYPOPARATHYROIDISM AND RELATIVES

HYPOPARATHYROIDISM

PSEUDO (RESISTANCE TO PARATHYROID HORMONE)

PSEUDOPSEUDO (BIOCHEMISTRY NORMAL)

Dystrophic

POST TRAUMATIC (includes PARALYSIS)

MULTIFOCAL

VASCULAR

  SCLERODERMA

  CREST

  DERMATOMYOSITIS

CRYSTALS

  CALCIUM PYROPHOSPHATE DIHYDRATE DEPOSITION DISEASE (CPPD)

  CALCIUM HYDROXYAPATITE DEPOSITION DISEASE (CHAD)

  TOPHACEOUS GOUT

FOCAL

FAT NECROSIS

INFECTION

INFLAMMATION

DEGENERATIVE CHANGE (esp TENDONS)

TUMOR

MYOSITIS OSSIFICANS

PARALYSIS

2.2.3 CALCIUM CRYSTALS
(types)

CPPD: Ca PYROPHOSPHATE DIHYDRATE

CHAD: Ca HYDROXYAPATITE DIHYDRATE

CaPO4: diCaPO4 DIHYDRATE

2.2.4 CHONDROCALCINOSIS

CPPD, HEMOCHROMATOSIS

DEGENERATIVE JOINT DISEASE

HYPERCALCEMIA

HYPERPARATHYROIDISM (primary)

GOUT

OCHRONOSIS

WILSON'S DISEASE

2.2.5 COARSE TRABECULATION

Focal

PAGET'S DISEASE

HEMANGIOMA

Diffuse

HEMOGLOBINOPATHIES

GAUCHER'S, OTHER STORAGE DISEASE

OSTEOPOROSIS

OSTEOMALACIA

MYELOMA

2.2.6 DENSE BONES – DIFFUSE [RSMOPMMPAF]

RENAL OSTEODYSTROPHY

SICKLE CELL DISEASE

METASTASES (and 1% of myeloma – POEMS)

OSTEOPETROSIS

PYKNODYSOSTOSIS

MYELOSCLEROSIS

MASTOCYTOSIS

PAGET'S

ATHLETES

FLUOROSIS

2.2.7 DENSE BONE: FOCAL DENSE LESION

Rule out treated lytic lesion then

Cortical

'HEALING' NON OSSIFYING FIBROMA

STRESS FRACTURE

OSTEOID OSTEOMA

OSTEOMYELITIS

OSTEOSARCOMA

Medullary

AVASCULAR NECROSIS/BONE INFARCT

DEGENERATING ENCHONDROMA

SCLEROTIC METASTASIS, HODGKIN'S DISEASE (see separate gamut)

MASTOCYTOSIS

OSTEOMA

OSTEOSARCOMA

Characteristic

MELORHEOSTOSIS

OSTEOPATHIA STRIATA

2.2.8 EPIPHYSEAL LYTIC LESION

CHONDROBLASTOMA (<30 years of age)

GIANT CELL TUMOR (closed physis)

ANEURYSMAL BONE CYST

INFECTION

METASTASIS

GEODE

2.2.9 ERLENMEYER FLASK DEFORMITY

HEMOGLOBINOPATHIES

GAUCHER'S DISEASE

METAPHYSEAL DYSPLASIA (Pyle)

FIBROUS DYSPLASIA AND DIAPHYSEAL ACLASIA

2.2.10 EROSIONS WITH OSTEOARTHRITIS (joints affected)

TEMPOROMANDIBULAR JOINTS (TMJ)

SACROILIAC JOINTS

SYMPHYSIS PUBIS

ACROMIOCLAVICULAR JOINTS

2.2.11 EXCESSIVE CALLUS

POOR IMMOBILIZATION ACROSS
FRACTURE SITE

NEUROPATHIC FRACTURE

STEROIDS OR CUSHING'S
SYNDROME

PARALYSIS

OSTEOGENESIS IMPERFECTA

CHILD ABUSE

2.2.12 FOCAL INDOLENT LYTIC LESION

RULE OUT GEODE (subchondral cyst)
then

MNEMONIC: IME FBE COAGS

I-NFECTION

M-YELOMA, METASTASIS,
LYMPHOMA

E-OSINOPHILIC GRANULOMA

F-IBROUS CORTICAL DEFECT (non
ossifying fibroma) AND F-IBROUS
DYSPLASIA

B-ROWN TUMOR

E-NCHONDROMA

C-HONDROBLASTOMA and
C-HONDROMYXOID FIBROMA

O-STEOBLASTOMA

A-NEURYSMAL BONE CYST

G-IANT CELL TUMOR

S-IMPLE (UNICAMERAL) BONE CYST

2.2.13 GEODES (occur in following arthritides)

CALCIUM PYROPHOSPHATE
DEPOSITION DISEASE

AVASCULAR NECROSIS

OSTEOARTHRITIS

RHEUMATOID ARTHRITIS

2.2.14 HANDS ARTHROPATHY GAMUTS

Symmetry and distribution

SYMMETRIC

RHEUMATOID ARTHRITIS, CREST
SYNDROME

CPPD/HEMOCHROMATOSIS

MULTICENTRIC RETICULOHISTIOCYTOSIS

ASYMMETRIC

PSORIASIS, REITER'S SYNDROME

OSTEOARTHRITIS

GOUT

PROXIMAL

RHEUMATOID ARTHRITIS,
CPPD/HEMOCHROMATOSIS

DISTAL

REITER'S, PSORIASIS, OSTEOARTHRITIS,
CREST SYNDROME

Cartilage loss late or not at all

GOUT

MULTICENTRIC RETICULOHISTIOCYTOSIS

SYSTEMIC LUPUS ERYTHEMATOSUS (SLE)

Ankylosis

PSORIASIS, CREST SYNDROME

RHEUMATOID ARTHRITIS (WRIST, LATE)

Erosions

MARGINAL (JUXTAARTICULAR)

RHEUMATOID ARTHRITIS, PSORIASIS,
REITER'S SYNDROME, CREST
SYNDROME

PERIARTICULAR

GOUT

Subarticular sclerosis, cysts

SCLEROSIS

PSORIASIS, REITER'S

OSTEOARTHRITIS

GOUT

CYSTS

RHEUMATOID ARTHRITIS

CPPD/HEMOCHROMATOSIS

Periarticular osteoporosis

RHEUMATOID ARTHRITIS, +/– CREST
SYNDROME, SLE

Proliferative bone formation/ proliferative erosions

PSORIASIS, REITER'S SYNDROME

OSTEOARTHRITIS

GOUT

Enthesopathy

PSORIASIS, REITER'S SYNDROME

Soft tissue calcification

CREST SYNDROME

GOUT

Soft tissue swelling

RHEUMATOID ARTHRITIS, PSORIASIS
(sausage digits), REITER'S
SYNDROME (sausage digits)

GOUT

Soft tissue deposits

GOUT

AMYLOID

MULTICENTRIC
RETICULOHISTIOCYTOSIS

2.2.15 IRREGULAR EPIPHYSES

see Ch 17

2.2.16 METAPHYSEAL BANDS – DENSE

see Ch 17

2.2.17 METAPHYSEAL LUCENCIES

see Ch 17

2.2.18 MISSING OUTER CLAVICLE

One

MYELOMA, METASTASIS

RESECTION

Both

PRIMARY HYPERPARATHYROIDISM

RHEUMATOID ARTHRITIS

CLEIDOCRANIAL DYSOSTOSIS

2.2.19 MULTIPLE LYTIC LESIONS

MNEMONIC: BEEFI M

B-ROWN TUMORS

E-NCHONDROMAS

E-OSINOPHILIC GRANULOMAS

F-IBROUS DYSPLASIA

I-NFECTION (multifocal)

M-YELOMA, METASTASES

2.2.20 OSTEOPENIA – GENERALIZED (adult)

'Osteoporosis'

PRIMARY OSTEOPOROSIS

STEROIDS, CUSHING'S SYNDROME

ALCOHOL

HYPERTHYROIDISM

HEPARIN

'Osteomalacia'

OSTEOMALACIA

PRIMARY HYPERPARATHYROIDISM

RENAL OSTEODYSTROPHY

'Myeloma'

MYELOMATOSIS

2.2.21 OSTEOPENIA – GENERALIZED (child)

see Ch 17

2.2.22 OSTEOPENIA – REGIONAL

RULE OUT PERMEATIVE LESION THEN

JOINT RELATED

MONO/OLIGO

TB

ATROPHY

NEUROPATHIC

IDIOPATHIC

POLY

RHEUMATOID ARTHRITIS

JUVENILE CHRONIC ARTHRITIS

AMYLOID

AVN LUCENT PHASE, TRANSIENT REGIONAL OSTEOPOROSIS

REFLEX SYMPATHETIC DYSTROPHY OR IMMOBILIZATION OSTEOPOROSIS

RADIATION OSTEONECROSIS

AND CONSIDER ENDOCRINOPATHIES ANYWAY!

2.2.23 PERIOSTEAL REACTION (neonate, infant)

see Ch 17

2.2.24 PERMEATIVE/AGGRESSIVE LESION

Adult

INFECTION

MYELOMA

METASTASIS

SMALL CELL LUNG CARCINOMA

RENAL CELL CARCINOMA

LYMPHOMA

OTHER

PRIMARY

MARROW ORIGIN

MYELOMA (very common!)

LEUKEMIA

PRIMARY BONE LYMPHOMA

EWING'S SARCOMA

NON CALCIFIED MATRIX

FIBROSARCOMA/MALIGNANT FIBROUS HISTIOCYTOMA

ANGIOSARCOMA (rare!)

Child

INFECTION

EOSINOPHILIC GRANULOMA (<30 years)

METASTASIS

NEUROBLASTOMA

LEUKEMIA

LYMPHOMA

RHABDOMYOSARCOMA

RETINOBLASTOMA

LYTIC OSTEOSARCOMA (<30 years)

PRIMARY

MARROW ORIGIN

EWING'S SARCOMA

LEUKEMIA

PRIMARY BONE LYMPHOMA

NON CALCIFIED MATRIX

FIBROSARCOMA/MALIGNANT FIBROUS HISTIOCYTOMA

ANGIOSARCOMA (rare!)

Beware hyperparathyroidism

2.2.25 POROTIC BALLOON JOINT (overgrown epiphyses)

see Ch 17

2.2.26 PSEUDOPERMEATIVE LESION

Cortically based

HEMANGIOMA

RADIATION NECROSIS

AGGRESSIVE OSTEOPOROSIS

2.2.27 SCLEROTIC METASTASES

TREATED METASTASIS OR

MNEMONIC: PBC SHOST

P-ROSTATE

B-REAST

C-ARCINOID

S-TOMACH

H-ODGKIN'S DISEASE

O-STEOSARCOMA

S-MALL CELL LUNG CANCER (but also other types)

T-RANSITIONAL CELL CARCINOMA

2.2.28 SEQUESTRUM

OSTEOMYELITIS

EOSINOPHILIC GRANULOMA

LYMPHOMA

FIBROSARCOMA, MALIGNANT
FIBROUS HISTIOCYTOMA

OSTEOID OSTEOMA (not a sequestrum,
but a calcified nidus)

2.2.29 SKULL GAMUTS

Microcephaly

ATROPHY, MALFORMATIONS

PRENATAL TORCH INFECTIONS

CHROMOSOMAL DISEASE

Macrocephaly

HYDROCEPHALUS

DYSPLASIAS,
MUCOPOLYSACCHARIDOSES

DYSMYELINATION

Wormian bones

MNEMONIC: I CHOP DOWN

I-DIOPATHIC

C-LEIDOCRANIAL DYSOSTOSIS

C-RETINISM

C-HROMOSOMAL DISORDERS

H-YPOPHOSPHATASIA

O-STEOGENESIS IMPERFECTA

P-YKNODYSOSTOSIS

DOWN'S SYNDROME

Enlarged or eroded pituitary fossa

MASS

EMPTY SELLA WITH
HYDROCEPHALUS

Enlarged vascular grooves

AV MALFORMATION, DURAL AV
FISTULA

MENINGIOMA

MOYA-MOYA SYNDROME

Basilar invagination

DIFFERENTIAL

MNEMONIC: ACHONDROPLASTIC PROOF

ACHONDROPLASTIC

P-AGET'S

R-HEUMATOID ARTHRITIS WITH 'CRANIAL
SETTLING'

O-STEOMALACIA

O-STEOGENESIS IMPERFECTA

F-IBROUS DYSPLASIA

MEASUREMENTS

CHAMBERLAIN

HARD PALATE TO FORAMEN MAGNUM

McGREGOR

HARD PALATE TO OCCIPUT BASE

LIMIT

dens no more than 5 mm in to skull (either line)

PLATYBASIA

BASAL ANGLE >140

Skull vault thickening

MNEMONIC: FAMPOD

F-IBROUS DYSPLASIA

A-NEMIAS (esp THALASSEMIA)

M-YELOFIBROSIS

P-AGET'S

O-VERSHUNTING

D-ILANTIN

2.3 MR

2.3.1 BLACK JOINT ON MR

(Plain film will help out)

PIGMENTED VILLONODULAR
SYNOVITIS

HEMOPHILIA

RHEUMATOID ARTHRITIS (low signal
pannus)

SYNOVIAL (osteo) CHONDROMATOSIS
(when calcified)

AMYLOID ARTHROPATHY

2.3.2 BONE MARROW CHANGES ON MR

Edema and replacement (low T1W, high T2W)

TRANSIENT EDEMA/REFLEX
SYMPATHETIC DYSTROPHY

AVASCULAR NECROSIS

BONE BRUISE, OCCULT FRACTURE,
STRESS FRACTURE

INFILTRATION

INFECTION

MODIC I ENDPLATE (by definition)

Reconversion (yellow to red) (mid T1W, mid T2W)

follows normal red marrow elsewhere;
equal or higher T1W signal than
muscle

Conversion (red to yellow) (high T1W)

RADIOTHERAPY CHANGE

MODIC II ENDPLATE (by definition)

Fibrosis (low T1W, low T2W)

MYELOPROLIFERATIVE DISEASE
including mastocytosis

STORAGE DISEASES, GAUCHER'S

AMYLOID

BURNT OUT PAGET'S

BONE MARROW IN DIABETICS AND
SMOKERS

MODIC III ENDPLATE (by definition)

2.3.3 DURAL ABNORMAL ENHANCEMENT

see Ch 10

2.3.4 FLUID–FLUID LEVELS ON MR/CT

ANEURYSMAL BONE CYST

UNICAMERAL (solitary) BONE CYST

GIANT CELL TUMOR

TELANGIECTATIC OSTEOSARCOMA

ANY NECROTIC TUMOR

FIBROUS DYSPLASIA (when cyst
present)

2.3.5 SPINAL CYSTS

SIMPLE SYNOVIAL CYST (from facet joint)

COMPLICATED SYNOVIAL CYST

ARACHNOID DIVERTICULUM

PERINEURAL (Tarlov) CYST

TRAUMATIC PSEUDOMENINGOCELE

2.3.6 SPINAL NERVE ROOT THICKENING (diffuse)

see Ch 10

2.3.7 T1W HIGH SIGNAL MATERIAL

BLOOD

FAT

THICK PROTEIN

MELANIN

DIFFUSE CALCIUM

GADOLINIUM

SLOW FLOW

2.3.8 T2W LOW SIGNAL MATERIAL

BLOOD

DENSE TISSUE
FIBROUS
CELLULAR
PROTEINACEOUS

IRON

CLUMPY CALCIUM

AIR

METAL (non iron)

FLOW VOID

2.4 NUC MED

2.4.1 COLD DEFECT OR 'DONUT' ON BONE SCAN

Non skeletal (overlying attenuation)

Skeletal
ARTICULAR
AVASCULAR NECROSIS (AVN)
JOINT EFFUSION
BLAND
SEPTIC
FOCAL BONY
EARLY BONE INFARCT
AGGRESSIVELY LYTIC TUMOR
METASTASIS
PRIMARY
INDOLENT TUMOR
HEMANGIOMA
SIMPLE (UNICAMERAL) BONE CYST
GIANT CELL TUMOR
RADIOTHERAPY (straight edge)
PROSTHESIS OR METAL
EARLY AGGRESSIVE OSTEOMYELITIS ('cold osteomyelitis')
ABSENT BONE (surgical or congenital)

2.4.2 HOT KIDNEYS

normal is less intense than lumbar vertebrae

OBSTRUCTION

NEPHROCALCINOSIS, HYPERCALCEMIA

ACUTE TUBULAR NECROSIS, CHEMOTHERAPY, NEPHRITIS

AMYLOID

2.4.3 SUPERSCAN

Appearance
loss of axial to appendicular differentiation, very low intensity kidneys and virtually invisible soft tissues

Differential
DIFFUSE PAGET'S

DIFFUSE METASTASES

MYELOFIBROSIS

METABOLIC BONE DISEASE
RENAL OSTEODYSTROPHY
OSTEOMALACIA
HYPERPARATHYROIDISM

2.4.4 INCREASED MDP/HDP NON SKELETAL UPTAKE

Urinary
CONTAMINATION

CALYX

URETER

BLADDER DIVERTICULUM

URINARY DIVERSION

Soft tissue
INJECTION SITE EXTRAVASATION

FREE PERTECHNETATE (THYROID, STOMACH)

NORMAL
BREAST
CALCIFYING CARTILAGE (e.g. ribs, thyroid)

TENDINOUS/ENTHESAL
e.g. rotator cuff
see articular uptake

TISSUE/BLOOD POOL
POSTOPERATIVE EDEMA (e.g. breast)
VENOUS STASIS
LYMPHATIC STASIS

DYSTROPHIC CALCIFICATION
VASCULAR
INFARCT/NECROSIS
BURNS/RHABDOMYOLYSIS
MYOSITIS OSSIFICANS
NECROTIC TUMOR
esp mucinous adenocarcinoma metastases with calcification
VIABLE TUMOR
PHEOCHROMOCYTOMA
NEUROBLASTOMA
BREAST CARCINOMA

METASTATIC CALCIFICATION
RENAL OSTEODYSTROPHY
HYPERPARATHYROIDISM
TUMORAL CALCINOSIS

2.4.5 INCREASED MDP/HDP SKELETAL UPTAKE

Specific appearance
DENTAL/SINONASAL

HYPEROSTOSIS FRONTALIS INTERNA

POST BIOPSY

PAGET'S DISEASE

Articular/enthesal

SINGLE OR FEW JOINTS (mono/oligo)

COALITION

'Hemophiliac SAINT'
see joint machine for mono/oligoarthropathy

SEVERAL OR MANY JOINTS (oligo/poly)

DEGENERATIVE JOINT DISEASE vs ALL ELSE
see joint machine for polyarthropathies

Focal bony

ONE OR FEW (mono/oligo)

FRACTURE

   ACUTE FRACTURE

   STRESS FRACTURE

   MICROFRACTURE/BONE BRUISE

OSTEOMYELITIS

SOLITARY METASTASIS

BONE INFARCT (AVN) OR TRANSIENT REGIONAL OSTEOPOROSIS

PAGET'S DISEASE

BONY PRIMARY (INCLUDING FIBROUS DYSPLASIA)

SEVERAL OR MANY (oligo/poly)

FRACTURES

METASTASES

MULTIFOCAL INFARCTS (AVN)

MULTIPLE PRIMARIES

MULTIFOCAL OSTEOMYELITIS

Linear bony

HYPERTROPHIC OSTEOARTHROPATHY

INSERTIONAL ENTHESOPATHY

STRESS FRACTURE

Diffuse

COALESCING METASTASES (superscan)

METABOLIC BONE DISEASE (superscan)

HYPERPARATHYROIDISM

RENAL OSTEODYSTROPHY

OSTEOMALACIA

SKELETAL DYSPLASIAS

BONE MARROW EXPANSION PATTERN

CHEMOTHERAPY

HEMOGLOBINOPATHIES

GAUCHER'S DISEASE

MYELOFIBROSIS

REGIONAL ONLY

REFLEX SYMPATHETIC DYSTROPHY

TRANSIENT REGIONAL OSTEOPOROSIS

2.4.6 INCREASED MDP/HDP THREE PHASE UPTAKE

Articular

ACUTE ARTHROPATHY

see Joint Machine

NEUROPATHIC JOINT

Solitary non specific

INTENSE

OSTEOMYELITIS

PAGET'S DISEASE

VASCULAR METASTASIS

VASCULAR PRIMARY TUMOR

   OSTEOID OSTEOMA

   FIBROUS DYSPLASIA

   EWING'S SARCOMA

   GIANT CELL TUMOR

LESS INTENSE

FRACTURE, STRESS FRACTURE

HEALING AVASCULAR NECROSIS

Diffuse

REFLEX SYMPATHETIC DYSTROPHY

2.4.7 SOLITARY LIMB DECREASED MDP/HDP UPTAKE

DECREASED VASCULARITY (usually arterial insufficiency)

DECREASED BONY TURNOVER

DISUSE/NON WEIGHTBEARING

PARALYSIS

RADIOTHERAPY

REFLEX SYMPATHETIC DYSTROPHY (rarely)

INCREASED MDP UPTAKE CONTRALATERALLY

2.4.8 SOLITARY LIMB INCREASED MDP/HDP UPTAKE

INCREASED VASCULARITY

CELLULITIS

AV SHUNT

REFLEX SYMPATHETIC DYSTROPHY, SYMPATHECTOMY

PARALYSIS

INCREASED BONY TURNOVER

See diffuse pattern, focal bony uptake several/many

TOURNIQUET ARTIFACT

DECREASED MDP UPTAKE CONTRALATERALLY

2.5 JOINT MACHINE

2.5.1 ARTHRITIS MACHINE (approach to arthritis)

Also see arthritis classification under joint overviews

Based on arthritis classification by Dr Graham Buirski

POLYARTHRITIS OR OLIGOARTHRITIS

SYNOVIOPATHY (erosive arthropathy)

OSTEOPOROTIC BONE DENSITY

RHEUMATOID ARTHRITIS

JUVENILE CHRONIC ARTHRITIS

SLE, MIXED CONNECTIVE TISSUE DISEASE, SCLERODERMA

NORMAL BONE DENSITY

PSORIASIS, REITER'S

ANKYLOSING SPONDYLITIS (and inflammatory bowel disease)

JUVENILE CHRONIC ARTHRITIS

ROBUST RHEUMATOID ARTHRITIS

CHONDROPATHY

(degenerative arthropathy)

MNEMONIC: NOAH'S CRYSTALS

N-EUROPATHIC

O-STEOARTHRITIS

A-VASCULAR NECROSIS

produces accelerated osteoarthritis

A-CROMEGALY

initially widened joint space

multiple other plain film signs of acromegaly

H-EMOPHILIA

produces accelerated osteoarthritis

CRYSTALS

GOUT

CALCIUM PYROPHOSPHATE DEPOSITION DISEASE, HEMOCHROMATOSIS

HYPERPARATHYROIDISM (primary)

WILSON'S DISEASE

ALKAPTONURIA

SOFT TISSUE DEPOSITION DISEASE

GOUT

AMYLOID

MULTIFOCAL RETICULOHISTIOCYTOSIS

HYPERCHOLESTEROLEMIA

CALCIUM HYDROXYAPATITE DEPOSITION

MONOARTHRITIS

MNEMONIC: HEMOPHILIAC SAINT

HEMOPHILIAC

WEIRD MONOARTHRITIS [S]

S-YNOVIAL CHONDROMATOSIS

PVNS

AMYLOID

ACCELERATED OSTEOARTHRITIS [AINT]

A-VASCULAR NECROSIS

I-NFECTION (pyogenic vs TB)

N-EUROPATHIC JOINT

T-RAUMA

or VERY FIRST INSTANCE OF POLYARTHRITIS

2 General musculoskeletal conditions

3. SYSTEMIC OR GENERAL BONE CONDITIONS

3.1 ACROMEGALY
(skeletal findings)

IMAGING

XR

HANDS
spade-like terminal tufts
bony widening
bony proliferation at entheses
widened cartilage space with premature
   degenerative changes

SKULL
large overpneumatized facial bones
prognathism and large mandible
may have enlarged pituitary fossa

3.2 AVASCULAR NECROSIS (AVN)

see osteochondritis dissecans, Ch 04, 3.11

CAVEAT

pathology and imaging sequences are
   variable and do not necessarily rigidly
   follow in order or correspond to each
   other

DEFINITION

ischemic death of bone cells with secondary
   change in bone matrix which leads to
   fatigue collapse of necrotic articular bone
   and cartilage with long term
   degenerative changes
other names: osteonecrosis, bone infarct

CLASSIFICATION

By location

3.2.1 ARTICULAR (SUBCHONDRAL)
NAMED (specific bone) vs NON NAMED
   (generic)
see named AVN overview Ch 03, 4.11

3.2.2 MEDULLARY (bone marrow)

By age

PEDIATRIC
'OSTEOCHONDRITIS DISSECANS'

ADULT
'BONE INFARCT/SPONTANEOUS
   OSTEONECROSIS'

ETIOLOGY (AVN)

commonest is idiopathic
other AVN causes [mnemonic: GESTALT]
   G-AUCHERS
   E-MBOLISM
   fat embolism (trauma or pancreatitis),
      rarely gaseous (decompression disease)
   S-TEROIDS
   second commonest, especially SLE
   both therapeutic corticosteroids and
      anabolic steroids
   T-RAUMA
especially femoral neck fractures
   A-LCOHOL
   L-UPUS (SLE) AND OTHER VASCULITIDES
      (including radiation necrosis)
   T-HROMBOSIS (esp SICKLE CELL DISEASE) and
      VENOUS THROMBOSIS/VENOUS
      HYPERTENSION

PATHOGENESIS

Avascularity
autolysis of osteocytes and bone marrow
   adipocytes
EXPECTED IMAGING FINDINGS
cold spot MDP, normal MR, normal XR

Reparative processes

MARGINAL HYPEREMIA, HYPEREMIC MARGINAL OSTEOPENIA
inflammation at margins of infarcted area
   with increased vascularity
osteoclastic resorption of dead bone
EXPECTED IMAGING FINDINGS
hot ring with cold center MDP, demarcating
   single or double line (with variable
   center) MR, normal XR (double line sign
   earliest appearance quoted at 48 hours)
later shrinking cold center MDP, double line
   (variable center) MR, osteopenic halo XR

CREEPING SUBSTITUTION
invasion of necrotic area by osteoclasts and
   osteoblasts

resorption of dead bone; formation of new
   woven bone over the scaffolding of
   remaining necrotic trabeculae
theoretically, eventual restoration of near
   normal bone architecture
EXPECTED IMAGING FINDINGS
hot ring with cold center progressing to hot
   area on MDP, double line (variable
   center) MR, sclerotic margin or diffuse
   sclerosis XR

Usual medullary infarct events
usually clinically silent unless extensive or
   severe (i.e. sickle cell disease or
   decompression disease)
cortical bone usually not affected because of
   preserved periosteal collaterals, and
   bone strength not compromised
infarcted area usually irregular or
   geographic
may resolve fully, or may leave behind
   permanently infarcted area with/without
   dense calcified margin

Usual articular AVN events
asymptomatic, or ill defined or dull pain on
   movement, restriction of motion
progressively increasing pain on movement
   and at rest

INFARCTION
infarcted area is often wedge shaped, with
   base on the articular surface and apex at
   depth (particularly so for femoral head)
articular cartilage remains alive (supplied
   via synovial fluid)

COLLAPSE OF NECROTIC BONE
fatigue collapse forms a subchondral
   crescent (fills with synovial fluid, myxoid
   material, debris) with covering flap of
   living cartilage
collapse of unsupported articular cartilage
   follows
EXPECTED IMAGING FINDINGS
classic imaging finding is a subchondral
   crescent: lucent on XR and usually fluid
   signal on MR

GROSS CHONDRAL AND SUBCHONDRAL COLLAPSE
EXPECTED IMAGING FINDINGS
hot spot MDP, variable appearance MR (see
   below), frank articular surface collapse
   with mixed sclerosis and lucency XR

OUTCOME
in children, complete remodelling or
   remodelling with residual deformity and
   early development of degenerative
   disease

in adults, collapse of weightbearing areas of joints leading to accelerated severe degenerative monoarthritis

IMAGING

Plain XR sequence

SUBARTICULAR BONE
I   NORMAL (avascularity, marginal hyperemia)
II OSTEOPENIA (hyperemic marginal osteopenia, early creeping substitution)
III SCLEROSIS, SUBCHONDRAL LUCENCY (collapse of necrotic subchondral bone)
IV COLLAPSE (gross chondral, subchondral collapse)
V   LATE DEGENERATIVE CHANGES

MARGINAL CONDENSATION (XR findings in spine)
occurs at vertebral endplates
collapse (due to softened bone) with increased sclerosis along endplates (due to microfractures with increased callus formation)

NUC MED

MDP
EARLY (AVASCULARITY)
cold area on all three phases (has to be sufficiently large) (BUT see steroid induced AVN findings)
LATER
hot ring on blood pool/tissue and delayed phases with cold center
HEALING
hot ring or hot spot on three phases
one side of joint only
ESTABLISHED DEGENERATIVE CHANGE
increased uptake on delayed phase only
one side of joint only which eventually evolves to both sides if arthritis advanced enough
STEROID INDUCED AVN
usually hot even at the time of presentation without a cold area
SICKLE CELL DISEASE
bone infarcts of multiple ages
background pattern of bone marrow expansion and increased skeletal MDP uptake
may see MDP uptake in autosplenectomy
RADIOTHERAPY CHANGE
CARDINAL SIGN: corresponds to radiotherapy portal
diffusely decreased MDP uptake

COLLOID (BONE MARROW SCAN)

ANY CAUSE OF BONE MARROW INFARCT
absent colloid uptake
sharp straight margin pathognomonic of radiation portal

MR findings

DEMARCATING LINE
serpiginous low signal in articular subchondral location
DOUBLE LINE SIGN
OUTER RIM low T1W, low T2W on spin echo sequences ('sclerosis')
INNER RIM low T1W, high T2W ('inflammation')
highly variable and inconstant

DIFFUSE HIGH T2W SIGNAL
may be only finding in early AVN
differential is transient (regional) osteoporosis

CHANGES IN CENTER
variable MR signal central to demarcating line, if any
these do not impart prognostic significance
ADIPOSE TISSUE SIGNAL
BLOOD SIGNAL
CLEAR FLUID SIGNAL (EDEMA)
DENSE SCLEROSIS SIGNAL (low T1W, low T2W)

RADIOTHERAPY CHANGE
very variable appearance
ESTABLISHED RADIOTHERAPY CHANGE
established radiotherapy change is red to yellow marrow conversion, with higher fatty signal than in normal yellow marrow
EARLY RADIOTHERAPY CHANGE
commonest early appearance is increased T2W signal and edema
does not necessarily indicate necrosis or persistent tumor infiltration
contrast enhancement (Gd) usually increased and variable; usually unhelpful
demarcating line and other changes of AVN are more specific findings

3.2.3 MIMICKER: TRANSIENT REGIONAL OSTEOPOROSIS

idiopathic and usually painful bone marrow edema; hips and knees common

IMAGING

XR
late changes, occur after MR changes become evident
diffuse osteopenia

NUC MED

MDP
regional bone marrow pattern (diffusely hot, not restricted to subarticular bone, one side of joint only)
hot on all three phases

MR
abnormal marrow signal with diffuse edema (high T2W)
no double line or geographic margin
does not extend past intertrochanteric line
joint effusion may be present

3.3 HEMOPHILIA

see Ch 03

3.4 HEMORRHAGE ON MR (MUSCULO-SKELETAL SYSTEM)

see musculoskeletal hematoma Ch 04

3.5 HYPERPARA-THYROIDISM

DEFINITION

elevated parathyroid hormone (PTH) levels with secondary manifestations mostly relating to hypercalcemia or bone disease

CLASSIFICATION AND ETIOLOGY

PRIMARY (PTH overproduction)
90% parathyroid adenoma, 10% parathyroid hyperplasia, parathyroid carcinoma rare

MIMICKER OF PRIMARY: PARATHYROID HORMONE RELATED PROTEIN
bronchogenic squamous cell carcinoma, other squamous cell carcinoma, renal cell carcinoma

SECONDARY (renal dysfunction)
either normal response or (eventually) parathyroid hyperplasia
parathyroid adenoma rare

TERTIARY (secondary that became autonomous)

MICRO (BONE DISEASE)

Generalized bone changes

increased osteoclast activity and number, trabecular resorption, peritrabecular fibrosis

Focal bone changes = brown tumor

bone removal en masse
osteoclast giant cells
fibrous tissue with spindle cells
hemorrhages, resulting hemosiderin pigment

IMAGING (BONE DISEASE)

XR/CT

RESORPTIVE CHANGES

GENERALIZED OSTEOPENIA

RESORPTION: GENERIC

subperiosteal, subendosteal, intracortical tunnelling
hands: tufts and radial periosteum of middle phalanges

RESORPTION: SPECIFIC

subchondral in specific joints: sacroiliac joints and symphysis pubis, acromioclavicular joints, temporomandibular joints
loss of lamina dura
subligamentous (clavicle, calcaneus at Achilles insertion)

BROWN TUMORS

see under bone tumor section

HYPERCALCEMIC CHANGES

SCLEROSIS (?MECHANISM)
generalized
rugger jersey spine

CHONDROCALCINOSIS

SOFT TISSUE CALCINOSIS

calcium hydroxyapatite deposition disease (CHAD)
tumoral calcinosis
vascular calcification

COARSENING OF PRIMARY TRABECULAE

MORE COMMON IN PRIMARY HYPERPARATHYROIDISM

brown tumors, chondrocalcinosis

MORE COMMON IN SECONDARY HYPERPARATHYROIDISM

sclerosis, soft tissue calcinosis

NUC MED

MDP
diffusely increased bone MDP uptake with decreased renal MDP clearance (superscan)
increased peripheral skeleton MDP uptake
soft tissue calcinosis may take up MDP (tumoral calcinosis; vascular calcification; lung MDP uptake (?calcinosis, ?other))
brown tumors may have increased tissue phase activity and focally increased uptake above background
may see shrunken or absent native kidneys or a renal transplant

3.6 HYPO-PARATHYROIDISM, PSEUDO, PSEUDOPSEUDO

3.6.1 HYPOPARATHYROIDISM

deficient parathyroid hormone (PTH) level (primary or secondary)
PRIMARY rare
SECONDARY usually surgical

3.6.2 PSEUDOHYPO-PARATHYROIDISM

genetically determined endorgan unresponsiveness to PTH

3.6.3 PSEUDOPSEUDO-HYPOPARATHYROIDISM

genetic syndrome of morphological changes of pseudohypoparathyroidism with normal biochemistry

IMAGING FINDINGS (entire group)

osteosclerosis (may have osteoporosis)
hypoplastic teeth if onset early
metastatic soft tissue calcification
basal ganglia calcification, falx calcification, calvarial thickening (rare in pseudopseudo)

IMAGING FINDINGS (pseudo, pseudopseudo ONLY)

short and obese

short metacarpals and metatarsals I, IV, V
cone epiphyses
growth deformities

3.7 LANGERHANS CELL HISTIOCYTOSIS

see Ch 05

3.8 LEUKEMIA AND LYMPHOMA

see Ch 05

3.9 MASTOCYTOSIS

see Ch 05

3.10 MODIC ENDPLATE CHANGES

see Ch 04 spine degenerative change

3.11 MYOSITIS OSSIFICANS

see Ch 05

3.12 OSTEOMALACIA AND RICKETS

DEFINITION

failure of osteoid ossification; rickets is resulting disease before epiphyseal closure, osteomalacia after epiphyseal closure

ETIOLOGY AND CLASSIFICATION

Vitamin D dependent

sunlight deficiency, nutritional deficiency or malabsorption, liver or renal disease

Vitamin D resistant

renal tubular rickets, hypophosphatemia

Renal osteodystrophy

combined hyperparathyroidism, osteomalacia/rickets and aluminum toxicity

Hypophosphatasia

inadequate levels of alkaline phosphatase producing failure of osteoid mineralization

MICRO

Rickets

failure of calcification in hypertrophic cartilage zone

widening of cartilage plate, chondrocyte column disorganization, poor primary trabeculae, widened osteoid seams

Osteomalacia

non mineralized osteoid lining Haversian canals

IMAGING – RICKETS

Plain XR

THREE METAPHYSEAL FINDINGS

LOSS OF JEANTET LAVAL COLLAR (thin layer of periosteally formed new bone around the metaphyseal aspect of a growth plate)

CUPPING, SPLAYING, FRAYING

WIDENING OF OSTEOID

EPIPHYSEAL FINDING

DELAY IN OSSIFICATION (DELAY IN RADIOGRAPHIC BONE AGE)

DIAPHYSEAL FINDING

LONG BONE BOWING AND SOFTENING

OTHER

RACHITIC ROSARY

LOSS OF LAMINA DURA AROUND TEETH

XR DIFFERENTIAL

HYPOPHOSPHATASIA

osteopenia

metaphyseal changes of rickets

craniostenosis, Wormian bones

markedly depressed alkaline phosphatase

METAPHYSEAL CHONDRODYSPLASIA

biochemically normal

metaphyseal pseudorickets

IMAGING – OSTEOMALACIA

Plain XR

OSTEOPENIA

CORTICAL TUNNELLING

TRABECULAR CHANGES

loss of secondary trabeculae, coarse and fuzzy primary trabeculae

LOOSER'S ZONES

insufficiency fractures healed by osteoid seams

LONG BONE BOWING AND SOFTENING

IMAGING – BOTH (NUC MED)

MDP

markedly increased delayed phase MDP skeletal uptake (metabolic superscan)

3.13 OSTEOMYELITIS (OM)

DEFINITION

bacterial, mycobacterial or fungal focus of bone infection with an inflammatory response, destruction and usually periosteal new bone formation

ETIOLOGY

BACTERIAL

Staphylococcus > Streptococcus > E coli > Hemophilus > Salmonella > other Gram negative rods

Neonates: organisms differ (Group B Streptococcus, Hemophilus, E coli)

FUNGAL

TUBERCULOUS

HYDATID

ACTINOMYCES, MADUROMYCES

PATHOGENESIS

Hematogenous spread

'spontaneous' (probably a transient bacteremia), spread from focus elsewhere, IV lines and IV drug use

Direct spread

surgical or traumatic inoculation; direct spread from soft tissue abscess (especially Actinomyces)

Location

actively growing bones, red marrow containing bones

75% long bones (femur > tibia > humerus > other), 25% flat bones

bacterial seeding in (hairpin) venous sinusoids, acute inflammatory exudate, markedly raised intraosseous pressure, focal thrombosis and ischemic necrosis or toxic necrosis

NEONATES

transphyseal vessels patent in neonates and up to 12 months old – metaphyseal osteomyelitis may spread to epiphysis and involve the joint cavity

CHILDREN: METAPHYSES AND EQUIVALENTS

vascular areas with increased blood supply

vessels form hairpin loops under proliferating cartilage zone – areas of potential stasis or thrombosis

ADULTS: EPIPHYSES, VERTEBRAE

no metaphyseal vascular loops to form a focus and no growth plate to prevent epiphyseal involvement

secondary septic arthritis therefore common

Spread along paths of least resistance

cortical, subperiosteal, soft tissue

medullary cavity

Spread to joint likely if

TB

adult, epiphyseal focus

high capsule attachment (capsule attaches further metaphyseally than growth plate)

transphyseal vascular anastomosis (neonate)

neglected metaphyseal osteomyelitis

CLINICAL

3.13.1 ACUTE OSTEOMYELITIS

focal pain, tenderness, redness, swelling

in toddler: refusal to weightbear or limping

fever

white cell count, inflammatory markers usually elevated

may give a history of recent injury – symptoms may be ascribed to it

SPINAL OSTEOMYELITIS

increasing back pain present on activity and at rest

fever (may or may not be present)

back pain in child – usually a significant symptom

differentiation from discitis is often impossible clinically (and on imaging grounds)

risk of epidural abscess with potential for paraplegia

3.13.2 CHRONIC OSTEOMYELITIS

indolent pain, swelling, discharge, sinus track

COMPLICATIONS

BRODIE'S ABSCESS (intraosseous abscess cavity)

SEQUESTRUM (dead fragment of bone central to mass of infected bone/inflammatory tissue)

INVOLUCRUM (outer sheath of periosteally formed new bone)

CLOACA/SINUS (perforation in involucrum/cortex and draining track)

PATHOLOGICAL FRACTURE

SQUAMOUS CELL CARCINOMA ALONG SINUS TRACK

GROWTH DISTURBANCE: DEFORMITY, TRANSPHYSEAL BAR, OVERGROWTH (secondary to hypervascularity)

SEPTIC ARTHRITIS WITH DESTRUCTION OF ARTICULAR SURFACES

AVASCULAR NECROSIS

SYSTEMIC SEPTIC COMPLICATIONS, AMYLOID (chronic osteomyelitis)

3.13.3 TUBERCULOUS OSTEOMYELITIS

indolent destruction without sequestration or involucrum formation

extensive tracking of caseous material with little containment

Classic pattern – spinal TB (Pott's disease)

paraspinal psoas abscesses (often bilateral)

tracking along psoas tendon into pelvis; may point in groin

vertebral body destruction, sharp kyphus deformity

IMAGING

XR

predominantly lytic destruction with late loss of cartilage, reactive osteopenia, little

periosteal new bone, large soft tissue mass and large joint effusion, extensive soft tissue calcification

3.13.4 ACTINOMYCOSIS AND MADUROMYCOSIS

mandible, maxilla, ribs

feet (maduromycosis especially)

chronic granulomatous inflammatory mass with network of sinuses and fistulae draining 'sulfur granules' (masses of Actinomyces bacteria)

IMAGING (OSTEOMYELITIS NOS)

XR

EARLY OSTEOMYELITIS

no findings

subtle displacement of soft tissue planes (usually recognized only in hindsight)

possibly a soft tissue mass (evident before bony changes)

main utility of XR is exclusion of alternative diagnoses when bone scan is positive

ESTABLISHED OSTEOMYELITIS

in general, earliest XR findings of bone destruction manifest at 2 weeks

can not see bony changes where there is no bone (e.g. neonatal epiphyses)!

permeative bone destruction

soft tissue mass may be present, not usually a dominant feature

early periosteal reaction

possibly, hypervascular osteopenia

CHRONIC OSTEOMYELITIS

differentiation from indolent tumor or eosinophilic granuloma not always possible on imaging alone

lytic bone destruction, usually well marginated with a narrow transition zone

variable amount of periosteal new bone formation: often considerable amount

indolent 'benign' periosteal new bone, often wavy unilamellar and thick

HELPFUL: cloaca (relatively small well defined cortical breach) with sinus track; sequestrum (loose bone fragment)

DISCITIS

see separate entry under joints

SEPTIC ARTHRITIS

see separate entry under joints

US

SUBPERIOSTEAL ABSCESS

reflective periosteal edge parallel to bone cortex

lens shaped or elongated fluid collection deep to it, of variable echotexture

irregular underlying cortical surface

SEPTIC ARTHRITIS

main utility is demonstration or exclusion of pediatric joint effusion

see separate entry under joints

CT

features similar to XR findings

bone marrow may be edematous and dense

may demonstrate large epidural collections

specific if shows gas

MR

suspected spinal or pelvic osteomyelitis or discitis is an absolute indication (only modality to reliably demonstrate or exclude significant epidural abscess formation (look for peripheral contrast enhancement))

OSTEOMYELITIS

use precontrast T1W for bone marrow; fat sat T2W (or STIR) for edema; post contrast (non fat sat) sequences to look for abscess/epidural collection

sensitive, non specific

relatively poor at showing bone destruction

cardinal finding is bone marrow edema (may be sharply delimited by the growth plate)

subperiosteal collections

soft tissue edema

epidural abscess: epidural fluid signal collection with marginal enhancement

soft tissue inflammatory mass/abscess may be outlined by contrast

NORMAL bone marrow rules out osteomyelitis with a high degree of confidence

FALSE POSITIVES

OTHER CAUSES OF BONE MARROW EDEMA

diabetic feet with neuropathic joints and secondary bone marrow changes

infiltrative tumor

DISCITIS, SEPTIC ARTHRITIS

see separate entry under joints

NUC MED

MDP

in general, requires a triple phase scan for specificity

need meticulous technique in children because of growth plates

specific at 2 days of symptoms

if plain film normal, highly sensitive and specific for osteomyelitis

if plain film abnormal, sensitive and not specific

may need to do a delayed image (fourth phase) if trying to differentiate retained tissue phase activity from bony uptake

USUAL FINDINGS IN OSTEOMYELITIS

increased vascularity

increased tissue phase activity

increased delayed uptake (may manifest as focal expansion of growth plate activity)

COLD OSTEOMYELITIS

area of infection and bone infarction

occurs early in timecourse, before osteoblastic reaction builds up

if suspected, repeat MDP (should turn to hot) or do a Ga scan or MR

CELLULITIS

increased vascularity

increased tissue phase activity (often diffuse)

mildly diffusely increased delayed phase activity, degree consistent with increased uptake secondary to increased vascularity only

helpful if uptake extensive and extends well beyond focal area under suspicion

FALSE NEGATIVES

spinal osteomyelitis

partly treated osteomyelitis

neonates

cold osteomyelitis

infected prosthesis (activity indistinguishable from normal bone reaction or loosening)

infected fracture (same as above)

FALSE POSITIVES

healing fracture

hypervascular tumor

cellulitis/soft tissue infection

GALLIUM

usually used in sequence after MDP (downscatter)

imaging at 48 hours

discordant gallium uptake (either in area: Ga uptake extending beyond MDP uptake; or in intensity: focally elevated Ga uptake without matching increased MDP uptake in same location) is positive

concordant Ga uptake indeterminate

WHITE CELL SCANNING

Cardinal sign: focus of white cell accumulation

FALSE POSITIVES

neuropathic joints

recent fractures or recent surgery or recent prostheses

bone marrow redistribution around prostheses (consider bone marrow scan)

FALSE NEGATIVES

particularly spine (do MR in preference)

chronic osteomyelitis (non neutrophilic)

granulomatous osteomyelitis (non neutrophilic)

partly treated OM

PET (FDG)

osteomyelitis (and soft tissue infection) is FDG avid (inflammatory cell uptake)

FDG uptake is not specific to infection (see Ch 25) and is also present in tumor, metastasis and healing scar

greatest utility is exclusion of osteomyelitis with a high degree of confidence if no uptake is present (i.e. high negative predictive value)

good positive predictive value if no alternative pathology (e.g. metastasis) is present

utility in diagnosing periprosthetic infection comparable to three phase MDP

3.14 OSTEOPOROSIS

DEFINITION

generalized reduction in bone mineral density with normal biochemistry and bone histology

CLASSIFICATION

Primary

WHO DEFINITIONS

T score: bone mineral density in standard deviations relative to gender matched young adults

OSTEOPOROSIS is $T < -2.5$

OSTEOPENIA is $-2.5 < T < -1.0$

Secondary

STEROIDS OR CUSHING'S SYNDROME

accelerated osteoporosis

accelerated osteoporotic fractures

abundant callus

combinations of fractures and callus: sclerotic vertebral endplates with fractures (marginal condensation); marginal fractures with callus

avascular necrosis (especially humerus and femur)

ALCOHOLISM

HYPERTHYROIDISM

ACROMEGALY

IMAGING

DEXA

bone mineral density (BMD) assessment

DEXA error 2%, QCT error 5%

serial monitoring most accurate in lumbar spine

measurement must be related to reference range

measurement given as T score (BMD in standard deviations relative to gender matched normal young adult mean)

RECOMMENDATIONS BY T SCORE

+1	do DEXA in 10 years
0	do DEXA in 5 years
−1	do DEXA in 2 years, consider treatment
−2.5	treatment imperative

XR

plain XR insensitive (need 50% BMD loss)

sharp primary trabeculae, picture frame vertebrae, biconcave or wedge compression fractures

INSUFFICIENCY FRACTURES

sacrum

pelvic ring (may be in one site only)

femoral neck

detection of undisplaced fractures may be very difficult with plain film because of reduced bony density

US

calcaneal ultrasound consistent with itself

not as accurate as DEXA

relevance of calcaneal density to lumbar and femoral fracture risk not fully determined

CT

quantitative CT has comparable accuracy to DEXA

BMD given in terms of volume rather than area density

assessment of lumbar spine only

useful in looking for fractures in osteopenic bone (especially sacrum)

MR

role in diagnosing undisplaced osteoporotic fractures (traumatic or insufficiency)

NUC MED

role in diagnosing undisplaced osteoporotic fractures

'honda sign' a classic finding in sacral fracture

PITFALL: poor or absent osteoblast reaction leading to false negative results (bedridden patient, or scan too early – scanning after 2 days is conservative and accurate but not infallible)

3.15 PAGET'S DISEASE

DEFINITION

focal or multifocal abnormal remodeling of bone with simultaneous osteoclast and osteoblast overactivity

EPIDEMIOLOGY

true incidence unknown

>40 years old, male > female

PATHOGENESIS

massive focal resorption followed by abnormal massive immature bone deposition (multiple cycles coinciding in all stages) resulting in bone softening, bowing, expansion and deformities (?viral)

CLINICAL

asymptomatic incidental finding or

bone pain, deformity and warmth (long bone bowing; skull expansion)

massively elevated alkaline phosphatase, elevated urine and serum hydroxyproline (varies with stage)

COMPLICATIONS:

arthritis, fractures, basilar invagination (30%) with hydrocephalus and spinal cord compression; cranial nerve compression

1% sarcomatous transformation (new pain, lytic lesion, soft tissue mass)

MORPHOLOGY

expanded softened bowed bone with thickened primary trabeculae, loss of secondary trabeculae, loss of corticomedullary junction, abnormal hypervascular soft tissue replacing bone marrow

LYTIC PHASE, MIXED PHASE, SCLEROTIC PHASE

IMAGING

XR/CT

LYTIC PHASE, MIXED PHASE, SCLEROTIC PHASE

frequency of bone involvement correlates with red marrow distribution

all bones can be affected, although fibula is rarely involved

75% SPINE

expanded dense vertebrae

picture frame margins, coarse vertical trabeculae

70% PELVIS

ileopectineal cortical thickening

coarsening, expansion

protrusio acetabuli

65% SKULL

osteoporosis circumscripta (frontal, occipital, both)

focal cotton wool sclerosis

expansion, loss of diploic space, sclerosis

basilar invagination

deformity of cranial foramina/temporal bone structures

35% LONG BONES

flame shaped osteoporosis starting in a subarticular location (except tibia which may start in diaphysis)

enlargement, coarsening, bowing

MR

differentiation from other causes of bone marrow change difficult in the absence of XR or other pointers

ACTIVE DISEASE

gross morphology (bowing, expansion) same as for XR/CT

bone coarsening hard to appreciate

marrow replaced by hypervascular fibrous tissue, low on T1W, mixed on T2W (high if active/edematous, low if fibrosed/sclerotic)

BURNT OUT DISEASE

marrow signal may return to fatty marrow (high T1W, low T2W) or remain that of fibrous tissue (low T1W, low T2W)

NUC MED

MDP

massively increased vascularity (increased perfusion and tissue phase activity)

increased early uptake, massively increased late phase uptake

pattern of abnormality analogous to XR change: involves only one side of a joint and may have an advancing 'edge'

vascularity correlates better with lytic disease, late uptake correlates better with sclerotic disease

'burnt out' quiescent Paget's may be cold

very useful monitor of disease activity especially if there is active treatment

COLLOID

bone marrow replacement with photopenic areas (see MR)

3.16 RENAL OSTEODYSTROPHY

DEFINITION

combination of several disorders of CaPO4 metabolism that occur in renal failure with/without dialysis

CLINICAL

secondary hyperparathyroidism, renal osteomalacia, aluminium overload

ASSOCIATED: articular amyloid of hemodialysis

IMAGING

see under each separate component

3.17 SARCOID (BONE)
(imaging findings)

see sarcoid in lung Ch 11 CNS, Ch 13 lungs

1–15% of sarcoid; lung and skin disease expected if bone involved

polyarthralgia – no XR changes

IMAGING

XR hands

osteopenia or sclerosis

lacy distal and middle phalanges

tuft sclerosis

3.18 SCHEUERMANN DISEASE

DEFINITION

abnormal ossification? AVN? of vertebral endplates

CLINICAL

adolescents, male:female 1.5:1
asymptomatic incidental finding or kyphosis or back pain

IMAGING

Plain XR

most frequent levels are T7–T10; possible at T4–L4
endplate sclerosis and irregularity
central Schmorl's nodes, marginal Schmorl's nodes
anterior wedging and kyphosis

3.19 SCOLIOSIS

see Ch 17

3.20 SCURVY

see Ch 17

3.21 SICKLE CELL DISEASE

see Ch 16

3.22 SPINAL INFECTION (overview)

also see osteomyelitis entry and septic arthritis and discitis entries in Ch 3

OSTEOMYELITIS, DISCITIS, SACROILIITIS

ETIOLOGY

BACTERIAL (usually Staphylococcus or Streptococcus); TUBERCULOUS/FUNGAL

IMAGING (all modalities)

Earliest changes
earliest detectable MDP uptake is at approximately 2 days
increased vascularity may occur earlier, but is usually not detected
bone marrow edema becomes visible on MR early, but exact time contentious

Established disease
BACTERIAL (usually discitis with later changes of vertebral osteomyelitis)
lytic bone destruction and paraspinal masses become visible at the earliest around 2 weeks
loss of disk height and later endplate destruction (XR)
increased T2W disk signal, loss of disk height, enhancement with Gd; endplate bone marrow edema
abnormal signal isocenter is on disk

TUBERCULOUS/FUNGAL (usually vertebral body infection with disk spared till late)
osteopenia, lytic vertebral destruction, collapse (XR)
paraspinal low density masses (CT)
eventual dystrophic calcification
changes of osteomyelitis with abnormal edema signal centered on vertebral body with disk spared till late (MR)

3.23 SYPHILIS (manifestations)

CONGENITAL

see Ch 17

ADULT (syphilis and yaws)

diffuse fibrosis, extensive sclerosis
irregular areas of destruction

3.24 TARSAL COALITION

see Ch 17

3.25 THALASSEMIA

see Ch 16

3.26 TRANSIENT REGIONAL OSTEOPOROSIS

see entry for avascular necrosis

4. SYNDROMES

4.1 ACHONDROPLASIA

DEFINITION

autosomal dominant non lethal failure of endochondral bone growth

MANIFESTATIONS

SKULL: large vault, short base, small foramen magnum
SPINE: bullet vertebrae with posterior scalloping; short pedicles with inferiorly narrowing interpedicular distance
PELVIS: squared iliac wings, small sciatic notch, flat acetabular angle
LONG BONES (including ribs): short and wide; trident hand (MC II, III, IV all same length)

4.2 CHONDRO-DYSPLASIAS

4.2.1 MULTIPLE EPIPHYSEAL DYSPLASIA

autosomal dominant
delayed, irregular, flattened epiphyses
delayed carpal and tarsal ossification
double layer patella
minimal vertebral wedging
early degenerative changes

4.2.2 DIAPHYSEAL ACLASIA

autosomal dominant
multiple sessile and pedunculated osteochondromas

may undergo sarcomatous degeneration
reverse Madelung deformity (radius longer
than ulna and bowed)

4.3 CLEIDOCRANIAL DYSOSTOSIS

autosomal dominant, variable penetrance
SKULL: multiple Wormian bones, late
sutural fusion, underdeveloped teeth,
hypertelorism
CLAVICLES: aplasia outside in
PELVIS: underdeveloped pubis, wide
symphysis, small iliac wings
HANDS: proximal accessory epiphyses of
metacarpals II and III

4.4 DOWN'S SYNDROME

see Ch 17

4.5 DWARFISM ASSESSMENT

see Ch 17

4.6 DYSOSTOSIS MULTIPLEX

see Ch 17

4.7 GAUCHER'S DISEASE

DEFINITION

sphingolipid storage disorder with
accumulation in reticuloendothelial
system

EPIDEMIOLOGY

?autosomal recessive, familial, male >
female, more frequent in Ashkenazi Jews

CLINICAL

Infantile form
hepatosplenomegaly, lymphadenopathy
CNS involvement with dementia and death
bone marrow replacement and anemia

Adult form
hepatosplenomegaly, ascites
bone pain, modeling deformities, bone
marrow expansion, multiple bone
infarcts

MICRO

bone marrow replaced by foamy binucleate
macrophages full of cerebroside (kerasin)

IMAGING

Marrow replacement
50% Erlenmeyer flask deformity
50% avascular necrosis (especially femoral
heads)
H shaped vertebrae (differential diagnosis is
sickle cell disease)
generalized osteopenia

MR
low T1W, low T2W marrow with expanded
marrow
T2W signal may be variable (?increases
reflect edema or infarction)

Hepatosplenomegaly

4.8 HYPER-PHOSPHATASIA

rare congenital disease with elevated
alkaline phosphatase and imaging
appearance of 'childhood Paget's'

4.9 HYPOPHOSPHATASIA

osteopenia
metaphyseal changes of rickets (rickets is
the differential diagnosis)
craniostenosis, Wormian bones
markedly depressed alkaline phosphatase

4.10 MARFAN'S SYNDROME

DEFINITION

autosomal dominant disorder of connective
tissue elastin with weakened aortic wall
and abnormally tall stature

CLINICAL

abnormal fibrillin gene (required for elastin
assembly); variable expressivity
tall stature, dolichocephaly, arachnodactyly
cystic medial necrosis of aorta, aortic root
ectasia with aortic valve incompetence,
aortic dissection
floppy mitral valve
ocular lens dislocation
hyperelasticity of joints, easy dislocations,
early joint degeneration

DIFFERENTIAL DIAGNOSIS
(on imaging)

HOMOCYSTINURIA
KLINEFELTER'S SYNDROME
TALL NORMAL

4.11 OSTEOGENESIS IMPERFECTA

see Ch 17

4.12 OSTEOPETROSIS

autosomal recessive or autosomal dominant
syndrome of osteoclastic failure with
dense brittle bones
SKULL: thick calvarium, stenosed foramina
VERTEBRAE: sandwich vertebrae
GENERAL: generalized sclerosis, bone in
bone appearance, increased fragility

4.13 PYKNODYSOSTOSIS

autosomal recessive syndrome of
generalized bone sclerosis and abnormal
morphology
SKULL: Wormian bones, persistently open
sutures, obtuse angle of mandible,
delayed, abnormal or incomplete dental
eruption
HANDS: pointed aplastic dense distal
phalanges
CLAVICLES: absent or hypoplastic distal
ends

3 Joint conditions

3. GENERAL

4. SPECIFIC CONDITIONS

3. GENERAL

3.1 ABBREVIATIONS

AS: ankylosing spondylitis

AVN: avascular necrosis (aseptic necrosis)

CHAD: calcium hydroxyapatite deposition disease

CPPD: calcium pyrophosphate deposition disease

CREST: calcinosis, Raynaud's phenomenon, Esophageal dysmotility, Scleroderma and Telangiectasia

DJD: degenerative joint disease

HPTH: hyperparathyroidism

IBD: inflammatory bowel disease

JCA: juvenile chronic arthritis (juvenile rheumatoid arthritis)

MCTD: mixed connective tissue disease

OA: osteoarthritis (osteoarthrosis)

OCD: osteochondritis dissecans (generic rather than eponymous)

RA: rheumatoid arthritis

Reiter's: arthropathy of Reiter's syndrome

SLE: systemic lupus erythematosus

3.2 ARTHROPATHY CLASSIFICATION AND DEFINITIONS

ACKNOWLEDGEMENT

this classification is based on the arthropathy classification by Dr Graham Buirski MD (St John of God Hospital, Ballarat, Australia)

3.2.1 SYNOVIOPATHY

DEFINITION

inflammatory (most likely autoimmune) arthropathy with synovial based inflammation and hypertrophy leading to synovial erosion of bone with relatively delayed loss of cartilage, and frequently with capsular or ligamentous inflammatory laxity or rupture

SIGNS

marginal erosions (located at areas of intracapsular bone not covered by articular cartilage = 'bare bone')

erosions start as focal reduction in density

progressive erosions show loss of cortex

cartilage loss may occur from margins in, but often cartilage space narrows more uniformly

sclerosis around erosion suggests reactive bone formation or healing of inactive synoviopathy

proliferative erosion has prominent periosteal new bone formation around erosion ('fluffy bone')

inflammatory effusion (may be dominant)

periarticular porosis

pannus (synovial proliferation – US, MR)

ASSOCIATED ABNORMALITIES

inflammatory tenosynovitis, synovial hypertrophy of tendon sheaths, tendon erosion, tendon rupture, deformities, contractures

PERIARTICULAR BONE DENSITY IS:

REDUCED IN

RA, JCA, SLE, CREST, MCTD

NORMAL IN

AS/IBD, PSORIASIS/REITER'S, JCA, ROBUST RA

3.2.2 CHONDROPATHY

DEFINITION

predominant or initial destruction of articular cartilage (idiopathic, mechanical, or due to crystal disease) with secondary bony reaction and possible secondary synovial reaction or inflammation

SIGNS

loss of cartilage (MR) or cartilage space (XR/CT), often but not necessarily in a predictable weightbearing distribution

reactive bony change: subarticular sclerosis, marginal osteophytes

degenerative change in cartilage: chondrocalcinosis

degenerative change in bone: irregularity and loss of articular cortical bone, articular surface erosions (central), subchondral cysts

DEGENERATIVE JOINT DISEASE

OA (primary or secondary), NEUROPATHIC ARTHROPATHY, HEMOPHILIAC ARTHROPATHY, post AVN, post traumatic

CRYSTAL DEPOSITION DISEASES

GOUT, CPPD/HEMOCHROMATOSIS, HPTH, WILSON'S DISEASE, ALKAPTONURIA

3.2.3 ENTHESOPATHY

DEFINITION

inflammatory (in inflammatory arthropathies) or degenerative (particularly in chronic sports injuries) abnormality of tendinous or ligamentous insertions into bone and the underlying cortical bone and periosteum

SIGNS

INFLAMMATORY

tendon or ligament swelling, loss of internal structure (US, MR)

bone erosion at or immediately adjacent to the insertion

proliferative new bone (marked in proliferative arthropathies i.e. AS, Reiter's, psoriasis)

possibly ankylosis

DEGENERATIVE

tendon or ligament attrition, loss of internal structure, degenerative calcification (chronic change on US, MR)

tendon or ligament swelling (acute superimposed injury or inflammation)

sclerosis, irregularity, new bone formation at tendon or ligament insertion

MAJOR CONDITIONS ASSOCIATED WITH ENTHESOPATHY

INFLAMMATORY: AS, Reiter's, psoriasis, RA

DEGENERATIVE: chronic overuse injuries (occupational, sporting) – anywhere, shoulder rotator cuff impingement

3.2.4 SOFT TISSUE DEPOSITIONAL DISEASE

DEFINITION

predominant deposition of crystalline or proteinaceous material in periarticular soft tissues, with joints involved secondarily

SIGNS

soft tissue density or calcified abnormal deposit masses around joints or in soft tissues (TOPHI in gout)

periarticular erosions: erosions away from articular surface, not directly related to intracapsular synovial covered bare bone, but rather occurring next to the soft tissue masses (a feature of gout especially)

MAJOR SOFT TISSUE DEPOSITIONAL DISEASES

GOUT, AMYLOID, MULTICENTRIC RETICULOHISTIOCYTOSIS, HYPERCHOLESTEROLEMIA

3.2.5 MONOARTHROPATHY

SYSTEMIC OLIGOARTHROPATHY IN ONE JOINT

(and history of prior manifestation or expectation of later manifestation in another joint)

ONLY SINGLE JOINT ABNORMAL

DAMAGE
TRAUMA
AVN
INFECTION
NEUROPATHIC

'TUMOR'
PVNS
SYNOVIAL CHONDROMATOSIS
AMYLOID

3.2.6 OLIGOARTHROPATHY

diagnostic watershed between 'mono' and 'poly' arthropathy

SINGLE JOINT ABNORMALITY OCCURRING IN SEVERAL JOINTS

MULTIFOCAL TRAUMA
MULTIFOCAL AVN
MULTIFOCAL INFECTION (esp TB)

CHONDROPATHIES WITH FEW JOINTS INVOLVED

NEUROPATHIC
HEMOPHILIA
GOUT
AMYLOID

EARLY POLYARTHROPATHY

3.2.7 POLYARTHROPATHY

systemic or multifocal joint disorder; by definition, all synoviopathies are oligo- or poly- arthropathies

SYNOVIOPATHY

OSTEOPOROTIC BONE DENSITY
RA, JCA, SLE, MCTD, CREST

NORMAL BONE DENSITY
PSORIASIS, REITER'S, AS (and IBD), JCA, robust RA, OA

CHONDROPATHY

DEGENERATIVE
PRIMARY OSTEOARTHRITIS
HEMOPHILIA

CRYSTAL DEPOSITION DISEASE
CPPD, HEMOCHROMATOSIS
HPTH
WILSON'S DISEASE
ALKAPTONURIA

3.3 HEMARTHROSIS

see under hemarthrosis and lipohemarthrosis Ch 04

3.4 JOINT XR: CHECKLIST

see Ch 27

3.5 JOINT EFFUSION
(site independent)

ETIOLOGY

Transudate
traumatic/overuse
nearby osteoid osteoma
nearby bone marrow edema (e.g. transient regional osteoporosis)

Exudate
inflammatory synoviopathy
crystal arthropathy
synovial (osteo)chondromatosis

Blood
trauma
hemophilia
other bleeding disorder
pigmented villonodular synovitis

Pus
septic arthritis

IMAGING

XR

SHOULDER
large effusion causes inferolateral humeral head displacement

ELBOW
ANTERIOR FAT PAD SIGN ('sail sign')
normal anterior fat pad margin may be visible running down at a steep angle from upper margin of coronoid fossa
displaced triangular anterior fat pad is 'elevated' by effusion

POSTERIOR FAT PAD SIGN
normal posterior fat pad never visible
displaced posterior fat pad runs diagonally down from upper margin of olecranon fossa

HIP
WIDENED MEDIAL JOINT SPACE ('TEARDROP SIGN')
requires radiographically otherwise normal hip joints and very symmetric film
>1 mm difference in the distance from medial femoral head to lateral margin of teardrop

KNEE

> 1cm of soft tissue between suprapatellar fat pad (behind quadriceps tendon) and anterior femoral fat pad

US

excessive joint fluid (>2 mm, or can compare with other side)

fluid may be clear, hypoechoic, echogenic; contain debris, clot, loose bodies

displaced/compressed articular fat pads

MR

straightforward diagnosis

NUC MED

MDP

blood pool/tissue phase photopenia (space occupying collection overlying a joint)

possibly delayed phase photopenia (?attenuation by large effusion vs ?decreased uptake in avascularity)

any increased uptake in either phase reflects soft tissue vascularity (usually inflammatory) and increased delayed uptake – not caused by the effusion itself

---

3.6 SYNOVITIS (imaging signs)

XR

effusion or no findings by definition

US

demonstrates effusion (see effusion) AND

synovium may be thickened or have frank masses of pannus (pannus can not be pushed away like fluid, and may have internal color flow)

articular cartilage loss suggests septic arthritis or prior chondropathy

marginal erosions with soft tissue masses suggest inflammatory synoviopathy or amyloid

MR

irregular synovial interface

thickened synovium

synovial masses (pannus) – enhances with Gd

abnormally intense or thickened synovial enhancement with Gd

NUC MED (MDP)

very mild increased blood pool/tissue phase uptake

normal or very minimal increased diffuse delayed phase uptake

---

4. SPECIFIC CONDITIONS

4.1 ALKAPTONURIA (OCHRONOSIS)

DEFINITION

absence of homogentisic acid oxidase leading to cartilage pigment deposits (abnormal homogentisic acid products) and premature cartilage wear

CLINICAL

usually presents with 'degenerative joint disease' in early adult life symmetrically involving spine and large joints (knee, hip, shoulder)

ear fibrocartilage and scleral pigmentation often visible

IMAGING

XR

symmetrical spondyloarthropathy (DJD distribution, but also involving shoulders)

dense hydroxyapatite chondrocalcinosis (hyaline cartilage, fibrocartilage, annulus fibrosus)

SPINE

progressive annulus calcification

CALCIFICATION OF NUCLEUS PULPOSUS

degenerative disk change and loss of height (lumbar > thoracic)

may progress to spinal ankylosis

PERIPHERAL JOINTS

chondrocalcinosis

marked changes of premature DJD

shoulders involved (unusual for primary OA)

4.2 AMYLOID (articular manifestations)

CLINICAL

amyloid deposition in synovium and in periarticular locations – inert but with erosions

particular association with dialysis amyloidosis (beta 2 microglobulin)

IMAGING

Distribution

carpal tunnel, elbow, shoulder, hip, cervical spine

XR

joint widened (infiltration)

well marginated erosions with deposits

cysts, diffuse osteoporosis

BULKY SOFT TISSUE DEPOSITS (extraarticular, intraarticular)

no enthesopathy, no periosteal reaction

US (dialysis related amyloid)

expanded hypoechoic tendons with loss of fibrillary structure

articular marginal soft tissue masses, may show frank bone erosion

soft tissue masses

joint effusion

MR

deposits low signal on both T1W and T2W sequences (differential: gout)

4.3 ANKYLOSING SPONDYLITIS (AS) AND ENTEROPATHIC ARTHROPATHY

DEFINITION

seronegative autoimmune inflammatory ankylosing spondyloarthropathy with extraarticular manifestations

CLINICAL

commonest seronegative arthropathy (0.04% of population), onset 15–35 years old, male:female 10–20:1

>90% HLA B27 (AS), 60% (IBD)

Early AS

insidious onset, usually of back pain

sacroiliitis (80%)

ascending spondylitis

hip, knee, shoulder pain in one third

small joints spared

Late AS

ankylosis with marked loss of range of motion

severe disability in 20%

PATHOLOGICAL FRACTURES (especially spine – may be multilevel)
PSEUDOARTHROSES

Extraarticular manifestations

UVEITIS (20%)

CARDIAC
pericarditis, conduction defects

AORTIC
aortitis, aortoannular ectasia, aortic valve insufficiency

PULMONARY
fibrosis – notably, of upper zone predominance
pleurisy

Enteropathic arthropathy

occurs in inflammatory bowel disease, and is radiographically indistinguishable from AS

DISTRIBUTION

SIJ, spine, hips, shoulders; with calcaneal and patellar enthesopathy

PATHOLOGY

early progression similar to RA, but no rheumatoid nodules; marked fibrotic response with obliteration of joint cavity and 'welding' of opposite articular surfaces followed by osseous ankylosis; deformity less marked

IMAGING

proliferative synoviopathy involving mainly large joints and spine
bone density normal
proliferative erosions and proliferative enthesopathy; ankylosis

XR – spine

sacroiliac changes usually already present
small endplate erosions
shiny corners (healing and proliferative bone at annulus to vertebral junctions)
bilateral symmetric syndesmophytes originating in lumbar spine and extending upwards in continuity
fusion of posterior elements (CHARACTERISTIC): ill defined early erosions with proliferative subchondral new bone formation and joint capsule ossification
bamboo spine

SYNDESMOPHYTE
ossification of annulus fibrosus with bridging of adjacent vertebral bodies
follows position and orientation of annulus (i.e. vertical, and arises from corners of discovertebral junction)
DIFFERENTIATION FROM DEGENERATIVE OSTEOPHYTE: osteophytes are wider, arise away from the very corner of the vertebral body, and tend to be horizontal in orientation

XR – pelvis

symmetrical sacroiliitis except very early in disease
loss of articular bone and subarticular osteoporosis
erosive changes, diffuse subarticular sclerosis
focal ankylosis progressing to involve entire joint
symphysis syndesmophytes, ischial whiskering, sacroiliitis proceeding to complete fusion

XR – large joints

hip ring osteophytes, erosive arthropathy (resembles RA), late fusion, late protrusio
lesser and greater trochanter enthesopathy
patellar enthesopathy
calcaneal enthesopathy
shoulder erosive and proliferative changes

NUC MED

MDP
early sacroiliitis shows on MDP (increased uptake) before plain film findings
sacroiliac joint to sacral ratios of over 1.5:1 abnormal
prominent demonstration of SI joints on anterior view of pelvis is abnormal
enthesopathy may show linear subligamentous increased MDP uptake in delayed phase
radiographically occult spinal fractures may have increased MDP uptake

4.4 BEHÇET'S SYNDROME

poorly understood syndrome of intermittent large joint oligoarthritis, oral and genital mucositis, uveitis and small vessel vasculitis

4.5 CPPD (CALCIUM PYROPHOSPHATE DEPOSITION DISEASE)

also see hemochromatosis

DEFINITION

calcium pyrophosphate deposition presenting as a spectrum of conditions (most common is pyrophosphate modified osteoarthropathy)

EPIDEMIOLOGY

male = female, elderly (30–60% of >85 year olds)

Associations
primary hyperparathyroidism, hypercalcemia
hypothyroidism, hypomagnesemia

CLINICAL

ASYMPTOMATIC CHANGES ONLY

LOW GRADE CHRONIC DISEASE (commonest, ~80%)
'pyrophosphate modified osteoarthropathy'
simulates degenerative joint disease
may or may not have intermittent flares
less commonly, symptoms mimic RA

INTERMITTENT ACUTE ATTACKS (20%)
clinically, 'pseudogout'
calcium pyrophosphate dihydrate crystal induced
crystals may be aspirated from joint fluid for diagnosis

DISTRIBUTION (ARTHRITIS)

patellofemoral, hip, wrist, shoulder, elbow, scapholunate, MCP joints II, III

DISTRIBUTION (CHONDROCALCINOSIS)

FIBROCARTILAGE: menisci, triangular fibrocartilage complex, symphysis pubis, annulus fibrosus, hip and shoulder labra
HYALINE CARTILAGE: knee, wrist, other

PATHOLOGY

milky white calcific deposits with little reaction, tending to fibrocartilage or hyaline cartilage (weakly positively birefringent crystals)

accelerated destruction of abnormal cartilage

IMAGING

chondropathy that resembles osteoarthritis, but also involves joints uncommon in OA

normal bone density

XR – any joint

cartilage loss

effusions

subarticular sclerosis

prominent subarticular cysts (larger and more frequent than in OA)

non weightbearing osteophytes

loose bodies

no ankylosis or periosteal bone formation or enthesopathy

DIFFERENTIATING SIGNS FROM OA

non weightbearing joints involved (see below)

cysts

chondrocalcinosis

gross destruction out of keeping with level of workload (if occurs: 'pseudoneuropathic arthropathy')

XR – hands/wrists

triangular fibrocartilage calcification

loss of radiocarpal cartilage space, subchondral cysts, destruction of scaphoid and lunate (may proceed to scapholunate advanced collapse)

drooping (hook) osteophytes of metacarpals II and III

XR – shoulders

chondrocalcinosis, degenerative change without history of trauma

XR – knees

meniscal chondrocalcinosis

patellofemoral disease

4.6 DIFFUSE IDIOPATHIC SKELETAL HYPEROSTOSIS (DISH)

DEFINITION

non degenerative, non inflammatory ossification of skeletal ligamentous structures usually defined radiographically

VARIANT: idiopathic sternocostoclavicular hyperostosis

CLINICAL

common, male > female

mild pain, stiffness, cervical osteophyte dysphagia

thoracic > cervical > lumbar spine

IMAGING

XR – spine

osteophytes progressing to flowing ossification of anterolateral vertebral bodies

minimal disk DJD, disk height preserved

anterior longitudinal ligament calcification, +/– post longitudinal ligament calcification/ossification

enthesopathy common, but no sacroiliitis or facet joint ankylosis

XR – pelvis, chest

associated findings include:

heterotopic bone formation and ligament ossification

non erosive pelvic enthesopathy

sternocostoclavicular hyperostosis

tendency to heterotopic bone formation post surgery

4.7 GOUT

DEFINITION

multiple episodes of urate crystal precipitation with acute neutrophilic crystal arthropathy progressing to chronic tophus formation and joint destruction

---

ETIOLOGY

Primary gout (90%)

PRIMARY HYPERURICEMIA (10% of population) – 1/100 get clinical gout

older individuals, male >> female (postmenopausal), white > black

family history, alcohol consumption, obesity

Secondary gout

myeloproliferative disease, leukemia, chemotherapy

renal failure

hyperparathyroidism

diuretics

congenital enzymatic defects

CLINICAL

Acute attacks

when precipitated in synovium or joint fluid, poorly soluble monosodium urate crystals induce an acute neutrophilic arthritis

single joint at a time

pain, swelling, purulent effusion (simulates acute septic arthritis)

negatively birefringent monosodium urate monohydrate crystals

Chronic tophaceous gout

follows ~12 years after first attack

tophi deposited in acral areas (colder) and around joints +/– in synovium (starts at capsule attachment)

soft tissue tophi deposit subcutaneously, around bursae and in ear pinnas

Gouty nephropathy

urate stones

urate nephropathy

hypertension

20% of nephropathy progress to endstage renal failure

DISTRIBUTION

acral (colder) parts: hands and feet, ankles and wrists

great toe MTP joint ('podagra')

knees, prepatellar bursa, elbows

MORPHOLOGY

Tophus

mass of crystals and chalky necrotic calcifying debris surrounded by foreign

body granulomas and a fibrotic cuff;
bone erosion from inflammatory response
urate strongly negatively birefringent

IMAGING

asymmetric acral polyarthropathy and soft
tissue deposition disease, normal bone
density

XR – any joint

periarticular well corticated erosions caused
by tophi
marginal erosions can occur
no cysts
overhanging edges at erosion margins
articular cartilage preserved until late
reactive sclerosis
tophi cause soft tissue deformity, and appear
as a dense mass
tophi occasionally calcify (amorphous
calcification)
bursal tophi can occur away from joints

MR

tophi low signal on both T1W and T2W

4.8 HEMOCHROMATOSIS
(skeletal manifestations)

*see CPPD arthropathy; hemochromatosis in
Ch 07*
about 1/2 of hemochromatosis patients have
some degree of arthropathy – identical to
CPPD

4.9 HEMOPHILIA

DEFINITION

progressive large joint arthropathy and
overgrowth secondary to repeated bleeds

EPIDEMIOLOGY

males only: factor VIII (hemophilia A), factor
IX (hemophilia B)
male and female: von Willebrand disease
(vW factor)

CLINICAL

Acute hemarthroses

repeated joint bleeds with pain and acute
deformity

Chronic arthropathy

HEMOPHILIAC SYNOVITIS
pannus with hemosiderin and fibrosis

HEMOPHILIAC ARTHROPATHY
cartilage loss, osteopenia, subchondral cysts,
collapse, secondary DJD

PHYSEAL OVERVASCULARITY
overgrowth and osteoporosis, premature
epiphysis closure, avascular necrosis

Soft tissue pseudotumors

DISTRIBUTION

knee > elbow > ankle > hip > shoulder
frequently asymmetrical; if symmetrical
often of different severity

MACRO

overgrown epiphysis with green (heme)
stained abnormally rigid cartilage that
rapidly wears down
hypertrophied green/brown synovium
(hemosiderin), fibrous tissue and
fibrocartilage ingrowth, contractures of
capsule

IMAGING

asymmetrical chondropathy; bone density
normal in adults, decreased in children

XR – any joint

cartilage loss, subchondral plate crenations,
subarticular cysts and clefts
secondary proliferative and sclerotic bone
changes of accelerated DJD

XR – child

overgrown epiphyses ('balloon epiphyses')
premature growth plate fusion
angulation, contractures

XR – specific joints

knee: squared femoral notch and patella
elbow: expanded radial head, larger notch
ankle: tibiotalar slant

US/CT

soft tissue pseudotumors
muscular hemorrhages and contractures

MR

synovial proliferation
irregular articular cartilage

subchondral cysts (fluid signal or
hemosiderin signal)
dark signal on T1W and T2W in joint
capsule and pannus from hemosiderin
deposition

4.10 JUVENILE CHRONIC ARTHRITIS (JCA)

DEFINITION

a group of juvenile autoimmune arthritides
with several overlapping patterns

CLINICAL

Early onset RA (5%)

female > male, rheumatoid factor positive
classic RA, marginal erosions, periosteal
reaction

Pauciarticular JCA (40%)

female > male, rheumatoid negative, ANA
positive
few large joints; iritis in 25%

Polyarticular JCA (25%)

female > male, rheumatoid factor negative
arthritis behaves as RA, but with mild
extraarticular manifestations

Still's disease (20%)

<5 years old, male = female, rheumatoid
negative
fever, anemia, raised white cell count, skin
rashes
hepatosplenomegaly, lymphadenopathy
pericarditis, myocarditis

Juvenile AS (rare)

male > female, rheumatoid factor negative,
HLA B27 positive
hips, knees > SIJ and spine

IMAGING

asymmetric synoviopathy with proliferative
periosteal reactions and ankyloses
deformities from marked growth
disturbances, subluxations and
contractures

XR – growth disturbance

'balloon joints' with epiphyseal overgrowth
gracile diaphyses

premature fusion with L/R asymmetry and
limb length discrepancies
knee: widened intercondylar notch
(differential: hemophilia)
hip: protrusio

XR – periarticular osteopenia

combination of hyperemia and disuse
periosteal reaction common (especially
hands and feet)
no enthesopathy
large effusions, soft tissue swelling
'growth arrest' lines

XR – erosions and cartilage loss

cartilage usually preserved till late
marginal erosions occur in classic RA,
juvenile onset
bony ankylosis can occur in small joints and
cervical spine even in JCA other than
juvenile AS

XR – deformity

synovitis with rupture of tendons and
ligaments
capsule fibrosis with contractures
bony ankylosis
atlantoaxial subluxation (not universal) –
>5 mm on lateral radiograph between
C1 anterior arch and odontoid process in
a child
cervical spine ankylosis (posterior elements
> vertebrae) with vertebral growth
disturbances

US

joint effusions
pannus
synovial cysts (especially Baker's cyst)
tendon attrition and tendonitis

NUC MED (MDP)

multifocal increased 3 phase MDP uptake
shows extent of disease
degree of hyperemia on flow phase and
tissue/blood pool activity reflects disease
activity

Monoarthritis differential

TB

REFLEX SYMPATHETIC DYSTROPHY

HEMOPHILIA

NEUROPATHIC JOINT

4.11 NAMED AVN/OCD/ OSTEOCHONDROSIS

TERMINOLOGY

*Osteochondritis dissecans (OCD): see Ch 4,
3.11*
eponymous OCD is usually osteochondral
AVN pre epiphyseal plate closure
eponymous AVN is usually small bone AVN
pre epiphyseal plate closure
eponymous apophysitis may or may not have
AVN as its cause
main plain film differential is an ossification
normal variant

4.11.1 LEGG–CALVÉ– PERTHES'

hip epiphyseal AVN, see Ch 17

4.11.2 KNEE OCD/SONK

traumatic or spontaneous medial condyle
osteochondral fragment
OCD if involves an unfused epiphysis
spontaneous osteonecrosis of the knee
(SONK) if occurs post growth plate fusion

4.11.3 OSGOOD–SCHLATTER

tibial apophysis AVN or traumatic avulsion

4.11.4 SINDING–LARSEN–JOHANSEN

inferior pole of patella

4.11.5 BLOUNT'S

medial tibial epiphysis delayed growth with
varus (see Ch 17)

4.11.6 TALAR DOME OSTEOCHONDRAL LESION (OCL)

traumatic; steroids; SLE

4.11.7 KOHLER'S

navicular AVN

4.11.8 SEVER'S

calcaneal apophysis traction apophysitis

4.11.9 FREIBERG'S INFRACTION

AVN of metatarsal heads II, III (female >
male)
related to pressure maldistribution and high
heels

4.11.10 PANNER'S

capitellum
usually post traumatic

4.11.11 TROCHLEAR OCD

4.11.12 KEINBOCH'S LUNATOMALACIA

lunate spontaneous or traumatic AVN

4.12 NEUROPATHIC JOINT

DEFINITION

disorganization, gross instability and
destruction of joints (by cumulative
microtrauma) secondary to neurosensory
and muscular proprioceptive/stability
failure

ETIOLOGY (six S's)

S-UGAR (DIABETES)
talonavicular, tarsometatarsal, MTP joints
!beware of superimposed osteomyelitis in
diabetic feet

S-YRINX
shoulders

S-YPHILIS
knee (tabes dorsalis)

S-PINA BIFIDA AND PARAPLEGIA
spine

S-CROFULA (lepromatous leprosy)
hands and feet

S-ENSELESSNESS (insensitivity to pain)
hands and feet

MORPHOLOGY

Hypertrophic (5 D's)

D-ISORGANIZATION

microfractures and osteochondral fractures, fragmentation

D-ISLOCATION

D-ENSE SCLEROSIS

D-EBRIS AND DETRITUS

D-ISTENSION BY EFFUSION

(imaging differential: OA, CPPD)

Mixed (imaging differential: Septic arthritis)

Atrophic

GROSS RESORPTION OF ARTICULAR ENDS WITH SHARP CUTOFF

FRAGMENTATION AND LOSS OF BONES (TARSUS, CARPUS)

'PENCIL–POINTING' OF METACARPALS, METATARSALS AND PHALANGES

IMAGING

XR

AS ABOVE

MR

fragmentation and disorganization as above

cortical and synovial thickening

joint effusions

sclerosis is low signal on both T1W and T2W

variable Gd enhancement is present

bone marrow edema (low on T1W, high on T2W) may occur, and can not be differentiated from edema of osteomyelitis

differentiation from superimposed septic arthritis/osteomyelitis is difficult, and is most helpful if there is no bone marrow edema

soft tissue abscesses or draining tracks indicate osteomyelitis

NUC MED

MDP

moderately increased perfusion, increased blood pool/tissue phase activity and markedly increased delayed MDP uptake (unless the foot is very ischemic)

amount of MDP uptake reflects reactive/proliferative/sclerotic changes

can not differentiate on its own from superimposed osteomyelitis, requires white cell or Ga scanning

cellulitis: more extensive tissue phase uptake than delayed phase uptake

GALLIUM

delayed Ga imaging combined with MDP

concordant Ga uptake is likely due to bone uptake alone

discordant Ga uptake suggests superimposed infection

focus of more intense Ga uptake than MDP in same location (compared with MDP and Ga uptake in the rest of the foot)

more extensive Ga than MDP uptake

WHITE CELL SCANNING

used to differentiate septic arthritis (see 4.17)

4.13 OSTEOARTHRITIS (OA)

4.13.1 OSTEOARTHRITIS NOT OTHERWISE SPECIFIED

DEFINITION

commonest single arthritis characterized by focal loss of weightbearing articular cartilage and secondary reactive changes

ETIOLOGY

Primary

female > male, incidence increases with age

affects hands (DIP joints especially) in females >60 years

Secondary

TRAUMA

isolated event

occupational repetitive

sporting repetitive

POST SEPTIC ARTHRITIS

GENETIC PREDISPOSITION – MECHANICAL

malformations

dysplasias

biomechanical problems

GENETIC PREDISPOSITION – CHEMICAL

alkaptonuria

CPPD/hemochromatosis

renal disease

POST AVASCULAR NECROSIS

NEUROPATHIC JOINT

POST INFLAMMATORY ARTHRITIS

CLINICAL

dull pain worsening with use, stiffness, crepitus, reduced range of motion, locking (loose bodies)

DISTRIBUTION

lower lumbar and lower cervical spine

first carpometacarpal joint, great toe MTP joint, scapho-trapezo-trapezoid joint, DIP joints

hips, knees

uncommonly shoulders and wrists and rarely elbows without an underlying cause or predisposing condition

IMAGING

asymmetrical or partly symmetrical chondropathy

bone density normal or increased

XR – spine

disk height loss and dessication

discogenic sclerosis

marginal osteophytes

facet/uncovertebral irregularity and osteophyte hypertrophy

displacement (anteroposterior, lateral, rotatory)

instability (abnormal excessive motion on flexion/extension views)

XR – hands + feet

(DIP, thumb carpometacarpal and scapho-trapezo-trapezoid joints)

cartilage loss

subchondral sclerosis and cysts with sclerotic margin

marginal osteophytes

XR – large joints

focal loss of weightbearing cartilage

subchondral sclerosis and cysts

marginal and periarticular osteophytes (may cover old subchondral line); loose bodies

enthesopathy
HIPS: superolateral joint space loss and narrowing (weightbearing surface)

MR

greatest utility is cartilage assessment
normal cartilage intermediate signal on T1W, PD and T2W images; isointense to synovial fluid on PD

PREFERRED MR SEQUENCES FOR EVALUATING CARTILAGE

3D FSPGR (fat suppressed)
FSE with fat suppression
GRE
T2W

CARTILAGE CHANGE

FLASH: loss of uniform high signal, areas of low signal
PD, T2W: focal areas of increased signal
surface erosions, full depth erosions
loose intraarticular cartilage bodies (in effusion or arthrography)

SUBCHONDRAL BONE CHANGE

sclerosis (focal low T1W, low T2W subchondral signal)
edema (low T1W, high T2W)
subchondral cysts
irregular subchondral cortex

NUC MED

MDP

focal areas of delayed phase MDP uptake
articular, frequently both sides of joint, frequently weightbearing or load transmitting surfaces
requires differentiation from other causes of focally increased MDP uptake (XR for correlation)

COMMON LOCATIONS:
facet joints of cervical spine
acromioclavicular joints (frequently greater on side of dominant hand)
sternoclavicular joints
mild thoracic facet joint irregularity
lumbar facet joints
lumbar linear peridiscal uptake (may be one side only)
superolateral hips
knees (medial and lateral compartments)
tarsal joints (often asymmetrical)
small joints of hands and feet

GALLIUM

a confounder for oncology and infection Ga studies
generally very low grade articular uptake only

PET (F-18 fluoride)
same findings as MDP

4.13.2 EROSIVE OSTEOARTHRITIS

CLINICAL

middle aged and older females
stiffness, pain and swelling of DIP joints
Heberden's nodes
serology negative

IMAGING

XR

changes of osteoarthritis (joint space narrowing, marginal osteophytes, subchondral sclerosis)
AND
articular surface sharp erosions (usually central articular)
may eventually ankylose

4.14 PSORIASIS AND REITER'S SYNDROME

DEFINITION

seronegative autoimmune inflammatory erosive arthropathy

EPIDEMIOLOGY

4.14.1 Psoriatic arthropathy

2–6% of young adults with psoriasis, male = female
HLA B27 in 60%, rheumatoid factor negative

4.14.2 Reiter's syndrome

young adults, male >> female
HLA B27 in 80%

CLINICAL

Psoriasis

2/3 slow onset, 1/3 rapid onset
asymmetric arthritis (hand + spine dominant)
uveitis, scleritis, conjunctivitis

Reiter's syndrome

arthritis + bursitis + tendonitis

urethritis (or cervicitis)
conjunctivitis
+/– keratoderma blenorrhagicum
few weeks following an episode of GIT or UGT infection
monoarticular or back pain
lower limb dominant
short duration, but recurrent episodes

IMAGING

asymmetrical proliferative synoviopathy with normal bone density

XR – spine

T-L junction spondyloarthropathy with bulky syndesmophytes
sacroiliitis with erosions, may ankylose

XR – hands + feet

psoriasis hand > foot, Reiter's foot > hand
DIP, PIP joint polyarthritis with severe marginal and subchondral erosions, cartilage loss, ankylosis, sausage digits
no cysts
enthesopathy, marginal osteophytes, periosteal new bone, proliferative bone
retrocalcaneal bursitis and plantar fasciitis with prominent erosions and periosteal new bone and spurs

XR – large joints

hip, knee, ankle arthritis
shoulder, wrist arthritis
erosions, no cysts
proliferative new bone

4.15 PIGMENTED VILLONODULAR SYNOVITIS (PVNS)/GIANT CELL TUMOR OF TENDON SHEATH (GCTTS)

DEFINITION

benign monoarticular synovial proliferative disease with a hemosiderin stained nodular synovial mass

CLINICAL

30–50 years old, male = female
high local recurrence rate, never metastasizes

4.15.1 Pigmented villonodular synovitis

KNEE (80%), HIP, ELBOW

monoarticular stiffness, bloody effusion, locking, pain

4.15.2 Giant cell tumor of tendon sheath

slow growing mass arising next to a tendon

mechanical obstruction, catching

macroscopically and histologically identical with PVNS

MORPHOLOGY

DIFFUSE FORM: thickened fronded synovium with hemosiderin

NODULAR FORM: brown 'seaweed' mass arising from synovium (hemosiderin stained)

synovial cells, macrophages and giant cells with hemosiderin +/− lipid

fibroblasts, variable amount of collagen

IMAGING

XR

erosions and subchondral cysts on both sides of joint

no cartilage loss or ankylosis

bone density normal, no productive changes, no periosteal reaction

differential diagnosis: infection, hemophilia, chondromatosis, gout

US

extensive synovial thickening and a large joint effusion

synovium nodular and hypoechoic

MR

synovial (joint or tendon) soft tissue mass with hemosiderin: signal is low T1W, low T2W

DIFFERENTIAL DIAGNOSIS

synovial osteochondromatosis (ossification on plain film)

hemophilia (overgrown characteristic epiphyses)

RA pannus (signal not low enough on T2W)

amyloid deposition (history of renal failure and dialysis)

4.16 RHEUMATOID ARTHRITIS (RA)

DEFINITION

autoimmune seropositive inflammatory polyarthropathy with extraarticular manifestations

EPIDEMIOLOGY

1% of population, female:male 3:1; onset 30–50 years old

95% rheumatoid factor positive at some time in disease

80% have HLA DR4 or DR1

CLINICAL

Early RA

morning stiffness, effusions, pain, boggy joints

soft tissue swelling, muscle wasting

20% have periods of remission

Late RA

joint deformities, tendon and ligament ruptures, loss of range of motion and power, loss of function, instability, fibrosis and contractures

Extraarticular manifestations

SUBCUTANEOUS NODULES (25%)

PAINLESS PLEURAL EFFUSIONS (common)

RHEUMATOID PLEURISY

INTERSTITIAL LUNG FIBROSIS (1%)

PULMONARY RHEUMATOID NODULES

RHEUMATOID VASCULITIS (rare)

Special variants

FELTY SYNDROME

RA, splenomegaly, leukopenia

SJÖGREN'S SYNDROME (with RA)

RA, xerostomia, keratoconjunctivitis sicca

KAPLAN SYNDROME

rheumatoid pneumoconiosis, cavitation common

PATHOLOGY

synovially based inflammation with secondary destruction (i.e. joints and tendon sheaths)

effusion, engorged synovium, tenosynovitis and bursitis

pannus (vascular inflammatory granulation tissue with iron deposited from small hemorrhages; starts in bare areas, erosive)

progressive erosion and loss of cartilage and bone

weakening and stretching of tendons, ligaments, joint capsule; eventual rupture

proliferative fibrotic response as pannus matures with contractures and ankylosis

resulting deformities (combination of subluxation, tendon rupture, fibrotic contractures)

IMAGING

symmetrical small and large joint synoviopathy with reduced bone density

XR – generic joint

symmetrical joint involvement, severity may differ side to side

marked periarticular osteoporosis

effusions, eventual cartilage space loss

late ankylosis (cervical spine and wrist)

marginal erosions then subchondral erosions

non sclerotic subchondral cysts

no proliferative bone until late secondary OA

soft tissue swelling

tenosynovitis with swelling and rupture

DEFORMITIES as above

XR – cervical spine

osteopenia then erosion of odontoid

atlantoaxial subluxation; atlantoaxial distance above 2–3 mm in flexion implies transverse ligament laxity or rupture

atlantoaxial impaction (atlas descending around dens)

erosions of cervical spine bodies

posterior element fusion occurs

XR – hands, feet

EARLY: periarticular osteoporosis, soft tissue swelling, soft marginal erosions (MCP and PIP joints)

LATE: carpus erosions and disorganization, loss of ulnar styloid, late fusion

MCP joint ulnar drift with volar subluxation

Z deformity of thumbs

interphalangeal subluxations

tendon laxity or ruptures with swan neck (PIP joint hyperextended) and boutonnière (PIP joint fixed flexed) deformities

MTP subluxations

XR – knees

large effusions, Baker's cysts
erosions may be difficult to identify
valgus deformity
three compartment cartilage/meniscal space
    loss
subchondral cysts
patellar pressure erosion of femoral shaft

XR – shoulders, elbows, hips

supraspinatus exit tunnel narrowing and
    rotator cuff rupture
high riding humeral head
marginal erosions, may have hatchet
    deformity
erosion of lateral clavicle, pressure
    resorption of acromial undersurface
pressure erosion of humeral shaft on
    inferior glenoid angle
elbow erosions with deep olecranon notch
hip concentric or irregular erosions with
    protrusio and superomedial migration
ankles affected relatively late

US

large joint effusion
Baker's cyst
rotator cuff attrition, long head of biceps
    tendon rupture
tenosynovitis, tendon inflammation and
    attrition elsewhere

MR

SYNOVITIS AND PANNUS

early: irregularity of synovial line
later: thickening of synovium, synovial
    irregular masses low on T1W,
    intermediate on T2W
pannus enhances with Gd
abnormal synovial enhancement with Gd

LARGE EFFUSIONS, SYNOVIAL
BURSAL CYSTS

CARTILAGE AND SUBCHONDRAL
BONE CHANGE

erosion and loss of articular cartilage
loss and irregularity of subchondral bone
subarticular cysts

TENOSYNOVITIS

NUC MED

MDP

protocol – whole body tissue/blood pool
    phase images, whole body delayed
    images
diffusely increased delayed phase uptake +/–
    tissue phase uptake

increased tissue phase uptake correlates
    with intensity of inflammation

4.17 SEPTIC ARTHRITIS

ETIOLOGY

same as osteomyelitis (Ch 02)

PATHOGENESIS

SPREAD FROM SUBARTICULAR
OSTEOMYELITIS

DIRECT HEMATOGENOUS SEEDING
OF SYNOVIUM

DIRECT INOCULATION (traumatic,
surgical)

RISK FACTORS: RA,
IMMUNOSUPPRESSION, IVDU

MORPHOLOGY

purulent inflammatory reaction with
    effusion
early chondrocyte death and cartilage loss
    from bacterial effects, inflammatory
    mediators, lack of synovial diffusion

CLINICAL

acutely hot, swollen, painful joint with
    effusion
fever (may not be present), high ESR
organisms on aspiration
fast progression with deformity, requires
    early aggressive treatment
gonococcal arthritis: often a multifocal
    arthritis +/– skin rash

IMAGING

Imaging workup

plain film signs late (irreversible destruction
    by time of signs)
MDP useful if positive, but negative scan
    may be false negative
white cell scan may be of help, but labeling
    and imaging are prolonged
MR – joint effusion, synovitis, bone marrow
    edema (non specific)
US – joint effusion (non specific)
JOINT ASPIRATION is specific

XR – early (still days after onset
and too late)

relatively fast progression of changes
effusion, early cartilage space and
    subchondral bone loss
marginal erosions, uneven endplate erosions
eventual periarticular osteoporosis

XR – late

growth plate disturbance, destruction of
    epiphysis, sclerosis, ankylosis of joint,
    periosteal metaphyseal reaction,
    secondary degenerative joint disease

XR – TB

slow progression, large effusion, marginal
    erosions, marked osteoporosis, little if
    any periosteal reaction; cartilage
    preserved till late
extensive soft tissue masses, calcification
    and tracking of caseous material
late: fibrous joint ankylosis
TB dactylitis (usually in children): periosteal
    reaction around lucent changes in an
    expanded phalanx

US

joint effusion
effusion may be clear, or contain debris (pus
    or hemorrhage)
synovium may be irregular or thickened or
    hypervascular on color Doppler
complex effusion makes septic arthritis more
    likely, but is not specific
at least in pediatric hips absence of joint
    effusion is good imaging evidence against
    septic arthritis
difficulty differentiating septic from non
    septic synovitis

CT

changes analogous to XR
not a major role in septic arthritis except for
    spine and SI joints

MR

joint effusion
synovitis (thickened and/or abnormally
    enhancing synovium)
cartilage destruction, later subchondral
    bone destruction
subchondral bone marrow edema
may show soft tissue abscesses with Gd
    (specific)
may show subcapsular focus of osteomyelitis
    or subperiosteal collection (specific)
difficulty differentiating septic from non
    septic synovitis

NUC MED

MDP

CLASSIC PATTERN

increased perfusion, increased periarticular tissue/blood pool activity, increased periarticular delayed phase uptake (both sides of joint)

OTHER PATTERNS

NORMAL

diffusely increased uptake both sides of joint

tissue/blood pool phase photopenia (large joint effusion)

decreased tissue and delayed phase periarticular uptake (attenuation by effusion vs infarction of bone)

GALLIUM

more suitable in spine than peripheries

usual criteria of discordant Ga vs MDP uptake (see osteomyelitis and neuropathic joint imaging entries)

WHITE CELL SCAN

more suitable in peripheries than spine (bone marrow in spine is a natural white cell reservoir and shows uptake)

focally elevated white cell accumulation combined with MDP, and more accurate than Ga

NEGATIVE STUDY EXCLUDES OSTEOMYELITIS

FALSE NEGATIVES IN GENERAL: partly treated osteomyelitis, granulomatous osteomyelitis (non neutrophilic), chronic osteomyelitis (non neutrophilic), spinal osteomyelitis (MR or Ga preferred)

false negatives other than partly treated osteomyelitis do not usually apply in neuropathic peripheral joints (i.e. diabetic feet)

CONCORDANT MILDLY INCREASED WHITE CELL ACCUMULATION IS CONSISTENT WITH NEUROPATHIC ARTHROPATHY OR YELLOW TO RED MARROW CONVERSION

pitfall: partly treated osteomyelitis

can use sulfur colloid scanning to map red marrow

if colloid scan concordant, likely marrow

if colloid scan cold, likely infection

MARKEDLY INCREASED WHITE CELL ACCUMULATION INDICATES INFECTION

false positives: healing fractures; recent surgery; recent prostheses; non infective acute inflammatory arthropathy

4.18 SPINAL DISCITIS

ETIOLOGY

same as osteomyelitis (Ch 02)

PATHOGENESIS

bacteremia seeding of vertebral endplate in adults, either endplate or possibly disk itself in children; or inoculation or direct spread from adjacent focus

bacterial destruction of disk, with secondary epidural and paraspinal abscesses

destruction of involved vertebral endplate (endplates), mechanical collapse, risk of paraplegia

Non septic 'discitis'

inflammatory arthropathy involvement of disk and vertebral endplates in a manner analogous to other joints (e.g. symphysis)

JCA, RA, AS, psoriasis, Reiter's

CLINICAL

lumbar > thoracic > cervical

progressive severe back pain and fever (not universal)

elevated white cell count, ESR

may present with neurological deficit as first manifestation

IMAGING

XR (signs late)

narrowing of disk space, often asymmetrical, and often greater than neighboring levels

destruction of one or both cortical endplates – often focal

angulation, collapse

TUBERCULOUS OSTEOMYELITIS/DISCITIS

large paraspinal calcifying soft tissue masses

disk spaces relatively preserved

CT

irregularity and narrowing of disk space

irregular destruction of vertebral endplate with focal patchy reparative sclerosis

paraspinal soft tissue masses

possibly epidural intraspinal soft tissue masses

MR (?discitis is an absolute indication)

peridiscal bone marrow edema (low on T1W, high on T2W) – mimics Modic I degenerative endplate change

possibly destruction of endplates

isocenter of change on disk itself

disk signal low on T1W, high on T2W with loss of normal lower signal T2W disk intranuclear cleft

T2W signal is often visibly higher than neighboring normal disks, and is definitely higher than dessicated disks

infected disk may also be relatively low on T2W (especially chronic osteomyelitis)

subligamentous collections (under anterior and posterior longitudinal ligaments)

paravertebral and intraspinal epidural abscesses (low T1W, high or mixed T2W)

abnormal enhancement of disk, endplates and paraspinal/epidural abscesses with Gd (enhancement usually peripheral, but may be patchy)

!MR is the only modality reliably showing intraspinal extent of infection

TUBERCULOUS OSTEOMYELITIS

disk destruction is late, and disks are relatively well preserved

gross vertebral body destruction and replacement with soft tissue collections/'cold' abscesses low on T1W and high on T2W

frequent involvement of multiple levels

posterior elements may be involved (risk of instability)

paraspinal abscesses with tracking

NUC MED

MDP

perfusion usually normal

increased blood pool/tissue activity centered on level of disk

increased delayed MDP uptake level with disk involving both endplates

may not involve entire width of endplate

useful if occurs at a radiographically normal disk (makes discitis likely)

early may have 'cold discitis' (photopenic area)

SPECT very helpful

GALLIUM

more successful in spine than white cell scanning

(postulated non neutrophilic chronic inflammation)

delay of 48 hours for imaging
discordantly increased Ga uptake at focus of
osteomyelitis/discitis

4.19 SYNOVIAL (OSTEO)CHONDRO-MATOSIS

DEFINITION

focal benign synovial metaplasia to cartilage
or bone that causes bone erosion and
loose bodies

CLINICAL

KNEE, HIP, SHOULDER, ELBOW
pain, swelling, locking, cracking
synovial surface studded with cartilage
nodules of various sizes and stages of
extrusion
may recur following excision

Primary

monoarticular disease; 30–50 years old,
male:female 2:1
cartilage metaplasia of synovium; growing
islands of cartilage with extrusion; loose
cartilaginous or osseocartilaginous bodies
(all same size)

Secondary

result of post traumatic or degenerative
change (not metaplasia)
loose bodies vary in size

IMAGING

XR/CT

multiple loose bodies: purely chondral
(invisible), chondral calcified, ossified
joint effusion
mechanical erosion (sclerotic margin) both
sides of joint
bone density normal; no periosteal reaction,
no enthesopathy
SECONDARY TYPE: evidence of degenerative
change

US

effusion usually not very large
intraarticular loose or capsule based solid
bodies: hypoechoic (?cartilage);
hyperechoic; may shadow (calcification,
ossification)

MR

multiple loose bodies
cartilaginous loose bodies tend to be low
T1W and intermediate T2W signal
(follow signal of cartilage)
calcified loose bodies tend to be low T1W
and T2W signal
ossified bodies can be of variable signal
depending on presence of marrow
joint effusion
bone erosion

4.20 SYSTEMIC LUPUS ERYTHEMATOSUS (SLE)

see Ch 15 vascular

3. GENERAL ACUTE, TRAUMA, SPORTING INJURIES AND DEGENERATIVE

3.1 ABSCESS (soft tissue)

IMAGING

US

variable appearance
thick walled fluid collection with increased through transmission (may have debris)
hypoechoic mass with increased through transmission
mixed echogenicity mass
by definition, no internal color flow
often a hypervascular ring
often a hyperechoic rim

CT

fluid density or soft tissue density mass
enhancing irregular wall of variable thickness
pockets of gas very helpful finding

MR

fluid collection with low T1W and high T2W signal
may be loculated
surrounding edema, possibly satellite abscesses
enhancing wall of variable thickness

3.2 BURSITIS

ETIOLOGY

trauma (including repeated overuse trauma)
septic bursitis
inflammatory synoviopathy (see joint gamuts)
crystal arthropathy with bursal deposition (gout, CPPD)

IMAGING

US

first sign is minimal separation of peribursal linear fat planes (if present)
accumulation of fluid within bursa
echogenicity of content variable (transudate, exudate, blood, pus, crystals)
!appearance does not indicate etiology

NUC MED

MDP

increased blood pool/tissue phase activity
rarely, increased perfusion (especially if very septic)
rarely, late phase uptake (dystrophic calcification, heterotopic bone)

MR

fluid in bursa
thickened bursal lining, may have abnormal enhancement

3.3 CRANIAL AND CNS TRAUMA

see Ch 11

3.4 ENTHESOPATHY

process analogous to tendinopathy but involving tendon insertion into bone, or occasionally ligament insertion into bone; may be traumatic/degenerative or inflammatory in inflammatory arthropathies
see Ch 03

3.5 FRACTURES AND MIMICKERS

PRINCIPLES OF IMAGING

Two orthogonal views (only need to see fracture in one of the views)
image both joints to assess rotation
coupled bones may fracture together or have fracture of one and dislocation of the other
beware direct neurovascular injury or compartment syndrome
in nuclear medicine imaging, both abnormally reduced and abnormally increased MDP uptake occurs, and is assessed relative to the normal side (need to know which is the normal side)

3.5.1 ACUTE FRACTURE

IMAGING

XR

non corticated margins
appearance and orientation of fracture lines consistent with mechanism of injury
may see soft tissue swelling, joint effusion or lipohemarthrosis

CT

soft tissue edema or hematoma blends into other soft tissues
particularly useful in multi-part fractures especially shoulder and pelvic girdles
3D and multiplanar reformats used in surgical planning

MR

bone marrow edema (low on T1W, high on T2W)
STIR or fat sat T2W particularly useful
cancellous bone fracture line itself may or may not be visible
cortical fracture line visible if displaced or filled with fluid exudate
allows assessment of articular cartilage in osteochondral fractures, tendons and ligaments, and soft tissues for discontinuity, edema or hematoma

NUC MED

MDP

mildly increased perfusion
moderately to prominently increased blood pool/tissue phase uptake
increased late phase uptake
beware of pathological fractures: may have no increased MDP uptake (e.g. myeloma)

REASONABLE TIMES AT WHICH A FRACTURE CAN BE EXCLUDED BY A NEGATIVE MDP SCAN
1 day in children
2 days in adults
3 days in elderly adults
up to 7 days in bed ridden elderly

HEALED FRACTURES
MDP may normalize completely (1 to 2 years)
or late phase uptake may persist indefinitely
non anatomically united fractures usually have persistent MDP uptake

GALLIUM

fractures show increased uptake and are a frequent cause of false positive Ga scans

3.5.2 OLD NON UNION

IMAGING

XR/CT

smoothly sclerotic margins

orientation of fracture lines consistent with mechanism of injury

variable amount of proliferative mature bone as periosteal bone, heterotopic bone or marginal osteophytes

no symmetrical accessory bones on other side

MR

variable bone marrow signal

sclerosis is low T1W, low T2W; edema is high T2W

NUC MED

MDP

increased delayed phase uptake, variable blood pool/tissue phase uptake, not increased or mildly increased vascularity

old avulsion fractures may eventually become cold

3.5.3 NON UNITED SECONDARY OSSIFICATION CENTER

IMAGING

XR

differential is avulsion fracture

smoothly sclerotic margins

appearance and orientation atypical for mechanism of injury

accessory ossicles or non united ossification centers may be present elsewhere (e.g. contralaterally)

lack of soft tissue swelling

NUC MED

often no increased uptake (helpful)

can not differentiate if uptake increased

3.5.4 BONE BRUISE

IMAGING

by definition, no displaced fracture present

microfractures possible

XR/CT

nil

MR

bone marrow edema, usually subarticular or related to area of impact

NUC MED

increased activity in all three phases acutely

progressively decreasing vascular then blood pool/tissue phase activity from 4–6 weeks onwards

rounded often subarticular/impact surface area of activity (dissimilar from stress fracture/periosteal uptake)

3.5.5 STRESS FRACTURE

IMAGING

XR

late and inconstant findings (delayed at least 2–4 weeks)

transverse or subcortical sclerotic band

periosteal reaction, endosteal reaction

CT

may show periosteal or endosteal callus earlier than XR

MR

bone marrow edema usually away from articular surfaces

NUC MED

increased uptake in all three phases acutely (0–4 weeks)

shape typically fusiform (along cortex) or rounded, and isocenter is often on bony cortex

perfusion and then blood pool/tissue phase uptake progressively disappear after 4–6 weeks of rest

late phase normalization with healing at approximately 12 months

persistent late phase uptake may be present beyond 12 months even in healed stress fractures

3.5.6 INSUFFICIENCY FRACTURE

stress fracture occurring in abnormally weak bone as a result of activities of daily living

ETIOLOGY: osteoporosis, other causes of osteopenia (see Ch 01)

IMAGING

Pelvis/sacrum

XR

usually completely unhelpful in sacrum

helpful in pelvis if displacement present

CT

do oblique coronal as well as axial study

may show minimally displaced fracture line

NUC MED

'Honda' sign of increased H shaped uptake in sacrum

MR

bone marrow edema around fracture; may see fracture line

Femoral neck

XR

may be totally normal

faint increased sclerosis extending towards medullary cavity from calcar femorale

NUC MED

same appearance as stress fracture

MR

low signal fracture line

bone marrow edema related to fracture (i.e. around calcar femorale)

Vertebral

XR

assess interpedicular distance

anterior wedge compression

biconcave fracture

uniconcave deformity of one endplate only

disk space characteristically preserved

kyphotic angulation at fractured segment

CT

usually non contributory unless looking for intraspinal canal fragments or position of fragments

NUC MED

may have difficulty differentiating from degenerative disease or old osteoporotic fractures

MR

bone marrow edema +/– hemorrhage in fractured vertebra

paraspinal hematoma, usually minor

allows intraspinal content assessment

old fractures have fatty bone marrow signal and can often be differentiated from acute fractures presence of fatty marrow helps exclude compression fractures secondary to metastatic disease

3.5.7 EFFECTS OF NON WEIGHT- BEARING/DISUSE

IMAGING

NUC MED (MDP)
reduced perfusion, blood pool/tissue phase activity and delayed uptake in non weightbearing or non used limb (includes growth plates)
may simulate reflex sympathetic dystrophy or other abnormalities on the normal comparison side
comparison normal side may have increased uptake due to increased loads

3.6 FRACTURES IN CHILD

see Ch 17

3.7 HEMARTHROSIS/ LIPOHEMARTHROSIS

IMAGING

XR/CT
hemarthrosis indistinguishable from effusion
lipohemarthrosis (fat–fluid levels on horizontal beam film) diagnostic of intraarticular fracture

US
hemarthrosis: increased amount of effusion debris, clot, and layering (cells dependent)
lipohemarthrosis: more echogenic fat floats on more hypoechoic blood

MR
ISOLATED HEMARTHROSIS
acute – indistinguishable from joint effusion, but may have fluid–fluid level
REPEATED HEMARTHROSES
hemosiderin deposition (low T1W, low T2W) and synovial proliferation

LIPOHEMARTHROSIS
fat–fluid level

3.8 HEMATOMA
(soft tissue, site independent)

IMAGING

US
EARLY
acutely, uniform hyperechoic collection with ill defined margins
no internal flow, but may find active bleeding on color Doppler

EVOLVING
collection of variable appearance
increasingly hypoechoic with dominant fluid component (liquefaction) and increasing through transmission
mixed echogenicity with hypoechoic and hyperechoic areas (clot, debris)
hyperechoic (organization)

MR
CNS rules for dating hemorrhage do not work well in the musculoskeletal system
major MR clue to subacute blood products is high T1W signal; and to hemosiderin is very low signal on T1W and T2W, with blooming on GRE

3.9 JOINT EFFUSION

see Ch 04

3.10 MUSCLE INJURIES

3.10.1 STRAIN

IMAGING

MR
increased perifascial T2W signal
diffuse swelling and increased T2W signal

3.10.2 TEAR

IMAGING

US
focal swelling and edema (partial tear)
cleft, deformity, discontinuity of fascial planes with defect
defect usually filled with hypoechoic fluid, but may have debris

MR
deformity, discontinuity, surrounding edema

3.10.3 HEMATOMA

IMAGING

US
intramuscular mass of variable echogenicity (see hematoma)

MR
mass with blood signal (see hematoma)

3.11 OSTEOCHONDRITIS DISSECANS (OCD)

see also AVN, Ch 2, 3.2

DEFINITION
focal articular osteochondral fracture, with overlap in clinical behavior and imaging findings with articular avascular necrosis (AVN)

ETIOLOGY
'ischemic theory' does not differentiate between OCD and focal articular AVN (which may be trauma induced)
'traumatic theory' holds that OCD is caused by local trauma (major trauma, shearing forces, repeated microtrauma, etc) and is determined by local factors; the corollary is that no systemic cause for AVN should exist in a case of OCD
if OCD and AVN are considered two separate entities, these are differentiated on lesion location and patient profile (e.g. knee OCD vs SONK)

CLINICAL

KNEE

classically non weightbearing medial femoral condyle, young adult, male > female

if non weightbearing surface ostechondral defect is regarded as OCD, weightbearing surface AVN is then considered spontaneous osteonecrosis of the knee (SONK)

TALUS

classically lateral or medial borders of the talar dome, young adult, male > female, sport related; tends to progress to fragment collapse

CAPITELLUM

typically sport related in adolescent; older age than capitellar AVN (Panner's disease)

MORPHOLOGY

range of findings from subchondral fracture with intact overlying articular cartilage to loose osteochondral fragment in an articular defect

Arthroscopy: Stage 1: intact articular cartilage; stage 2: cartilage defect, no loose body; Stage 3: partially detached fragment; Stage 4: loose osteochondral body in a crater

IMAGING

also see AVN, Ch 2

MR

low T1W and low or high T2W signal in bone fragment

subchondral high T2W crescent

may have surrounding marrow edema

overlying cartilage varies from normal to abnormal signal to fissured to absent

interface between fragment and bed enhancing with Gd suggests loose fragment

fluid filled cleft between fragment and its bed (high on T2W) indicates undisplaced loose fragment

intraarticular Gd tracking around a fragment is an unequivocal sign of loose fragment

displaced fragment is unequivocal

low signal interface between fragment and bed usually indicates stability

---

3.12 REFLEX SYMPATHETIC DYSTROPHY

CLINICAL

poorly understood vascular syndrome triggered by an injury

hyperemic, hot, swollen, painful limb distal to the site of injury, atrophic skin

slowly resolves/stabilizes over many months

IMAGING

XR

changes occur late

peripheral osteopenia involving entire limb

osteopenia most prominent in periarticular distribution

NUC MED (MDP)

diffusely markedly increased MDP activity in all three phases

hypervascular limb, increased blood pool/ tissue activity

classically, periarticular increased delayed MDP uptake

more or less uniformly involves entire limb distal to the site of injury

---

3.13 TENDINOPATHY
(site independent)

3.13.1 TENOSYNOVITIS

DEFINITION

inflammation of synovial tendon sheath

IMAGING

US – tenosynovitis

tendon sheath fluid, possibly synovial thickening

+/– tendonitis

MR – tenosynovitis

normal size tendon

low signal (black) on T1W, T2W

increased fluid around tendon/within tendon sheath

NUC MED (MDP) – tenosynovitis

see tendonitis

3.13.2 TENDONITIS

DEFINITION

abnormal tendon with a prominent inflammatory component

often in context of septic or autoimmune inflammatory arthritis

IMAGING

US – tendonitis

(in general; differentiation from tendinopathy difficult)

hypoechoic swelling of tendon/enthesis

preservation or obscuration of fibrillary structure

synovial fluid with variable amount of debris

direct tenderness

MDP – tendonitis

tissue phase linearly increased uptake along known course of a particular tendon

normal or minimally increased (secondary to hyperemia) late phase uptake

indicates active hyperemia and correlates with inflammatory change

MR

MR can not distinguish 'tendinopathy' (see below) from 'tendonitis', and 'tendinopathy' also blends into partial tears on MR

diagnosis of 'tendonitis' is usually not made on MR, with the preferred MR diagnosis being 'tendinopathy'

see MR findings for tendinopathy and partial tear below

3.13.3 TENDINOPATHY/ TENDINOSIS/DEGENERATIVE CHANGE

DEFINITION

intrasubstance degeneration and healing response in variable proportions with inflammatory component minor or absent

IMAGING

US – tendinopathy

(in general; differentiation from tendonitis difficult)

hypoechoic intrasubstance change without swelling

hypoechoic intrasubstance change with swelling

tendon thinning or contour irregularity

hyperechoic areas (?granulation tissue)

loss of fibrillary structure

partial thickness tears

intrasubstance tears or splits

peritendinous/synovial fluid possible

intratendinous calcification (chronic)

irregularity of bony cortex at insertion (chronic)

MR – tendinopathy

(in general; forms a spectrum with partial tears)

swollen tendon

no disruptions or tendon discontinuities

high signal on PD, increased T2W and T1W signal (gray)

3.13.4 PARTIAL THICKNESS TEAR

IMAGING

US – partial thickness tear

loss of fibrillary structure with contour deficiency

may be filled with fluid (hypoechoic, hyperechoic)

may be filled with bright solid (?granulation)

thinning or thickening

intrasubstance cleft without contour disruption

MR – partial thickness tear

(in general; forms spectrum with tendinopathy)

'tendinopathy' and 'partial thickness tear' may be indistinguishable on MR

swollen tendon or attenuated tendon

longitudinal split/heterogeneous signal

high signal on PD, high signal on T2W

3.13.5 FULL THICKNESS TEAR

IMAGING

US – full thickness tear

tendon discontinuity or enthesis avulsion by definition

gap contains fluid or debris

MR – full thickness tear

empty fluid filled sheath

retracted tendon ends

atrophic muscle belly if longstanding

3.13.6 MUSCULOTENDINOUS JUNCTION TEAR

IMAGING

US

position closer to muscle belly than tendon itself

usually filled with hematoma (see hematoma)

4. SPINE ACUTE TRAUMA

4.1 CERVICAL SPINE FRACTURES BELOW C2

abbreviations: anterior longitudinal ligament: ALL; posterior longitudinal ligament: PLL

classification adapted from Harris

4.1.1 FLEXION INJURIES – STABLE

4.1.1.1 Clay shoveler's fracture

no spinal cord injury

avulsion of tip of spinous process, most commonly C7, rarely C6, not diagnosed above that

fracture line that extends through spinolaminar line indicates serious unstable injury and is not a clay shoveler's fracture

4.1.1.2 Simple wedge compression fracture

no spinal cord injury

impaction fracture of superior endplate (anterior column only)

possible tear of PLL with delayed instability

4.1.2 FLEXION INJURIES – UNSTABLE

4.1.2.1 Flexion subluxation

may have spinal cord injury

torn posterior ligament, posterior facet joint capsules, +/– PLL, +/– posterior disk (two column)

vertebral body translated, angulated anteriorly

facets uncovered, non congruent

spinous processes widened

deformity worst in flexion

DO: flexion/extension views (acute, delayed), MR for ligamentous and spinal cord injury

50% fail to heal – delayed instability

4.1.2.2 Bilateral facet dislocation

often has spinal cord injury

all column ligamentous tear

vertebral body displaced anteriorly (>50% its depth)

locked facets always have neuro deficit

perched facets may have neuro deficit

distracted facets

oblique views helpful for confirmation

4.1.2.3 Flexion teardrop

spinal cord injury present

torn posterior ligament, facet capsules, PLL, ALL, disk AND a fracture dislocation of vertebral body above disk (anteroinferior corner fragment)

anterior cord syndrome (loss of all motor and sensory tracts except dorsal columns)

kyphosis at site of fracture, soft tissue tears

triangular teardrop fragment

4.1.3 FLEXION ROTATION INJURIES – STABLE

4.1.3.1 Unilateral facet dislocation

usually no spinal cord injury

unilateral tear post ligament, facet capsule, PLL, +/– disk +/– ALL; locked inferior facet of vertebra above +/– subluxation or perching of contralateral facet

ROTATION of spinous process on AP view to side of injury

ANTERIOR DISPLACEMENT of body (lateral view)

dislocated ipsilateral facet (obliques, lateral view)

subluxed not dislocated contralateral facet

4.1.4 LATERAL FLEXION INJURIES – STABLE

4.1.4.1 Uncinate process fracture

usually no spinal cord injury

4.1.5 VERTICAL COMPRESSION INJURIES – UNSTABLE

4.1.5.1 Burst fracture

spinal cord injury present
straight spine at impact
nucleus driven into body – mechanism of
    burst
disruption of vertebral body (two column
    fracture)
neuro deficit variable
alignment straight
fracture of both endplates, vertical fracture
    limbs
widened interpedicular distance,
    neurocentral joints, articular pillars on
    AP view
often multilevel fractures
CT shows intracanal fragments

4.1.6 EXTENSION INJURIES – STABLE

4.1.6.1 Isolated laminar fracture

spinal cord injury possibly present
compression fracture of lamina +/– spinous
    process of level above
usually no neuro deficit
CT for possible intracanal fragment

4.1.7 EXTENSION INJURIES – POSSIBLY UNSTABLE

4.1.7.1 Extension teardrop

usually no spinal cord injury
avulsion of anteroinferior vertebral body by
    intact ALL (anterior column injury)

4.1.8 EXTENSION INJURIES – UNSTABLE

4.1.8.1 Hyperextension dislocation

spinal cord injury present

(2/3) avulsion fracture of inferior endplate of
    verterbral above OR
(1/3) tear through ALL and disk AND tear
    through posterior disk with PLL stripped
    off vertebra below
+/– tear of posterior ligament (two or three
    column injury)
central cord syndrome
usually have normal alignment +/– disk
    space widened anteriorly
100% prevertebral hematoma
anteroinferior endplate avulsion wide > tall
    (differential extension teardrop)

4.1.9 EXTENSION ROTATION INJURIES – STABLE

4.1.9.1 Isolated pillar fracture

no spinal cord injury
articular mass fracture with intact pedicle
    and lamina and with abnormal rotation
AP: defect in articular mass, open facet joint
    below
LAT: posterior lying fragment discontinuous
    with pillar contour

4.1.10 EXTENSION ROTATION INJURIES – UNSTABLE

4.1.10.1 Pedicolaminar fracture

may have spinal cord injury
unilateral injury of articular pillar +
    ipsilateral lamina and pedicle + anterior
    column/disk +/– contralateral facet joint
rotated articular mass fragment as above
anterolisthesis on side of injury
disruption of contralateral facet joint
fracture line that extends through
    spinolaminar line indicates serious
    unstable injury – and is not a clay
    shoveler's fracture
!mimics a flexion injury

4.2 CERVICAL SPINE FRACTURES C2 AND ABOVE

abbreviations: anterior longitudinal
    ligament: ALL; posterior longitudinal
    ligament: PLL
classification adapted from Harris

4.2.1 EXTENSION INJURIES – STABLE

4.2.1.1 Fracture of posterior arch C1

no spinal cord injury
isolated compression injury to C1 posterior
    arch (and as a result no prevertebral
    swelling)
no neuro deficit
differential is Jefferson fracture (which has
    prevertebral swelling)
CT evaluates position of fragments

4.2.2 EXTENSION INJURIES – POSSIBLY UNSTABLE

4.2.2.1 Avulsion C1 tubercle

no spinal cord injury

4.2.3 EXTENSION INJURIES – UNSTABLE

4.2.3.1 Hangman's fracture

spinal cord injury may be present
traumatic spondylolisthesis of C2 at pars
    interarticularis +/– disk tear +/– facet
    dislocations
neuro damage uncommon or minor
vertebral body displaced anteriorly +/– facet
    joints dislocated
VARIANTS
pars interarticularis fracture, C2/3 disk
    intact
C2/3 disk torn with vertebral body
    displacement
with facet joint dislocations or locking
fracture line that runs through posterior C2
    body not pars

4.2.4 VERTICAL COMPRESSION INJURIES – UNSTABLE

4.2.4.1 Jefferson fracture

spinal cord injury may be present
burst fracture of C1 ring in at least 2 places
open mouth view: C1 lateral masses
    separated, not aligned with C2 shoulders
lateral view: fracture posterior arch of atlas
    + prevertebral hematoma
CT evaluates extent of fractures and position
    of fragments

4.2.5 OTHER INJURIES – STABLE

4.2.5.1 Rotatory C1–C2 subluxation

no neuro symptoms or spinal cord injury
persistent asymmetry on open mouth view
not fully correctable by position
CT allows definitive assessment

4.2.6 OTHER INJURIES – POSSIBLY UNSTABLE

4.2.6.1 Occipital condyle fracture

neurological injury may or may not be present
may require CT with sagittal or coronal reconstructions

4.2.7 OTHER INJURIES – UNSTABLE

4.2.7.1 Occipitocervical dislocation

spinal cord/brainstem injury present
tip of clivus not aligned with odontoid process
HARRIS'S POSTERIOR AXIAL LINE
basion within 12 mm anterior (or 4 mm posterior) of C2 PLL line AND basion to odontoid interval <12 mm

4.2.7.2 Odontoid fractures

spinal cord/brainstem injury may be present
HIGH (BASE OF ODONTOID): 50% delayed non union (traumatic os odontoideum)
LOW (ARC THROUGH C2 BODY): disruption of 'axis ring', prevertebral hematoma

4.3 CERVICAL SPINE MEASUREMENTS

see Ch 01 normal

4.4 COLUMN CONCEPT

ANTERIOR COLUMN: anterior margin of vertebra to nucleus pulposus
MIDDLE COLUMN: nucleus pulposus to pedicles
POSTERIOR COLUMN: articular pillar and neural arches

Rules

middle column fractured = unstable
two or more columns fractured = unstable

4.5 SPINAL LINES OF ALIGNMENT AND MEASUREMENTS

see Ch 01 normal

4.6 THORACIC AND LUMBAR SPINE INJURIES

! paravertebral hematoma implies fracture (differential is aortic injury with hematoma)

4.6.1 SIMPLE WEDGE FRACTURE

anterior column only disrupted; stable, no spinal cord injury
superior endplate injury, height loss, mild kyphosis
paravertebral hematoma
posterior cortex remains concave; no retropulsed fragments

4.6.2 COMPLEX COMPRESSION/BURST FRACTURE

anterior and middle column disruption; unstable; may have spinal cord injury
crush injury, vertical coronal fracture, anterior–posterior fragment separation, angulation
retropulsed segments, posterior cortex convex
widened interpedicular distance
paravertebral hematoma

4.6.3 FRACTURE DISLOCATION

flexion rotation; unstable; spinal cord injury present

4.6.4 CHANCE FRACTURE

named after Dr Chance, not after the probability of the fracture!
classic 'lap only' seatbelt injury at thoracolumbar junction

distraction of posterior and middle columns, compression of anterior column
fracture passes through: pedicles +/– laminae +/– spinous processes; vertebral body (crush anteriorly) – may exit through disk
widened neural foramina, separation of posterior elements
widened interpedicular distance if lateral fragment separation
unstable, may have conus injury
50% have intraabdominal injuries (classically duodenal rupture/hematoma)
variant: bilateral facet joint dislocation

5. SPINE DEGENERATIVE CHANGE

5.1 DISK DEGENERATIVE DISEASE (without protrusions)

5.1.1 MATURING LUMBAR DISK

decreasing H_2O content
increasing collagen concentration
development of fibrous 'cleft' (low signal on T1W and T2W)

5.1.2 ANNULUS FIBROSUS TEARS

Concentric

delamination of layers
thin cleft high on T2W visible in sagittal (vertical cleft) and axial (circumferential cleft) planes

Transverse

tear at attachment of Sharpey fibers

Radial

associated with disk protrusions, extrusions
thin cleft high on T2W visible in axial plane (radial cleft)

5.1.3 MODIC ENDPLATE CHANGES

MODIC I
inflammatory, endplate marrow low T1W, high T2W

disk low on T2W = degenerated disk

disk high on T2W ?calcified disk, ?discitis

disk high on T1W ? calcified disk

MODIC II

fatty change, endplate marrow high T1W, follows fat on T2W

MODIC III

fibrosis, endplate marrow low T1W, low T2W

5.2 DISK PROTRUSIONS/EXTRUSIONS

CLASSIFICATION BY LOCATION

POSTERIOR MIDLINE (central)

POSTEROLATERAL (paracentral)

NEURAL EXIT FORAMINAL

FAR LATERAL

CLASSIFICATION BY TYPE

5.2.1 Broadbased bulge

bulging of entire disk including annulus fibrosus

annulus fibrosus may be attenuated but overlies bulge by definition

clearly broader than deeper, continuous with disk overall contour

5.2.2 Protrusion

focal in continuity penetration of disk contents through annulus fibrosus

by definition, no annulus fibrosus overlying

usually base broader than protrusion deeper

5.2.3 Extrusion

focal penetration of disk contents through annulus fibrosus with loss of continuity but not contiguity

by definition, outside annulus fibrosus (and outside its projected contour)

5.2.4 Sequestration = sequestered fragment

focal penetration of disk contents through annulus fibrosus with loss of contact with parent disk material

5.2.5 Migratory fragment

migration of sequestered segment away from its level of origin

DIFFERENTIALS

Rim enhancing intraspinal mass

SEQUESTERED FRAGMENT

CYST

CONJOINED ROOT

Solidly enhancing intraspinal mass

SCAR

SCHWANNOMA

TUMOR NOS

5.3 SPINAL CANAL STENOSIS

ETIOLOGY

Congenital

CONGENITAL SHORT PEDICLES

ACHONDROPLASIA

MORQUIO'S SYNDROME

Acquired

HYPERTROPHIC FACET JOINT DEGENERATIVE DISEASE

DISK BULGES, LIGAMENTOUS BUCKLING

SPONDYLOLISTHESIS (with canal narrowing)

when pedicles are congenitally short the canal is more susceptible to stenosis from relatively minor degenerative change

CLINICAL

Lumbar

spinal claudication, back pain, myelopathy

commonest lumbar levels are L2 to L5

5.3.1 CENTRAL TYPE LUMBAR CANAL STENOSIS

concentric narrowing of spinal canal

5.3.2 LUMBAR LATERAL RECESS STENOSIS

narrowing of lateral recesses of the spinal canal (gutters between superior facets of vertebra below and body of vertebra above that contain transiting nerve roots of the level below); usually compress the nerve roots of the level caudal to the stenosis

5.3.3 LUMBAR NEURAL EXIT FORAMINAL STENOSIS

narrowing of the neural exit foramen (canal) by osteophytes or posterolateral/far lateral disk bulges; compress the exiting nerve at the level of the stenosis

Cervical

compressive myelopathy (pain, slowly progressive sensory and motor deficits)

radiculopathy

5.3.4 CENTRAL CERVICAL CANAL STENOSIS

discogenic osteophytes and ligamentous buckling; worse with short pedicles; infrequently caused by posterior longitudinal ligament ossification

5.3.5 CERVICAL FORAMINAL STENOSIS

uncinate process osteophytes

IMAGING

Modality utilization (degenerative spine disease)

MR is the modality of choice for assessment of canal stenosis, cord compression and neural foraminal stenosis

CT is adequate in lumbar spine for disk protrusions and canal stenosis and is preferred for evaluation of purely osseous pathology (e.g. pars defects)

CT is inadequate in cervical spine for anything other than bony canal stenosis

CT myelography is invasive, and is reserved for patients who can not have MR

with the exception of fine bone detail, MR provides the same or more information than CT or CT myelography

CT/CT myelogram/MR (central cervical canal stenosis)

reduced anteroposterior canal diameter (<11 mm)

reduced subarachnoid space

rotated, compressed or deformed cord

MR: compressive myelopathy has high T2W cord signal

causative factors: disc protrusions, discogenic osteophytes, ligamentous buckling; vertebral displacement; combinations of multiple factors

CT/CT myelogram/MR (central type lumbar canal stenosis)

anteroposterior diameter reduction <12 mm

concentrically narrowed thecal sac, compressed and lost epidural fat

crowded, stretched nerve roots
engorged spinal veins
causative factors: facet joint osteophytes;
    disk bulges and protrusions; buckled
    ligamenta flava
other: synovial cysts, sequestrated fragments

CT/CT myelogram/MR (lumbar
lateral recess stenosis)

reduced lateral recess <4 mm
loss of epidural fat in lateral recess
causative factors: hypertrophic facets,
    posterolateral disk bulging with/without
    osteophytes

CT/CT myelogram/MR (neural
exit foraminal stenosis)

narrowed neural exit foramen (canal)
loss of foraminal fat
possibly high T2W signal within compressed
    exiting nerve root
causative factors: posterolateral/far lateral
    disk bulge, hypertrophic facet, discogenic
    osteophytes, uncinate process
    osteophytes

5.4 SPINAL CANAL CYSTS AND MIMICKERS

5.4.1 SIMPLE SYNOVIAL CYST

fluid contents, arises from facet joint

IMAGING

closely related to degenerate facet joint
fluid density and MR signal (may be different
    from CSF)

5.4.2 COMPLICATED SYNOVIAL CYST

inspissated protein or blood contents
arises from facet joint

IMAGING

closely related to degenerate facet joint
complex signal on MR, dense on CT, possibly
    fluid–fluid level

5.4.3 ARACHNOID DIVERTICULUM

NOT A TARLOV CYST
arises from root sleeve, contains CSF

IMAGING

density and MR signal same as CSF
fills with subarachnoid contrast

5.4.4 TARLOV (PERINEURAL) CYST

NOT AN ARACHNOID ROOT SLEEVE
    DIVERTICULUM
arises from root sleeve at dorsal ganglion
has nerve fibers in wall

IMAGING

density and MR signal same as CSF

5.4.5 TRAUMATIC PSEUDOMENINGOCELE

empty root sleeve
cervical > thoracic or lumbar

5.4.6 MENINGOCELE

5.4.6.1 Multilevel dural ectasia
Ehlers–Danlos syndrome, neurofibromatosis
    1, Marfan's syndrome
thoracic > lumbar > cervical

5.4.6.2 Anterior sacral meningocele
see Ch 20

5.4.6.3 Dorsal meningocele, myelomeningocele, spina bifida
see Ch 20

6. UPPER LIMB ACUTE TRAUMA

6.1 AC JOINT INJURY

6.2 CARPUS TRAUMA

6.2.1 NORMAL MEASUREMENTS

Scapholunate interval 2 mm

Scapholunate angle (lateral film)
(axis of lunate runs through centers of distal
    and proximal articular surfaces)
long axis of scaphoid to axis of lunate
30–60 degrees is normal
increased in DISI (see below)
decreased in VISI (see below)

Lunate–capitate angle
long axis of capitate to axis of lunate
normal is <20 degrees

6.2.2 ISOLATED ROTATORY SUBLUXATION OF SCAPHOID

6.2.3 (TRANSSCAPHO/) PERILUNATE DISLOCATION

6.2.4 AS ABOVE + HAMATE/TRIQUETRAL FRACTURE OR DISLOCATION

6.2.5 (TRANSSCAPHO/) LUNATE DISLOCATION

6.2.6 SCAPHOID FRACTURES

APPROACH

scaphoid views looking for
    displaced/undisplaced fracture
look for scaphoid fat pad displacement (not
    always present)
must immobilize until there is proof of no
    fracture

OPTIONS FOR DIAGNOSIS OF
    OCCULT FRACTURES
immobilize, repeat films in 7–10 days
3 phase MDP scan
CT
MR (recommended)

COMPLICATIONS
non union
avascular necrosis (proportional to proximal
    location of fracture)

IMAGING

NUC MED

95% of scaphoid fractures have increased 3 phase MDP uptake

CT

need scans along scaphoid long axis fracture line, cortical step

MR

scaphoid edema, cortical displacement, fracture line

6.2.7 TRIQUETRAL FRACTURE

6.2.8 HOOK OF HAMATE FRACTURE

XR: carpal tunnel view, hook of hamate (glass holding) view
CT diagnostic

6.2.9 LUNATE INSTABILITY (DISI, VISI)

6.2.9.1 Dorsal intercalated segment instability (DISI)

commoner consequence of ligamentous injury than VISI
associated with disruption of scapholunate ligaments
lunate distal articular surface rotates DORSAL
scapholunate angle increased, lunate–capitate angle decreased or reversed

6.2.9.2 Volar intercalated segment instability (VISI)

lunate distal articular surface points VOLAR
decreased scapholunate angle, increased lunate–capitate angle

6.2.10 CARPOMETACARPAL FRACTURE OR FRACTURE/ DISLOCATION

XR: reverse oblique for bases of MC IV and V

6.2.11 BENNETT FRACTURE
(2 part fracture of MC I)

fracture through articular surface
proximal fragment pulled proximally by abductor pollicis longus
(reverse Bennett fracture occurs at MC V)

6.2.12 AVULSION FRACTURES

6.2.13 RADIOGRAPHICALLY OCCULT FRACTURES

scaphoid (beware of avascular necrosis)
lunate
hook of hamate
triquetral

6.3 ELBOW TRAUMA

also see Ch 17

6.3.1 AVULSION INJURIES

6.3.1.1 Medial epicondyle
medial capsule may be torn
avulsed medial epicondyle with its flexor origin may be caught in joint (and hence missing from its normal position medially and relatively posteriorly)

6.3.1.2 Lateral epicondyle

6.3.2 SUPRACONDYLAR FRACTURE

most common childhood elbow fracture
consider injury to neurovascular bundle in angulated fractures
joint effusion usually present
fracture line may not be visible on XR
assess anterior humeral line

6.3.3 LATERAL CONDYLAR FRACTURE

6.3.4 RADIAL HEAD FRACTURE

most common occult adult elbow fracture
joint effusion usually present

6.3.5 OLECRANON FRACTURE

6.3.6 MONTEGGIA FRACTURE

ulnar fracture with dislocated radial head

6.3.7 GALEAZZI FRACTURE

radial fracture with dislocated distal ulna

6.3.8 JOINT EFFUSION

see Ch 04
in trauma, suspicious of underlying occult fracture

6.4 FOREARM TRAUMA

6.4.1 TORUS (pediatric fracture)

buckle fracture often with minimal angulation
may be visible in only one of the two bones

6.4.2 GREENSTICK
(pediatric fracture)

angulation of one cortex with distraction fracture of the opposite cortex; may be present in one bone only

6.4.3 SALTER–HARRIS I, II, LESS FREQUENTLY III, IV, V

see Ch 17

6.4.4 COLLES FRACTURE

distal radial fracture with impaction and dorsal angulation +/– dorsal displacement
ulnar styloid process may be avulsed by the triangular fibrocartilage or triangular fibrocartilage itself may be damaged
fracture limbs may extend to radiocarpal joint
flexor tendons 'bowstring' over the fracture with carpal volar flexion and 'dinner fork' deformity on lateral view

6.4.5 DISTAL RADIAL FRACTURE NOS

6.4.6 SMITH'S FRACTURE

'reverse Colles'
distal radius angulated volar, impacted, may be displaced volar
infrequent

6.4.7 ULNAR DISLOCATION

6.4.8 ULNAR FRACTURE DISLOCATION

6.4.9 GALEAZZI

radius fracture, ulnar dislocation

6.4.10 ISOLATED ULNAR FRACTURE ('NIGHTSTICK FRACTURE')

result of direct force on the mid ulna

6.4.11 MID FOREARM FRACTURE

fracture of both mid radius and mid ulna
usually requires open reduction to preserve
pronation and supination

6.5 SHOULDER JOINT INJURIES

6.5.1 GLENOHUMERAL DISLOCATIONS

6.5.1.1 Anterior

6.5.1.2 Posterior

XR
classic trap if only one view (AP) taken
'light bulb' sign in AP view (severe internal
rotation makes humeral head look
relatively symmetrical)

6.5.1.3 Luxatio erecta
rare inferior dislocation of humeral head
with humerus (and arm) fixed in vertical
position

6.5.2 FRACTURES ASSOCIATED WITH SHOULDER DISLOCATIONS

6.5.2.1 Hill Sachs fracture

6.5.2.2 Bankart fracture

6.5.2.3 Reverse Hill Sachs (trough) fracture

6.5.2.4 Reverse Bankart

6.5.3 UPPER HUMERAL FRACTURE

Neer's humeral fracture classification
number of fragments and their relationship
more important than classification
helical CT with 3D and multiplanar
reconstruction very useful

Physeal plate vs fracture
physeal plate parallel sclerotic (rises
posteriorly)
fracture line non parallel non sclerotic

6.5.4 LABRAL TEARS

6.5.4.1 Anterior
commonly associated with anterior
dislocation
fluid under anterior labrum on CT
arthrography or MR arthrography
may see labral deformity or sublabral fluid
on plain MR
variant: ALPSA (anterior labrum periosteal
sleeve avulsion)

6.5.4.2 SLAP (superior labrum anterior to posterior)
tear of superior labrum with avulsed labrum
carrying biceps insertion; multiple types
described; variable appearance; labral
and biceps origin displacement or defect
on MR arthrography

6.5.4.3 Buford complex – normal variant (beware)
absent anterosuperior labrum and thickened
middle glenohumeral ligament inserting
close to biceps origin

6.5.5 BICEPS TENDON DISLOCATION

always medial, over medial lip of bicipital
groove

7. UPPER LIMB DEGENERATIVE CHANGE

7.1 CARPAL TUNNEL SYNDROME

DEFINITION

compression of median nerve in carpal
tunnel with sensory +/– motor
neurological deficit

IMAGING

US

NORMAL MEDIAN NERVE
hypoechoic tubular structure with sharply
defined margin superficially located in
carpal tunnel and less mobile than
tendons

ABNORMAL MEDIAN NERVE
flattening (width:depth >3:1) in carpal tunnel
swelling of nerve proximal to tunnel
perineural edema (loss of sharp margins)
+/– bowing of flexor retinaculum outward
(effect of pressure)

MR

may demonstrate cause, especially synovitis
or soft tissue deposition
enlargement of median nerve at level of
pisiform, median nerve flattening
median nerve edema (increased T2W signal)
bowing of flexor retinaculum

FIBROLIPOMATOUS HAMARTOMA
(pathognomonic on MR)
probably congenital proliferation of fibrofatty
mesenchymal cells in nerve sheath
'coaxial cable' appearance

7.2 ROTATOR CUFF DEGENERATIVE CHANGE

7.2.1 ROTATOR CUFF IMPINGEMENT

DEFINITION

idiopathic or post traumatic impingement (virtually always supraspinatus) between humeral head and acromion or acromioclavicular ligament

mechanism is poor humeral head depression by the rotator cuff as the deltoid lifts the humerus

CLASSIFICATION

BY LOCATION

acromion (lateral or anterior)
acromioclavicular ligament (anterior)

BY IMPINGING STRUCTURE

Bursal only
Tendinous (supraspinatus)
Bony

IMAGING

XR

acromial undersurface types: type I flat, type II curved, type III hooked
type III acromion (?acquired, ?congenital) associated with impingement
acromial undersurface spur

US – dynamic observation

bunching or squeezing of bursa
bunching of tendon
tendon jammed between greater tuberosity and acromion
greater tuberosity impacts on acromion

US – secondary signs

isolated bursal thickening/bursitis

MR signs of impingement

NORMAL

normal subacromial fat (fat plane surrounding subacromial subdeltoid bursa)

EARLY IMPINGEMENT (indirect signs)

loss of subacromial fat plane
irregularity of superior contour of supraspinatus

7.2.2 TENDINOPATHY/ TENDINOSIS

DEFINITION

degenerative tendon change, grossly preserved continuity
frequent age related incidental finding in asymptomatic individuals
only clinically relevant if correlates with presentation

IMAGING

XR

variable amount of supraspinatus tunnel narrowing
sclerosis of greater tuberosity at rotator cuff insertion with small spurs (enthesophytes)
sclerosis of acromial undersurface, acromial spur

US

focal hypoechoic area of loss of fibrillary structure; no discontinuity
thinning of tendon suggests chronic low grade surface tearing or degeneration
irregularity of greater tuberosity bone at insertion common (enthesopathy)
joint or bursal fluid a sensitive but not specific finding

MR

preservation of tendon contour
diffusely increased signal on short TR/TE and PD sequences
increased T2W signal with appearance merging into that of partial tear

INCIDENTAL ASYMPTOMATIC DEGENERATIVE CHANGE

age related asymptomatic increased signal is common, and of clinical relevance only if it correlates with presentation
no increasing signal with increasing T2 weighting

OTHER NON PATHOLOGICAL CAUSES OF INCREASED SIGNAL

partial voluming on adjacent fat or cartilage
extension of muscle bundles into tendon (distal musculotendinous junction)

NUC MED (MDP)

frequent incidental finding on bone scans
increased uptake involving greater tuberosity at rotator cuff insertion
occasionally increased blood pool/tissue phase activity involving superolateral shoulder (tendonitis)

7.2.3 TENDONITIS

DEFINITION

degenerative or traumatic change with a prominent inflammatory component (and responding to appropriate treatment)

IMAGING

US

generally not an US diagnosis; presence of pain on direct pressure, diffuse tendon swelling and increased vascularity suggest inflammatory component
joint effusion or bursal effusion/bursitis also suggestive

7.2.4 CALCIFIC TENDINOSIS

DEFINITION

intratendinous calcification – may or may not be symptomatic

IMAGING

XR

clumpy calcification overlying greater tuberosity, and moving with rotator cuff in internal and external rotation

US

focal areas of (usually curvilinear) echogenic shadowing or smaller echogenic foci

7.2.5 INTRASUBSTANCE TEAR

DEFINITION

arthroscopically occult tear deep within tendon

IMAGING

US

usually hypoechoic area within confines of tendon contours

7.2.6 PARTIAL THICKNESS TEAR

DEFINITION

tear with some normal fibers remaining, and no retraction of torn ends

IMAGING

US

focal contour discontinuity with loss of all fibrillary structure in two planes

may be filled with fluid (hypoechoic) or granulation tissue (hyperechoic)

bursal surface more common than articular surface

some fibers remain by definition

bursal fluid/joint fluid may be present

if acute with an inflammatory component, tendon may be swollen

if chronic with atrophy, tendon usually thinned

MR

focal defect in tendon with high T1W and T2W (long TR/TE) signal

may involve either bursal or articular surface or be entirely within tendon contours (intrasubstance)

MR arthrography outlines undersurface defects and irregularities

7.2.7 FULL THICKNESS TEAR

DEFINITION

traverses thickness of the cuff by definition
retraction of torn ends occurs if tear wide

FOCAL (PARTIAL WIDTH)

usually anterior supraspinatus fibers tear first

supraspinatus: anterior, mid, posterior

subscapularis: superior, mid, inferior

FULL WIDTH

IMAGING

XR

loss of supraspinatus exit tunnel width

ultimately, humeral head impacted against acromial undersurface

Arthrography

entry of contrast into subacromial/subdeltoid bursa (specific)

defect size may be directly shown

US

major discontinuity of tendon contour and fibrillary structure

reproducible in two planes

deltoid (+ bursa and its fat) dip into the tear

filled with synovial fluid (may have echogenic debris) or prolapsed bursa (with two fat planes around it)

tear moves with the tendon

proximal tendon may retract, increasing length of tear; retracted muscle may atrophy

joint effusion together with bursal fluid

MR

defect extending full thickness of tendon filled with fluid or with high T1W, high T2W signal

signal brightens with increasing T2 weighting

bursal and joint fluid, loss of peribursal fat

superior humeral head subluxation

thin atrophic tendon (chronic tear likely)

retraction of torn tendon edges (large tear)

MR arthrography: outlines extent and shape of defect

7.2.8 LONG HEAD OF BICEPS PROBLEMS

7.2.8.1 Dislocation

medially placed tendon

empty bicipital groove

7.2.8.2 Rupture

retracted distal +/– proximal ends

empty bicipital groove

7.2.9 ADHESIVE CAPSULITIS

CLINICAL

reduced range of motion

follows injury or less well described causes

IMAGING

Arthrography

small volume restricted joint space

MR

synovial thickening of >4 mm from humerus to inferior portion of joint space (easier to measure with fluid in joint)

---

8. PELVIS (AND HIP) ACUTE TRAUMA

classification of pelvic ring fractures is adapted from Harris

8.1 APPROACH TO PELVIC FRACTURES

Pelvis

if in doubt: do caudal and cranial angulation views, and CT

assess sacral arcs and sacral ala

assess SI joints ?vertical displacement ?diastasis

lateral hip views: cross table, frog leg lateral

8.2 ACETABULAR FRACTURES (LETOURNEL)

8.2.1 POSTERIOR COLUMN FRACTURE (ILIOISCHIAL)

8.2.1.1 Posterior acetabular lip

8.2.1.2 Posterior column

Pitfall

posterior column fracture may look like a superposition shadow – do CT

evaluate for round foci of air in joints – this suggests hip dislocation (crescentic 'vacuum phenomenon' is normal)

8.2.2 ANTERIOR COLUMN FRACTURE (ILIOPUBIC)

8.2.2.1 Anterior acetabular lip

8.2.2.2 Anterior column

8.2.3 TRANSVERSE

8.2.4 T SHAPED

8.2.4.1 Transverse, extension to anterior column

8.2.4.2 Transverse, extension to posterior column

8.2.5 CENTRAL

8.3 FEMORAL NECK FRACTURES

8.3.1 INTRACAPSULAR

8.3.1.1 Subcapital

8.3.1.2 Transcervical

8.3.2 EXTRACAPSULAR

8.3.2.1 Intertrochanteric (2, 3, 4 part)

8.3.2.2 Peritrochanteric

IMAGING (femoral neck fractures)

IMAGING

XR

diagnosis usually a problem in osteopenic elderly when there is no obviously displaced fracture and an undisplaced fracture has to be confirmed or ruled out

irregular medial femoral sclerotic density (near horizontal density at calcar femorale) strongly suggests an insufficiency or stress fracture

irregular density extending across femoral neck suggests an impacted minimally displaced fracture

discontinuity or angulation of primary and secondary trabecular lines in femoral neck suspicious for fracture

serial XR may show angulation or further impaction

CT

may need to do fine slice CT with coronal reconstruction as fracture often is in the axial plane

shows subtle cortical steps and trabecular disruption

NUC MED (MDP)

see entry on fracture, stress fracture, insufficiency fracture earlier in this chapter

classically, increased three phase MDP uptake (particularly increased blood pool/tissue phase uptake more than perfusion)

late phase MDP uptake may take days to increase above background, particularly in bed ridden elderly; in this case, blood pool/tissue phase uptake is only clue (imaging differential is then soft tissue injury in isolation)

at 1 week, absence of MDP uptake rules out fracture

may effectively diagnose femoral head devascularization immediately (if shows cold femoral head on all phases)

MR

normal femoral head epiphysis contains yellow marrow; normal metaphysis contains red marrow well into adult life

fracture has surrounding bone marrow edema

fracture line itself may be visible

MR changes of avascular necrosis occur 2–5 days post fracture

8.4 HIP DISLOCATIONS AND FRACTURE DISLOCATIONS

8.4.1 HIP DISLOCATION WITHOUT FRACTURE

8.4.1.1 Posterior

8.4.1.2 Anterior

8.4.1.3 Obturator

into the obturator foramen

8.4.2 HIP FRACTURE DISLOCATION

8.4.2.1 Femoral head Hill Sachs (accompanies anterior dislocation)

8.4.2.2 Femoral head split (accompanies posterior dislocation)

8.4.2.3 Acetabular lip fractures

8.5 PELVIC FRACTURE WITHOUT PELVIC RING DISRUPTION

8.5.1 AVULSION INJURIES

8.5.1.1 Anterior superior iliac spine (sartorius)

8.5.1.2 Anterior inferior iliac spine (straight head rectus femoris, iliofemoral ligament)

8.5.1.3 Ischial tuberosity (hamstrings)

8.5.1.4 Lesser trochanter (psoas/iliacus)

8.5.2 ISOLATED FRACTURES

8.5.2.1 Vertical iliac wing (Duverney)

8.5.2.2 Sacrum/coccyx

8.5.2.3 Teardrop

8.5.3 STRESS AND INSUFFICIENCY FRACTURES

see general entry on stress and insufficiency fractures

allowed to be at one point in the pelvic ring

diagnosis of insufficiency pelvic/sacral fracture in osteoporotic elderly is often impossible on plain film and may require CT (for pelvic ring fracture), MR/CT (for sacral fracture) or NUC MED (MDP)

8.6 PELVIC RING DISRUPTION (HARRIS)

pelvic ring tends to fracture in at least two places at any one time

unless proven otherwise, need to identify companion fractures to an isolated fracture (or dislocation)

fracture is a disruption by definition

dislocation of sacroiliac joint or pubic symphysis is a disruption

RULES

Common posterior sites

sacral ala or sacroiliac joint or both counts as one site

Common anterior sites

pubis/both pubic rami or symphysis counts as one site; if both this counts as two sites

8.6.1 TYPE I (Malgaigne)

ipsilateral anterior and posterior disruption (Malgaigne)

8.6.2 TYPE II (bucket handle)

contralateral anterior and posterior disruption

8.6.3 TYPE III AND IIIA (three places)

III: one disruption posteriorly, two anteriorly
IIIa: one disruption anteriorly, two posteriorly

8.6.4 TYPE IV (four places)

bilateral anterior and posterior disruptions

8.6.5 OPEN BOOK

disruption of symphysis with separation of hemipelves
can be type I, III or IV injury

8.7 PELVIC SOFT TISSUE TRAUMATIC INJURIES

see Ch 08

9. PELVIS AND HIP DEGENERATIVE CHANGE

9.1 PUBIC SYMPHYSITIS

IMAGING

XR

increased sclerosis or erosions around symphysis
narrowed symphysis space
secondary degenerative change

NUC MED

diffusely increased MDP uptake around symphysis

9.2 TROCHANTERIC BURSITIS

IMAGING

US

thickened bursa or fluid in bursa

MR

increased T2W signal adjacent to greater trochanter (may not be well defined)

NUC MED

increased tissue phase uptake over greater trochanter
diffuse increased mild late phase uptake in underlying greater trochanter

10. LOWER LIMB ACUTE TRAUMA

10.1 ANKLE

10.1.1 FRACTURE CLASSIFICATION

By stability

STABLE = BELOW PLAFOND

UNSTABLE = AT OR ABOVE PLAFOND

By extent

10.1.1.1 UNIMALLEOLAR (?contralateral ligament rupture)

10.1.1.2 BIMALLEOLAR

10.1.1.3 TRIMALLEOLAR

10.1.1.4 PYLON (i.e. COMMINUTED PLAFOND FRACTURE)

(BEWARE TALAR DOME INJURIES)

Weber classification

10.1.1.5 WEBER A (usually an inversion injury)
AVULSION FRACTURE OF LATERAL MALLEOLUS BELOW PLAFOND
+/− IMPACTION FRACTURE OF MEDIAL MALLEOLUS

10.1.1.6 WEBER B (usually an eversion injury)
IMPACTION FRACTURE OF LATERAL MALLEOLUS AT LEVEL OF PLAFOND
+/− AVULSION FRACTURE MEDIAL MALLEOLUS
UNSTABLE, REQUIRES INTERNAL FIXATION

10.1.1.7 WEBER C (usually an eversion injury)
IMPACTION FRACTURE OF FIBULA ABOVE PLAFOND
+/− AVULSION FRACTURE OF MEDIAL MALLEOLUS
UNSTABLE, REQUIRES INTERNAL FIXATION

Fracture position and tibiofibular diastasis

fractures that disrupt the tibiofibular interosseous ligament (normally fractures above the level of the plafond) usually require repair with internal fixation (diastasis screw)

10.2 TALUS OSTEOCHONDRAL INJURIES AND FRACTURES

10.2.1 TALUS ACUTE FRACTURES

incidence of talar head avascular necrosis increases with severity of injury

10.2.1.1 Talar neck fracture without dislocation

10.2.1.2 Talar neck fracture with posterior talocalcaneal dislocation

10.2.1.3 Talar neck fracture with posterior talocalcaneal and talocalcaneonavicular dislocation

10.2.2 TALUS OSTEOCHONDRAL INJURY

acute traumatic injury or osteochondritis dissecans

IMAGING (chondral injury only)

XR/CT
no findings

MR
cartilage defect or high signal

NUC MED
no findings or mild changes

IMAGING (osteochondral fracture)

XR
may see lucent line or irregular articular surface; possibly no findings

CT
subchondral step, fracture line, sclerosis, subarticular cysts, loose bodies

MR
subchondral bone marrow edema
signal changes of avascular necrosis if osteochondritis dissecans
loose chondral or osseous bodies
secondary degenerative change
MR SIGNS OF UNSTABLE OSTEOCHONDRAL FRAGMENT
loose fragment
high T2W signal cleft completely surrounding the fragment
high signal in the fragment or its bed

NUC MED
increased MDP uptake in all three phases

10.3 HINDFOOT INJURIES

10.3.1 CALCANEAL COMPRESSION FRACTURE

IMAGING

XR
loss of calcaneal angle (Bohler's angle)
cortical step
trabecular sclerosis

NUC MED
see fracture under general
increased activity centered on calcaneal body

10.3.2 CALCANEAL INSUFFICIENCY FRACTURE

XR
nil or sclerotic line

NUC MED
see insufficiency fracture under general
increased activity centered on calcaneal body

10.4 FOREFOOT INJURIES

10.4.1 LISFRANC FRACTURE DISLOCATION

IMAGING

XR
fracture dislocation through the tarsometatarsal joint
loss of alignment of metatarsal bases and their cuneiforms
fractures through bases of metatarsals or through cuneiforms may require CT to confirm
HOMOLATERAL: all metatarsals shift laterally
DIVERGENT: first metatarsal moves medially, rest move laterally

NUC MED
usually not required and an incidental finding in neuropathic feet

CT
definitive assessment of tarsometatarsal alignment
(axial and coronal acquisition, multiplanar and 3D reconstruction)

10.5 KNEE INJURIES

Abbreviations
ACL: anterior cruciate ligament
PCL: posterior cruciate ligament
MCL: medial collateral ligament
LCL: lateral collateral ligament

10.5.1 'LARGE' FRACTURES AROUND THE KNEE

Tibia
10.5.1.1 PLATEAU
10.5.1.2 INTERCONDYLAR (Y)

Femur
10.5.2.1 CONDYLAR
10.5.2.2 INTERCONDYLAR
10.5.2.3 SUPRACONDYLAR

Fibula
10.5.3.1 HEAD/NECK

Patella
10.5.4.1 BURST
10.5.4.2 TRANSVERSE

Secondary signs of fracture
EFFUSION
LIPOHEMARTHROSIS

10.5.2 'SMALL' FRACTURES AROUND THE KNEE

Tibia
10.5.2.1 INTERCONDYLAR SPINE
MEDIAL SPINE AVULSION (ACL AVULSION)
   MINIMALLY DISPLACED
   HINGED
   FULLY DISPLACED
LATERAL SPINE (ISOLATED)
10.5.2.2 OSTEOCHONDRAL FRAGMENT
10.5.2.3 SEGOND FRACTURE
lateral capsule avulsion fracture (fragment avulsed off the lateral tibia)
associated with ACL injuries

10.5.3 PATELLAR DISLOCATION

always lateral, may spontaneously relocate
more common in females (greater carrying angle)
more common in patella alta

10.5.4 SALTER–HARRIS FRACTURES

see Ch 17

11. LOWER LIMB DEGENERATIVE CHANGE AND SPORTS INJURIES

11.1 KNEE DEGENERATIVE CHANGE

11.1.1 DISCOID MENISCUS

IMAGING

almost always the lateral meniscus

MR (intact discoid meniscus)
normal signal meniscus that extends too far medially
too many 'bow-ties' (more than three with 5 mm sections)
abnormal meniscal cross section
may completely divide joint space (thick meniscus separating femoral and tibial articular surfaces)

MR (degenerating discoid meniscus)
increasing meniscal signal
prone to tears and degeneration
abnormal intrameniscal signal or meniscal cyst–evaluate for a tear

11.1.2 MENISCAL DEGENERATION

IMAGING (MR)

11.1.2.1 Normal meniscus
black on all sequences; width (in general) 10–12 mm
lateral meniscus cross section uniform throughout
medial meniscus cross section: posterior horn size is greater than anterior horn, which is greater than body
evaluate on short TE images

11.1.2.2 Grade I
amorphous rounded intrasubstance increased signal
clinically usually asymptomatic myxoid degeneration

11.1.2.3 Grade II
linear intrasubstance increased signal not reaching a surface
linear myxoid degeneration

11.1.2.4 Grade III (tear)
linear intrasubstance increased signal extending to and involving at least one articular surface

11.1.3 MENISCAL TEARS

IMAGING (MR)

abnormal meniscal surface (blunting, truncation)
linear intrasubstance high signal with extension to at least one surface
parameniscal cyst

11.1.3.1 Longitudinal vertical tear

UNDISPLACED TEAR

BUCKET HANDLE TEAR
long horizontal tear with displacement of inner portion of meniscus
more common in medial meniscus
remaining peripheral meniscus truncated, with too few 'bow ties' (too many slices with anterior and posterior horns separate)
SIGNS OF MEDIAL MENISCUS BUCKET HANDLE TEAR
too few 'bow ties'
double posterior cruciate ligament
extra linear low signal intercondylar structure (torn half flipped into medial gutter)
SIGNS OF LATERAL MENISCUS BUCKET HANDLE TEAR
too few 'bow ties'
flipped meniscus (posterior horn detaches and lies along anterior horn) – anterior horn too long, posterior horn absent
extra linear low signal intercondylar structure (if ACL intact, the torn half can not get past it)

11.1.3.2 Longitudinal horizontal (cleavage)
run horizontally from inner angle or distal inner margin to periphery
associated with parameniscal cysts

11.1.3.3 Oblique
starts on free edge of meniscus and curves obliquely into meniscus

vertical and horizontal components
PARROT BEAK TEAR, FLAP TEAR

11.1.3.4 Radial
vertical tear running outward from free meniscal edge
may show as focal absence of meniscus

11.1.4 MIMICKERS OF MENISCAL TEARS

IMAGING (MR)

11.1.4.1 Meniscofemoral ligaments
arise from surface of posterior horn of lateral meniscus and insert on medial femoral condyle

LIGAMENT OF HUMPHREY (ANTERIOR MENISCOFEMORAL LIGAMENT)
runs anterior to posterior cruciate ligament
present in 1/3 of patients

LIGAMENT OF WRISBERG (POSTERIOR MENISCOFEMORAL LIGAMENT)
runs posterior to posterior cruciate ligament
present in 1/3 of patients
may be well shown in coronal images

11.1.4.2 Transverse meniscal ligament
joins anterior horns of menisci, runs in Hoffa's (infrapatellar) fat pad where no menisci present

11.1.4.3 Popliteus tendon
runs deep to lateral collateral ligament and inserts into posterior horn of lateral meniscus

11.1.5 SURGICAL MANAGEMENT OF MENISCAL TEARS

Repair
peripheral longitudinal tears close to capsule
large bucket handle tears

Resection
oblique tears, tears in inner avascular zone of meniscus
horizontal tears

11.2 KNEE SPORTS INJURIES AND RELATED CONDITIONS

ABBREVIATIONS

ACL: anterior cruciate ligament
PCL: posterior cruciate ligament
MCL: medial collateral ligament
LCL: lateral collateral ligament

11.2.1 OSGOOD–SCHLATTER DISEASE

CLINICAL

avulsion injury of tibial tubercle or apophysis

IMAGING

XR

late inconstant sclerosis
soft tissue swelling may be present

NUC MED

increased uptake at tubercle, greater than other side

11.2.2 PELLEGRINI–STIEDA LESION

part avulsion/tear of MCL with calcification/ossification

11.2.3 OSTEOCHONDRITIS DISSECANS (OCD)/SONK

11.2.4 PATELLAR TENDINOSIS

(jumper's knee)

see its own entry

IMAGING

non inflammatory degenerative process

US

fibrillar disruption, focal hypoechoic swelling
focal hypoechoic defect
+/− calcification

NUC MED

increased uptake at inferior patellar pole
degree of tissue phase uptake correlates with acuteness of injury

MR

high on T1W and T2W; very high on GRE T2W, high on STIR
swollen tendon

11.2.5 CRUCIATE AND COLLATERAL LIGAMENT TEARS

IMAGING

11.2.5.1 PCL tears (MR)

NORMAL
fully black curved (not under tension) ligament
originates in a wide posterior intercondylar tibial attachment and extends up to the posterolateral inner aspect of medial femoral condyle (anteroposterior attachment)

TEAR
increased GRE and PD signal
hematoma (less prominent than with ACL)
discontinuity, gap (complete tear, unusual)
avulsion (with possibly visible bony fragment)

ASSOCIATED INJURIES
MCL, ACL, other

11.2.5.2 ACL tears (MR)

NORMAL
alternating black and gray diagonal bands parallel to roof of intercondylar tunnel
originates in anterior tibial intercondylar area and extends up to the posteromedial inner aspect of lateral condyle

TEAR
loss of internal structure, increased GRE, PD and T2W signal
discontinuity, 'fallen' ACL (complete tear)
intercondylar blood or fluid
avulsion (with possibly visible bony fragment)

ASSOCIATED INJURIES
O'Donoghue's triad: ACL, MCL, medial meniscus
bone bruises (lateral femoral condyle and posterior lateral tibial plateau)

11.2.5.3 MCL tears

US
Sprain: thickened hypoechoic ill defined but continuous ligament surrounded by edema
Tear: discontinuity of ligament with hematoma (variable echogenicity) filling gap with surrounding edema

MR
NORMAL
thin black line with thin fibrofatty layer between MCL and medial meniscus outer margin
GRADE I SPRAIN
edema and hemorrhage parallel and superficial to MCL
GRADE II PARTIAL TEAR
ligament attenuation, displacement of ligament from bone, variable amount of high GRE, PD, T2W signal
surrounding edema and hemorrhage
GRADE III FULL THICKNESS TEAR
complete discontinuity of ligament fibers, replacement by hematoma

ASSOCIATED INJURIES
ACL, medial meniscus, lateral compartment bone bruises

SPECIFICALLY LOOK FOR SUBTLE INJURIES

intrasubstance tears
ligament partial tears
occult fractures, bone bruises
missing cartilage (best is FSE with fat sat)

11.3 LOWER LIMB SPORTS INJURIES

11.3.1 ANKLE POSTERIOR IMPINGEMENT

CLINICAL

impingement of posterior tibial lip on an os trigonum
occupational/sporting ankle plantar flexion or extreme plantar flexion

IMAGING

XR

os trigonum – in itself a normal variant

MR

abnormal signal in os trigonum and around
flexor hallucis longus tendon

NUC MED

increased MDP uptake in os trigonum
degree of tissue phase uptake reflects how
acute the syndrome is

11.3.2 ANKLE ANTERIOR IMPINGEMENT

IMAGING

XR

talar neck degenerative spur

MR

low T1W and T2W signal in lateral gutter
(scar)

NUC MED

increased three phase uptake centered on
the spur

11.3.3 SHIN SPLINTS

IMAGING

XR

early and late: nil
very late: benign periosteal new bone,
usually symmetrical and bilateral

NUC MED

normal perfusion, normal or near normal
tissue phase
linear delayed uptake along tibial surface
classically posterior mid tibia (soleus
attachment) and symmetrical left–right

11.3.4 SESAMOIDITIS, SESAMOID FRACTURE

MDP: increased 3 phase activity (differential
bipartite sesamoid is cold)

11.4 TARSUS AND FOOT DEGENERATIVE CHANGE

11.4.1 TARSAL COALITION

see Ch 17

11.4.2 PLANTAR FASCIITIS

IMAGING

XR

nil or calcaneal spur or calcaneal spur with
soft tissue swelling

US

thickened hypoechoic tender plantar fascia
(4 mm is normal thickness)

MR

increased T2W signal in plantar fascia
and/or adjacent soft tissues

NUC MED

increased MDP uptake in three phases, with
extension into plantar fascia on tissue
phase and delayed uptake centered on
plantar fascia insertion

5 **Musculoskeletal tumors**

3. GENERAL

3.1 ASSESSMENT OF BONE TUMOR

AGGRESSIVITY (plain XR and CT)

Features to assess

PATTERN

LYTIC

SCLEROTIC

MIXED

PERMEATIVE

ill marginated patchy diffusely decreased bone density (implies an aggressive process)

DESTRUCTIVE

EXPANSILE

LOCATION

TRANSITION ZONE AND MARGIN

narrow transition zone: indolent process

wide imperceptible transition zone: aggressive process

well defined vs ill defined margin

MATRIX

osteoid: amorphous ossification as dense as or less dense than bone

chondroid: heavy clumped calcification (popcorn) denser than cortical bone

fibrous: no calcific/ossific density

vascular: no calcific/ossific density (phleboliths can occur in hemangioma)

fibrous dysplasia: ground glass

CORTICAL BREACH

cortical breach implies aggressivity (unless clearly an established cloaca of chronic osteomyelitis)

SOFT TISSUE MASS

extraosseous soft tissue mass may be apparent on XR and is visible on CT, MR, US

extraosseous soft tissue: generally aggressive, often malignant

intraosseous soft tissue mass best shown on MR or CT (replacement of marrow fat by soft tissue)

PERIOSTEAL REACTION

'BENIGN' or 'INDOLENT'

expanded remodeled cortex

single thick layer of new cortical bone

expanded single thin layer of new bone ('shell')

multiple ('soap bubble') expanded shells

'MALIGNANT' or 'AGGRESSIVE'

thick Codman's triangles with some preserved bone

thin Codman's triangles in association with soft tissue mass

multilayered ('onion skin') periosteal reaction

spiculated periosteal reaction ('sunrise')

Resulting descriptor

AGGRESSIVE

INDETERMINATE

INDOLENT

MULTIPLICITY (NUC MED – MDP)

LOCAL EXTENT (MR and/or CT)

Compartments

staging involves assigning muscular compartment of origin and compartments involved

Neurovascular bundle

location of principal compartment neurovascular bundle (or another transiting bundle) relative to the mass

INVASION

ENCASEMENT

ABUTMENT

DISPLACEMENT

CLEAR

DISTANT SPREAD (CXR vs CT)

staging for distant metastases – particularly lungs

HISTOLOGY

imaging used to direct biopsy

biopsy may not be representative of entire tumor

transgressing compartments not involved by tumor may compromise subsequent limb preservation surgery

PITFALLS OF IMAGING

MR post biopsy or surgery (biopsy or surgical edema resolves between 6 hours

(for small caliber needle biopsy) and up to 2 years (for open surgery))

4. BENIGN TUMORS

4.1 ANEURYSMAL BONE CYST (ABC)

DEFINITION

expansile highly vascular tumor arising in another lesion in 30–50%

CLINICAL

PRIMARY TYPE: <25 years old, male = female

SECONDARY TYPE: usually older individual, evidence of underlying lesion

knee, femur, tibia–fibula; proximal humerus; neural arches of vertebrae; pelvis

non endothelialized blood filled cavities lined by giant cells and fibrous tissue

50% recur with curettage

IMAGING

XR/CT

lytic highly expansile often multiloculated

eccentric metaphyseal

narrow transition zone, fine sclerotic rim

lucent matrix

no soft tissue mass

periosteal reaction if fractured

may have periosteal reaction even without fracture

CT/MR

mass composed of cystic spaces with fluid–fluid levels

5% appear solid

Angio

central portion avascular

NUC MED (MDP)

hypervascular flow and increased blood pool/tissue phase activity

photopenic center with increased activity rim on delayed phase

4.2 BENIGN FIBROUS CORTICAL DEFECT/NON OSSIFYING FIBROMA

DEFINITION

non neoplastic cortical defect filled with fibrous tissue

CLINICAL

95% <20 years old; usually converts to cortical mature bone ('healing')
80% in lower limb and 90% monostotic, may fracture
BFCD is defined <2 cm and NOF >2 cm
whorls of mature fibrous tissue and foamy histiocytes

IMAGING

XR/CT

metaphyseal intracortical lucent indolent lytic defect
parallel to long axis of bone
narrow transition zone, sclerotic margin
lucent matrix slowly filling in with bone
densely sclerotic where 'healing' (filling in)
no soft tissue mass (by definition)
no periosteal reaction
follows cortex contours on CT

MR

low on T1W and T2W; may enhance with Gd

NUC MED (MDP)

cold defect with thin rim of increased uptake
may be totally cold
once 'healed' can not be distinguished from normal bone

4.3 BENIGN FIBROUS HISTIOCYTOMA (BFH)

benign fibrous tumor with a histiocyte component (storiform pattern)

IMAGING

XR

lytic septated indolent tumor
central metaphyseal
narrow transition zone, sclerotic margin

lucent matrix
no apparent soft tissue mass
no periosteal reaction

4.4 BROWN TUMOR
(of hyperparathyroidism)

see Ch 02 hyperparathyroidism
NOT a tumor (focal collection of active osteoclasts in hyperparathyroidism)

IMAGING

XR/CT

MUST HAVE OTHER SIGNS OF HYPERPARATHYROIDISM
multiple lucent lytic lesions of variable appearance and variable aggressivity
commonly narrow transition zone, no matrix calcification, little periosteal reaction
if healing, can have periosteal reaction, sclerotic margins, shrinks, and may eventually disappear
may present with pathological fracture

NUC MED (MDP)

increased MDP uptake on a background of metabolic bone disease

4.5 CHONDROBLASTOMA

CLINICAL

rare benign solitary epiphyseal chondroid tumor, pre-epiphyseal closure
usually presents with painful joint
proximal humerus; femur; tibia; talus; calcaneus
polyhedral chondroblasts in amorphous matrix with chickenwire calcification

IMAGING

XR

indolent lytic epiphyseal lesion
central epiphyseal but may cross growth plate with skeletal maturity
narrow transition zone
50% of chondroblastomas have finely stippled calcified matrix
50% have metaphyseal periosteal reaction

MR

low T1W signal and usually low T2W signal with surrounding marrow edema

NUC MED (MDP)

always increased MDP uptake

NUC MED (DMSA (V))

increased pentavalent DMSA uptake occurs in malignant or high grade chondroid tumors (see comments under enchondroma)

4.6 CHONDROMYXOID FIBROMA

rare tumor of mixed myxoid cartilage and primitive mesenchymal fibrous tissue

IMAGING

XR

metaphyseal eccentric lytic well defined tumor
matrix not mineralized
transition zone usually well defined

4.7 CYSTIC ANGIOMATOSIS

multiple lytic pseudopermeative cortically based (hem)angiomas in axial and peripheral skeleton

4.8 ENCHONDROMA

CLINICAL

benign usually asymptomatic chondral tumor
incidental finding in 20–40 year olds; male = female
60% occur in digits (purely lytic)
other: femur, tibia, proximal humerus (always have chondroid matrix)
grade rises with more proximal tumors
arise from remnants of growth plate that persist in medullary cavity
mature hyaline cartilage with abundant extracellular matrix; clumps of chondrocytes
probably <10% undergo malignant degeneration

Multiple enchondroma syndromes

OLLIER'S

unilateral; non hereditary

MAFUCCI'S

also hemanigomas; non hereditary, non
familial; risk of malignancy 100%

IMAGING

XR

central medullary metaphyseal
lytic expansile (in hands)
chondroid calcification in long bones
(differential bone marrow infarct)
endosteal scalloping may be present
no soft tissue mass, no cortical breach
no periosteal reaction unless fractured

CT

well circumscribed ovoid soft tissue mass
within medullary cavity replacing fat
density of marrow
chondroid clumpy calcification may be
present

MR

well circumscribed medullary ovoid mass
low homogenous or heterogeneous signal on
T1W
heterogeneous high/low signal on T2W
(clumpy or lobulated or rounded or
speckled) from mixture of lobules of
chondroid high water matrix and
calcification

NUC MED (MDP)

typically increased MDP uptake in delayed
phase
may have increased uptake in blood
pool/tissue phase
not hypervascular
may have no MDP uptake
allows identification of further tumors

NUC MED (DMSA (V))

taken up in malignant or high grade
chondral tumors, not low grade chondral
tumors

NUC MED (Thallium)

generally no or low grade uptake

PET (FDG)

cold, possibly warm if very metabolically
active

4.9 FIBROMATOSIS
(including desmoids)

DEFINITION

heterogeneous group of soft tissue fibrous
proliferative tumors with benign natural
history

MORPHOLOGY

firm white infiltrative transcompartmental
mass
does not respect tissue planes
mature fibroblasts and abundant collagen
not malignant but recurs

IMAGING (muscular desmoid tumors)

CT

soft tissue mass blending with muscle and
other soft tissue structures
does not calcify (unless dystrophic
postoperative calcification)

MR

80% low T1W, low T2W (densely fibrous)
enhances with Gd but this does not help
predict behavior
transcompartmental mass, low on T1W, low
or intermediate on T2W that may be
difficult to distinguish from surrounding
muscle
may have an infiltrative edge that
interdigitates with muscle bundles
frequently multiple
treated desmoids have increased T2W signal
(radiotherapy change)

NUC MED (MDP)

may show increased vascularity in blood
pool/tissue phase
otherwise unhelpful unless bone or
periosteum involved

NUC MED (Thallium)

desmoids take up and retain Tl
treated desmoids wash out to the degree of
cell damage

PET (FDG)

very FDG avid unless post therapy

4.10 FIBROUS DYSPLASIA (FD)

DEFINITION

metaplastic replacement of bone by various
admixtures of bone and fibrous tissue

CLINICAL

fishhook trabeculae in fibrous spindle cell
stroma, cartilage, cystic areas

Monostotic 70%

Polyostotic 30%

Location

ribs, pelvis (bubbly), femur (with neck of
femur deformity)
tibia (can be confused with adamantinoma)
sclerotic at skull base

Craniofacial type

10% of monostotic FD, 50% of polyostotic FD
*see Ch 20 pediatric CNS facial dysmorphic
syndromes*

McCune–Albright syndrome

3% of polyostotic FD
females, polyostotic FD, café-au-lait spots,
precocious puberty

IMAGING

XR/CT

expansile, ground-glass, bubbly, variable
appearance mass
sclerotic at skull base
transition zone usually well defined but can
be variable
matrix lucent to ground-glass ('groundglass' characteristic of FD)
no soft tissue mass outside of bone contours
(which may be expanded)
no periosteal reaction

MR

heterogeneous on both T1W and T2W with
mixed areas of high, intermediate and
low signal
bone marrow replaced by FD
enhances more or less uniformly with Gd
with sharply delineated margins

NUC MED (MDP)

markedly increased MDP uptake on all three phases

very rarely warm rather than hot

4.11 GANGLION

also see subchondral cyst, synovial cyst

cyst postulated to result from degeneration of extracellular matrix with no synovial lining by definition, but which nonetheless may communicate with joint or tendon

IMAGING

XR/CT

INTRAOSSEOUS GANGLION

subarticular lucent rounded mass with sclerotic rim

may or may not see radiographic communication with joint cavity

usually unicompartmental

US

cystic or hypoechoic structure with clear fluid or occasionally debris

related to joint cavity or tendon sheaths

ganglion cysts non compressible or partly compressible, may be lobulated

compressibility of a clear fluid cyst suggests a synovial cyst, but non compressibility does not exclude a synovial cyst

'tail' extending to joint may be seen

can not always distinguish synovial from ganglion cysts

MR

SOFT TISSUE GANGLION

periarticular well marginated mass low on T1W and high on T2W

INTRAOSSEOUS GANGLION

subarticular well marginated mass with low T1W, high T2W signal

may communicate with a soft tissue ganglion

4.12 GEODE

see subchondral cyst

4.13 GIANT CELL TUMOR (GCT)

DEFINITION

predominantly benign tumor with characteristic radiology, histology and behavior

CLINICAL

occurs post epiphyseal fusion

female > male

5% of all bone primaries

5% have lung deposits (benign behaving), 5% show malignant behavior

50% at knee; distal radius, tibia and fibula, vertebral bodies, metacarpals

tendency to recur and to undergo malignant transformation following irradiation

BIPHASIC HISTOLOGY: mononuclear round and spindle clonal cells; and osteoclast like giant cells

IMAGING

XR/CT

found in mature skeleton

lucent expansile indolent mass

eccentric epiphyseal (or apophyseal) location extending to subarticular bone

'fills corners' adjacent to articular surfaces

narrow transition zone without sclerotic margin

lucent matrix

no periosteal reaction unless fractured

MR

low T1W signal and mixed T2W signal due to blood products

Angio

vascular blush

NUC MED (MDP)

hypervascular on flow and increased blood pool/tissue phase activity

increased delayed phase uptake (may have photopenic areas)

4.14 HEMANGIO-ENDOTHELIOMA (skeletal)

vascular lesion of intermediate malignant potential, often polyostotic and with a variable natural history

IMAGING

lytic lesion

cortical diametaphyseal

transition zone narrow but no sclerotic margin

matrix lucent, soft tissue mass possible

no periosteal reaction

CT or MR: no fat

4.15 HEMANGIOMA

4.15.1 CAPILLARY HEMANGIOMA

4.15.2 CAVERNOUS HEMANGIOMA

4.15.3 SKELETAL CAVERNOUS HEMANGIOMA

CLINICAL

common benign tumor composed of vascular spaces lined by normal endothelium

usually thoracic or lumbar vertebral (occurs in 15% of normals), also skull

rarely underlies pathological fracture

very rare aggressive growing hemangioma may have mass effect with e.g. cord compression

synovial hemangioma (knees, elbows) has repeated single joint hemarthroses (pseudohemophilia)

IMAGING

XR

lytic geographic or lytic pseudopermeative lesion

narrow transition zone, often sclerotic margin

SKULL: coarse 'sunburst' trabeculae

VERTEBRAL: focal area of coarser primary vertical trabeculae with rarefaction of secondary trabeculae

CT

well circumscribed mass with narrow transition zone

characteristic 'polka dot' appearance of coarse remaining trabeculae within mixed fat and soft tissue density stroma

MR

amount of fat present determines T1W signal; typically high on T1W

high signal on T2W (fat and blood on FSE, blood on SE)

atypical hemangiomas may be low on T1W

enhance with Gd like any other hemangioma

NUC MED (MDP)

asymptomatic 'quiet' hemangiomas are cold with no increased uptake

increased uptake if fractured

NUC MED (RBC)

if large enough, visible on RBC labeled scan as focal RBC collection

4.15.4 DEEP SOFT TISSUE CAVERNOUS HEMANGIOMA

CLINICAL

deep mass which may have phleboliths (characteristic)

MAY PRESENT WITH

muscle atrophy, fat replacement

pain on movement

may be confused with sarcoma

IMAGING

XR/CT

possibly soft tissue mass; rounded phleboliths quite suggestive

US

heterogeneous mass of mixed echotexture with ill defined margins

phleboliths shadow; may see serpiginous vascular channels

usually no visible color Doppler or pulse Doppler flow

MR

irregular mass replacing muscle

does not respect compartment boundaries

low or heterogeneous on T1W (high signal due to fat)

heterogeneous multicystic, stippled or serpiginous on T2W, with blood filled spaces that have fluid signal, fat and fibrosis following their respective T2W characteristics; flow voids and calcifications have low signal

vascular spaces enhance slowly with Gd

may have fluid fluid levels

no surrounding edema

NUC MED (RBC)

if large enough, visible on RBC labeled scan as focal RBC collection

4.15.5 SYNDROMES WITH HEMANGIOMAS

Mafucci

enchondromas and hemangiomas

Kasabach Merritt

consumption coagulopathy and hemangiomas

Blue rubber bleb nevus

vascular GIT lesions and cutaneous hemangiomas

4.16 INTRAOSSEOUS GOUT

periarticular lucent intraosseous mass with sclerotic rim

4.17 JUXTACORTICAL CHONDROMA

benign chondroid tumor centered subperiosteally, and behaving like an enchondroma

IMAGING

XR

digits, metacarpals, metatarsals, rare in long bones

focal lytic paracortical mass

narrow transition zone, sclerotic margin

cortical erosion

50% have chondroid matrix calcification

periosteal reaction

4.18 LANGERHANS CELL HISTIOCYTOSIS (overview)

also see Ch 11 CNS, Ch 13 lungs

DEFINITION

neoplastic disorder of Langerhans cell histiocytes with some features of a reactive process and with several distinct clinical presentations

Langerhans histiocyte: antigen presenting cell of macrophage origin, has Birbeck ('tennis racquet') granules on electron microscopy

4.18.1 EOSINOPHILIC GRANULOMA (EG)

('granuloma' like behavior)

children and young adults, <30 years old

unifocal or oligofocal indolent bone lesion

presents with pain or fracture

reddish gray fleshy mass with reactive features ('granuloma'); inflammatory infiltrate, giant cells, fibroblasts, fibrosis

4.18.2 HAND–SCHULLER–CHRISTIAN DISEASE (multifocal histiocytosis)

('metastases' like behavior)

children and adolescents

systemic disorder of acute onset with fever and Hand–Schuller–Christian triad (HSC triad)

HSC triad: pituitary involvement producing diabetes insipidus, exophthalmos, multiple skull lesions

mild hepatosplenomegaly, lymphadenopathy

multifocal pulmonary nodules (late)

multiple bony nodules (marrow replacement confers poor prognosis)

scalp and external ear infections

4.18.3 LETTERER–SIWE DISEASE (acute disseminated histiocytosis)

('leukemia' like behavior)

infants <2 years

systemic disorder of abrupt onset with fever and generalized skin eruptions

marked hepatosplenomegaly, lymphadenopathy, bone marrow replacement, cytopenia

pulmonary nodules late, bone lesions uncommon

IMAGING (EG)

XR/CT

lytic variably aggressive (from permeative to well defined)

variable transition zone from wide to sclerotic (in healing EG)

50% in skull, 30% in spine, pelvis, proximal femur, floating teeth (erosion of lamina dura with no visible bony support for teeth); multifocal in 10%

calvarium: beveled diploe

vertebrae: body (may collapse leading to vertebra plana)

(VERTEBRA PLANA: purely descriptive term where there is a flat collapsed vertebral body with preserved posterior elements)

long bones: central metadiaphyseal

matrix lucent +/– sequestra

soft tissue mass common

periosteal reaction of variable aggressivity

SEE Ch 13 FOR LUNG IMAGING FINDINGS

MR

mass low on T1W and high on T2W or STIR

possible surrounding shell of expanded bone

NUC MED (MDP)

variable appearance (photopenic, hot, donut)

50% not visible on bone scan

4.19 LIPOMA

totally benign mass of mature fat cells

IMAGING

XR

uniform fat density mass

US

uniform, ovoid, hyperechoic well defined deformable non tender mass

has same echo pattern as subcutaneous fat

frequently has a smooth capsule

most frequently subcutaneous, often intermuscular, but may be intramuscular

CT

fat density uniform mass

no hemorrhagic or solid components

minimal mass effect

MR

follows normal fat on all sequences (high T1W, T2W depends on sequence i.e. FSE high, SE low, STIR low)

uniformly fully loses signal with fat suppression

no appreciable enhancement

smooth capsule

thin internal septations may be visible

no soft tissue solid, hemorrhagic or cystic components

minimal or mild mass effect

4.20 LYMPHANGIOMA

see Ch 17

4.21 MORTON'S NEUROMA

perineural fibrosis around a plantar digital nerve produced by entrapment presenting with pain +/– mass

IMAGING

US

ovoid or dumbbell soft tissue mass between metatarsal heads

MR

ovoid or dumbbell mass between metatarsal heads, low or intermediate T1W and T2W signal

enhances with Gd

4.22 MYOSITIS OSSIFICANS (heterotopic bone formation)

4.22.1 MYOSITIS OSSIFICANS CIRCUMSCRIPTA

CLINICAL

postulated hematoma ossification sequence, cause unknown

Zonal architecture

external atrophic muscle

thin sheath of fibrous tissue

peripheral mature bone

intermediate cartilage zone, immature woven bone

central immature fibroblastic tissue, granulation tissue and hematoma

IMAGING

XR/CT

soft tissue mass with peripheral ossification

avoid biopsy (misleading because of increased mitoses)

progressively increasing mature appearing bone

US

(usually starts with appearance of hematoma)

EARLY

central hypoechoic core, ill defined outer ring of higher echogenicity, hypoechoic ill marginated periphery (separates mass from surrounding muscle)

ADVANCED

slow increase in echogenicity of hyperechoic ring until it shadows (ossification)

surrounding edema slowly resolves

MR

high T2W signal centrally with possible areas of hemorrhagic signal, low or heterogeneous T1W signal

low signal rim corresponding to peripheral ossification

variable degree of surrounding edema

NUC MED (MDP)

of prognostic use when planning excision

pattern of MDP uptake indicates activity of myositis and maturity of bone

active myositis has prominent hyperemia and increased blood pool/tissue phase activity

mature bone has progressively late only uptake that slowly decreases in intensity with time

4.22.2 MYOSITIS OSSIFICANS PROGRESSIVA (fibrodysplasia ossificans progressiva)

autosomal dominant pathologic progressive ossification of intermuscular fibrous septa producing severe disability

4.23 OSTEOBLASTOMA

rare benign osteoblastic tumor with histology same as osteoid osteoma

IMAGING

XR/CT

lytic expansile (resembles an ABC), >2 cm by definition

diaphyseal or metaphyseal, central or eccentric

narrow transition zone, thin sclerotic rim

matrix ranges from lucent to calcified

no cortical breach, may expand overlying cortex

mild periosteal reaction

NUC MED (MDP)

increased uptake in all three phases (usually very hot)

4.24 OSTEOCHONDROMA (exostosis)

CLINICAL

displaced island of growth plate producing a bony proboscis covered by a cartilaginous cap

common, male > female; presents at 10–20 years with lump or pain

40% around knee; 95% in limbs (metaphyseal)

growth stops at maturity

pain may be related to development/inflammation of bursa, mechanical problems or malignant transformation (<1% risk)

DIAPHYSEAL ACLASIA has multiple mostly sessile exostoses with growth deformities, mechanical problems and sarcomatous degeneration (total risk 20%)

IMAGING

XR/CT

exophytic continuation of cortical bone and bone marrow

cartilaginous cap may calcify (chondroid matrix)

pedunculated osteochondroma has a characteristic 'cauliflower on stalk' appearance

sessile osteochondroma may be difficult to characterize

no periosteal reaction unless fractured

MR

evaluates state of cartilage cap

proboscis same characteristics as parent cortex and bone marrow

cartilage cap low on T1W, high on T2W; in general follows cartilage elsewhere on variable sequences

overlying bursa may be a potential space, or be thickened/contain fluid (high T2W)

WORRISOME FEATURES FOR MALIGNANT CHANGE

cartilage cap >2 cm

frank invasion

heterogeneity and irregularity of cap

NUC MED (MDP)

'warm' on MDP delayed phase (comparable uptake to normal epiphyseal plates in childhood and normal bone in adulthood)

cartilage cap may have thin line of higher uptake

discordantly increased uptake may occur in trauma or malignant transformation

NUC MED (DMSA (V))

pentavalent DMSA taken up in malignant or high grade chondral tumors, not low grade chondral tumors

NUC MED (Thallium)

generally no or low grade uptake (benign osteochondroma)

PET (FDG)

warm, reflecting both contained marrow activity and cartilage cap activity

increased uptake suspicious for malignant transformation

4.25 OSTEOID OSTEOMA

CLINICAL

benign osteoid line tumor causing intense reactive sclerosis

2% of all bone primaries

usually <30 years old, male > female

night pain relieved with aspirin

painful scoliosis in spine

femur, acetabulum, spine neural arches, tibia, talus

plump osteoblasts rimming immature osteoid; vascular elements; nerve endings

IMAGING

XR

indolent lytic lesion, <2 cm by definition

cortical, subperiosteal, intramedullary or intracapsular (especially hip)

narrow transition zone

matrix may calcify (better shown by CT)

massive benign periosteal reaction or sclerosis

CT

shows both the lucent nidus and any intranidal calcification – diagnostic

otherwise similar to plain XR

MR

nidus has increased T2W signal

extensive surrounding bone marrow edema (high on T2W, low on T1W) and often a joint effusion if related to capsule

NUC MED (MDP)

may have increased flow and blood pool/tissue phase uptake

classically, double density uptake in late phase: very intense uptake at nidus, and surrounding cuff of more diffusely increased uptake

4.26 OSTEOMA/ ENOSTOSIS (bone island)

abnormal overgrowth and overmaturation of intramembranous bone (includes subperiosteal region of long bones)

IMAGING

XR/CT

area of increased bony density with preserved normal architecture

if elongated, long axis parallels long bone axis

continuation of trabeculae into surrounding bone

in paranasal sinuses: mature rounded bony lump projecting into sinus space (especially frontal sinus); very rarely causes obstruction of drainage

MDP

same uptake as normal bone

MR

same signal as normal cortical bone

4.27 SOLITARY (unicameral, simple) BONE CYST (SBC or UBC)

CLINICAL

benign expansile fluid filled medullary cavity cyst

<30 years, male > female

usually presents with fracture, and may heal spontaneously

50% proximal humerus, 20% femoral neck

distal femur, proximal tibia and fibula, calcaneus, pelvis

50% recur with curettage and packing if cyst active

IMAGING

XR/CT

expansile lytic indolent, totally lucent matrix

metaphyseal: starts at growth plate and migrates to diaphysis

sharp transition zone, sclerotic margin

no soft tissue mass

no periosteal reaction unless fractured

fallen fragment sign: in fractured SBC a fractured fragment settles to bottom of cyst implying fluid content and indicating diagnosis

MR

fluid filled sharply marginated expansile cyst

may show blood products in wall

may show fracture fragments

4.28 SUBCHONDRAL CYST (GEODE)

also see ganglion and synovial cyst

intraosseous fluid or myxoid material containing cyst occurring beneath articular cartilage and cortex in degenerative joint disease

IMAGING

XR/CT

sharply marginated lucent rounded mass immediately beneath articular surface

related to weightbearing or force transmitting surfaces

evidence of degenerative joint disease (articular cartilage loss, reactive subchondral sclerosis, reactive osteophytes)

MR

fluid density subarticular mass related to a joint with degenerative change

Arthropathies associated with geodes

osteoarthritis (primary or secondary)

rheumatoid arthritis (late)

calcium pyrophosphate deposition disease (CPPD)

4.29 SYNOVIAL CYST

also see ganglion and subchondral cyst

outpouching of joint synovial cavity, lined by synovial cell and at least originally in communication with the parent joint

CLINICAL

commonest location is Baker's cyst, especially in rheumatoid arthritis

others – dorsum of wrist, ankle

IMAGING

US

cystic structure containing clear fluid or small amount of debris

regular thin wall

no hematoma/blood unless traumatized or ruptured

track to joint line may be visible

compressibility suggests synovial cyst, but may also be non compressible

location may be characteristic (e.g. Baker's cyst)

CT

fluid density soft tissue mass related to joint capsule

MR

fluid signal mass with thin sharp wall related to joint

communication to joint space may be demonstrated

5. MALIGNANT TUMORS

5.1 BONE ANGIOSARCOMA

aggressive and often multifocal vascular sarcoma

IMAGING

XR/CT

permeative and expansile lytic mass

metaphyseal location

wide transition zone

lucent matrix

large soft tissue mass

minimal periosteal reaction

NUC MED (MDP)

increased MDP uptake

5.2 CHONDROSARCOMA (CS)

CLINICAL

malignant chondroid tumor usually with initially slow progression

Primary (central skeleton)

male:female 2:1, 40–70 years old

asymptomatic until late, presents with pain or mass

femur, knee, shoulder, ribs, sternum, iliac
crest, pelvis
THE MORE CENTRAL, THE MORE
MALIGNANT

Secondary (appendicular skeleton)

develops from enchondroma,
osteochondroma, Paget's disease, fibrous
dysplasia
male > female, younger
usually low grade initially

HISTOLOGICAL TYPES

Conventional

plump multinucleated malignant
chondrocytes permeating bone marrow

Dedifferentiated (e.g. to MFH)

Mesenchymal (20–40 years old)

(Clear cell)

IMAGING

XR/CT

lytic permeative or indeterminate
primary: central metaphyseal
secondary: on top of other chondroid mass
transition zone indeterminate or variable
light to heavy chondroid calcification (well
shown with CT)
tumor itself forms ST mass with cortical
breach
periosteal reaction

Biopsy

in consultation with the treating surgeon, as
limb salvage surgery may require
particular limb compartments are not
transgressed by the biopsy track

MR

low grade tumor follows cartilage signature
high grade tumor variable
in general, low T1W, high T2W (variable and
heterogeneous)
lobulated 'chondroid' matrix unless dedifferentiated
soft tissue extent well shown with MR,
particularly in pelvis

NUC MED (MDP)

hot on all three phases

NUC MED (DMSA (V))

increased uptake and retention of
pentavalent DMSA (compared to normal
bone and cartilage)

PET (FDG)

increased FDG uptake, areas of higher FDG
uptake correlate well with areas of
higher grade on histology
useful in guiding biopsy
may have areas of necrosis (low FDG
uptake)

5.3 CHORDOMA

CLINICAL

uncommon malignant tumor of notochord
remnant origin occurring in vertebral
column with locally aggressive behavior
and very late metastases
usually >40 years
50% sacral, 30% sphenooccipital, rest
vertebral
present with pain or neurological deficit
tend to grow slowly and recur
invade spinal canal and extend along it
midline avascular gelatinous/myxoid mass,
calcifies; PHYSALIFEROUS (vaculolated)
cells

IMAGING

vertebral roughly midline mass

XR

bony destruction main finding
presacral or retrosacral large soft tissue
mass (may not always be visible on plain
film)
variable zone of transition
periosteal reaction not a major feature
matrix lucent or contains dystrophic
calcification (in 50%)

CT/MR

large vertebral based soft tissue mass with
dystrophic calcification
encasement, compression, invasion of spinal
canal and contents
in continuity invasion of paravertebral
muscle and other structures
low or intermediate signal on T1W
high T2W signal often with septated or
lobulated structure
enhances following contrast

5.4 EWING'S SARCOMA

CLINICAL

highly aggressive small round blue cell
skeletal tumor of children and young
adults related to neuroectodermal tumors
male > female, white > black
t(11,22) shared with primitive
neuroectodermal tumor (PNET)
presents with bone pain, mass and systemic
symptoms (fever, elevated white cell
count and ESR, anemia)

IMAGING

XR

permeative lytic diaphyseal or flat bone
lesion with lamellated ('onion skin')
periosteal reaction +/– endosteal reaction
center on medullary cavity
very wide zone of transition, possible
cortical breach, large soft tissue mass, no
matrix calcification or ossification by
definition
extraosseous soft tissue mass may be
considerable and out of proportion to the
relatively little gross cortical destruction
or periosteal reaction (beware especially
in pelvis and spine)
pathological fracture possible

CT/MR

cardinal finding is soft tissue mass on CT
and soft tissue mass and bone marrow
edema/replacement on MR (high T2W)
soft tissue usually low on T1W, high on T2W
but may have hemorrhagic or apparent
cystic areas
CT shows cortical and medullary bone
destruction well especially in pelvis

NUC MED

MDP

hot on perfusion and blood pool/tissue phase
increased delayed phase MDP uptake or a
rim of osteoblastic reaction, but rarely
may show only mild diffuse uptake or no
uptake in delayed phase

THALLIUM

intact tumor is vascular and thallium avid
(with retention); may have necrotic
center

PET (FDG)

very FDG avid, often with a necrotic center

5.5 FIBROSARCOMA

malignant fibrous tumor WITHOUT osteoid or cartilage by definition
in many pathological classifications no distinction made between fibrosarcoma and malignant fibrous histiocytoma

IMAGING

XR/CT

lytic permeative
central diametaphyseal
wide zone of transition
lucent matrix (occasional dystrophic calcification)
may have sequestration
large ST mass +/– pseudocapsule
malignant periosteal reaction

MR

T1W signal similar to muscle, T2W signal low (50%) but can also be high

5.6 HEMANGIO-PERICYTOMA

rare malignant tumor of capillary pericyte origin forming vascular channels

5.6.1 SKULL HEMANGIOPERICYTOMA

5.6.2 DEEP SKELETAL HEMANGIOPERICYTOMA

5.7 KAPOSI'S SARCOMA (KS)

see Ch 13 lung, Ch 08 GIT

5.8 LEUKEMIA AND LYMPHOMA (skeletal)

leukemia, Hodgkin's disease, non Hodgkin's lymphoma: see Ch 16 hematology

5.9 LIPOSARCOMA

CLINICAL

malignant adipocyte tumor
usually >50 years old
large soft tissue mass in retroperitoneum (presents late)
less commonly, deep limb mass
overall, 50% recur

IMAGING

CT

large mass with displacement or encasement of adjacent structures
density varies from fat density to solid density
often has heterogeneous areas of solid and fat density
may have a relatively minor solid component marginal to a larger fatty mass

MR

large mass with displacement or encasement of adjacent structures
signal may not follow fat faithfully
variable admixtures of solid, cystic and hemorrhagic components; thick septa; soft tissue nodules

5.10 LYMPHOMA
(primary bone lymphoma)

DEFINITION

aggressive primary bone lymphoma
'reticulum cell sarcoma' in older texts

CLINICAL

30–60 years old, male > female
spread to lymph nodes and bone, hematogenous uncommon
long bones, scapula, pelvis, spine; more common in lower than upper limb
overall, 50% 5 year survival

IMAGING

XR/CT

lytic permeative or mixed lytic/sclerotic lesion
central diaphyseal
wide transition zone
lucent matrix (may have sequestra)
huge soft tissue mass
extensive cortical breach
aggressive periosteal reaction

MR

may be low signal on both T1W and T2W sequences (cellularity)

NUC MED (MDP)

increased MDP uptake (reactive bone)

PET (FDG)

FDG avid

5.11 MALIGNANT FIBROUS HISTIOCYTOMA (MFH)

CLINICAL

commonest single malignant soft tissue tumor; commonest fibrous primary bone tumor
primary or secondary
20–70 years old; male:female 1:1 or 1.5:1
more common than fibrosarcoma (4:1)
aggressive (5 year survival is 25%)
whorls and storiform bundles of spindle cells, histiocytes present, cartilage and osteoid absent by definition
hematogenous metastases to lungs, bone, viscera
local lymphatic metastases

Bone MFH

knee, pelvis, proximal humerus

Soft tissue MFH

limbs (thigh commonest)
high grade deep (muscular or extramuscular)
low grade more superficial
lower limb 50%, upper limb 20%, retroperitoneum 20%

IMAGING

XR/CT

lytic permeative mass
central diametaphyseal
wide transition zone
lucent matrix (occasional dystrophic calcification)
large soft tissue mass +/– pseudocapsule
malignant type periosteal reaction

MR

similar to muscle signal on T1W, high on
T2W

5.12 MASTOCYTOSIS

rare proliferative disorder of mast cells with
focal, multifocal (skin, gut, bone marrow)
or generalized deposits

5.13 METASTASES TO BONE

GENERAL

metastatic tumor:primary tumor is 25:1
prostate, breast, kidney, thyroid, lung, gut,
lymphoma

IMAGING

XR/CT

PURELY LYTIC
renal always lytic
metastases from other primaries commonly
lytic
prostate rarely lytic

MIXED
1. treated metastasis
2. breast > prostate > lung > bladder

SCLEROTIC
1. treated metastasis
2. prostate, breast, carcinoid, stomach,
Hodgkin's lymphoma, osteosarcoma,
small cell lung carcinoma, transitional
cell (urothelial) carcinoma (PBC SHOST)

NUC MED (MDP)

degree of uptake reflects reparative
osteoblastic reaction
very aggressive destructive metastases have
little MDP uptake
prostate metastases incite massive
osteoblastic response and have massive
MDP uptake

COLD METASTASES
renal cell
breast
thyroid

VERY HOT METASTASES
prostate

FLARE RESPONSE

successfully treated metastases have
increased healing reaction with increase
in intensity of MDP uptake in the first
approximately 6 months following
treatment
uptake then decreases again
new foci of MDP uptake not meant to appear
(very few metastases go from
subscintigraphic to scintigraphic with
flare response alone)

PITFALLS

METASTASES vs DEGENERATIVE CHANGE
distinction made on location for each
individual focus and on distribution of
foci whether characteristic of
degenerative joint disease or not; then
XR

METASTASIS vs FRACTURE
distinction made on location (especially
typical for rib fractures), appropriately
timed history; XR

CHANGING INTENSITY OF METASTATIC
UPTAKE
may be spurious because two successive
scans have not been displayed with
thresholds set on the same standard

MR

well circumscribed masses, but may have
surrounding edema
may break through black signal of cortex
low on T1W (outlined by fatty marrow, may
contrast less with red marrow), high or
variable on T2W
mixed/sclerotic metastases may be low
signal on T2W

PET (F18- fluoride, F-)

analogous to MDP bone scanning
F- is a bone tracer
more sensitive than MDP, and provides
automatic volumetric acquisition
subject to same rules as MDP

PET (FDG)

normal red bone marrow has mild FDG
uptake
red marrow recovering from chemotherapy
or on colony stimulating factor treatment
has increased FDG uptake
irradiated marrow has no FDG uptake
metastases in general have the same
metabolic characteristics as primary
tumor
if metabolically active, contrast with red
marrow high

if metabolically low grade, may not be
visible
small metastases are subject to partial
volume effects

5.14 OSTEOSARCOMA AND VARIANTS

GROUP DEFINITION

malignant sarcoma defined by its formation
of tumor osteoid; usually has early
hematogenous metastases and
transcompartment spread

CLASSIFICATION

Central osteosarcoma (75%)
most are high grade

CONVENTIONAL OSTEOSARCOMA
(high grade)
HISTOLOGICAL VARIANTS
OSTEOBLASTIC (1/2)
CHONDROBLASTIC (1/4)
FIBROBLASTIC (1/4)
TELANGIECTATIC
ROUND CELL (differential: Ewing's)

CENTRAL OSTEOSARCOMA (low
grade)

Peripheral osteosarcoma (25%)
most low grade osteosarcomas are
peripheral

SURFACE OSTEOSARCOMA (high
grade)

PERIOSTEAL OSTEOSARCOMA
(intermediate grade)

PAROSTEAL OSTEOSARCOMA (low
grade)

5.14.1 CONVENTIONAL CENTRAL HIGH GRADE OSTEOSARCOMA

CLINICAL

20% of all bone primaries, 75% of all
osteosarcomas
<30 years old, male:female 2:1

Risk factors (primary)

retinoblastoma (RB) change on chromosome 13q (retinoblastomas and osteosarcomas associated)
Gardner's syndrome

Risk factors (secondary)

PAGET'S DISEASE
POST RADIOTHERAPY
DEDIFFERENTIATED CHONDRAL TUMORS
CHRONIC OSTEOMYELITIS

Location

2/3 at knee; other – proximal femur, humerus, ilium and pelvis

Spread

transcompartmental (relationship to neurovascular bundle important)
early hematogenous metastases
20% have lung metastases at diagnosis
lymph node metastases late

MORPHOLOGY

MUST HAVE TUMOR OSTEOID
50% osteoblastic, 25% chondroblastic, 25% fibroblastic
variable macro appearance; gritty gray-white mass invading and destroying bone; areas of necrosis, cystic change, hemorrhage
micro: primitive osteoid in trabeculae; anaplastic cells with mitoses; extensive pleomorphism
vascular invasion, tumor thrombi

Histological subtypes

defined by other forms of matrix formed beside tumor osteoid
osteoblastic, chondroblastic, fibroblastic, telangiectatic, round cell

NATURAL HISTORY

treatment is commonly induction chemotherapy and surgery (limb salvage or amputation)
overall 5 year survival 50%; relapses usually occur within 2 years (80% lung, 20% bone elsewhere)
20% 5 year survival with lung metastases

IMAGING

XR/CT

lytic permeative
90% metaphyseal, 75% involve growth plate
start centrally, replace fatty bone marrow
wide transition zone
90% have amorphous osteoid tumor matrix
large ST mass, extensive cortical breach
sunray spiculation, Codman triangles
CXR or chest CT for lung metastases (and pneumothoraces)

MR

large soft tissue mass engulfing and breaching cortex
heterogeneous signal, usually low on T1W and variable on T2W
areas of hemorrhagic change have blood signature
areas of cystic change are high on T2W
calcified or ossified areas low on T1W and T2W
extensive surrounding edema high on T2W
differentiation of surrounding edema (no mass effect) from direct tumor infiltration (theoretically, mass effect) very difficult
shows skip metastases to bone marrow in same bone
shows relationship to neurovascular bundle (not related, displacement with preserved fat planes, contiguity, compression, encasement)
shows relationship to joint capsule and epiphyseal growth plate

Biopsy

in consultation with the treating surgeon, as limb salvage surgery may require particular limb compartments are not transgressed by the biopsy track

NUC MED

MDP

increased three phase uptake
may have central photopenia (necrosis, cystic change)
in treated osteosarcoma maintained increased MDP uptake may be reactive bone and does not indicate failure of treatment
detects bony metastases elsewhere
may show ossifying lung metastases

THALLIUM

thallium avid with uptake and late retention
damaged tumor shows variable degree of washout

PET (FDG)

FDG avid
variable FDG uptake reflects areas of metabolic differentiation or necrosis
allows monitoring of chemotherapy and radiation therapy

5.14.2 PAROSTEAL OSTEOSARCOMA (low grade)

CLINICAL

15–40 years old, male = female, same sites as conventional osteosarcoma
slow growing (5 year survival 90%) but can dedifferentiate

MORPHOLOGY

macro: circumscribed or lobulated tumor on stalk arising from cortex and separated from cortex by periosteum; adherent and grows external to periosteum; bony, cartilaginous and fibrous areas with dense center
little periosteal reaction
micro: mass of well differentiated trabecular bone, low grade fibrosarcomatous stroma

IMAGING

XR/CT

well defined ossifying mass on stalk wrapping around bone (densest in center)
differential diagnosis is myositis ossificans (densest peripherally)

5.14.3 TELANGIECTATIC OSTEOSARCOMA (high grade)

CLINICAL

rare
totally lytic and massively vascular

MORPHOLOGY

hemorrhagic multiloculated mass
vascular channels, spaces, cysts

IMAGING

XR/CT/MR
aggressive permeative soft tissue mass
fluid–fluid levels

5.15 PLASMACYTOMA, MULTIPLE MYELOMA

DEFINITION

indolent or aggressive focal/multifocal/diffuse plasma cell neoplasm with tendency to fractures, renal failure and amyloid

EPIDEMIOLOGY

commonest adult bone primary
>40 years old, male > female
70% multiple myeloma (MM), peak incidence >50 years
30% solitary plasmacytoma (evolves to MM)
1% POEMS (P-olyneuropathy, O-rganomegaly, E-ndocrinopathy, M-yeloma (SCLEROTIC), S-kin lesions)
ASSOCIATION: monoclonal gammopathy of uncertain significance, Waldenstrom's macroglobulinemia, benign monoclonal gammopathy

CLINICAL

Presentation
most commonly presents with fracture or bone pain; possibly hypercalcemia, proteinuria
uncommon presentation with soft tissue only plasmacytoma (e.g. upper respiratory tract)
in general, follows red marrow distribution

Complications
FRACTURES

RENAL FAILURE
Bence Jones protein renal toxicity commonest
also: direct cell infiltration, metastatic calcinosis, renal amyloid (10%)

BONE MARROW FAILURE, ANEMIA, INFECTIONS

THROMBOEMBOLISM

MORPHOLOGY

sheets of monoclonal plasma cells, secreted IL-1 leads to osteoclast activation and osteoblast inhibition ('cold holes' on imaging)

IMAGING

XR/CT
plasmacytoma is focal, MM is multifocal or permeative

LYTIC EXPANSILE LESION
lucent expansile 'punched out' tumor
centered on bone marrow (including diploic space)
transition zone may be narrow, usually not sclerotic (unless treated and healing)
no matrix calcification or ossification
reactive sclerosis and periosteal reaction in 1%
usually no soft tissue mass outside of bone

PERMEATIVE LESIONS
permeative pattern with ill defined wide transition zone
no periosteal reaction in 99%
'osteopenia' only in 20%
central medullary mass with extension to cortex
'pepper pot' skull

US

MYELOMA NEPHROPATHY
bilaterally enlarged kidneys
may be hypoechoic, with lost corticomedullary differentiation

MR
most sensitive modality
bone marrow replacement

FOCAL/MULTIFOCAL PATTERN
bone marrow based masses, follow red marrow in distribution (spine especially)
low on T1W, high on T2W
produce little mass effect (replace, do not displace)

DIFFUSE PATTERN
'speckled' bone marrow, best shown on T1W

NUC MED

MDP
hot in 10% only
may see persistent MDP uptake in renal parenchyma or no renal excretion of MDP at all

MIBI
active myeloma may be hot on MIBI
used in determining activity in structurally unchanged treated lesions (therapeutic monitoring)
loss of MIBI retention associated with tumor developing drug resistance

PET (FDG)
FDG avid

5.16 RHABDO-MYOSARCOMA

CLINICAL

malignant embryonal mesenchymal neoplasm with rhabdoid differentiation
10% of all pediatric solid tumors; male = female

Embryonal

HEAD AND NECK
orbit, nasopharynx, ear
tendency for skull base invasion and perineural spread
common in masticator space, with trigeminal (third division) involvement
may have deep cervical nodal metastases

BODY
COMMON LOCATIONS: bladder, prostate, vagina
invasive mass with hemorrhage
BOTRYOID variant: dense submucosal (cambium), polypoid grape like mass with loose core
spreads by lymphatics and hematogenously

HISTOLOGY
small round blue cells and tadpole rhabdomyoblasts in variably myxoid stroma

Alveolar/pleomorphic
aggressive muscular mass, lymphatic and hematogenous spread
small round blue cells, giant cells, rhabdomyoblasts

IMAGING

XR
usually unhelpful
soft tissue mass
bone destruction

US

soft tissue mass of variable vascularity

may show bladder masses well

CT

may be used for local staging (MR better)

soft tissue aggressive destructive mass with ill defined or invasive edge

shows skull base bony destruction well

need to identify space of origin by isocenter and stage local (see head and neck chapter)

use in whole body metastasis staging

intravesical portion of bladder rhabdomyosarcoma may be obscured by dilute contrast – also do US

MR

main local staging modality

defines local extent and invasion of adjacent tissues

in large pelvic rhabdomyosarcomas, US, CT and MR may be unable to identify the organ of origin

no specific MR characteristics

usually low T1W, high T2W, may have cystic or hemorrhagic areas

enhances patchily or diffusely with Gd

NUC MED

MDP

assessment of focal bony destruction/erosion

GALLIUM

rhabdomyosarcoma is gallium avid

PET

FDG

avid

5.17 SYNOVIAL SARCOMA

CLINICAL

soft tissue tumor with biphasic histology perhaps originating from primitive synovial precursors, resembles sinovial cells, but very rarely arising directly from joints

10% of all soft tissue sarcomas

70% around large joints

presents with mass and pain

BIPHASIC HISTOLOGY (NOT synovial): epithelium in cords, surrounding spindle cells

IMAGING

XR/CT

soft tissue mass often with speckled or amorphous calcification

bone or joint destruction if invasion in continuity

MR

non specific low on T1W and high on T2W; OR

low on T1W and mimics fluid on T2W

T2W signal may be very intense and difficult to tell from fluid

diffusely enhances with Gd (fluid does not)

(and solid rather than fluid on US)

5.18 TIBIAL ADAMANTINOMA

rare slow growing malignant tumor of uncertain histogenesis with an epithelial component

IMAGING

XR/CT

lytic expansile intermediate aggressivity mass

eccentric cortical diaphyseal location

90% in tibia

variable transition zone

lucent matrix

may have soft tissue mass or cortical breach

Abdominal

1. NORMAL

1.1 MEASUREMENTS

Air–fluid levels

up to 5 (<2.5 cm long) including colon is normal

always abnormal in dilated bowel

Size

LB normal <5.5 cm; imminent perforation if >9 cm

jejunum <4 cm, ileum <3 cm, valves <2 mm thick (enteroclysis)

jejunum <3 cm (small bowel series)

Thickness

esophageal wall <3 mm (distended)

stomach wall <4 mm (distended)

LB wall <3 mm (distended)

presacral space <1.5 cm at S4 (double contrast enema)

1.2 NORMAL SUPINE SCINTISWALLOW

pharynx to esophagus transit: 0.5–1s

esophageal transit time: 5–10s

normal amount of reflux once all activity is cleared from esophagus 3% or less (background corrected)

1.3 BARIUM SWALLOW TERMINOLOGY

Rings

A RING

transient muscular contraction ring (top of vestibule)

B RING

transient muscular contraction (bottom of vestibule)

may transiently move above C ring during swallowing

C RING

diaphragmatic impression on esophagus

Z LINE

squamocolumnar junction

anywhere between A and B rings

SCHATZKI RING

fixed hypertrophied B ring (an imaging finding)

overgrown muscularis mucosae at Z line (histology)

Hiatus hernia

(definition from Grainger and Allison)

B ring 2 cm above C ring or 5+ mucosal folds above C ring

1.4 NUC MED GASTRIC EMPTYING

Liquids

emptying is monoexponential or linear; faster than solid

Solids

lag phase, emptying phase, late slow emptying phase (sigmoidal curve)

normal T1/2 30–60 min

delay in emptying completely non specific and does not identify the cause

1.5 NUC MED SMALL BOWEL TRANSIT STUDY

leading edge of radiotracer column reaches cecum at approximately 3 hours (wide variation: 90 min – 4.5 hours)

1.6 NUC MED Ga-67 COLON TRANSIT STUDY

50% of dose is excreted by 24 hours, 75% by 72 hours, and 90% by 96 hours (protocol from The Alfred Hospital, Melbourne)

1.7 ESOPHAGEAL NORMAL HISTOLOGY

stratified squamous non keratinizing mucosa

lamina propria, muscularis mucosae, submucosa

submucosal mucin secreting glands

muscularis with myenteric plexus (vagus endings, sympathetic endings)

columnar gastric epithelium below squamocolumnar junction

striated muscle in upper esophagus merges into smooth muscle in lower esophagus

1.8 GASTRIC NORMAL HISTOLOGY

Layers

lamina propria

muscularis mucosae

Meissner plexus

submucosa

muscularis (oblique layer, circular layer, Auerbach plexus, longitudinal layer)

serosa

Mucosa

MUCOUS GLANDS

ACID/PEPSIN GLANDS

AREAE GASTRICAE

fine line pattern of normal gastric mucosa on double contrast air distended study forming a 'meshwork of cells'

normal 1–2 mm

hypertrophy 4–5 mm

1.9 BOWEL NORMAL HISTOLOGY

Mucosa

villi to crypt height ratio 3:1

regeneration time 6 days with cells rising from crypt up to tip of villus

EPITHELIUM: enterocytes, goblet cells (secrete mucus), stem cells, APUD cells

large bowel: crypts only, no villi; more goblet cells

lamina propria, muscularis mucosae

Submucosa

duodenum only: Brunner's glands (serous alkaline glands secreting alkaline)

submucosal neural plexus

Muscularis

inner layer circular, myenteric plexus, outer layer longitudinal

large bowel: outer layer bunched into three taeniae

Serosa

1.10 ULTRASOUND GUT SIGNATURE

SURFACE OF MUCOSA: ECHOGENIC INTERFACE

DEEP MUCOSA/MUSCULARIS MUCOSAE: HYPOECHOIC

SUBMUCOSA: ECHOGENIC

MUSCULARIS: HYPOECHOIC

SEROSA, FAT: ECHOGENIC INTERFACE

1.11 MR RECTAL WALL SIGNATURE

(THIN SECTION FSE T2W IMAGES)

EITHER ENDORECTAL OR SURFACE PELVIC COIL

MUCOSA	LOW SIGNAL
SUBMUCOSA	HIGH SIGNAL
MUSCULARIS	LOW SIGNAL (intramuscular neural plexus high)
SEROSAL FAT	HIGH SIGNAL

2. GAMUTS

2.1 GENERIC
(all modalities, all regions)

2.1.1 AIR–FLUID LEVELS, NO OBSTRUCTION

Mnemonic: 4ID

I-LEUS
see ileus gamut

I-NFECTION (gastroenteritis)

I-SCHEMIC GUT

I-ATROGENIC (procedures, fluids)

D-IVERTICULOSIS (jejunal)

2.1.2 BILIARY GAS VS PORTAL VENOUS GAS

see Ch 07

2.1.3 CALCIFICATION

Hepatic

INFECTION

GRANULOMATOUS FOCUS
may be multiple punctate
  TB
  FUNGUS
  SARCOIDOSIS
HYDATID
curvilinear
OLD ABSCESS

TUMOR

METASTASES

HEPATOMA

Splenic

INFECTION

GRANULOMATOUS FOCUS
  TB
  FUNGUS
  SARCOIDOSIS
HYDATID

VASCULAR

SPLENIC ARTERY ANEURYSM

OLD INFARCT

Pancreas

DIFFUSE

CHRONIC PANCREATITIS

CYSTIC FIBROSIS

HYPERCALCEMIA, METASTATIC CALCIFICATION

FOCAL

HEMATOMA

PSEUDOCYST

ANEURYSM

ISLET CELL TUMOR, CARCINOMA

Gallbladder

STONES

PORCELAIN GALLBLADDER
increased risk of malignancy

Renal

FOCAL

LUMPY
  STONE OR PAPILLA
  TB OR SCAR
  HEMATOMA OR ABSCESS
  ABSCESS OR XANTHOGRANULOMATOUS PYELONEPHRITIS
  CARCINOMA
CURVY
  CYST
  HYDATID
  ANEURYSM

DIFFUSE

CORTICAL
  (TRANSPLANT REJECTION)
  CORTICAL INFARCT
  MICROVASCULAR THROMBOSIS

DISSEMINATED INTRAVASCULAR COAGULATION OR PREECLAMPSIA

CHRONIC GLOMERULONEPHRITIS

MEDULLARY
  HYPERCALCEMIA
    IDIOPATHIC
    PRIMARY HYPERPARATHYROIDISM
    PARATHYROID HORMONE related PROTEIN
    SARCOIDOSIS
    VITAMIN D OVERDOSE
  SECONDARY HYPERPARATHYROIDISM
  RENAL TUBULAR ACIDOSIS (distal or type 1), VITAMIN D RESISTANT RICKETS
  HYPERCALCURIA
  OXALOSIS
  MEDULLARY SPONGE KIDNEY

Adrenal

HEMATOMA

TB, FUNGUS

TUMOR

PHEOCHROMOCYTOMA

NEUROBLASTOMA

METASTASIS

ADDISON'S DISEASE (rare)

Gynecological

UTERUS

LEIOMYOMA

SQUAMOUS CELL CARCINOMA

TB

OVARY

TERATOMA
look for teeth!

TB

Appendicolith

Non visceral

INFECTION

HYDATID

CYSTICERCOSIS

TB
  PERITONEAL
  PSOAS

VASCULAR

VENOUS OR HEMANGIOMA PHLEBOLITHS

ARTERIAL OR ANEURYSMAL

LYMPHATIC

TUBERCULOUS OR FUNGAL NODES

TUMOR

PERITONEAL CARCINOMATOSIS

CALCIFYING OR OSSIFYING PRIMARY

GLUTEAL INJECTION SITES

Skeletal

2.1.4 CYSTIC ABDOMINAL MASSES ON IMAGING

TRAUMATIC (rupture, duct transsection)

PANCREATIC PSEUDOCYST, OTHER INFLAMMATORY

HYDATID, OTHER INFECTIVE

DEVELOPMENTAL

ENTERIC

DUPLICATION

LYMPHANGIOMA SPECTRUM

VASCULAR

NEOPLASMS FORMING CYSTS

NEOPLASMS LOOKING LIKE CYSTS

LOW DENSITY OR EDEMATOUS CORE

HEMANGIOMA ON MR

NEOPLASMS DEGENERATING INTO CYSTS

NECROSIS AND LIQUEFACTION

HEMORRHAGE

SUPERINFECTION AND ABSCESS FORMATION

NEOPLASMS OBSTRUCTING DUCTS

CYSTIC SPACE FORMING BEHIND TUMOR

2.1.5 DILATED SMALL VS LARGE BOWEL

Small bowel

CENTRAL MULTIPLE LOOPS OF (usually) SMALLER CALIBER (up to 5 cm)

TIGHT COILS, CLOSE TOGETHER

MUCOSAL FOLDS ACROSS ENTIRE BOWEL (jejunum)

Large bowel

FORMED FECAL SHADOWS

PERIPHERAL 'PICTURE FRAME' LOOP OF LARGER (5 cm and over) CALIBER DIRECTLY AGAINST PROPERITONEAL FAT

HAUSTRAE NOT COMPLETELY ACROSS BOWEL

SIGMOID COLON MAY BE HARD TO DISTINGUISH FROM SMALL BOWEL ON POSITION, CALIBER, ETC

2.1.6 FREE AIR PITFALLS

Pseudo free air

BELOW DIAPHRAGM

COLONIC INTERPOSITION (CHILAIDITI SYNDROME)

SUBPHRENIC FAT

SUBPHRENIC ABSCESS

PNEUMATOSIS INTESTINALIS

ABOVE DIAPHRAGM

LINEAR LUNG COLLAPSE

Non pathological free air

POSTOPERATIVE

PERITONEAL DIALYSIS

IATROGENIC (VENTILATION)

UTERINE INSTRUMENTATION

RUPTURED PNEUMATOSIS INTESTINALIS

2.1.7 FREE INTRAPERITONEAL FLUID

Ascites
see its own entry

Blood

TRAUMA

ECTOPIC PREGNANCY

ANEURYSM (WITH LEAK)

Pus

APPENDICITIS

DIVERTICULITIS

NECROTIZING ENTEROCOLITIS

PERITONITIS INCLUDING TB

PELVIC INFLAMMATORY DISEASE

Cells

MALIGNANT ASCITES

Urine

Chyle

LYMPHATIC DUCT INJURY

LYMPHATIC OBSTRUCTION

LYMPHANGIECTASIA

Chyme (small bowel contents)

Bile

Pseudomyxoma peritonei

SIMPLE

RUPTURED APPENDIX OR GALLBLADDER MUCOCELE

MALIGNANT

APPENDIX CYSTADENOCARCINOMA

GALLBLADDER CARCINOMA

OVARIAN CARCINOMA

2.1.8 GASLESS ABDOMEN

HIGH GASTROINTESTINAL OBSTRUCTION

EXCESSIVE VOMITING OR PANCREATITIS

FLUID FILLED BOWEL

EXTREME ASCITES

2.1.9 ILEUS

Trauma

POSTOPERATIVE

TRAUMA

RENAL COLIC

Infection

GENERALIZED PERITONITIS

FOCAL PERITONITIS

APPENDIX

GALLBLADDER

PANCREAS

PELVIC INFLAMMATORY DISEASE

GENERALIZED SEPSIS

Ischemia

THROMBOTIC OR EMBOLIC

VASCULITIS

Neuromuscular

DIABETIC GASTROPARESIS

SCLERODERMA

ACUTE SPINAL ILEUS

OPIOIDS

HYPOKALEMIA

Large bowel pseudoobstruction

Beware local ileus (sentinel loop)

2.1.10 INTRAMURAL AIR

Necrotizing enterocolitis (in premature newborn)

Emphysematous enteritis (adult)

GALLBLADDER (emphysematous cholecystitis)

STOMACH (emphysematous gastritis)

APPENDIX (usually with infarction)

COLON (typhlitis, ischemic colitis with superinfection)

Ischemic gut/volvulus

Retroperitoneal emphysema

Vomiting

Iatrogenic

Pneumatosis intestinalis
idiopathic and harmless intramural air, particularly in colon

2.1.11 OMENTAL THICKENING OR INFILTRATION

Focal

INFLAMMATORY

CHOLECYSTITIS

DIVERTICULITIS

CROHN'S DISEASE

SEALED PERFORATION OF GASTRIC ULCER

APPENDICITIS (IF PERITONEAL)

NEOPLASTIC

ADJACENT TO DIRECTLY INVASIVE TUMOR

Diffuse (omental cake)

INFLAMMATORY

PERITONITIS INCLUDING TB

NEOPLASTIC

PERITONEALLY SPREADING TUMOR

GASTRIC, OVARIAN, COLONIC CARCINOMA

MESOTHELIOMA

PERITONEAL CARCINOMATOSIS

VASCULAR TUMOR SEEDING

ANY ADENOCARCINOMA

LYMPHATIC TUMOR SPREAD

LYMPHOMA

2.2 COMMONLY USED DESCRIPTORS

2.2.1 BARIUM STUDY FINDINGS

Mucosal changes

ULCERATION

EROSIONS

APHTHOUS ULCERS

lymphoid hyperplasia with overlying ulcer

FOCAL ULCERS

CONFLUENT ULCERS

SLOUGHING AND PSEUDOMEMBRANE

REACTIVE CHANGES

GRANULARITY AND FOCAL EDEMA

GENERALIZED EDEMA

REGENERATIVE PLAQUES AND REGENERATIVE PSEUDOPOLYPS

ARCHITECTURAL CHANGES

FOLD APPEARANCE

FOLD THICKNESS
(normal is 2 mm)

FOLD ORIENTATION

Deep wall changes

ULCERATION

DEEP FOCAL ULCERS

DEEP FISSURING

FISTULATION

REACTIVE CHANGES

GRANULATION TISSUE AND FIBROSIS

STRICTURES

SHORTENING

ARCHITECTURAL CHANGES

LOSS OF FOLD OR HAUSTRAL PATTERN

RIGIDITY

MOTILITY CHANGES

LOSS OF PERISTALSIS

SPASM

2.2.2 MASS POSITION DESCRIPTORS

Isocenter

INTRALUMINAL
within the confines of the expected lumen
sharp angles with wall

INTRAMURAL
within the confines of the expected wall
90 degree angles with wall

EXTRAMURAL
outside the expected lumen
obtuse angles with wall

2.2.3 OBSTRUCTION BY TYPE

Simple mechanical obstruction

INTRALUMINAL

EXTRALUMINAL

STRICTURE

INTUSSUSCEPTION

Closed loop obstruction

Functional obstruction

Complete vs partial obstruction

2.2.4 POLYP BY TYPE

a framework for classification

Non neoplastic

INFLAMMATORY – REGENERATIVE

HYPERPLASTIC

HAMARTOMATOUS – RETENTION
(juvenile)

HAMARTOMATOUS – CHORISTOMATOUS

VASCULAR

Neoplastic

EPITHELIAL

MESENCHYMAL

LYMPHOID

Sporadic vs syndromic

2.2.5 POLYP – RISK OF MALIGNANCY VS SIZE

Type	<5mm	5–10mm	1–2cm	>2cm
Tubular adenoma	<<1%	1%	10%	40%
villious adenoma	?	10%	12%	>60%

2.2.6 STRICTURE BENIGN/MALIGNANT STATUS VS APPEARANCE

Benign

SMOOTH AND GRADUAL

SYMMETRICAL

MUCOSA INTACT

Malignant

SHORT SHARP AND SHOULDERED

IRREGULAR

MUCOSA ULCERATED

2.2.7 ULCER BENIGN/MALIGNANT STATUS VS APPEARANCE

Benign ulcer

PROTRUDES BEYOND WALL

ROUND + DEEP

SYMMETRICAL MOUND

SMOOTH COLLAR +/– HAMPTON'S LINE

(Hampton's line: thin line of overhanging normal mucosa)

SMOOTH THIN FOLDS

HEALS COMPLETELY

Ulcerating malignancy

NOT BEYOND WALL

IRREGULAR + SHALLOW

IRREGULAR RIGID MOUND

NO COLLAR

THICK IRREGULAR FOLDS

DOES NOT HEAL COMPLETELY

2.3 ESOPHAGUS GAMUTS

2.3.1 AIR IN ESOPHAGUS ON PLAIN FILM

Normal esophagus

AIR SWALLOWING

Abnormal esophagus

ACHALASIA

STRICTURE OF OTHER CAUSE

SCLERODERMA (reflux, reduced motility)

EXTRINSIC COMPRESSION

Another structure simulating esophagus

STOMACH PULLUP OR COLONIC INTERPOSITION

2.3.2 ESOPHAGEAL MUCOSAL ABNORMALITIES

Webs and rings

Glycogenic acanthosis

Erosions, ulcers, edema

LOWER ONLY

REFLUX ESOPHAGITIS, PEPTIC ULCER

MULTIFOCAL/DIFFUSE

INFECTIVE ESOPHAGITIS

CORROSIVE ESOPHAGITIS (at holdup points)

RADIATION ESOPHAGITIS (correlates to portal)

Tears

Varices

Tumors (usually carcinoma)

2.3.3 ESOPHAGEAL STRICTURE

Schatzki ring <13 mm produces dysphagia (Grainger and Allison)

Benign

PEPTIC

POST SEVERE ESOPHAGITIS

POST SURGICAL OR FROM NASOGASTRIC TUBE

CORROSIVES

RADIOTHERAPY

CROHN'S DISEASE

ACHALASIA

Malignant

ESOPHAGEAL SQUAMOUS CELL CARCINOMA

BARRET'S CARCINOMA

STOMACH CARCINOMA

LYMPHOMA

METASTASES (melanoma, lung, breast)

2.3.4 ESOPHAGEAL WALL THICKENING

Focal wall thickening, but not a mass

TRAUMA

INTRAMURAL HEMATOMA

POST PROCEDURAL

IATROGENIC

RADIATION

INFILTRATING TUMOR

CARCINOMA

LYMPHOMA

AUTOIMMUNE

CROHN'S DISEASE

Diffuse

TRAUMA/INFLAMMATORY

CORROSIVE INGESTION (chronic stage)

SEVERE ESOPHAGITIS OF ANY CAUSE

AUTOIMMUNE

ACHALASIA

SCLERODERMA

2.3.5 ESOPHAGEAL WELL MARGINATED MASS

FOREIGN BODY

FIBROEPITHELIAL POLYP

INTRAMURAL HEMATOMA

VARICES (change appearance with Valsalva)

PAPILLOMA

NEUROFIBROMA

LEIOMYOMA

ADENOMA

WELL MARGINATED CARCINOMA

2.3.6 PROLONGED SCINTIGRAPHIC ESOPHAGEAL TRANSIT

can quantify severity, can not determine etiology

Mechanical holdup
does not wash out with water

PEPTIC STRICTURE

MALIGNANT STRICTURE

BENIGN STRICTURE – OTHER ETIOLOGY

ACHALASIA

Pseudoholdup

HIATUS HERNIA

LOW DIVERTICULUM

Aperistalsis
washes out with water

SCLERODERMA

PRESBYESOPHAGUS

NEUROPATHY: DIABETIC, AUTONOMIC, ALCOHOLIC

Disordered peristalsis, fragmentation, retrograde motion

DIFFUSE ESOPHAGEAL SPASM

2.4 STOMACH GAMUTS

2.4.1 RAPID GASTRIC EMPTYING

POSTOPERATIVE

PARTIAL GASTRECTOMY

PYLOROPLASTY

PEPTIC ULCER

HYPERTHYROIDISM

CARCINOID SYNDROME INCLUDING ZOLLINGER–ELLISON SYNDROME

DRUGS

DOMPERIDONE

CISAPRIDE

ERYTHROMYCIN

2.4.2 STOMACH FOLD HYPERTROPHY

HYPERGASTRINEMIC HYPERTROPHY (multifocal ulceration)

MÉNÉTRIER'S DISEASE

IDIOPATHIC HYPERTROPHIC GASTRITIS

UNUSUAL MANIFESTATION OF ANY GASTRITIS

VARICES

LYMPHOMA OR PSEUDOLYMPHOMA

INFILTRATING CARCINOMA

AMYLOIDOSIS

2.4.3 STOMACH LINITIS PLASTICA PATTERN

Neoplastic linitis plastica

CARCINOMA

LYMPHOMA

METASTASES (melanoma, breast)

Corrosives (acids > alkali)

Radiation

Granulomatous gastritis

TB

SARCOIDOSIS

SYPHILIS

CROHN'S DISEASE

EOSINOPHILIC GASTRITIS

Amyloidosis

2.4.4 STOMACH MASS

Polyp
see polyps entry

Neoplastic mass

ADENOMA/CARCINOMA

LEIOMYOMA

NEUROFIBROMA

LIPOMA

SARCOMA

LYMPHOMA AND PSEUDOLYMPHOMA

METASTASIS AND KAPOSI'S SARCOMA

Bezoar

Mimickers

EXTRINSIC COMPRESSION SIMULATING MASS

POSTOPERATIVE PSEUDOMASS (HEAPED UP MUCOSA)

MURAL HEMATOMA SIMULATING MASS

2.4.5 STOMACH OBSTRUCTION/DILATION

Simple mechanical obstruction

ULCER AND SCARRING

TUMOR

EXTRINSIC COMPRESSION

BEZOAR OR FOREIGN BODY

HYPERTROPHIC PYLORIC STENOSIS (INFANT)

Closed loop obstruction

GASTRIC VOLVULUS (mesenteric or organoaxial)

Functional: gastroparesis

NON SELECTIVE VAGOTOMY WITHOUT PYLOROPLASTY

TRAUMA, SURGERY, VERY ILL PATIENT, PERITONITIS

PANCREATITIS

DIABETES, AUTONOMIC NEUROPATHY

HYPOTHYROIDISM

DRUGS

NICOTINE

ANTICHOLINERGICS (INCLUDING PSYCHOTROPICS)

2.4.6 STOMACH TARGET LESION

Mass with central ulceration

MELANOMA METASTASIS

BREAST METASTASIS

LUNG METASTASIS

CARCINOID

KAPOSI'S SARCOMA

HETEROTOPIC PANCREAS (duct opening is the umbilicus)

2.5 SMALL BOWEL GAMUTS

2.5.1 DUODENAL FILLING DEFECT

Mnemonic: ABCD POLYP

A-MPULLARY MASS

B-LEED OR B-LOOD FILLED VARIX

C-OMPRESSION FROM OUTSIDE

D-IVERTICULUM OR D-UPLICATION CYST

POLYP

2.5.2 DUODENAL OBSTRUCTION

Adult: mnemonic B CUPS

B-LEED

C-ANCER

U-LCER

P-ANCREATITIS

S-MA COMPRESSION SYNDROME

Newborn: mnemonic DAMP (from vomiting)

D-UODENAL ATRESIA, D-UPLICATION CYST

A-NNULAR PANCREAS

M-ALROTATION, VOLVULUS, LADD BANDS

P-REPYLORIC PORTAL VEIN, OTHER ABERRANT VEIN

2.5.3 SMALL BOWEL BARIUM DILUTION

This gamut and small bowel fold thickening gamut cover most entities!

Findings

WALL

DILATION

LOSS OF FOLDS

FOLD PATTERN REVERSAL

BARIUM COLUMN

DILUTION

SEGMENTATION

FLOCCULATION

MOULAGE

Gamut (mnemonic: TAIL CRAWL)

T-ROPICAL SPRUE

A-IDS

I-SCHEMIA

ADULT

THROMBOTIC, EMBOLIC

VENOUS

PEDIATRIC

HENOCH–SCHÖNLEIN PURPURA

HEMOLYTIC UREMIC SYNDROME

L-YMPHOMA

C-ELIAC DISEASE

R-ADIATION

A-MYLOID

W-HIPPLE'S DISEASE (CHILD: W-ORMS)

L-YMPHATIC FAILURE, L-YMPHANGIECTASIA

2.5.4 SMALL BOWEL FOLD THICKENING

This gamut and small bowel barium dilution gamut cover most entities!

Mnemonic: HILL WAVE

H-EMORRHAGE AND H-YPOPROTEINEMIA

I-SCHEMIA

L-YMPHOMA

L-YMPHANGIECTASIA, L-YMPHATIC FAILURE

W-ORMS AND W-HIPPLE'S

A-MYLOID AND A-NGIONEUROTIC EDEMA

V-ASCULITIS AND V-ENOUS OBSTRUCTION

E-OSINOPHILIC E-NTERITIS

2.5.5 SMALL BOWEL NODULES

Mnemonic: KLMNOP

K-APOSI'S SARCOMA

L-YMPHOMA

M-ETASTASES, M-ASTOCYTOSIS

N-ODULAR LYMPHOID HYPERPLASIA

O-THER: CROHN'S DISEASE

P-OLYPS

2.5.6 SMALL BOWEL OBSTRUCTION

Mnemonic: SHAVE IT – 4ID

S-TRICTURE, S-TONE (for the exams)

H-ERNIA

A-DHESIONS

V-OLVULUS

E-XTRINSIC MASS

I-NTUSSUSCEPTION

T-UMOR

(4ID)

I-LEUS

I-SCHEMIA

I-NFECTION

I-ATROGENIC

D-IVERTICULOSIS

2.5.7 SMALL BOWEL STRICTURE

INCLUDES TERMINAL ILEUM

Mnemonic: CT LICORICE

C-ROHN'S DISEASE

T-B (AND YERSINIA)

L-YMPHOMA

I-SCHEMIA

C-ARCINOID

O-PERATIVE COMPLICATION (anastomotic stricture)

R-ADIATION STRICTURE, ALSO CORROSIVES (NSAIDs, potassium tablets)

I-NFECTION

TERMINAL ILEUM: GRANULOMATOUS INFECTION

  TUBERCULOSIS

  YERSINIA

  FUNGI

  SYPHILIS

TERMINAL ILEUM: OTHER INFECTION

  APPENDICITIS

  TYPHLITIS

C-ARCINOMA, (LEIOMYO)SARCOMA, METASTASES

E-XTRINSIC COMPRESSION AND E-NDOMETRIOSIS

2.6 LARGE BOWEL GAMUTS

2.6.1 LARGE BOWEL OBSTRUCTION

Signs

AXR

dilated large bowel proximal to and collapsed large bowel distal to obstruction

air–fluid levels in large bowel (always abnormal if dilated)

completely fluid filled cecum or colon may appear to be a soft tissue mass (rare)

transition zone implied at point where dilated pockets of gas stop

if ileocecal valve patent, no small bowel distension until late (build-up of small bowel gas and content)

if ileocecal valve incompetent, air decompresses into small bowel with reduction in cecal size and small bowel dilation

volvulus has its own signs (see volvulus)

FLUORO

usually a water soluble single contrast enema

demonstrates transition zone (usually carcinoma)

CT

particularly if collimation of 5 mm or less

demonstrates transition zone (see small bowel obstruction entry)

may demonstrate cause directly

Differential

left colon obstruction more common than right colon

STRICTURE (see large bowel stricture gamut)

MALIGNANT

DIVERTICULAR

VOLVULUS

HERNIA

OBSTRUCTION BY TUMOR FROM OUTSIDE

e.g. prostate carcinoma

PSEUDOOBSTRUCTION

CHILD: HIRSCHSPRUNG'S DISEASE (Ch 18)

2.6.2 LARGE BOWEL STRICTURE

Mnemonic: CT LICORICE

Note that the gamut is very similar to small bowel stricture, but carcinoma takes first place ahead of Crohn's disease

C-ARCINOMA

T-B, PSEUDOTB

L-YMPHOMA

I-SCHEMIA

C-ROHN'S DISEASE

O-PERATIVE COMPLICATION (ANASTOMOTIC STRICTURE)

R-ADIATION STRICTURE

I-NFECTION

DIVERTICULAR ABSCESS

AMEBIC STRICTURE

C-ARCINOID

E-XTRINSIC COMPRESSION INCLUDING PERIDIVERTICULAR ABSCESS, ENDOMETRIOSIS

2.6.3 LARGE BOWEL THUMBPRINTING

Mnemonic: ICU MILK

I-SCHEMIA

C-ROHN'S DISEASE

U-LCERATIVE COLITIS

M-ETASTASES

I-NFECTION INCLUDING TYPHLITIS

L-YMPHOMA

K-APOSI'S SARCOMA

2.6.4 PRESACRAL SPACE >1.5 cm

Mnemonic: MAP PRESS

M-ESORECTUM

A-BSCESS

P-RESACRAL

P-ROCTITIS

R-ECTAL TUMOR

E-NDOMETRIOMA

S-ACRAL TUMOR

S-ACRAL MALFORMATION

2.6.5 POLYP VS DIVERTICULUM

Location

INTRALUMINAL HAT (POLYP) VS EXTRALUMINAL HOLE (DIVERTICULUM)

Morphology

STALK OR TARGET (POLYP) VS AIR–FLUID LEVEL (DIVERTICULUM)

Edge (meniscus)

SHARP INNER (POLYP) VS SHARP OUTER (DIVERTICULUM)

2.6.6 ULCERATIVE COLITIS VS CROHN'S DISEASE

Helpful signs

LIKELY CROHN'S DISEASE

APHTHOUS ULCERS

COLLARSTUD ULCERS

DEEP FISSURING ULCERS

THICKENED BOWEL WALL

FISTULAS

SKIP LESIONS

ONLY ONE SIDE OF BOWEL INVOLVED

MESENTERY, LYMPH NODE, FAT INVOLVEMENT

LIKELY ULCERATIVE COLITIS

FILIFORM POLYPS

Less helpful signs

MORE LIKELY ULCERATIVE COLITIS

CONFLUENT ULCERS

PSEUDOPOLYPS

SHORTENING, HAUSTRAL LOSS

DISEASE IN CONTINUITY

2.7 NEONATE AND CHILD GAMUTS

see Ch 18

CONDITIONS OF THE GASTROINTESTINAL TRACT

3. CONDITIONS OF THE ESOPHAGUS

3.1 ACHALASIA

DEFINITION

idiopathic loss of esophageal neural plexus with tonic lower esophageal sphincter contraction and secondary dilation above

CLINICAL

megaesophagus, food retention, aspiration, lung abscess or basal fibrosis, weight loss

squamous cell carcinoma in distal esophagus (relative risk x7)

treatment: balloon dilation, Heller's myotomy (risk: perforation)

MACRO/MICRO

short narrow hypertrophic distal segment

loss of myenteric plexus and wall sclerosis

proximal gross dilation, wall atrophic to hypertrophic

crocodile leather with ulceration, leukoplakia, papillomas, squamous carcinomas

IMAGING

CXR, AXR

dilated esophagus with air–fluid level

NUC MED

marked prolonged retention of bolus in distal esophagus

no washout

Fluoro

dilated amotile megaesophagus with barium level

no peristalsis from at least mid esophagus distally

contracted vestibule with 'beak' configuration

intermittent low volume opening (with passage of small amounts of barium)

may have findings of complications

CT

grossly dilated lower thoracic esophagus with air–fluid level, possibly thickened wall and retained debris

Achalasia vs other conditions

PEPTIC STRICTURE

peristalsis preserved

MALIGNANT STRICTURE

features of mass

peristalsis preserved above mass

CHAGAS DISEASE

identical findings to achalasia

3.2 BENIGN ESOPHAGEAL TUMORS

3.2.1 FIBROEPITHELIAL POLYP

benign vascular fibroblastic tissue covered by esophageal mucosa

3.2.2 PAPILLOMA

3.2.3 NEUROFIBROMA

3.2.4 LEIOMYOMA

benign focal tumor of smooth muscle
lobulated or smooth mucosal/submucosal
   mass
may calcify or have patchy necrosis; may
   occasionally ulcerate

IMAGING

Fluoro

sharply marginated intramural mass

CT

variably enhancing intraesophageal soft
   tissue mass

3.3 DEVELOPMENTAL ANOMALIES

see Ch 18

3.4 DIVERTICULA

3.4.1 PHARYNGEAL POUCH

CLINICAL

pulsion diverticulum through the two parts
   of cricopharyngeus (oblique and circular)
   at Killian's dehiscence
associated with cricopharyngeal dysfunction
contains a thin layer of muscle
presents with halitosis, mass, dysphagia
complications – perforation, stasis
   carcinoma (rare)

IMAGING

XR

cervical air–fluid level

Fluoro

variable size posterolateral pouch at level of
   cricoid, internal debris

CT

if filled with fluid or content, produces a
   cervical mass in visceral compartment

MR

may effectively simulate a soft tissue tumor
   if filled with semisolid content

creates a signal void if filled with air
air–fluid level most reliable sign (differential
   is an abscess)
walls enhance with Gd

3.4.2 MID ESOPHAGEAL DIVERTICULUM

PATHOGENESIS

?traction diverticulum from adherence to
   retracting fibrosing nodes
may be present in achalasia or diffuse
   esophageal spasm

IMAGING

All modalities

irregular perhaps angular expansion of
   esophagus, often level with carina

3.4.3 EPIPHRENIC DIVERTICULUM

PATHOGENESIS

rare pulsion diverticulum
associated with disordered peristalsis, e.g.
   diffuse spasm

IMAGING

All modalities

small outpouching above diaphragm

3.4.4 ESOPHAGEAL PSEUDODIVERTICULA

MORPHOLOGY

dilated mouths of submucosal mucinous
   glands
collar–stud shaped pseudodiverticula
do not extend beyond submucosa
symptoms probably arise from associated
   conditions (usually chronic esophagitis)

IMAGING

Fluoro

small (1–2 mm) collarstud pseudodiverticula
   filled with barium

3.5 ESOPHAGEAL CARCINOMA

DEFINITION

aggressive malignancy with several
   histological types and uniformly poor
   prognosis once invasive

EPIDEMIOLOGY

~1/10 000, wide geographic variation,
   occurs usually >60 years old
male: female 3:1 except if Plummer–Vinson
   syndrome present

ETIOLOGY

Personal carcinogens
smoking, alcohol, substance chewing

Dietary carcinogens
smoked foods, nitrosamines, moulds; trace
   elements deficiency

Industrial carcinogens (ingested)
especially rubber and petroleum industries

Focal factors
STASIS
STRICTURE
ACHALASIA
incidence of carcinoma is approximately 7x
   baseline
CHRONIC INFLAMMATION
CHRONIC ESOPHAGITIS
BARRETT'S ESOPHAGUS

CLINICAL

Presentation
dysphagia and weight loss
pain, local symptoms (involvement of nerves,
   bronchi)
nodal metastases with compression of
   adjacent structures (e.g. SVC)
distant metastases

Location
50% mid, 30% low, 20% high esophagus
cardia (gastric adenocarcinoma, spread up)

Barrett's esophagus (adenocarcinoma, low esophagus)

Spread

no serosal barrier, usually advanced at diagnosis

invades in continuity, forms fistulas to trachea/bronchi

rapid lymphatic spread (cervical, mediastinal, gastric, celiac nodes)

Staging

TNM

T1	mucosa, submucosa (US layers 1–3)
T2	muscularis propria (US layers 1–4)
T3	adventitia (US layers 1–5)
T4	adjacent structures
N1	regional lymph nodal metastases
M1	distant metastases (including celiac lymph nodes)

GROUPED TNM STAGES

S0	T in situ N0 M0
SI	T1 N0 M0
SIIa	up to T3 N0 M0
SIIb	N1 up to T2
SIII	T3 N1 or T4 any N
SIV	M1

MACRO

white/gray firm invasive mass, necrosis, hemorrhage, ulceration

stenosing (circumferential with central irregular residual channel)

polypoid less common

verrucous (exophytic exuberant mass) occurs in achalasia

MICRO

Squamous carcinoma

WELL DIFFERENTIATED to ANAPLASTIC

Adenocarcinoma

Barrett's carcinoma (10%, incidence increasing)

Gastric carcinoma, spread up from cardia

Adenocarcinoma arising in submucosal glands

IMAGING

Fluoro

CARDINAL SIGNS

fixed mucosally based abnormality

loss of normal distensibility and peristalsis under abnormality

NEOPLASTIC PLAQUE

eccentric fixed irregular plaque

mucosal isocenter +/– sharp angle with wall

CIRCUMFERENTIAL CARCINOMA

irregular focal 'applecore' stricture shouldered, centered on mucosa, short irregular central lumen

VARICOID CARCINOMA

irregular longitudinal involvement of mucosa with fold thickening

may mimic varices

ULCERATING CARCINOMA

large shallow malignant ulcer with tumor edges (see stomach)

POLYPOID CARCINOMA

exophytic masses

SCLEROSING/INFILTRATING CARCINOMA

preservation of smooth mucosa

more uniform tapered stricture from tumor infiltrating muscle coat in preference to destroying the mucosa

CT

use Buscopan to reduce peristalsis and on table water to outline mucosa of esophagus

focally or circumferentially thickened esophageal wall

murally based abnormal soft tissue mass or circumferential mass, may be ulcerated

may clearly invade adjacent organs

edema of periesophageal fat planes indeterminate (edema vs infiltration)

enlarged paraesophageal, diaphragmatic, celiac, superior mesenteric, lesser curve and renal hilar nodes

MR

morphology similar to CT

low T1W and high T2W signal

PET (FDG)

most esophageal carcinomas are FDG avid

focal or elongated increased uptake in position of esophagus corresponding to the endoscopic, fluoroscopic or CT position of the carcinoma

very thin mucosal only disease is usually invisible

may have difficulty distinguishing paraesophageal nodes as anatomically separate

differential: physiological lower esophageal sphincter uptake (low grade and regular uptake)

differential: reflux esophagitis (usually relatively low grade uptake)

post treatment esophagitis: extensive lower grade diffuse uptake conforming to radiation portal and extending beyond the position of the original tumor

3.6 ESOPHAGEAL TRAUMA

3.6.1 EMETOGENIC TEAR
(Mallory–Weiss tear)

DEFINITION

lower esophageal mucosal and submucosal laceration resulting from vomiting without relaxation of the lower esophageal sphincter

CLINICAL

strong association with alcoholism

classically middle aged and older males

presents with upper GI hemorrhage (may be massive)

IMAGING

USE WATER SOLUBLE CONTRAST NOT BARIUM

single contrast swallow: mucosal linear tear, intramural hematoma, varices or rupture

3.6.2 EMETOGENIC RUPTURE
(Boorhaave syndrome)

CLINICAL

spontaneous rupture of the esophagus, usually during vomiting, with high risk of mediastinitis

presents with severe unremitting chest pain

IMAGING

USE WATER SOLUBLE CONTRAST NOT BARIUM

CXR

mediastinal loculated air or air–fluid level

mediastinal free air (differential: medial pneumothorax)

surgical emphysema

pleural effusion or pneumothorax (left >
   right)

Fluoro

loculated extravasation

esophagopleural fistula

differential: perforated peptic ulcer

CT

periesophageal hematoma/fluid (differential:
   edema and hemorrhage without
   perforation)

pleural effusion

mediastinal free air or air/fluid levels

pathognomonic if intraesophageal contrast
   extravasates

3.6.3 SPONTANEOUS INTRAMURAL HEMORRHAGE (esophageal apoplexy)

CLINICAL

non traumatic spontaneous intramural
   hemorrhage

associated with anticoagulation or vomiting

presents with severe unremitting chest pain

IMAGING

CXR

usually no findings by definition

may have evidence of obstruction (air–fluid
   level)

Fluoro

smooth intramural mass with luminal
   narrowing

(unless cavitates into lumen)

CT

intramural non enhancing (or ring
   enhancing once resorption/organization
   starts) smooth mass

may have evidence of mediastinal
   hemorrhage

3.6.4 IATROGENIC INJURY

any combination of any of the above imaging
   findings, history of endoscopic
   manipulation is paramount

3.7 ESOPHAGEAL VARICES

GROUP DEFINITION

abnormally dilated venous channels from
   high venous pressure; 'downhill' varices
   result from SVC obstruction and 'uphill'
   varices result from portal venous
   hypertension

CLINICAL

asymptomatic OR

presents with hematemesis and melena

dysphagia exceedingly rare

3.7.1 UPHILL VARICES

by definition, the etiology of uphill varices is
   the etiology of portal venous
   hypertension (Ch 07)

beware varicoid lymphoma or carcinoma
   simulating varices (does not alter with
   respiration or position)

3.7.2 DOWNHILL VARICES

a less common and less well defined entity
   caused by SVC obstruction and azygous
   system recruitment; varices more
   prominent around upper esophagus

IMAGING (GROUP)

Fluoro

thick compressible serpiginous vertical folds
   of mucosa that change shape and degree
   of distension

shows submucosal varices only

CT

portal phase enhancing tortuous vessels
   extending from lesser curve and lesser
   sac area around lower esophagus to pass
   through diaphragmatic hiatus

many do not indent the esophagus

signs of portal hypertension

3.8 GLYCOGENIC ACANTHOSIS

incidental intraepithelial glycogen plaques

IMAGING

Fluoro

granularity or 1–4 mm ovoid or rounded
   nodules

3.9 HIATUS HERNIA (HH) AND GASTRIC VOLVULUS

GROUP DEFINITION

abnormal herniation of lower esophageal
   segment or part of stomach into the chest

3.9.1 SLIDING HH (90%)

esophageal B ring 2 cm above C ring or 5 or
   more mucosal folds >2 cm above
   diaphragm

INTERMITTENT

INCARCERATED (FIXED)

3.9.2 ROLLING HH (paraesophageal) (10%)

small part of stomach herniates next to
   esophagus

potential complications of obstruction and
   ischemia

3.9.3 INTRATHORACIC STOMACH

usually incarcerated

3.9.4 GASTRIC VOLVULUS

DEFINITION

abnormal rotation of the stomach on one of
   its two free axes; involves herniation of
   part or all of the stomach through the
   diaphragmatic hiatus

3.9.4.1 ORGANOAXIAL VOLVULUS

rotation around long axis of stomach
   (gastroesophageal junction to pylorus)

part of greater curve herniates into chest

3.9.4.2 MESENTEROAXIAL VOLVULUS (RARE)

rotation around the long axis of the mesentery (vascular pedicle, right angles to long axis)

CLINICAL

asymptomatic incidental finding
pain, dysphagia, gastric outlet obstruction
venous obstruction and gastric infarction

IMAGING (GROUP)

CXR/AXR

abnormal air–fluid level behind heart (or a completely fluid filled mass behind heart)
gastric air bubble may be absent or displaced

Fluoro

sliding hiatus hernia readily demonstrated
rolling hiatus hernia may not fill
non obstructed volvulus readily demonstrated
obstructed volvulus has a 'twisted' termination of lower esophagus, leading towards a soft tissue density mass possibly containing an air–fluid level

CT

hiatus hernia is a fluid, contrast or air filled mass behind the heart and passing through the diaphragmatic hiatus
in volvulus, the body of the stomach is displaced from its usual position, the lower esophagus and the first part of duodenum are stretched and displaced (more in mesenteroaxial than organoaxial volvulus)
stomach may be very distended (if obstructed) or thick walled (if ischemic)

3.10 MOTILITY DISORDERS

3.10.1 CRICOPHARYNGEAL SPASM

3.10.2 TERTIARY CONTRACTIONS SPECTRUM

3.10.2.1 TERTIARY CONTRACTIONS (tertiary peristalsis)

IMAGING

non propulsive multifocal swinging contractions distorting esophageal lumen (corkscrew esophagus)
scintigraphic bolus fragmentation, delay in esophageal transit and disordered bolus movement (supine scan)

3.10.2.2 PRESBYESOPHAGUS

broad term for age related motility changes

IMAGING

spectrum from normal to tertiary peristalsis
loss of primary peristalsis
failure of lower esophageal sphincter relaxation
tertiary contractions
delay in esophageal transit

3.10.2.3 DIFFUSE ESOPHAGEAL SPASM

CLINICAL

circular smooth muscle hypertrophy in mid esophagus
presents with dysphagia, pain

IMAGING

irregular disordered tertiary contraction waves

3.10.2.4 NUTCRACKER ESOPHAGUS

an ill defined entity
usually a manometric diagnosis of abnormally high intraluminal pressure

3.10.3 ACHALASIA

see its own entry

3.10.4 CHAGAS DISEASE

infection with Trypanosoma cruzi with cardiomyopathy, and megaesophagus, megaureter and megacolon secondary to toxin induced denervation; differential of achalasia

3.10.5 LATE STAGE SCLERODERMA/CREST

IMAGING

incompetent lower esophageal sphincter, poor peristalsis and clearing
dilated immobile esophagus with free reflux
lower esophageal stasis on scintigraphy (supine scanning)
may develop complications of peptic esophagitis
may have dilated relatively immotile duodenum

3.10.6 ESOPHAGEAL REFLUX

see reflux esophagitis

3.10.7 SECONDARY MOTILITY DYSFUNCTION

DIABETIC NEUROPATHY

AUTONOMIC NEUROPATHY

ALCOHOLIC NEUROPATHY

MOTOR NEURON DISEASE

3.11 REFLUX ESOPHAGITIS

DEFINITION

abnormal consequences of gastroesophageal reflux, comprising clinical symptoms, or histologic changes, or both

CLINICAL

Infant

immature lower esophageal sphincter – improves with age
reflux, ulceration, aspiration, failure to thrive

Adult

incompetent lower esophageal sphincter or hiatus hernia
OTHER: pregnancy, nasogastric tube, previous surgery, scleroderma
reflux, ulceration, inflammation, metaplasia
late strictures, late chronic ulcers, carcinoma

MACRO/MICRO

distal esophageal location predominates

NO HISTOLOGICAL CHANGE

REACTIVE CHANGE
reddened glistening mucosa

MUCOSAL ULCERATION
reactive change plus shallow scattered
ulcers

DEEP ULCERATION
usually a focal deep punched out ulcer
(gastric ulcer histology)

METAPLASIA (Barrett's esophagus)
velvety red mucosa ascending from Z line
gastric or intestinal metaplasia with or
without atypia

FOCAL OR MULTIFOCAL STRICTURES

IMAGING

Fluoro

NO FINDINGS

REFLUX (with or without evidence of
esophagitis)
spontaneous
elicited (water, coughing, rolling,
compression)

MUCOSAL CHANGES
distal esophageal location
mucosal granularity, mucosal edema
focal erosions, confluent erosions

ARCHITECTURAL CHANGES
fold thickening
transverse folds (feline esophagus)

COMPLICATIONS
STRICTURES
lower esophagus
short, occasionally long in continuity
usually circumferential
+/– proximal dilation above stricture
DEEP ULCERS
usually unifocal or oligofocal
lower esophagus
deep punched out regular ulcers

NUC MED

REFLUX SCAN
reappearance of tracer in esophagus
very sensitive; clinical relevance varies
'milk scan' in infants (tracer in milk or
formula)
tracer in lungs implies reflux with aspiration

3.12 SPECIFIC ESOPHAGITIS

diverse conditions causing esophageal
inflammation
no single fluoroscopic finding can reliably
distinguish between the different entities

3.12.1 INFECTIVE ESOPHAGITIS

mid and upper esophagus predominates

ETIOLOGY

HSV, HZV, CMV
Candida
all occur in AIDS or immune
suppression/neutropenia

IMAGING

viral: focal ulcers, normal intervening
mucosa
CMV: focal giant ulcer
Candida: granularity, shaggy adherent
plaques, cobblestoning
eventual loss of normal peristalsis

3.12.2 CORROSIVE ESOPHAGITIS

CLINICAL

focal destruction and inflammation at bolus
holdup points
early perforation, late stricture

IMAGING (FLUORO)

granularity, confluent ulcers, long strictures
that occur late

3.12.3 AUTOIMMUNE ESOPHAGITIS

ETIOLOGY

Crohn's disease
Behçet's disease

IMAGING (Crohn's)

mucosal aphthous ulcers
deep fissures and fistulas

3.12.4 RADIATION ESOPHAGITIS

CLINICAL

appropriate history and time interval
conforms to radiation portals

IMAGING

early – mucosal changes only
late–may produce strictures

3.13 WEBS AND RINGS

3.13.1 WEBS (UPPER ESOPHAGUS)

thin gray elastic transverse membrane
anterior wall or circumferential

IMAGING

Barium swallow
thin fixed impression on Ba column
usually based on anterior wall
differential: post cricoid impression or
pharyngeal venous plexus (neither fixed)

3.13.2 RINGS (lower esophagus)

*see normal section for description of
physiological rings*

Schatzki ring (acquired)
thin annular membrane at Z line
overgrown muscularis mucosae and
connective tissue
lined by esophageal or gastric mucosa
<13 mm produces dysphagia (Grainger and
Allison)

4. CONDITIONS OF THE STOMACH

4.1 ACUTE GASTRITIS

ETIOLOGY

Infective
immune suppresion

Chemical
alcohol, irritants, corrosives, NSAIDs

Hemorrhagic

burns, trauma, sepsis, raised intracranial
    pressure
multiple shallow mucosal 'stress' erosions

IMAGING

Fluoro

no findings or multiple erosions

NUC MED (RBC) –
hemorrhagic gastritis

requires NO FREE TcO4 IN LABELED RED
    CELLS
diffuse outline of gastric wall (usually entire
    gastric wall) that slowly increases with
    time, and eventually begins to fill
    stomach
unlike bleeding from an ulcer, no focal
    accumulation of activity and no early
    migration distally
must confirm location (imaging for long
    enough; imaging with markers)

4.2 CHRONIC GASTRITIS

GROUP DEFINITION

histological definition based on infiltrate of
    chronic inflammatory cells

4.2.1 HELICOBACTER GASTRITIS

ETIOLOGY

Helicobacter pylori (HP, Gram negative
    microaerophilic urease positive acid
    sensitive rod) attached to gastric mucosa

MORPHOLOGY/CLINICAL

HP attached to mucosa but not invasive
slow epithelial and gland destruction
    (?modified autoimmune)
gastric and duodenal ulcers
chronic inflammatory infiltrate in mucosa
    +/– lymphoid follicles
low grade lymphoproliferative disorders
    (may reverse with HP eradication)
full spectrum of symptoms with poor
    correlation with histology
C-14 breath test positive
gastritis reverses if HP eliminated

4.2.2 CHRONIC AUTOIMMUNE GASTRITIS

MORPHOLOGY/CLINICAL

thyrogastric cluster of autoimmune disease,
    pernicious anemia
circulating autoantibodies to parietal cells
    and intrinsic factor
hypochlorhydria with hypergastrinemia
gland destruction, thin atrophic mucosa,
    chronic lymphocytic infiltrate, intestinal
    metaplasia
gastritis itself asymptomatic; increased
    incidence of dysplasia and carcinoma

4.2.3 CHRONIC REFLUX GASTRITIS

duodenogastric bile reflux (usually
    postoperative)

4.2.4 GRANULOMATOUS GASTRITIS

ETIOLOGY

TB/HISTOPLASMOSIS
CROHN'S DISEASE (1% of all Crohn's)
SARCOIDOSIS
SYPHILIS

4.2.5 EOSINOPHILIC GASTRITIS

usually asymptomatic
associated with allergic or parasitic disease
diffuse eosinophilic infiltrate with peripheral
    eosinophilia

4.2.6 HYPERTROPHIC GASTRITIS

GASTRIC MUCOSAL HYPERTROPHY, NOT A
    GASTRITIS

IMAGING (chronic gastritis)

Fluoro

loss of areae gastricae
thinning or loss of folds
ulcer
narrowed stomach, scarring

EARLY CROHN'S DISEASE

aphthous ulcers (not specific to Crohn's
    disease)

disorganization of folds
more confluent ulceration

LATE APPEARANCE OF ANY
GRANULOMATOUS GASTRITIS

LINITIS PLASTICA pattern (see its gamut)
signs: see gastric carcinoma entry

4.3 GASTRIC CARCINOMA

DEFINITION

malignant neoplasm of gastric epithelium
    with outcome critically dependent on
    stage

EPIDEMIOLOGY

wide geographic variation in incidence and
    type
particularly common in Japan (?dietary
    associated)
incidence increases with age, blood group A,
    male > female
falling incidence overall, but still 3rd leading
    cause of cancer death in the USA
early gastric cancer found in screening
    programs (e.g. Japan)

ETIOLOGY

Dietary

nitrosamines and precursor compounds
    (smoked and pickled foods)

Chronic gastritis

CHRONIC AUTOIMMUNE GASTRITIS
    (via intestinal metaplasia)
MÉNÉTRIER'S DISEASE
HELICOBACTER GASTRITIS (via
    dysplasia or intestinal metaplasia)

Partial gastrectomy

PATHOGENESIS

evolution from dysplasia to in situ to
    invasive carcinoma

Precancerous states

INTESTINAL METAPLASIA
EPITHELIAL DYSPLASIA (I TO III)

Early gastric cancer

DEFINED AS MUCOSAL AND SUBMUCOSAL
INVOLVEMENT ONLY

Advanced gastric cancer

INVASION INTO MUSCULARIS BY
DEFINITION

CLINICAL

Presentation

at screening
as ulcer
as gastritis
locally advanced disease (pain, weight loss,
obstruction)
with disseminated metastases

Spread

LOCAL

LYMPHATIC

very common once cancer invades
muscularis (~90%)

HEMATOGENOUS

occurs early (e.g. ~40% at diagnosis)
liver, lung, bone

TRANSCELOMIC

ascites, diffuse peritoneal seeding
Krukenberg tumors (ovarian deposits of
gastric carcinoma)

Staging – TNM

TUMOR

T1	lamina propria, submucosa
T2	muscularis, subserosa
T3	through serosa
T4	adjacent organs

NODES

N1	1 to 6 nodes (in a lymphadenectomy specimen)
N2	6 to 15 nodes
N3	>15 nodes

GROUPING BY STAGE

STAGE Ia	T1 N0 M0
STAGE Ib	T stage + N stage = 2
STAGE II	T stage + N stage = 3
STAGE IIIa	T stage + N stage = 4
STAGE IIIb	T3 N2 M0
STAGE IV	T4 or N3 or M1

MACRO

FUNGATING (large irregular bulky mass)
ULCERATING (classic malignant ulcer)

DIFFUSE/SCIRRHOUS (classic linitis plastica
pattern)
antrum > lesser curve > cardia

MICRO

Adenocarcinoma (most)

INTESTINAL: forms islands and glands
DIFFUSE: clumps or separate cells
SIGNET RING: diffuse carcinoma with cells
distended with mucin and nucleus
pushed to one side

Neuroendocrine

TYPICAL or ATYPICAL CARCINOID

Grading

WELL DIFFERENTIATED (forms glands) TO
ANAPLASTIC
GROWTH PATTERN EXPANSILE (better) VS
INFILTRATIVE (worse)

IMAGING

Fluoro – early gastric cancer

focal elevation, depression or irregularity of
mucosa
rearrangement of mucosal folds
focal erosion/ulcer (malignant ulcer)

Fluoro

classic malignant ulcer (see gamuts)
large mucosally based irregular mass, may
have a shoulder, may ulcerate

LINITIS PLASTICA PATTERN

featureless contracted stomach, particularly
distally ('funnel')
loss of mucosal architecture
loss of distensibility
loss of peristalsis
see linitis plastica gamut

CT

use water to distend stomach +/– Buscopan
roll patient to outline tumor with water

stomach wall thickening, usually focal;
smooth or nodular or irregular or
ulcerated
infiltration and soft tissue strands extending
into surrounding fat implies transserosal
spread
invasion may be present if no fat between
stomach and adjacent organs
tumor may enhance differently from healthy
stomach wall
nodes >1 cm are likely to be involved

PET (FDG)

NORMAL PHYSIOLOGICAL FDG
GASTRIC UPTAKE

normal stomach muscle often has enough
physiological uptake FDG to be visible –
beware of calling stomach carcinoma as
an incidental finding on PET
uniform, diffuse, low grade and outlines all
of stomach or extends from cardia
distally

CARCINOMA

markedly increased gastric wall uptake
clearly focal increased FDG uptake relative
to rest of stomach
PET extremely useful in locoregional nodal
staging (increased uptake at celiac, SMA,
peripancreatic locations indicates nodal
metastases – beware of diaphragmatic
crura simulating nodes)
recurrence (hot) differentiated from
postoperative fibrosis

4.4 GASTRIC DIVERTICULUM

true wide mouthed diverticulum
usually occurs near gastroesophageal
junction
may peristalse, may have normal mucosal
surface
differential is a large ulcer!

4.5 GASTRIC LEIOMYOMA/ LEIOMYOSARCOMA

IMAGING

Fluoro

focal mass, isocenter in wall
may ulcerate

CT

rounded focal mass with enhancement,
centered on wall
multifocal massive thickening of stomach
wall
leiomyosarcoma may be low density
irregular enhancement with areas of non
enhancement implying necrosis

PET (FDG)

FDG avid

4.6 GASTRIC LYMPHOMA

see Ch 16

4.7 GASTRIC POLYPS
(overview)

CLASSIFICATION

Non neoplastic

HYPERPLASTIC

<2 cm sessile or pedunculated, common accompanies chronic gastritis

FUNDIC GLAND RETENTION CYST

HAMARTOMATOUS CHORISTOMATOUS

HETEROTOPIC PANCREAS

PEUTZ–JEGHER'S SYNDROME

sessile or pedunculated, branching smooth muscle core, loose connective tissue stroma, non dysplastic epithelium

VASCULAR

HEREDITARY HEMORRHAGIC TELANGIECTASIA

Neoplastic – mucosal origin

ADENOMA (tubular, villous)

POLYPOID CARCINOMA

CARCINOID

Neoplastic – wall origin

LEIOMYOMA

LIPOMA

NEUROFIBROMA

LYMPHOMA

SARCOMA (including KAPOSI'S SARCOMA)

METASTASIS

IMAGING

Definitely benign on imaging

stomach wall lipoma on CT: uniform fat density mass

Likely benign

small, smooth, regular, on stalk

Likely malignant

sessile, large, irregular, ulcerated

4.8 GASTRIC VOLVULUS

see hiatus hernia entry in esophageal section

4.9 MÉNÉTRIER'S DISEASE

DEFINITION

idiopathic hyperplasia of surface epithelium with thickened folds and increased mucus production

CLINICAL

triad of hypochlorhydria, protein losing enteropathy and giant mucosal hypertrophy; increased incidence of carcinoma

IMAGING

differentiation from lymphoma difficult
see stomach fold hypertrophy gamut

Fluoro

massively thickened relatively mobile folds
wall relatively distensible, with preserved peristalsis
diffuse change more prominent in body/greater curve
antrum usually spared

CT

massively thickened gastric wall even with water distension
relatively sharp boundary between normal and abnormal mucosa

4.10 PEPTIC ULCERS

DEFINITION

chronic benign (by definition) acid/pepsin destructive ulcer into or through the visceral wall

EPIDEMIOLOGY

Gastric ulcer (GU)

male:female 2:1
older, lower socioeconomic class, NSAIDs, alcohol
Helicobacter pylori present in ~70%

Duodenal ulcer (DU)

male:female 3:1
middle age, upper socioeconomic class, blood type O
Helicobacter pylori present in ~100%

ETIOLOGY

Hyperacidity

smoking, coffee, stress, hypercalcemia
Zollinger–Ellison syndrome (multifocal, distal, recurrent ulcers)

Mucosal damage

GU: NSAIDs, alcohol, H pylori present in ~70%
DU: H pylori in almost 100%, eradication gives high cure rate

Unusual ulcers

MECKEL'S DIVERTICULUM ULCER

ANASTOMOTIC ULCER

PATHOGENESIS

initiating injury to mucosa, chronic balance between damage and healing

CLINICAL

silent or non specific symptoms
classic symptoms (burning pain related to meals exacerbated by coffee, food, etc and relieved by antacids; nocturnal pain)

Complications

BLEED (can be catastrophic)
BLOCK (DU – acquired pyloric stenosis; GU – hourglass stomach)
BURST (GU and anterior DU)
BURROW (fistulas, pancreatitis)

MACRO

focal deep punched out crater <2 cm (rarely, giant ulcer)
clean sharp edge and base, mucosal overhang
fibrotic walls, reactive fibrosis

MICRO

NECROTIC SURFACE LAYER
EXUDATE
GRANULATION TISSUE
FIBROSIS, ENDARTERITIS OBLITERANS

IMAGING

Fluoro

see ulcer: benign vs malignant gamut
DU is virtually always benign, and in cap or
pyloric canal
benign GU classically along lesser curve and
in antrum
malignant GU anywhere

ULCER DESCRIPTORS

crater (floor, walls)
collar = constriction of neck of crater
mound = fixed elevation of contour around
ulcer (edema or neoplastic mass)
Hampton's line = thin overhang of normal
mucosa
incisura = fixed indentation opposite ulcer,
?fixed spasm; affects greater curve

HEALED SCAR

scar pattern: dot or line or depression or
bump with radiating gastric folds;
scarring in antrum may be concentric

NUC MED (RBC)

requires NO FREE TcO4 IN LABELED RED
CELLS
focal gastric or duodenal non vascular
accumulation of labeled RBC that
increases with time, outlining gastric or
duodenal shape and migrating distally
must confirm location (imaging for long
enough; imaging with markers)
confirmation of duodenum is also by relation
to vascular anatomy (renal pedicles,
aorta, IVC)

5. CONDITIONS OF THE SMALL BOWEL

5.1 AFFERENT LOOP SYNDROME

CLINICAL

following roux-en-Y surgery peristalsis
directs upper GI (e.g. stomach) content
into the afferent loop, resulting in
functional obstruction

IMAGING

Fluoro

roux-en-Y anastomosis (e.g. Polya
gastrectomy)

may show preferential transit of barium into
the afferent loop

5.2 CELIAC DISEASE

DEFINITION

abnormal immune response to gluten
leading to small bowel mucosal damage,
secondary malabsorption and late
lymphoma

EPIDEMIOLOGY

northern Europeans 1/2000; familial
incidence
associations: small bowel carcinoma, breast
carcinoma

CLINICAL

CHILD: failure to thrive, growth retardation,
bloating, diarrhea
ADULT: diarrhea, abdominal pain, weight
loss, symptoms of malabsorption

Complications
enteropathy associated T cell lymphoma
MALABSORPTION COMPLICATIONS

MACRO

flattened mucosa, small bowel dilation
proximal bowel to distal bowel gradient of
disease severity, reversal of fold height
proximal to distal

MICRO

Early

crypt hyperplastic villous atrophy,
lymphocytic infiltrate
proximal bowel to distal bowel gradient of
disease severity

Late (refractory sprue)
collagenosis, fibrosis

IMAGING

FLUORO

loss of mucosal folds (may be more severe
proximally, with proximal to distal bowel
severity gradient)

thickening of mucosal folds
abnormal bowel dilation
barium segmentation, flocculation, moulage
(featureless barium column)
non obstructing intussusception

CT

abnormal mild diffuse wall thickening,
dilation
focal severe thickening or aneurysmal
dilation suggests lymphoma

PET (FDG)

small bowel is usually unapparent on fasted
FDG scans
focal intense accumulation is indicative of
supervening lymphoma

5.3 CONGENITAL SMALL BOWEL DISEASE

see Ch 18

5.4 CROHN'S DISEASE

*see Crohn's disease entry in large bowel
section*

5.5 CYSTIC FIBROSIS (CF)

also see Ch 13
malabsorption, steatorrhea, malnutrition
secondary to pancreatic insufficiency
meconium ileus in neonates (Ch 18)
meconium ileus equivalent in adults
(obstruction by viscous bowel content)
biliary cirrhosis (Ch 07)
duodenum often has smooth mucosal
surfaces without folds
jejunum may have mucosal fold thickening
and dilation (20%)

5.6 EOSINOPHILIC GASTROENTERITIS

CLINICAL

strong association with allergy and atopy
eosinophilic infiltration of GI tract
presents with pain and malabsorption

IMAGING

Fluoro

diffuse mucosal fold thickening
loss of bowel folds
if involvement of wall – rigid wall
ascites possible if serosa involved

5.7 GALLSTONE ILEUS

rare condition except in exams!
gallstone eroding a gallbladder to enteric
    fistula and causing bowel obstruction

IMAGING

AXR

partial or complete small bowel obstruction
    WITH
biliary air
may see calcification in stone

Barium

classically, outlines gallstone AND shows
    fistula!

CT

partial or complete small bowel obstruction,
    biliary air AND
shows stone directly at small bowel
    transition zone

5.8 INTUSSUSCEPTION
(manifestations)

see Ch 18
must seek lead point in adults – usually
    polyp or tumor unless there has been a
    roux-en-Y loop (anastomotic
    intussusception)

IMAGING

AXR

small bowel obstruction
soft tissue mass at transition zone may be
    visible
may see crescent of gas or fat (rare)

Fluoro

classic 'coiled spring' appearance with
    barium tracking between intussusceptum
    (inner bowel) and intussuscipiens
    (receiving bowel)
for reduction see Ch 18

US

concentrically layered mass with crescent of
    echogenic fat (US crescent sign) – rarely
    a complete circle of fat
can usually identify transverse and
    longitudinal orientations
may see peristalsis into the intussusception
may see gut wall signature in outer and
    inner bowel; more commonly too
    edematous to discern
color flow confirms (at least arterial)
    vascular integrity

CT

focal mass at transition point with crescent
    of mesenteric fat separating inner soft
    tissue mass from outer bowel
may see mesenteric edema and distortion of
    mesenteric vessels

5.9 ISCHEMIA

ETIOLOGY

INFANT
NECROTIZING ENTEROCOLITIS
VOLVULUS (VENOUS INFARCT)

CHILD
SMALL BOWEL VASCULITIS
    (Henoch–Schönlein purpura)

YOUNG ADULT
SYSTEMIC LUPUS ERYTHEMATOSUS
    VASCULITIS
POLYARTERITIS NODOSA VASCULITIS
PORTAL VEIN THROMBOSIS

OLDER ADULT (atherosclerosis)
MESENTERIC ANGINA
ISCHEMIC COLITIS
CATASTROPHIC NECROSIS

ANY AGE
TRAUMATIC
HYPOTENSIVE WATERSHED MUCOSAL
    SLOUGHING
EMBOLIC

PATHOGENESIS

Rules

1. non diseased arterial collaterals are
   excellent – compensate for chronic
   arterial insufficiency
2. most vulnerable area is tips of villi due to
   vascular countercurrent and high
   metabolic needs

Depth of injury determines outcome

SUPERFICIAL MUCOSA
crypts intact – full regeneration

ENTIRE MUCOSA
wall intact – fibrotic healing with strictures

TRANSMURAL
rupture
sepsis
portal gas, portal pyemia
disseminated intravascular coagulation (DIC)

MACRO

Mucosal damage only
edematous dull red mucosa which sloughs
    (pseudomembrane)
denuded muscularis with reactive hyperemia

Transmural infarct
atonic blood filled dilated red/black bowel
    loops

IMAGING

AXR

no findings or
abnormal air–fluid levels
abnormal bowel dilation
abnormal mucosal thickening or
    thumbprinting
intramural gas
portal venous gas
perforation

Fluoro

early no findings
mucosal and valvular edema and ulceration
chronic ischemic strictures

Angio

not a common investigation for acute bowel
    ischemia, as laparotomy supervenes
may be done looking for atherosclerotic
    causes of chronic ischemia

ACUTE ISCHEMIA
complete cutoff of a mesenteric artery or
    branch
absent mucosal blush in subtended territory
may be a prelude to thrombolysis

CHRONIC ISCHEMIA
stenoses or occlusions of major mesenteric
    vessels (celiac axis, SMA, IMA)
extensive arterial collateralization from
    remaining vessels (marginal artery of
    Drummond)

US

in mesenteric angina, Doppler US is used to look for celiac artery or SMA stenosis (same Doppler criteria as for arterial stenoses elsewhere: Ch 15)

CT

PORTAL PEDICLE

SMA thrombosis, SMV thrombosis
portal gas

ABNORMAL BOWEL WALL

differential in enhancement may indicate the ischemic to normal junction (especially in arterial ischemia)

extremely thick bowel wall

gas in bowel wall

arterial phase uniform mucosal enhancement makes significant ischemia unlikely

presence of bowel enhancement as such does not rule out bowel ischemia (slow influx or re-flow to infarcted bowel occurs, but shows a 'late stain')

later in ischemia may have rings of enhancement (extravasation of contrast)

ABNORMAL BOWEL MORPHOLOGY

dilation
appearance of obstruction
mesenteric edema, ascites

5.10 LYMPHOMA

see Ch 16

5.11 MALABSORPTION

DEFINITION

1. failure to absorb enough for metabolic needs and/or
2. failure to clear osmotic or caloric load leading to symptoms

ETIOLOGY

'Too little'

not enough nutrients or enzymes
PANCREATIC INSUFFICIENCY
BILE ACID INSUFFICIENCY
BACTERIAL OVERGROWTH (DIVERTICULA, BLIND LOOPS)

'Too short'

not enough bowel length
SHORT GUT SYNDROME
SURGICAL BYPASSES
ISOLATED LOSS OF TERMINAL ILEUM (loss of bile acids)
CROHN'S DISEASE

'Too fast'

overfast small bowel transit
VIPoma
CARCINOID SYNDROME
ZOLLINGER–ELLISON SYNDROME

Brush border failure

DISACCHARIDASE DEFICIENCY

Crypt hyperplastic villous atrophy

destruction of villi with intact regeneration mechanism
CELIAC DISEASE
INFECTIONS (TROPICAL SPRUE, WHIPPLE'S DISEASE)

Crypt hypoplastic villous atrophy

loss of regeneration mechanism with secondary loss of villi
RADIATION, CHEMOTHERAPY

Vascular failure

AMYLOIDOSIS
CHRONIC VASCULAR INSUFFICIENCY

Lymphatic failure

LYMPHOMA (?MECHANISM)
LYMPHANGIECTASIA (rare malformation of lymphatics with failure of chyle absorption)
FILARIASIS

CLINICAL MANIFESTATIONS

Calorie/protein deficiency

weight loss, lethargy, hypoproteinemia, amenorrhea

Fe/B12/folate deficiency

anemia, other B12 complications

DEAK (fat soluble vitamins D, E, A, K) deficiency

osteomalacia, hypocalcemia, secondary hyperparathyroidism
bleeding dyscrasias
skin, epithelial, retinal changes

Intestinal symptoms

bloating, pain, diarrhea, steatorrhea

IMAGING

generally unrewarding

Major conditions with imaging findings

celiac disease
radiation enteritis (chronic)
Crohn's disease
all short bowel/diverticular/blind loop syndromes
Whipple's, tropical sprue and mimics
amyloidosis
Henoch–Schönlein purpura
lymphoma, lymphangiectasia

5.12 MECKEL'S DIVERTICULUM

see Ch 18

5.13 POLYPS – SMALL BOWEL (overview)

Retention

CRONKHITE–CANADA SYNDROME

Hamartomatous

PEUTZ–JEGHERS SYNDROME

Neoplastic – adenoma

AMPULLA OF VATER
CARCINOID

Neoplastic – connective tissue

LIPOMA
LEIOMYOMA/LEIOMYOSARCOMA
NERVE SHEATH TUMOR

5.14 RADIATION ENTERITIS

5.14.1 EARLY RADIATION ENTERITIS

MUCOSAL DAMAGE: edema, swelling, ulceration, sloughing

5.14.2 LATE RADIATION FIBROSIS

ENDARTERITIS OBLITERANS: fibrosis, stenosis, strictures; neovascular telangiectasia

IMAGING

Fluoro
ulceration (early)
mucosal fold thickening (may conform to radiation field)
loss of mucosal pattern
wall thickening, strictures, stenoses, fistulas
fixity of loops implying adhesions

5.15 SMALL BOWEL INFECTIONS (overview)

5.15.1 VIRAL

5.15.2 BACTERIAL/FUNGAL

Luminal/toxigenic

5.15.2.1 Invasive (pseudoCrohn's)
TB

YERSINIA PSEUDOTUBERCULOSIS

ACTINOMYCOSIS, BLASTOMYCOSIS

5.15.3 PARASITIC

5.15.3.1 Protozoan
GIARDIA LAMBLIA
CRYPTOSPORIDIUM (classic AIDS defining illness)

5.15.3.2 Nematodal (roundworm)
ASCARIS LUMBRICOIDES
TOXOCARA CANIS
ANKYLOSTOMA DUODENALE, NECATOR AMERICANIS

5.15.3.3 Cestodal (tapeworm)

ADULT FORM (ingested larvae)

LARVAL FORM (ingested eggs, larval deposition in the body)
HYDATID DISEASE
CYSTICERCOSIS

5.16 SMALL BOWEL OBSTRUCTION (SBO)

ETIOLOGY

see SBO, ileus and SB stricture gamuts

Intraluminal
polyp, foreign body, worms, even stone

Mural
hemorrhage, acute edema, mass
STRICTURE (benign or neoplastic)

Extraluminal
ALL OF THESE MAY CAUSE CLOSED LOOP OBSTRUCTION
adhesions (main cause overall)
external hernia (inguinal, incisional, femoral, Spigelian)
internal hernia
volvulus
intussusception
abscess, inflammatory mass
peritoneal tumor

Functional (ileus)
not meant to have a transition zone!
can demonstrate bowel continuity and normal caliber

CLINICAL

Acute
abdominal pain, swelling, vomiting, increased peristalsis (audible or visible)
lesser degree of small bowel dilation

Chronic
chronic or intermittent or grumbling abdominal pain
may have weight loss, malabsorption
bowel dilation greater than in acute SBO

IMAGING

AXR
dilated loops of small bowel with air–fluid levels
STRING OF BEADS SIGN: largely fluid filled bowel with small pockets of air trapped under mucosal folds
number and position of loops guide to level of obstruction
distal bowel collapsed and empty including large bowel (takes hours)
transition point may be evident in a hernia, at an abdominal mass or abdominal stone; rarely (especially Crohn's disease) air may outline strictured or spasmed loop
size of loops guide to duration and severity of obstruction, but in partial chronic obstruction may be misleadingly large
partial obstruction: signs may be absent or minor
complete obstruction: AXR changes develop over 6–12 hours
MAY SHOW A CLOSED LOOP ESPECIALLY AT HERNIAL ORIFICE

Fluoro
delayed small bowel transit and then failure of contrast to progress
shows degree of small bowel dilation
if outlines cecum – rules out complete small bowel obstruction
leading edge of contrast may outline cause of obstruction
if passes obstruction point proves a transition zone (dilated above to collapsed below)
differential of delayed small bowel transit is ileus
advantage of thin barium over gastrograffin: does not dilute out with distance (can find transition point)
gastrograffin often used by surgeons anyway; advantage over barium: mild osmotic cathartic
MAY EVENTUALLY FILL CLOSED LOOP

CT
particularly if 5 mm collimation or thinner
dilated loops of small bowel with fluid, air–fluid or oral contrast
oral contrast may reach transition zone if left for sufficiently long
distal small bowel collapsed (change in caliber significant even if transition point not evident)
may show cause of obstruction (e.g. mass or internal hernia)

MR
fast heavily T2 weighted sequences used to show fluid filled dilated loops of bowel
signs analogous to small bowel contrast study

Differentiation from ileus

ILEUS
clinical findings of no bowel sounds, relevant history
uniform dilation, uniform air–fluid levels
no transition zone

no peristalsis

MECHANICAL OBSTRUCTION

clinical findings of cramps, increased
  peristalsis
CARDINAL SIGN: transition zone
different level air–fluid levels in same bowel
  loop (implies active peristalsis, but not
  reliable)
empty distal bowel
CLOSED LOOP INDICATES MECHANICAL
  OBSTRUCTION

5.17 TB (small bowel)

also see Ch 13, Ch 08

DEFINITION

primary or secondary TB infection of bowel
  with ulcerative or ulceroconstrictive forms

PATHOGENESIS

localizes in lymphoid tissue particularly
  terminal ileum
PRIMARY GIT (TB in milk, food)
SECONDARY GIT (50%) swallowed sputum
common in Asia; commonest cause of small
  bowel stricture in India

MORPHOLOGY

Ulcerative

more likely to be active disease
annular raised mucosal ulcers
lymphoid patches and lymph nodes enlarged
  and caseating
caseating granulomas, few acid fast bacilli
  (AFB)

Ulceroconstrictive

ulcerated mucosa
hypertrophic fibrotic response
thick wall, strictures (variable length and
  number)
pseudoCrohn's
conical cecum, strictured or dilated terminal
  ileum
muscularis replaced by massive fibrosis
AFB hard to find

IMAGING

Fluoro

same features on barium study as
  morphology

---

generally can not differentiate from Crohn's
  disease or other invasive infections

CT

concentric wall thickening and deformity
classically right iliac fossa but may be
  multifocal
ring enhancing lymphadenopathy with low
  density core
may have ascites (peritoneal TB)
may have evidence of urogenital
  involvement (Ch 08)
may have tuberculous retroperitoneal
  abscesses or psoas/iliacus abscesses
  (much more likely to originate from
  spinal TB)

5.18 TRAUMA OVERVIEW (bowel)

ETIOLOGY

BLUNT TRAUMA VS PENETRATING TRAUMA

Location

DUODENUM

involved in blunt trauma much more
  commonly than mobile bowel

SMALL BOWEL

MESENTERY, VASCULAR PEDICLE

COLON (UNCOMMON)

Morphology

5.18.1 CONTUSION

5.18.2 INTRAMURAL HEMATOMA

5.18.3 LACERATION,
  RETROPERITONEAL PERFORATION

5.18.4 LACERATION,
  INTRAPERITONEAL PERFORATION

5.18.5 ARTERIAL DISSECTION,
  ISCHEMIC BOWEL

5.18.6 TRAUMATIC SMV OCCLUSION

IMAGING

AXR

duodenal injury incidence is high if a Chance
  vertebral fracture is present
retroperitoneal gas in retroperitoneal
  duodenal perforation
free intraabdominal gas in bowel perforation

---

ileus, dilated loops of bowel, possibly a
  transition zone

CT

NON SPECIFIC SIGNS

free intraperitoneal fluid
free fluid at base of mesentery
omental and mesenteric stranding

SIGNS OF DUODENAL INJURY

intramural hematoma: irregularly or
  circumferentially thickened duodenal
  wall, obliteration of luminal contrast
periduodenal edema or fluid
extravasation of duodenal contents, contrast
  or air into retroperitoneum (oral contrast
  and air very specific)

SIGNS OF BOWEL INJURY

edematous bowel wall
dilated small bowel, mid small bowel
  transition zone
bowel intramural hematoma
free intraperitoneal air
edematous mesentery

SIGNS OF MESENTERIC INJURY

hematoma at base of mesentery
non opacification of superior mesenteric
  vein or artery
non enhancement of a segment of bowel
  wall
uniformly dilated bowel

5.19 TROPICAL SPRUE

celiac disease like syndrome, of presumed
  infective origin
treated with broad spectrum antibiotics

5.20 TYPHOID FEVER

systemic infection by Salmonella typhi, with
  a gut entry portal (typically terminal
  ileum Peyer's patches) and chronic
  biliary reservoir leading to a carrier state

5.21 WHIPPLE'S DISEASE

DEFINITION

multisystem bacterial infection by
  Trophyrema whippelii (an actinomycete)
  with malabsorption the most pronounced
  manifestation

CLINICAL

male:female 10:1, 30–60 years old
malabsorption
lymphadenopathy (50%)
hyperpigmentation
migratory polyarthralgia
CNS infection (rare, often mass-like, may be
    multifocal)
macrophages full of organisms at sites of
    disease

6. CONDITIONS OF THE LARGE BOWEL

6.1 ANGIODYSPLASIA

DEFINITION

acquired dilation of colonic mucosal/
    submucosal veins presenting with GIT
    bleeding

ETIOPATHOGENESIS

intermittent venous obstruction by muscular
    contraction producing ectatic venous,
    venulous, capillary mucosal and
    submucosal channels

CLINICAL

common: 20% of GIT bleeds; occurs in over
    60 year olds, incidence rises with age
painless massive bleed or chronic GIT blood
    loss
more common in cecum/ascending colon
    than left colon

IMAGING

Fluoro

usually no findings

Angio

if brisk bleeding during angio, nidus and
    intraluminal contrast show on selective
    colic artery injection
may proceed to embolization

NUC MED (RBC)

RBCs labeled preferably in vitro to avoid
    free pertechnetate
dynamic imaging for at least 30 min and
    then spot views
non anatomical non vascular appearance
    and accumulation of activity that follows
    the contour and position of bowel and
    demonstrates peristalsis
activity in feces is proof of GIT hemorrhage
    (calibrate against patient soft tissue
    activity to avoid false positive diagnosis)
need to observe accumulation of activity to
    prove bleeding point
of use only if bleeding at the time
    (continuously or intermittently)

POTENTIAL TRAPS

INTRAVASCULAR SPACES
portal vein
IVC
liver, spleen
penis blood pool
uterine blood pool
accessory spleen
aneurysms and varices

FREE/DETACHED PERTECHNETATE
kidneys, collecting systems, ureters, bladder
urine contamination

INTERVAL BLEED
bowel filled with RBCs, but no point of
    accumulation is evident
proves bleed but does not localize
in general, SB blood suggests SB
    hemorrhage, and LB blood is unhelpful

6.2 APPENDICITIS

ETIOPATHOGENESIS

single commonest cause of acute abdomen
    in 1–30 year olds
requires both obstruction (edema, lymphoid
    hyperlasia, fecolith, worms, acute
    kinking) AND infection (bowel flora)

Stages of inflammation

mucosal then transmural; thrombosis of
    vascular pedicle (endarteries, endveins)
    leading to gangrene and rupture
low grade inflammation may resolve if
    obstruction spontaneously relieved

Complications

portal pyemia
mesenteric vein septic thrombosis
liver abscess
septicemia
right iliac fossa or retroperitoneal abscess
generalized peritonitis

Unusual types

TUBERCULOUS

APPENDICEAL CROHN'S DISEASE

'GRUMBLING APPENDICITIS'
ill defined entity
intermittent self-limiting acute episodes

IMAGING

AXR (KUB)

most commonly no findings
fecolith
sentinel loop (terminal ileum)
localized fluid or localized abscess
generalized ileus
free air

Fluoro

normal appendix on barium enema
    effectively excludes (if entire appendix
    fills)

US

requires direct demonstration of either
    normal or abnormal appendix to be
    diagnostic, and limited by bowel gas and
    patient's tenderness

NORMAL
entire appendix thickness (Kirks) 6 mm or
    less
normal US gut signature
non tender and compressible
may have mobile intraluminal air
can be followed out to tip (hopefully)

ABNORMAL
edematous appendix, surrounding edema
fecolith (shadowing edge, does not move)
non compressible and tender
increased vascularity on color (subjective
    call)

CT

requires direct demonstration of appendix
various maneuvers include thinner slices,
    rectal contrast and decubitus scanning
best for retrocecal (and therefore fixed and
    visible) appendix

APPENDICITIS
thickened non filling appendix with evidence
    of surrounding fat edema or infiltration
fecolith
may have localized ileus, or draining vein
    thrombosis (expanded non enhancing
    cord like)

APPENDIX ABSCESS

right iliac fossa complex mass with ring
   enhancement, likely air–fluid level and
   thickened wall
differential is Crohn's abscess

NUC MED

white cell scanning may be used where US
   or CT inconclusive
see under Crohn's disease

6.3 APPENDIX MUCOCELE

6.3.1 SIMPLE OBSTRUCTIVE MUCOCELE

non infected obstruction of appendix neck
   leading to accumulation of mucus
if ruptured, leads to simple pseudomyxoma
   peritonei

6.3.2 CYSTADENOMA, CYSTADENOCARCINOMA

obstruction of appendix with a neoplasm
when ruptured, causes malignant
   pseudomyxoma peritonei, often with
   peritoneal seeding

IMAGING

CT/US

absent normal appendix
mass centered on appendix, often with a
   visible wall and internal non enhancing
   complex fluid content

6.4 CARCINOID TUMOR

DEFINITION

benign or malignant tumor of visceral
   neuroendocrine cells originally of neural
   crest origin, often retaining endocrine
   activity

CLINICAL

Distribution

APPENDIX (~95% benign) then
ILEUM (~25% of all carcinoids, ~60% are
   malignant) then
RECTUM (~20% of all carcinoids, ~15% are
   malignant) then

STOMACH (most malignant) then
COLON (most malignant)
multiple in up to 25%

Presentation

local obstruction
bleeding (especially rectal)
carcinoid syndrome (if liver metastases)
other hormonal syndrome (especially
   Zollinger–Ellison syndrome)
lymph nodal or distant metastases
bowel obstruction (reactive fibrosis)

Spread

uncommon when <1 cm
LATE SPREADING: appendix and rectum
EARLY SPREADING: ileum, stomach, colon
LYMPHATIC SPREAD induces desmoplastic
   reaction
LIVER and DISTANT metastases

Carcinoid syndrome

results from systemic release of serotonin
   from carcinoid metastases to liver
intestinal rushes, great tricolor blushes, hot
   flushes
asthma attacks, vasomotor instability
systemic fibrosis, cardiac fibrosis
   (pulmonary and tricuspid)

MORPHOLOGY

mural nodule or mass with desmoplastic
   reaction and fibrosis
nests, cords of well differentiated
   neuroendocrine argentaffin and
   argyrophil positive cells
malignancy unequivocal only if distant
   metastases or massive direct and
   vascular invasion

IMAGING

Fluoro

mucosally based mass with no specific
   features

CT (gut carcinoids)

vascular enhancing mural mass or
   thickening, or primary may not be visible
mesenteric lymphadenopathy
straight radiating mesenteric or
   retroperitoneal fibrosis (characteristic,
   non specific)
hypervascular, arterial phase enhancing
   liver metastases, often with central
   necrosis or cystic change
occasionally calcifies

NUC MED

In-111 OCTREOTIDE

more carcinoids take up octreotide than
   MIBG, many take up both
abdominal SPECT and planar images at 24
   and 48 hours post injection
need to differentiate from normal bowel
   uptake

NORMAL In-111 OCTREOTIDE DISTRIBUTION

spleen (more intense), liver (less intense)
bone marrow (low grade)
kidneys and urine
blood pool, mediastinum
bowel
pituitary, thyroid

CARCINOID UPTAKE

persistent focal uptake which does not
   change position with time
location commonly in right iliac fossa, root
   of mesentery, pancreas, other
liver metastases may be masked by liver
   uptake, but usually exceed liver
   background

GRADING
0   no uptake
I   equivocal
II   less than normal liver
III equal to or greater than normal liver
IV   greater than spleen

I-123 or I-131 MIBG: see adrenal
   nuclear medicine Ch 08

6.5 ISCHEMIC COLITIS

see small bowel ischemia – mechanism and
   pathology analogous

IMAGING

Acute ischemic colitis

most common cause is watershed ischemia,
   therefore usual location is around splenic
   flexure

AXR

no findings
thickened fuzzy mucosa
'thumbprinting'
narrowed lumen, proximal dilation

CT

same as for small bowel ischemia
thickened wall, may have ring enhancement
may correspond to a watershed or other
   vascular territory
differential is other causes of colitis

6.6 COLONIC ADENOMA

DEFINITION

premalignant epithelial neoplasm with adenoma to carcinoma progression and malignant risk proportional to size

ETIOPATHOGENESIS

SPORADIC: geography, age, diet; family history, male = female
SYNDROMIC: familial polyposis coli and variants: gene 5q21 (dysplastic field change, innumerable adenomas)
DYSPLASIA–ADENOMA–CARCINOMA SEQUENCE
risk depends on size (see gamuts entry), villous histology, degree of dysplasia
invasion is first intramucosal then frankly invasive

CLINICAL

Presentation
asymptomatic at screening
coexisting with other pathology (e.g. carcinoma)
anemia, GIT blood loss

Distribution
ascending 25%
descending/sigmoid 25%
rectosigmoid 25%
often multiple

MICRO

TUBULAR (most)
>75% tubular histology
usually pedunculated
tubular glands lined by dysplastic epithelium
non neoplastic lamina propria
transition zone usually on stalk

Tubulovillous
25–50% villous histology

Villous
>50% villous histology
favors rectosigmoid, tends to be sessile
thin leafy growths of dysplastic epithelium on thin lamina propria
dysplasia up to carcinoma in situ

IMAGING

see polyps entry

6.7 COLORECTAL CARCINOMA

DEFINITION

colorectal epithelial malignancy with a long premetastatic window

EPIDEMIOLOGY

Sporadic (majority)
as for adenomas
arises in adenoma (lag time 10–15 years)
female = male (rectum male > female)

Syndromic

ULCERATIVE COLITIS
in foci of dysplasia, often flat

FAMILIAL POLYPOSIS COLI

GARDNER'S SYNDROME, TURCOT'S SYNDROME

HEREDITARY NON POLYPOSIS COLORECTAL CANCER

LYNCH SYNDROME I
elevated incidence of colorectal cancer only

LYNCH SYNDROME II
elevated incidence of colorectal cancer
increased risk of endometrial, ovarian, pancreatic cancer

CLINICAL

Presentation
1. see adenoma entry
2. with altered bowel habit, large bowel obstruction, metastases

Distribution – same as adenomas

Spread
LYMPHATIC – late, as no mucosal lymphatics
HEMATOGENOUS – late, liver, lungs, brain, bone

Staging (Dukes)

10% DUKES A
not beyond muscularis, lymph nodes -ve
100% 5 year survival

35% DUKES B
beyond muscularis, lymph nodes -ve
70% 5 year survival

50% DUKES C
node +ve
35% 5 year survival

DISTAL METASTASES (NOT IN DUKES)

Staging (TNM)

T STAGE
T1 submucosa
T2 muscularis
T3 subserosa or through rectal wall into non peritonealized tissues
T4 perforates visceral peritoneum or invades surrounding organs or structures

N STAGE
N1 3 regional nodes or fewer
N2 more than 3 regional nodes

NOTE
tumor nodule in perirectal fat up to 3 mm is classified as discontinuous extension (T3), and over 3 mm as a regional lymph node metastasis

STAGE GROUPING
I   T1 or T2 N0 M0
II T3 or T4 N0 M0
III any T N1 or N2 M0
IV any T any N M1

MACRO

FUNGATING (cecum > other)
ANNULAR STENOSING (left colon > other)
RECTAL TUMOR has no serosa – spreads in continuity

MICRO

98% ADENOCARCINOMA
WELL DIFFERENTIATED (malignant mucous glands) to POORLY DIFFERENTIATED (sheets of cells)

IMAGING

Fluoro/CT colography
can not differentiate adenoma from carcinoma
pedunculated polyp unlikely to be malignant, sessile large mass is likely
MASS: persistent elevation of mucosal contour, fixed on many views; may ulcerate; may have shoulders; may be cauliflower-like

STRICTURE: classically an applecore stricture with sharp shoulders and irregular carcinoma inner lumen

CT

focal murally based mass (beware of normal but collapsed and folded mucosa or adherent feces)

focal circumferential thickening with stricture

may enhance (then unequivocally not feces)

evidence of local spread: permeation/masses in perirectal or mesenteric fat; invasion of adjacent organs definite only if invading or distorting contour; contiguity suspicious

LYMPHADENOPATHY: based on size criteria (1 cm cutoff); pelvic, mesenteric, retroperitoneal, celiac, portal nodes

LIVER METASTASES: classically low density multiple rounded masses more obvious with contrast, may show portal phase ring enhancement

RECURRENCE: difficult; need baseline and serial CT for growth; else unequivocal invasion of normal structures (e.g. sacrum)

US

endorectal US may demonstrate local stage (hypoechoic irregular mass disrupting normal gut wall layers)

LIVER METASTASES: classically hypoechoic masses with evidence of distortion or displacement of normal liver vascular architecture

MR (rectal carcinoma)

thin section multiplanar FSE T2W, with/without Buscopan

tumor: low signal mass with shoulders or focal thickening of the mucosa and with disruption and loss of normal MR rectal wall signature (signal is higher than the low T2W signal of muscularis propria)

transmural spread shown by spiculation, nodules and infiltration of surrounding fat (if unequivocal, upstages to T3)

intramural extent may show as mass disrupting normal wall layers with loss of dark T2W signal of muscularis propria

sensitive for pelvic and retroperitoneal lymphadenopathy; may see small presacral space nodes of uncertain significance

LIVER METASTASES: Ch 07

RECURRENCE: difficult; high T2W signal may indicate post surgical or post radiotherapy change, and enhancement does not differentiate; growth on serial MR required, else unequivocal invasion of normal structures (e.g. sacrum)

PET (FDG)

primary carcinoma usually FDG avid (beware uptake in normal bowel wall)

RECURRENCE: most sensitive non invasive test for local recurrence, with FDG avid uptake indicating recurrence

postoperative scar and post radiotherapy changes have mildly increased FDG uptake for weeks–months

colostomy has increased FDG uptake

differential of rectal recurrence: early postoperative change vs bladder diverticulum or ureter vs abscess vs cervical or prostate tumor

LYMPHADENOPATHY: increased FDG uptake usually highly suggestive; should have direct correlation with CT to locate site of increased FDG uptake

LIVER METASTASES: many are FDG avid, but may be relatively 'cold' and difficult to see in metabolically active liver parenchyma

6.8 CROHN'S DISEASE

DEFINITION

chronic granulomatous enteritis of uncertain etiology

EPIDEMIOLOGY

geography, family history, white, female, Jewish, young adult > other ages

PATHOGENESIS

progressive non phasic regional segmental transmural granulomatous inflammation with fissures and fibrosis

CLINICAL

pain, weight loss, malabsorption
subacute partial small bowel obstruction
perianal fistulas

Location

terminal ileum commonest (30–50%), appendix
colon, anorectum (10–30%)
both (30%)
anywhere else

Complications

SMALL AND LARGE BOWEL OBSTRUCTION

FISTULAS
VAGINA, BLADDER
SKIN, PERIANAL
BETWEEN SMALL BOWEL LOOPS

Extraintestinal manifestations
MNEMONIC: [2-ITIS 3-UM]
ARTHR-ITIS ('enteropathic arthropathy')
UVE-ITIS
ERYTHEMA NODOS-UM
PYODERMA GANGRENOS-UM
DIRECT INVOLVEMENT PERIAN-UM

MORPHOLOGY

multiple skip lesions
metachronous lesions
entire bowel wall edematous and thickened, not hyperemic
lumen irregular and narrow
abnormal hypertrophic fat, mesenteric lymphadenopathy
loss of peristalsis
deep fissures through all wall layers, fistulas
non necrotizing granulomas (70%): DIAGNOSTIC ONCE TB RULED OUT
TOXIC MEGACOLON

IMAGING

Fluoro
see ulcerative colitis vs Crohn's disease gamut

EARLY
aphthous ulceration
lymphoid hyperplasia
cobblestone mucosa

LATE
segmental involvement
collarstud ulcers, deep ulcers
fissuring (may have 'rose thorn ulcers')
narrowed lumen (concentric or eccentric)
pseudodiverticula (scarred wall deformity)
fistulas (to bowel, skin, bladder, vagina)
'string sign' (separation of diffusely narrowed involved loop from other loops by thickened wall)
conical featureless cecum with involved ileocecal valve
may see sinus track into an abscess

CT

segmental wall thickening, luminal
    narrowing
stranding and edema of surrounding fat
surrounding edema
abscess formation (retroperitoneal,
    mesenteric)
proliferation of mesenteric fat surrounding
    diseased bowel – characteristic
may show ring enhancement when acutely
    inflamed
fistula tracks may be visible

NUC MED

WBC scan (In-111 or HMPAO or colloid
    labeled)
early (1 hour) uptake in involved bowel wall
may excrete WBC into bowel lumen later
differential is Crohn's disease, ulcerative
    colitis, infective colitis, ischemic colitis

6.9 DIVERTICULAR DISEASE

DEFINITION

DIVERTICULOSIS: formation of diverticula
    secondary to abnormal muscular activity
    and low fiber diet
DIVERTICULITIS: infective complications

CLINICAL

silent diverticula
diverticulum superinfection
diverticular abscess
perforation and peritonitis
fistulas to vagina, bladder, small bowel
complex inflammatory mass
massive bleed

IMAGING

Fluoro

sigmoid > left > transverse > right colon
need to differentiate diverticula from polyps
saw tooth colon (mostly sigmoid) with
    rounded diverticula at apices of saw teeth
normal colon but with diverticula
mucosal irregularity and lumen narrowing –
    diverticulitis
barium tracking from diverticulum –
    peridiverticular abscess
may show fistulas
differential of diverticular stricture is
    carcinoma

CT

characteristic small pockets of gas following
    colon wall on each side

DIVERTICULITIS

focal stranding and edema of pericolic fat
focal wall thickening, focal paracolic fluid
    collection
paracolic abscess (fluid with enhancing wall
    adjacent to colon)
free intraperitoneal gas and fluid from
    perforation

NUC MED

see angiodysplasia (RBC scan)

6.10 INFECTIVE COLITIS

MUST DIFFERENTIATE INFECTIVE COLITIS
    FROM INFLAMMATORY BOWEL
    DISEASE

6.10.1 BACTERIAL COLITIS

CLINICAL

usually immunocompetent host and virulent
    organism
crampy pain, small volume frequent
    diarrhea with mucus and/or blood

IMAGING

ileus, dilation
mucosal edema and ulceration

6.10.2 PSEUDOMEMBRANOUS COLITIS

CLINICAL

Clostridium difficile (Gram +ve rod which
    produces exotoxin)
classically hospitalized patient on antibiotics
raised yellow plaques becoming confluent
    into a pseudomembrane (comprising
    mucosa, upper submucosa)

IMAGING

Fluoro

ragged sloughing mucosa

CT

as for other colitides
thickened wall, may have edematous inner
    layer
may have ring enhancement peripherally
may be dilated

6.10.3 NEUTROPENIC COLITIS (typhlitis)

CLINICAL

immunosuppressed patients, bone marrow
    transplant patients, AIDS patients

IMAGING

as for other colitides
segmental or pancolitis
edema and ulceration of entire bowel wall;
    necrosis and perforation possible

6.10.4 AMEBIC COLITIS

CLINICAL

Entameba histolytica
encysted forms swallowed with
    contaminated food or water

MORPHOLOGY

proximal colon > distal colon
yellow raised plaques, transverse ovoid
    ulcers with undermined edges
COMPLICATIONS: perforation, amebic liver
    abscess

IMAGING

FLUORO

as in other forms of colitis
segmental or diffuse
mucosal granularity or ulceration
late masses (amebomas), strictures, fistulas

6.10.5 TUBERCULOUS COLITIS

see small bowel TB
can not differentiate from Crohn's colitis on
    imaging alone

6.11 POLYPOSIS SYNDROMES

Name	Type	Polyp type	Polyp sites	Extra GI manifestations	Ca risk
Juvenile polyposis	?AD	hamartomatous – retention	colon, often single; stomach >50%		not elevated
Cronkhite–Canada	sporadic	inflammatory polyps	stomach 95–100%; colon near 100%, small bowel 50%	alopecia, onycholysis, clubbing, hyper-pigmentation	not elevated
Peutz–Jeghers	AD	hamartomatous	small bowel 95%, colon/rectum 30%, stomach 25–50%; may have colonic adenomas	mucosal and skin pigmentation	elevated (breast, ovary, uterus, lung, pancreas, GIT)
Cowden	?AD	hamartomatous	esophagus to rectum; stomach in 20%	labial papillomatosis and gingival hyperplasia; breast, thyroid, skin carcinomas	elevated (breast, thyroid)
Osler–Weber–Rendu	AD	vascular	commonest SB	mucosal angiomas	not elevated
Familial adenomatous polyposis coli	AD	adenomatous	colon; uncommonly stomach + duodenum		near 100% colon
Gardner	AD	adenomatous	colon; uncommonly stomach + duodenum	mesenteric desmoid fibromas, soft tissue tumors, osteomas; 10% ampullary carcinoma	near 100% colon
Turcot	AR	adenomatous	colon	CNS gliomas	very high risk of gliomas and colorectal carcinoma

6.12 POLYPS

also see polyposis syndromes

Non neoplastic

INFLAMMATORY REGENERATIVE
inflammatory pseudopolyps: islands of residual mucosa
post inflammatory pseudopolyps: filiform mucosal tags

HYPERPLASTIC
very common; 5 mm or less hemispheric; 50% rectosigmoid
serrated infolded non neoplastic epithelium

HAMARTOMATOUS – RETENTION
JUVENILE POLYP
1–3 cm rounded on long stalk, solitary, 80% rectal
abundant dilated cystic glands, no dysplasia, normal lamina propria

HAMARTOMATOUS – CHORISTOMATOUS
PEUTZ–JEGHERS POLYP

VASCULAR
HEREDITARY HEMORRHAGIC TELANGIECTASIA

Neoplastic
ADENOMA-CARCINOMA
CARCINOID
LYMPHOMA

IMAGING

see polyp vs diverticulum gamut

Fluoro/CT colography
pedunculated mobile rounded filling defect attached by stalk
sessile mass elevating mucosal contour
may ulcerate centrally
can not distinguish sessile adenoma from carcinoma

CT
focal mucosal mass with projection into lumen
difficult to distinguish from collapsed wall or adherent feces in unprepared colon
if unequivocally enhances then vascular polyp

PET
adenomas often accumulate FDG
carcinomas are mostly FDG avid (see colorectal carcinoma)
differential is focal wall contraction or folding

6.13 PSEUDO-OBSTRUCTION

DEFINITION
functional stasis and dilation of large bowel without mechanical obstruction

CLINICAL
often elderly, institutionalized, bed ridden or psychiatric patients
if acute, causes similar to ileus
presents with absent bowel actions and increasing distension
may perforate

IMAGING

AXR

mimics large bowel obstruction

may use prone lateral shoot through to demonstrate air migrating into rectum implying no obstruction (proof is still with fluoro)

Fluoro

by definition, no obstruction

must demonstrate cecal pole or ileal reflux for proof

can accept passage of contrast beyond postulated transition zone if can not demonstrate cecal pole

6.14 RADIATION COLITIS/RADIATION PROCTITIS

CLINICAL/IMAGING

Acute

acute mucosal injury with ulceration/sloughing

Chronic

endarteritis, fibrosis

loss of normal mucosal architecture

loss of normal motility and haustration

wall thickening (CT differential is local recurrence), may enhance

radiation strictures

rarely, radiation fistulas

conforms to radiation field

6.15 TOXIC MEGACOLON

CLINICAL

acute massive dilation of large bowel, usually due to transmural infection with neuromuscular paralysis; progresses to perforation

causes: ulcerative colitis > Crohn's disease > infective colitis

IMAGING

DO NOT PERFORM BARIUM ENEMA

CARDINAL SIGN: acute massive dilation of part (less commonly all) of large bowel, most commonly cecum

acutely, cecum >9–10 cm is about to rupture

acutely, colon >5–6 cm may rupture

may have thickened irregular mucosa

may have mucosal sloughing/tags

6.16 ULCERATIVE COLITIS

DEFINITION

chronic inflammatory relapsing–remitting proctocolitis involving mucosa only, with high risk of late neoplasia

EPIDEMIOLOGY

geographic variation, young adult > other, family history, female > male

ankylosing spondylitis and HLA B27

CLINICAL

acute inflammation of colonic mucosa only, postulated autoimmune

fluctuant disease with remissions and recurrences

ulcerative proctitis (more indolent)

fulminant episode, TOXIC MEGACOLON

risk of carcinoma increases with time (arises in flat dysplasia)

Extraintestinal manifestations

MNEMONIC: 3ITIS 2UM

ARTHR-ITIS ('enteropathic arthropathy')

UVE-ITIS

SCLEROSING CHOLANG-ITIS

ERYTHEMA NODOS-UM

PYODERMA GANGRENOS-UM

MORPHOLOGY

Acute phase

rectum involved, with spread proximally in continuity

backwash ileitis 10%

granular friable congested mucosa, shallow to confluent ulceration

crypt abscesses with neutrophils passing into lumen

inflammatory pseudopolyps (surviving edematous mucosa)

muscularis uninvolved, serosa normal

Quiescent phase

shortened teniae and muscularis

flat or hyperplastic mucosa, regenerative pseudopolyps

LATE DYSPLASTIC FOCI IN REGENERATIVE BACKGROUND

IMAGING

see ulcerative colitis vs Crohn's disease gamut

see toxic megacolon

Fluoro

ACUTE

granular mucosa from rectum proximally

shallow ulceration, confluent ulceration, sloughing

undermined mucosal tags

CHRONIC

shortened featureless colon ('lead pipe') with loss of haustrae and narrowing

regenerative pseudopolyps: worm-like elongated filiform polyps projecting from mucosa

may have macroscopic neoplasia

CT

similar to other colitides

thickened wall, may show ring enhancement

wall thickening less prominent than in Crohn's disease

6.17 VOLVULUS

6.17.1 CECAL VOLVULUS

IMAGING

AXR

grossly distended cecum in left upper quadrant, or elsewhere

pathognomonic if appendix outlined by gas

may have 'two gastric air–fluid levels'

small bowel obstruction

no normal cecum in right iliac fossa

collapsed and empty large bowel

CT

grossly distended cecum which may be traced to hepatic flexure; ileocecal junction displaced with cecum

Fluoro

distal large bowel fills with barium, with a twisting obstruction at level of volvulus

6.17.2 SIGMOID VOLVULUS

IMAGING

AXR

grossly distended closed loop ('coffee bean' shape) arising out of left iliac fossa

loop classically lies in right upper quadrant (overlaps liver) but may lie under left hemidiaphragm

may have large bowel obstruction proximally

distal large bowel empty and collapsed

normal (or distended) cecum and flexures present and overlapped

Fluoro

barium fills distal large bowel with a smooth beak-like twist at point of volvulus – pathognomonic

7. CONDITIONS OF THE PERITONEUM

7.1 ASCITES

ETIOLOGY

Low protein

CIRRHOTIC (TRANSUDATE)

High protein

HEPATIC
BUDD–CHIARI SYNDROME
RIGHT HEART FAILURE
CONSTRICTIVE PERICARDITIS

INFECTIVE
BACTERIAL PERITONITIS
TB PERITONITIS

PANCREATITIS

Blood stained

HEPATOMA
PERITONEAL METASTASES
OVARIAN CARCINOMA

IMAGING

AXR

fluid density opacity in pelvis

separation of colon from properitoneal fat stripes

loss of hepatic outlines

separation of small bowel loops

diffuse swelling and haze without gaseous distension

US

shifting free intraperitoneal fluid

places where small volume ascites may 'hide' include rectovaginal or rectovesical pouch, hepatorenal pouch, very lateral flanks and between liver and right hemidiaphragm

CT/MR

fluid density/signal triangular material (unless hemorrhagic or purulent)

pouch of Douglas; paracolic gutters; between bowel loops; around liver (hepatorenal, perihepatic, subphrenic), around spleen, in lesser sac, around omentum

if bowel not opacified, may be difficult to confirm

7.2 HERNIAS

also see inguinal hernia entry in Ch 09

7.2.1 BOCHDALEK

CLINICAL

hernia through diaphragm between crus and posterior rib attachments (posteriorly located)

right or left sided

commonly contains fat only; may contain kidney, liver or bowel

CONGENITAL DIAPHRAGMATIC HERNIA IS A BOCHDALEK HERNIA (Ch 18)

IMAGING

posterior costophrenic angle mass

cross sectional imaging pathognomonic

7.2.2 HIATUS

see esophagus section

7.2.3 MORGAGNI

CLINICAL

hernia through diaphragm between attachment to sternum and anterior ribs (retrosternal foramen)

right or left sided (right more common)

can contain fat, omentum, colon; often contains liver if right sided

IMAGING

AXR/CXR

cardiophrenic mass with obtuse angles

differential is of anterior mediastinal mass but hernia has a diaphragmatic base

Fluoro

pathognomonic if colon or bowel in hernia

CT

good demonstration of liver herniation

7.2.4 TRAUMATIC

CLINICAL

early (1/3) or late (2/3) sequelae of traumatic diaphragmatic rupture (90% left diaphragm)

usually contains stomach; may cause strangulation of stomach or left colon

IMAGING

CXR

absent/abnormal contour of diaphragm

stomach or colon extend above diaphragm (classically in lateral costophrenic angle)

Fluoro

usually pathognomonic (differential is diaphragm eventration)

CT

may be difficult as diaphragm may be difficult to define

classically lateral extension of stomach or colon with a very thin interface to lung (viscus wall only)

if right sided, liver protrudes through defect

MR

allows coronal imaging, and may be only modality to show liver protrusion through the defect (with a constricting 'waist')

NUC MED

Tc-99m colloid injected into pleural or peritoneal space appearing in the other space

7.2.5 EPIGASTRIC

painful protrusion of fat through linea alba defect

IMAGING

US

may show fatty mass above line of linea alba with a defect if reducible

7.2.6 FEMORAL

CLINICAL

rare compared to inguinal hernia (may be difficult to distinguish)
commoner in females
hernia through femoral canal with hernial mass forming a bulge in medial thigh
tends to obstruct or strangulate

IMAGING

AXR

gas outside of expected peritoneal contours +/− bowel obstruction

CT

difficult if small
pathognomonic if bowel runs through femoral canal

7.2.7 INCISIONAL

may incarcerate, rarely strangulates (if neck narrow)

IMAGING

easiest with cross sectional imaging

7.2.8 UMBILICAL/ PARAUMBILICAL

also see Ch 18
protrusion of omentum or bowel through umbilical ring
may strangulate

IMAGING

US

fat or bowel pushing through rectus sheath

CT

pathognomonic if present

7.3 INFECTION
(manifestations)

7.3.1 NON SPECIFIC PERITONITIS

IMAGING

CT

free intraperitoneal fluid
variable amount of peritoneal enhancement
may be indistinguishable from ascites

PET

cause of peritoneal FDG activity (differential of peritoneal carcinomatosis)

7.3.2 PERITONEAL TB

IMAGING

CT

dense ascites
linear peritoneal enhancement
omental cake, ring enhancement
thickened mesentery, surface enhancement
TB adenopathy (low density core, ring enhancement)

7.4 MESENTERIC CYST

CLINICAL

contains serous, chylous or hemorrhagic fluid
often asymptomatic or may present with mass effect, bleed, tort, cause bowel obstruction
ENTERIC CYST: enteric epithelium only
DUPLICATION CYST: complete enteric wall; mesenteric side of bowel
LYMPHANGIOMA
MESOTHELIAL CYST

IMAGING

unilocular or multilocular fluid filled mass
thin wall except for enteric duplication cyst

ENTERIC DUPLICATION CYST has a thick wall resembling bowel wall, may enhance
content density and MR signal varies

7.5 SOLID MASS (overview)

Metastasis

7.5.1 Mesothelioma

7.5.2 Peritoneal/ retroperitoneal primary

7.5.2.1 NEUROFIBROMA

7.5.2.2 LEIOMYOMA/ LEIOMYOSARCOMA

7.5.2.3 LIPOMA/LIPOSARCOMA

7.5.2.4 FIBROUS TUMOR SPECTRUM
AGGRESSIVE FIBROMATOSIS = DESMOID TUMOR
MALIGNANT FIBROUS HISTIOCYTOMA/FIBROSARCOMA

7.6 PNEUMO-PERITONEUM

ETIOLOGY

Spontaneous
PERFORATION OF VISCUS (DU, GU, colonic diverticulum)

Other
see free air pitfalls gamut

IMAGING

AXR

ERECT/CXR
allow sufficient time for gas to migrate (e.g. 5–10 min)
subdiaphragmatic gas (differential interposed colon)
gas outlining falciform ligament
extramural air–fluid levels

LATERAL DECUBITUS/SUPINE LATERAL SHOOT THROUGH
free gas underlying lateral or anterior abdominal wall
particularly useful if between liver and body wall (i.e. use left lateral decubitus)

SUPINE AXR

gas around liver including hepatorenal gas

Rigler's sign: demonstration of single wall thickness by air inside and outside bowel (beware two loops containing air next to each other)

gas outlining extramural ligaments (usually only falciform ligament)

triangular air trapped between loops of bowel

non–anatomic rounded central air collection (football sign)

CT

extramural gas; use lung windows if in doubt

collects at highest points unless loculated

need to track bowel if in doubt

may identify source of perforation

7.7 RETROPERITONEAL FIBROSIS

see Ch 15

8. AIDS ABDOMEN OVERVIEWS

8.1 ESOPHAGUS

Acute HIV infection
giant usually solitary ulcer

Candida
diffuse ulceration, shaggy plaques

Herpes
multiple scattered shallow mucosal ulcers, may have edematous edge

Cytomegalovirus
discrete ulcers/giant ulcers

TB
usually by direct extension from mediastinal nodes (therefore focal extrinsic compression or focal mucosal thickening/stricture/ulceration/fistula)

Kaposi's sarcoma
discrete submucosal masses

8.2 STOMACH

Cytomegalovirus
edematous thick mucosa and wall, may be nodular

Kaposi's sarcoma
flat mucosal plaques; smooth submucosal nodules with or without central ulceration (umbilication) but normal mucosa elsewhere; involvement of muscularis; polypoid or sessile masses

8.3 SMALL BOWEL

Cryptosporidium
thick folds, dilation, fragmentation (malabsorption pattern)

Mycobacterium avium complex
mucosal change resembling Whipple's disease, wall thickening, MAC nodes

TB

Cytomegalovirus
thick nodular mucosa (esp ileum)

Kaposi's sarcoma
mucosal/submucosal nodules or wall thickening, may have umbilication; intervening mucosa normal

8.4 COLON

TB

Cytomegalovirus
colitis with variable ulceration and wall thickening (on CT, may enhance); may proceed to toxic megacolon

Lymphoma
bulky mass, no lymphadenopathy

Kaposi's sarcoma
nodular submucosal masses, malignant strictures

8.5 LIVER

Non specific hepatosplenomegaly

AIDS cholangitis
Cytomegalovirus (CMV) or Cryptosporidium; looks like sclerosing cholangitis; may have gallbladder wall thickening

TB
focal or multifocal masses

Mycobacterium avium complex
diffuse hepatomegaly, lymphadenopathy; may have focal low density masses

Candidiasis
part of disseminated candidiasis; multiple small abscesses

Kaposi's sarcoma/bacillary angiomatosis
multifocal periportal infiltrate; small intraparenchymal nodules; hyperechoic on US, low density possibly enhancing masses on CT; may be vascular on angio

Cytomegalovirus
tiny hypoechoic and later calcified foci

Pneumocystis
tiny calcified foci

Lymphoma
usually aggressive non Hodgkin's lymphoma; solitary or multiple hypoechoic small or large low density masses in liver and spleen; lymphadenopathy (differential: reactive only, MAC/TB, KS)

8.6 SPLEEN

Microabscesses
usually bacterial

TB/Mycobacterium avium complex/fungi
usually granulomatous masses; may have low density diffuse splenomegaly; associated lymphadenopathy

Disseminated CMV

tiny calcified foci

Disseminated pneumocystis

tiny calcified foci

Lymphoma

8.7 KIDNEYS

HIV nephropathy

increased echogenicity

Microabscesses

as for liver/spleen

Lymphoma

8.8 LYMPHADENOPATHY

SPECIFIC CAUSE CAN NOT BE DIAGNOSED
ON IMAGING ALONE

**Persistent generalized
lymphadenopathy ('reactive')**

RETROPERITONEAL ONLY, <1.5 cm

TB

low density core, ring enhancing

**Mycobacterium avium
complex**

soft tissue density

Lymphoma

soft tissue or low density

Kaposi's sarcoma

vividly enhancing

8.9 KAPOSI'S SARCOMA

also see Ch 13

ETIOLOGY

Human herpes virus 8

Non HIV

rare, elderly males

HIV (50% overall)

SKIN 90%
LYMPH NODES 70%
LUNGS 50%
GUT 50% (duodenum most common, but
 may occur anywhere)
LIVER/SPLEEN 30%

MACRO

vascular mass
appearance depends on location

MICRO

spindle epithelial cells
slit-like vessels
lymphocytic infiltrate

1. NORMAL

1.1 NORMAL IDA SCAN

Tracers

IDA: imino-diacetic acid (basic molecule forming core part of Tc-99m biliary tracers)

HIDA: 'hepatic' IDA (dimethyl IDA, lidofenin)

DISIDA: disopropyl IDA, disofenin

BrIDA: bromotriethyl IDA, mebrofenin

Time at which structures become visible

LIVER at 5 min
BILIARY TREE by 10 min
GALLBLADDER by 30 min
DUODENUM by 30 min
KIDNEYS <2–3% of dose

If no gallbladder showing

?not fasted

see discussion under acute cholecystitis – further maneuvers

1.2 NORMAL SULFUR COLLOID (LIVER/SPLEEN) SCAN

UPTAKE INTENSITY: LIVER > SPLEEN > BONE MARROW

1.3 NORMAL LIVER DOPPLER US

Portal vein

gently phasic, up to 30 cm/s hepatopetal

Hepatic vein

triphasic (atrial filling with dicrotic notch due to ventricular relaxation; transient reversal during atrial contraction)

difference reduced at Valsalva

NB tricuspid regurgitation: biphasic with reversal

Normal transjugular portocaval shunt

up to 200 cm/s

1.4 NORMAL LIVER MR

Sequences

T1W FSE, T2W FSE, chemical shift (in phase out of phase), Gd contrast, ferrumoxides (RESOVIST)

Normal liver appearance

brighter than spleen on T1W sequences

darker than spleen on T2W sequences

in phase out of phase detects fatty change

Gd functions similarly to CT contrast

20–30s is hepatic arterial phase

70s is portal venous phase

ferrumoxides function similarly to sulfur colloid: demonstrate presence of normal Kupffer cells

1.5 NORMAL PANCREAS MR

high T1W signal (remains high with fat sat, due to proteinaceous content), isointense T2W signal

adenocarcinoma is hypovascular, islet cell tumors hypervascular

therefore, suggest fat sat T1W, T2W, and fat sat dynamic contrast enhanced sequences

1.6 NORMAL DUCTS

Duct diameters
After R.N. Gibson (1995)
INTRAHEPATIC 2–5 mm
CBD <60 years old: 5 mm (SD 2 mm)
CBD 60–70 years old: 6 mm (SD 3 mm)
CBD >70 years old: 8 mm (SD 4 mm)
PANCREATIC DUCT <60 years old: 3 mm (SD 1 mm)
PANCREATIC DUCT >60 years old: 3.5 mm (SD 1 mm)

1.7 LIVER SEGMENTAL ANATOMY (Couinaud segments)

Division planes

HORIZONTAL IS PLANE OF PORTA HEPATIS

on sectional imaging this is the axial slice with the two branches of the portal vein originating from the portal vein itself

VERTICAL PLANES ARE THE HEPATIC VEINS

middle hepatic vein separates functional right lobe from the functional left lobe

right hepatic vein separates the right anterior sector from the right posterior sector

left hepatic vein separates the functional left lobe medial sector (towards the midline of the LIVER, comprises quadrate lobe) from the left lobe lateral sector (the tip of the left lobe)

CAUDATE LOBE is not a part of either lobe

Segmental numbering

numbering starts at caudate lobe, descends along left lobe, crosses to right lobe, ascends to under the dome

1 caudate lobe
2 left lobe lateral upper segment
3 left lobe lateral lower segment
4a left lobe medial upper segment = quadrate lobe upper segment
4b left lobe medial lower segment = quadrate lobe lower segment
5 right lobe anterior lower segment
6 right lobe posterior lower segment
7 right lobe posterior upper segment
8 right lobe anterior upper segment

Biliary drainage

CONVENTIONAL PATTERN

right anterior and posterior sectorial ducts form the right lobar duct (right posterior sectorial duct arches over the right portal vein)

left medial and lateral sectorial ducts (left medial sectorial duct drains the quadrate lobe) form the left lobar duct

caudate drains to left side, or both

COMMON VARIANTS

right anterior, right posterior and left lobar
    ducts form a three way confluence
right anterior sectorial duct inserts into the
    left lobar duct
right posterior sectorial duct inserts into the
    left lobar duct

IMPORTANT VARIANT

sectorial or segmental duct (often right
    sided) inserts directly into the common
    hepatic or common bile duct

2. GAMUTS

2.1 GENERIC (all modalities)

2.1.1 BEADED BILE DUCTS

BACTERIAL CHOLANGITIS

AIDS CHOLANGITIS

PRIMARY SCLEROSING
    CHOLANGITIS

PARASITIC CHOLANGITIS

MULTIFOCAL
    CHOLANGIOCARCINOMA

NO RELIABLE DIFFERENTIATOR
    BETWEEN DOMINANT BENIGN
    STRICTURE AND
    CHOLANGIOCARCINOMA!

2.1.2 BILIARY DILATION VS OBSTRUCTION

Signs

BIOCHEMICAL

rising conjugated bilirubin and cholestatic
    liver enzymes do not differentiate
    intrahepatic cholestasis from biliary tree
    obstruction

MORPHOLOGICAL

! dilation does not equal obstruction !
CARDINAL SIGN: BILIARY TREE DILATION
if smooth and involving entire tree,
    probability of obstruction depends on size
    of ducts
if sharp transition zone, obstruction likely
ALWAYS ABNORMAL IF
segmental
a high transition zone
double duct sign present (dilation of both
    CBD and pancreatic duct implying
    obstruction at level of ampulla)

FUNCTIONAL

evidence of obstruction with IDA, CT
    intravenous cholangiogram (CTIVC) or
    ERCP (not MRCP)

CTIVC

delay in contrast excretion AND an
    obstructive level
study may also demonstrate cause

IDA

good uptake by liver
no biliary opacification (high grade
    obstruction)
delay in opacification of biliary tree, dilated
    biliary tree, delay in biliary to bowel
    transit
progressive hepatocyte dysfunction and
    rising bilirubin levels eventually make
    differentiation from intrahepatic
    cholestasis impossible

Differential

HIGH OBSTRUCTION

BENIGN
IATROGENIC
MIRIZZI'S SYNDROME
PARASITES, INFECTIVE CHOLANGITIS
SCLEROSING CHOLANGITIS
COMPRESSION BY LIVER MASS

MALIGNANT
GALLBLADDER CHOLANGIOCARCINOMA
KLATZKIN CHOLANGIOCARCINOMA
METASTASES OR PORTAL NODES

MID LEVEL OBSTRUCTION

BENIGN
IATROGENIC
GALLSTONES
HEMOBILIA AND CLOT
PARASITES, INFECTIVE CHOLANGITIS
SCLEROSING CHOLANGITIS
CHRONIC PANCREATITIS

MALIGNANT
CHOLANGIOCARCINOMA
LYMPH NODES

LOW (AMPULLARY) OBSTRUCTION

BENIGN
GALLSTONES
IATROGENIC STRICTURE
CHOLEDOCHAL CYST
PANCREATITIS

MALIGNANT
PANCREATIC CARCINOMA
AMPULLARY CHOLANGIOCARCINOMA

DILATION WITHOUT OBSTRUCTION

by definition, no functional evidence of
    biliary obstruction

RELIEVED OBSTRUCTION

spontaneous passage of stone
surgical or endoscopic intervention

AGE RELATED NORMAL

REFLUX

usually following biliary to enteric
    anastomoses

ECTASIA

choledochal cyst and related conditions

BENIGN VS MALIGNANT STRICTURE

*probability of a stricture being benign versus
malignant is analogous to intestinal stricture
– see Ch 06*

2.1.3 HEPATOMEGALY

Metabolic

FATTY LIVER CHANGE AND EARLY
    CIRRHOSIS

Infective

VIRAL HEPATITIS (hepatitic viruses, EBV)

HYDATIDS

MALARIA

Syndromic

POLYCYSTIC LIVER

Vascular

PASSIVE CARDIAC CONGESTION

Tumors and mimickers

METASTASES

LYMPHOMA

HEPATOCELLULAR CARCINOMA

EXTRAMEDULLARY HEMOPOIESIS

MYELOFIBROSIS

HEMOGLOBINOPATHIES

Storage disorders

AMYLOID

GAUCHER'S

GLYCOGEN AND LIPID STORAGE
    DISEASES

2.1.4 ISOLATED GALLBLADDER MASS

STONE

ADENOMYOSIS

POLYP

CARCINOMA

2.1.5 ISOLATED LIVER MASS

See section 5 for imaging differentiation of these!

Non tumoral mass

CYST

FOCAL FATTY CHANGE – not a true mass

FOCAL FATTY SPARING – not a true mass

ABSCESS

FOCAL NODULAR HYPERPLASIA

REGENERATING NODULE

Premalignant mass

DYSPLASTIC NODULE

Benign tumor

HEMANGIOMA

HEMANGIOENDOTHELIOMA (CH 18)

HEPATOCELLULAR ADENOMA

Malignant tumor

METASTASIS

HEPATOCELLULAR CARCINOMA

HEPATOBLASTOMA (CH 18)

CHOLANGIOCARCINOMA

ANGIOSARCOMA

2.1.6 ISOLATED PANCREATIC MASS

Non tumoral mass

PANCREATITIS, NECROSIS

RETENTION CYST

PSEUDOCYST

ABSCESS

Tumor

ADENOCARCINOMA NOS

'CYSTIC TUMOR'

ISLET CELL TUMOR

METASTASIS, LYMPHOMA

2.1.7 ISOLATED SPLENIC MASS

LYMPHOMA, METASTASIS (especially melanoma)

HEMATOMA, ABSCESS

HEMANGIOMA

2.1.8 JAUNDICE

with increasing jaundice there is deteriorating uptake of IDA tracers and CTIVC contrast by the liver, eventually making these examinations non diagnostic

Unconjugated

INCREASED BILIRUBIN PRODUCTION
ACUTE HEMOLYSIS, HEMOLYTIC ANEMIAS
HEMOGLOBINOPATHIES
RESORPTION OF MASSIVE HEMATOMAS
DRUGS

DECREASED LIVER UPTAKE OF BILIRUBIN
DRUGS

DECREASED CONJUGATION
PREGNANCY PHYSIOLOGIC
NEONATAL PHYSIOLOGIC
BREAST MILK JAUNDICE
CRIGLER–NAJJAR SYNDROME, GILBERT SYNDROME
HEPATOCYTE INJURY

Conjugated

DECREASED HEPATOCYTE EXCRETION
DRUGS
DUBIN–JOHNSON SYNDROME, ROTOR SYNDROME
HEPATOCYTE INJURY

INTRAHEPATIC OBSTRUCTION
PRIMARY BILIARY CIRRHOSIS
SCLEROSING CHOLANGITIS
CONGENITAL BILIARY CIRRHOSIS

EXTRAHEPATIC OBSTRUCTION
see biliary obstruction gamut

2.1.9 SPLENOMEGALY

see Ch 16

2.2.1 BILIARY GAS VS PORTAL VENOUS GAS

Biliary gas
central and vertical

IATROGENIC
CHOLEDOCHOENTEROSTOMY
CHOLECYSTOENTEROSTOMY
ENDOSCOPIC SPHINCTEROTOMY

FISTULA
MALIGNANT
BENIGN (gallstone ileus, peptic)

SPONTANEOUS
INCOMPETENT SPHINCTER

Portal venous gas
peripheral and horizontal

ALWAYS OF GRAVE PROGNOSTIC SIGNIFICANCE
mesenteric ischemia/bowel infarction
intestinal gas gangrene
necrotizing enterocolitis – neonates

2.2.2 CALCIFICATION

see Ch 06

2.3 US

2.3.1 DIFFUSE LIVER CHANGE ON US

Bright
ACUTE FATTY LIVER
CHRONIC HEPATITIS
CIRRHOSIS (look for nodules)
MALIGNANT INFILTRATION
STORAGE DISEASE

Dark
ACUTE HEPATITIS
MALIGNANT INFILTRATION

2.3.2 ISOLATED CYSTIC LESION

! ensure there is no continuation with biliary tree and no vascular flow !

CYST

HYDATID CYST

BILOMA

HEMATOMA

ABSCESS

CYSTIC TUMOR

2.3.3 ISOLATED (FOCAL) LIVER CHANGE ON US

Bright

FOCAL FATTY CHANGE

HEMANGIOMA

FOCAL NODULAR HYPERPLASIA, ADENOMA, HEPATOCELLULAR CARCINOMA

GIT, UGT METASTASIS

HEMATOMA, ABSCESS

Dark

METASTASIS, LYMPHOMA

HEPATOCELLULAR CARCINOMA

HEMATOMA, ABSCESS

HEMANGIOMA

FOCAL FATTY SPARING

FUNGAL ABSCESS (has a central bright spot)

2.3.4 THICK GALLBLADDER WALL

defined as >3 mm

Contracted gallbladder

Cholecystitis

Other

CIRRHOSIS

NEPHROTIC SYNDROME

CONGESTIVE CARDIAC FAILURE

HYPOALBUMINEMIA

TUMOR

2.4 CT

2.4.1 ABDOMINAL TRAUMA CT CHECKLIST

Soft tissue windows

FREE BLOOD

RETROPERITONEAL BLOOD

PANCREATIC/DUODENAL INJURY

BLADDER INJURY

Lung windows

RUPTURED DUODENUM

FREE INTRAPERITONEAL GAS

Bone windows

RIB FRACTURES

SPINAL AND PELVIC FRACTURES

Liver windows

LIVER + SPLEEN LACERATIONS

Check area: diaphragm

2.4.2 ARTERIAL PHASE ENHANCING MASS (adult)

ANEURYSM AND RELATED CONDITIONS
arterialized hemangioma
arteriovenous malformation

FOCAL NODULAR HYPERPLASIA

ADENOMA

HEPATOCELLULAR CARCINOMA
including FIBROLAMELLAR variant

HYPERVASCULAR METASTASIS

2.4.3 CYSTIC NEOPLASMS ON IMAGING

see Ch 06

2.4.4 DIFFUSE LIVER CHANGE ON CT

Low density

FATTY LIVER

AMYLOID

STORAGE DISEASES

High density

HEMOCHROMATOSIS

HEMOSIDEROSIS

GLYCOGEN STORAGE DISEASES

AMIODARONE THERAPY

GOLD THERAPY (in rheumatoid arthritis)

2.4.5 PERIPORTAL TRACKING

Signs
low density (CT) or hypoechoic (US) cuffing surrounding portal structures

Differential diagnosis

TRAUMA

CONGESTIVE HEPATOMEGALY

MALIGNANT LYMPHATIC OBSTRUCTION

2.4.6 VASCULAR MASS WITH CENTRAL SCAR

FOCAL NODULAR HYPERPLASIA

FIBROLAMELLAR HEPATOCELLULAR CARCINOMA

HYPERVASCULAR METASTASIS WITH SCAR

HEMANGIOMA WITH SCAR
DIFFERENT ENHANCEMENT FROM REST OF THIS GROUP

2.5 MR

2.5.1 DIFFUSE LOW T1W LOW T2W SIGNAL

HEMOCHROMATOSIS

HEMOSIDEROSIS

MILD ALCOHOLIC CIRRHOSIS

2.5.2 ISOLATED AREA OF HIGH T1W SIGNAL

BLOOD (especially in adenoma)

FAT IN FOCAL FATTY CHANGE

FATTY CHANGE IN ADENOMA

FATTY CHANGE IN HEPATOCELLULAR
CARCINOMA

MELANIN

REGENERATING NODULE IN
CIRRHOTIC LIVER

2.5.3 ISOLATED (FOCAL) MASS

see isolated liver mass gamut in generic
gamuts and section 5 for MR findings for
each of these!

2.6 NUC MED

2.6.1 GALLIUM

2/3 of hepatomas hot, rest isointense or cold
adenomas and focal nodular hyperplasia
may be hot
lymphoma and melanoma usually hotter
than background liver

2.6.2 IDA

Hot mass
mechanism is late trapping with impaired
washout
FOCAL NODULAR HYPERPLASIA
ADENOMA
HEPATOCELLULAR CARCINOMA

Isointense mass
FOCAL NODULAR HYPERPLASIA
ADENOMA
HEPATOCELLULAR CARCINOMA
FATTY CHANGE OR SPARING – not a true
mass

Cold mass
CYST
HEMANGIOMA
METASTASIS
HEPATOCELLULAR CARCINOMA
CHOLANGIOCARCINOMA
ANY NON HEPATOCYTE CONTAINING
TUMOR

2.6.3 RBC

Hot mass
HEMANGIOMA

Isointense mass
FATTY CHANGE OR SPARING – not a true
mass

Cold mass
ALL OTHER MASSES

2.6.4 SULFUR COLLOID

**Diffuse nodular uptake,
colloid shift**
reduced liver uptake, increased splenic and
bone marrow uptake
CIRRHOSIS

Hot mass
FOCAL NODULAR HYPERPLASIA (this is
helpful)
CAUDATE LOBE IN BUDD–CHIARI
SYNDROME

Isointense mass
FATTY CHANGE OR SPARING – not a true
mass

Cold mass
no perfusion or no Kupffer cells
CYST
HEMANGIOMA
FOCAL NODULAR HYPERPLASIA
METASTASIS
ADENOMA
HEPATOCELLULAR CARCINOMA
CHOLANGIOCARCINOMA

HEPATO-PANCREATOBILIARY CONDITIONS

3. DIFFUSE LIVER DISEASE

3.1 ACUTE HEPATITIS

DEFINITION

acute diffuse inflammatory disorder of
hepatic parenchyma with direct or
immune mediated hepatocyte injury

ETIOLOGY

VIRAL HEPATITIS (HAV, HEV, HBV, HDV,
HCV)
VIRAL DISEASE, LIVER INVOLVED (EBV,
CMV, HSV)
DRUG INDUCED AUTOIMMUNE
ACUTE TOXIC INJURY (ALCOHOL, TOXINS)
ACUTE EXACERBATION OF METABOLIC
LIVER DISEASE

MORPHOLOGY

diffuse hepatocyte injury, random patchy
necrosis
reactive infiltrate, regenerative response

IMAGING

US
commonly normal or hepatomegaly
spectrum from diffuse fatty change to diffuse
hypoechoic liver
often hepatomegaly
no biliary tree dilation by definition

CT
spectrum from diffuse fatty change to
normal

NUC MED
IDA
normal or evidence of hepatic insufficiency
(poor uptake, poor biliary excretion,
increased renal excretion)

3.2 ALCOHOLIC LIVER DISEASE

CLINICAL

ACUTE ALCOHOLIC HEPATITIS

CHRONIC ALCOHOLIC HEPATITIS

CIRRHOSIS

ACUTE LIVER DECOMPENSATION
HEPATIC ENCEPHALOPATHY
PORTAL HYPERTENSIVE BLEED
! spontaneous bacterial peritonitis

HEPATOMA (15% of cirrhosis)

MORPHOLOGY

Fatty liver
large droplet/small droplet

Chronic alcoholic hepatitis
focal necrosis, attempted regeneration

CHARACTERISTIC FEATURES

Mallory bodies
megamitochondria
increased hepatocyte iron
pericellular neutrophils
pericellular active fibrosis

Alcoholic cirrhosis

shrinking liver, large caudate and left lobes
micro then macronodular cirrhosis

Portal hypertension

IMAGING

see fatty change, acute hepatitis, cirrhosis, portal hypertension

3.3 ALPHA 1 ANTITRYPSIN (alpha 1 AT) DEFICIENCY

see Ch 18

3.4 ASCITES

see Ch 06

3.5 AUTOIMMUNE HEPATITIS

DEFINITION

hepatitis secondary to clearly documented autoimmune processes in the PROVEN ABSENCE of viral markers and underlying metabolic abnormalities

CLINICAL

female > male, young or middle aged
80% have autoantibodies: antinuclear, anti smooth muscle cell, antimicrosomal

Associated conditions

ULCERATIVE COLITIS
RHEUMATOID ARTHRITIS/SJÖGREN'S SYNDROME
AUTOIMMUNE THYROID DISEASE
IMMUNE PULMONARY FIBROSIS

3.6 CHRONIC HEPATITIS

DEFINITION

chronic (by definition >6 months) diffuse inflammatory disorder of hepatic parenchyma commonly with immune mechanism involvement

ETIOLOGY

Chronic viral hepatitis

HBV, HDV, HCV

Drug induced autoimmune hepatitis

isoniazid, alpha methyldopa, etc

Autoimmune hepatitis

see its own entry

Non immune hepatitis

ALCOHOLIC OR TOXIC LIVER DISEASE

METABOLIC LIVER DISEASE

ADULT
HEMOCHROMATOSIS, HEMOSIDEROSIS
WILSON'S DISEASE
MUCOPOLYSACCHARIDOSES, GAUCHER'S, STORAGE DISORDERS

CHILD
CYSTIC FIBROSIS
STORAGE DISORDERS
SUGAR METABOLISM ERRORS

BILIARY CIRRHOSIS

ADULT
PRIMARY BILIARY CIRRHOSIS
SECONDARY BILIARY CIRRHOSIS
SCLEROSING CHOLANGITIS

CHILD
ALPHA 1 ANTITRYPSIN DEFICIENCY
NEONATAL HEPATITIS SPECTRUM
BILIARY ATRESIA SPECTRUM
BILIARY DILATION SPECTRUM

PATHOGENESIS

fluctuating or progressive destruction of individual cell groups with slow fibrosis and variable regeneration
underlying process ranges from clearly extrinsic injury (non immune hepatitis) through interaction of external and immune factors to clearly autoimmune

merges into cirrhosis
increased risk of hepatoma, very increased in HBV, HDV, HCV

MORPHOLOGY

range from hepatomegaly to normal to shrunken liver
similar for different etiologies, graded on histological activity

Chronic persistent hepatitis

lymphocyte and mononuclear infiltrate limited to portal tracts
occasional focal parenchymal necrosis
preservation of liver architecture

Chronic active hepatitis (five features)

severe form that often progresses to cirrhosis

I. NECROSIS
degeneration, piecemeal necrosis, focal necrosis, confluent necrosis

II. IMMUNE INFILTRATE
portal or parenchymal

III. FIBROSIS
active fibrosis
passive fibrosis (through parenchymal collapse)

IV. REGENERATION

V. BILIARY LESIONS (epithelial hyperplasia)

IMAGING

see fatty change, cirrhosis, portal hypertension

3.7 CIRRHOSIS

DEFINITION

global and diffuse PROGRESSIVE destruction of hepatocytes and reticulin skeleton with IRREVERSIBLE architectural and vascular disorganization together with fibrosis and regeneration

ETIOLOGY

see chronic hepatitis

Western adults

ALCOHOL 60%
VIRAL HEPATITIS 15%
BILIARY (1RY OR 2RY) 10%
IRON OVERLOAD 5%
METABOLIC DISEASE 1%

PATHOGENESIS

Nature of mechanism

underlying process ranges from clearly
extrinsic injury (non immune hepatitis)
through interaction of external and
immune factors to clearly autoimmune

Parenchymal disease

loss of hepatocytes
collapse and loss of reticulin skeleton
inflammatory infiltrate (except
hemochromatosis)
abnormal fibrosis (bridging fibrosis allows
shunts)
regeneration by hepatocytes (regenerative
hyperplastic nodule–adenomatous nodule
–dysplastic nodule–hepatocellular
carcinoma sequence)
persistence and chronicity

Architectural distortion

irreversible loss of histoarchitecture
(bridging fibrosis, loss of ordered flow,
bypassed hepatocyte islands)
altered flow dynamics (shunts, increased
resistance)
reduction in metabolic exchange surface
area
increase in diffusion distance

CLINICAL

metabolic liver failure
synthetic liver failure
portal hypertension, thrombosis, varices
infection (especially spontaneous bacterial
peritonitis)
hepatoma

MORPHOLOGY

typical sequence is of enlarged liver with
islands and patches of fatty change
progressing to eventual shrunken hard
nodular liver
MACRONODULAR CIRRHOSIS (nodules
>3 mm)
MICRONODULAR CIRRHOSIS (nodules
<3 mm)
hyperplasia of lobes with preserved venous
drainage and/or portal inflow: caudate
and left lobes

IMAGING (cirrhosis and regenerating nodules)

*see fatty change and portal hypertension
separately*

AXR

no findings or hepatomegaly

US

ARCHITECTURE

small liver, relatively enlarged caudate and
left lobes
irregular nodularity (macro or micro)
nodular edge (use linear array)
fibrotic bands with distortion of architecture
disorganized portal tree, loss of portal
architecture
lost hepatic veins
large nodules often have mass effect on
vasculature

ECHOGENICITY

generally increased, may be patchy

CT

ARCHITECTURE

as in US

ENHANCEMENT

non contrast: nodules usually isodense to
fibrosis
any fatty change readily visible
post contrast: nodules enhance variably
depending on degree of hepatic arterial
versus portal venous supply; fibrous scar
enhances less
geographic areas of arterial enhancement
where portal vein branches are
thrombosed
rounded mass like area of arterial
enhancement is suspicious for HCC
dominant mass is suspicious for HCC

MR

ARCHITECTURE

better contrast between nodules and scarred
septa than CT
cirrhotic background: diffuse decrease in
T1W signal and increase in T2W signal

REGENERATING NODULES AND DYSPLASTIC NODULES

non siderotic nodules higher on T1W and
lower on T2W than scar
siderotic nodules low on both T1W and T2W
(regenerating nodules accumulate iron)
central focus of high T2W inside a
regenerating nodule suspicious for an in
situ HCC

absence of change of signal in a nodule does
not rule out a small focus of HCC

ENHANCEMENT PATTERNS

similar to CT (arterial versus portal venous
phase)

NUC MED

IDA

eventual hepatic parenchymal failure with
prolonged uptake time, reduced
parenchymal uptake, decreased biliary
secretion and increased renal excretion

COLLOID

shunting of uptake to spleen and bone
marrow ('colloid shift')
clumpy heterogeneous poor liver uptake

3.8 FATTY CHANGE AND FATTY SPARING

DEFINITION

diffuse or focal reversible accumulation of
intracellular fat as a result of impaired
metabolic capacity

ETIOLOGY

ALCOHOL
DIABETES
ULCERATIVE COLITIS/CROHN'S DISEASE
STEROID TREATMENT
RIGHT HEART FAILURE

3.8.1 IMAGING (focal fatty change)

NO MASS EFFECT ON ANY MODALITY
frequent position: adjacent to gallbladder,
falciform ligament

AXR

no findings or hepatomegaly

US

DIFFUSE FATTY CHANGE

diffusely increased echogenicity
+/– coarse echotexture, loss of brighter
portal tract walls, obscuration of smaller
vessels
no mass effect
preserved vascular architecture, no
displacement of vessels

FOCAL FATTY CHANGE

same echotexture as in diffuse fatty change
geographic margins

may conform to vascular territory

no mass effect, no distortion of vessels passing through

CT

geographic area (as above)

precontrast, decreased liver density compared to normal liver

hepatic and portal veins show as denser structures in low density parenchyma

still lower density post contrast, but may be masked by contrast

MR

geographic area (as above)

increased T1W signal, no change in T2W signal relative to rest of liver

can use fat saturation sequences (decreases signal of focal fatty change towards that of normal liver)

in phase–out of phase imaging most sensitive (signal drops towards normal liver)

Ferrumoxides sequences show normal loss of signal (normal Kupffer cell function)

NUC MED

normal liver colloid scan (normal Kupffer cell function)

very helpful in larger areas of focal fatty change or sparing

3.8.2 IMAGING (focal fatty sparing)

NO MASS EFFECT ON ANY MODALITY

common position: adjacent to gallbladder, falciform ligament, caudate lobe

AXR

no findings or hepatomegaly

US

DIFFUSE FATTY CHANGE

diffusely increased echogenicity

+/– coarse echotexture, loss of brighter portal tract walls, obscuration of smaller vessels

no mass effect

preserved vascular architecture, no displacement of vessels

FOCAL FATTY SPARING

lower echotexture relative to diffuse fatty change elsewhere

geographic margins

may conform to vascular territory

no mass effect, no distortion of vessels passing through

CT

geographic

precontrast, increased liver density compared to diffusely fatty liver elsewhere

hepatic and portal veins show as hypodense in higher density parenchyma of focal fatty sparing, and as hyperdense in fatty liver elsewhere

greater density of sparing preserved with contrast, but may be masked

MR

geographic

decreased T1W signal (relative to rest of liver), no change in T2W signal

can use fat saturation sequences (decrease signal of rest of liver towards the signal of the fatty sparing area)

in phase–out of phase imaging most sensitive (rest of liver signal drops to that of focal area)

Ferrumoxides sequences show normal loss of signal (normal Kupffer cell function) in focal fatty sparing and rest of liver

NUC MED

normal liver colloid scan (normal Kupffer cell function)

very helpful in larger areas of focal fatty change or sparing

3.9 FULMINANT HEPATIC NECROSIS

DEFINITION

severe acute destruction of hepatic parenchyma (by definition, progression over 2–3 weeks)

ETIOLOGY

Toxic

DRUGS (Acetaminophen/paracetamol)

INDUSTRIAL (CCl_4)

POISONING

Infective

VIRAL HEPATITIS

Vascular

TRANSPLANT ISCHEMIA

?Immune

HALOTHANE

ECLAMPSIA

CLINICAL

tender hepatomegaly, then rapidly shrinking liver

acute liver failure

encephalopathy and death

3.10 GLYCOGEN STORAGE DISEASE

deficiency or dysfunction of a glycogen metabolism enzyme leading to abnormal accumulation of glycogen and glycogen products typically with hepatomegaly and liver failure, myocardial involvement and cardiomyopathy

EPONYM (Type): Von Gierke (I), Pompe (II), Cori (III), Andersen (IV), McArdle (V), Hers (VI)

3.11 HEMOCHROMATOSIS

DEFINITION

abnormally increased intestinal iron absorption leading to iron toxicity in target organs

EPIDEMIOLOGY

autosomal recessive, chromosome 6, 1/250 Europeans

male >> female (menstrual loss); usually over 50 years old at presentation

ETIOLOGY

loss of feedback control over gut iron absorption

symptoms after total 20 g body iron (normal is 5 g)

CLINICAL ('bronze diabetes')

hepatocyte hemosiderin accumulation and micronodular cirrhosis (cell loss WITHOUT inflammation) with 200x risk of hepatoma

80% diabetes mellitus + pancreatic atrophy
80% iron and melanin skin pigmentation
AND
accelerated CPPD and synovial deposits
myocardial hemosiderosis + fibrosis
(cardiomyopathy and arrhythmias)
testicular atrophy

IMAGING

GOLD STANDARD: total unfixed liver iron
content

CT

increased liver density (need precontrast
scans); HU 100–140
signs of cirrhosis
eventual multifocal hepatocellular
carcinomas

MR

increased liver iron leads to decreased T2W
signal, mildly decreased T1W signal
GRE sequences more sensitive than FSE
eventual multifocal hepatocellular
carcinomas – tend to have less iron and
therefore more T2W signal

DIFFERENTIAL

Hemosiderosis (deposition of iron in liver
and spleen macrophages – spleen
changes also present; spleen is normal in
hemochromatosis)

3.13 LIVER DISEASE IN PREGNANCY

3.13.1 ACUTE FATTY LIVER OF PREGNANCY

3.13.2 INTRAHEPATIC CHOLESTASIS

3.13.3 PREECLAMPSIA WITH HELLP SYNDROME

see preeclampsia Ch 22
H-EMOLYSIS, E-LEVATED L-FTs, L-OW
P-LATELETS

3.14 LIVER FAILURE

DEFINITION

residual functional capacity insufficient for
metabolic needs (<10%)
independent of portal hypertension and the
two can occur separately or together

ETIOLOGY AND CLASSIFICATION

Acute

TOXIC
DRUGS (e.g. Acetaminophen/paracetamol)
INDUSTRIAL (e.g. CCl_4, phosphorus)
TOXINS/POISONS
HALOTHANE, REYE HEPATITIS

ECLAMPSIA (MICROVASCULITIS)

INFECTIVE
FULMINANT INFECTIVE HEPATITIS

Chronic

FINAL COMMON PATHWAY OF CIRRHOSIS,
METABOLIC OR STORAGE DISEASE

MANIFESTATIONS

Metabolic failure

ascites
conjugated jaundice (intrahepatic excretion
deteriorates ahead of conjugation)
hyperestrogenism (gonads, gynecomastia,
liver palms, spider nevi)
hyperammonemia
hepatorenal syndrome
hepatic encephalopathy (portosystemic
shunts contribute)

Synthetic failure

hypoalbuminemia, coagulopathy,
(hypoglycemia)

IMAGING

see imaging section of cirrhosis entry
IDA scans and CTIVC show no liver uptake

3.15 MAJOR HEPATITIS VIRUSES

CLINICAL

HAV

fecal–oral spread, acute epidemic disease
fulminant disease 0.1%

3.12 LIPID STORAGE DISEASES

Disease	Enzyme defect	Lipid	Tissue involved	Clinical	Microscopy
Tay–Sachs	hexosaminidase A	GM2 gangliosde	brain, retina	cherry red macula	foamy cytoplasm
Gaucher	glucocerebrosidase	gluco-cerebroside	liver, spleen, bone, brain	hepatomegaly, splenomegaly	fibrillary cytoplasm
Niemann–Pick	sphingomyelinase	sphingomyelin	brain, liver, spleen		parallel lamellas (zebra bodies)
Metachromatic leukodystrophy	arylsulfatase A	sulfatide	brain, kidney, liver, nerves		
Fabry	A-galactosidase	ceramide trihexoside	skin, kidney		
Krabbe	Galacto-sylceramidase	galacto-cerebroside	brain		

HEV
fecal–oral spread, acute epidemic disease
20% mortality in pregnancy

HBV
parenteral/sexual spread
vertical transmission at birth (gives carrier
    status)

ACUTE DISEASE
subclinical disease 60%, acute disease 25%,
    fulminant disease 1%

PERSISTENT DISEASE – INCREASED INCIDENCE OF HEPATOMA
persistent infection 5%, healthy carrier 5%
    (most of vertical), frank cirrhosis 1%,
    ???% with DNA integration

HDV

COINFECTION WITH HBV
90% recover with immunity
5% fulminant disease

SUPERINFECTION OF HBV
80% chronic disease with cirrhosis

HCV
parenteral
sexual transmission less important ??
75% SUBCLINICAL DISEASE, 25% MILD
    ACUTE DISEASE, 1% FULMINANT
    DISEASE
50% PROGRESS TO CHRONIC DISEASE AND
    CIRRHOSIS WITH HEPATOMA
    (controversial statistic)

3.17 PORTAL HYPERTENSION

DEFINITION

abnormally elevated portal venous system
    pressure (see normal liver ultrasound
    and portal hypertension on US gamut for
    criteria of portal hypertension)

ETIOLOGY

Adult

3.17.1 POSTHEPATIC
BUDD–CHIARI SYNDROME

3.17.2 HEPATIC
CIRRHOSIS (see etiology of chronic hepatitis)
ALCOHOLIC
VIRAL
AUTOIMMUNE
METABOLIC
BILIARY CIRRHOSIS

HEPATOCELLULAR CARCINOMA

METASTASES

3.17.3 PREHEPATIC
BLAND THROMBOSIS
COAGULOPATHY
COMPRESSION
IDIOPATHIC

SEPTIC THROMBOSIS

TUMOR THROMBOSIS

SCHISTOSOMIASIS

Child

3.17.4 POST HEPATIC
IVC WEBS
BUDD–CHIARI SYNDROME

3.17.5 HEPATIC
CIRRHOSIS (see etiology of chronic hepatitis)
  VIRAL
  AUTOIMMUNE
  METABOLIC
  CYSTIC FIBROSIS
  STORAGE DISORDERS
  SUGAR METABOLISM ERRORS
  BILIARY CIRRHOSIS
HEPATOCELLULAR CARCINOMA,
    HEPATOBLASTOMA etc

3.17.6 PREHEPATIC
BLAND THROMBOSIS
COAGULOPATHY
DEHYDRATION
COMPRESSION

SEPTIC THROMBOSIS
UMBILICAL PYEMIA
PORTAL PYEMIA

TUMOR THROMBOSIS

SCHISTOSOMIASIS

PREPYLORIC PORTAL VEIN

IMAGING

GENERAL (all modalities)

FINDINGS OF CIRRHOSIS
see cirrhosis

ASCITES (transudate)
see Ch 06

CONGESTIVE SPLENOMEGALY

ENLARGEMENT OF PORTAL VEIN (PV)
see below

VARICES
ligament teres (in free edge of falciform
    ligament) and periumbilical vein
    (eventually caput medusae)
esophageal – submucosal or periesophageal
gastric – submucosal, serosal (lesser curve,
    greater curve)
perihepatic, perisplenic, perirenal
enhance in portal venous phase or may
    enhance earlier

PORTAL VEIN (PV) THROMBOSIS
failure of enhancement (CT) or flow void (MR)
altered perfusion to areas supplied by
    thrombosed PV

3.16 MUCOPOLYSACCHARIDOSES

Type	Enzyme	Saccharide stored	Tissue	Inheritance	Severity
I Hurler	a-L-Iduronidase	heparan sulfate, dermatan sulfate	skin, cornea, bone, heart, brain, liver, spleen	AR	severe
II Hunter	L-Idurinosulfate sulfatase	heparan sulfate, dermatan sulfate	skin, bone, heart, ear, retina	X-linked	moderate
III Sanfilippo	many types	heparan sulfate	brain, skin	AR	moderate
IV Morquio	N-Acetyl-galactosamine 6-sulfatase	keratan sulfate, chondroitin sulfate	skin, bone, heart, eye	AR	mild

prominent hepatic artery and branches; arterial phase enhancement corresponding to a vascular territory (may be a wedge with thrombosed vein at apex)

possible cavernous transformation (leash of recanalized veins at porta)

Ultrasound
after R.N. Gibson

CIRRHOSIS, ASCITES
heterogeneity, irregular liver edge
large left and caudate, small right lobes
abnormal hepatic venous architecture

VARICES
ligament teres hepatofugal flow >5 cm/s OR recanalized vein >2.5 mm diameter
coronary vein >5 mm diameter
gastroesophageal or perisplenic varices

PORTAL VEIN (PV)
main portal vein >13 mm diameter (50% specificity)
splenic vein or SMA >10 mm diameter
PV flow reversal (high specificity, low sensitivity)
PV thrombosis (and large hepatic artery)

CORONAL SPLENOMEGALY (>13 cm)

3.18 PRIMARY BILIARY CIRRHOSIS

DEFINITION

progressive autoimmune destruction of intrahepatic bile ducts

CLINICAL

90% are middle aged females
60% have antimitochondrial antibody
lymphocyte and macrophage mediated granulomatous destruction of small bile ducts, reparative ductular proliferation

Associated conditions
CREST, rheumatoid arthritis, Sjögren's syndrome, membranous glomerulonephritis

Early
cholestasis dominates, malabsorption, cholesterol retention

Late
stigmata of chronic liver disease; osteomalacia, cirrhosis, portal hypertension, bleeds; death of liver failure, infection, bleeding

IMAGING

see cirrhosis

3.19 SCHISTOSOMIASIS

CLINICAL

infestation of portal vein and branches by Schistosoma species with deposition of ova
(bladder schistosomiasis: Ch08)
obliteration of PV branches, portal fibrosis (pipe stem fibrosis) but no cirrhosis
portal hypertension
liver function remains normal

IMAGING

see portal hypertension

3.20 SCLEROSING CHOLANGITIS

DEFINITION

probably autoimmune inflammation of large bile ducts leading to focal sclerosis, strictures and eventual biliary cirrhosis with disappearing ducts

EPIDEMIOLOGY

male:female 2:1, 30–50 years old
ulcerative colitis (UC) in 70% (4% of all UC), HLA B27
Crohn's disease in 5%
AIDS CHOLANGITIS MACROSCOPICALLY SAME

PATHOGENESIS

lymphocytic infiltrate, onion skin fibrosis around duct
progressive multifocal strictures (beaded ducts)

secondary biliary cirrhosis from cholestasis with portal–portal fibrous septa
cholangiocarcinoma 10%

IMAGING

Contrast studies

ERCP, PERCUTANEOUS CHOLANGIOGRAM
early: shallow or deep small ulcerations
established: multifocal strictures, interposed dilation (beaded ducts)
dominant stricture in 15%
90% intra and extra hepatic, 10% only intrahepatic
progressive irregular dominant stricture suggests malignant transformation
may form stones proximal to strictures

DIFFERENTIAL
bacterial cholangitis
AIDS cholangitis
parasitic cholangitis
multifocal cholangiocarcinoma
radiotherapy stricturing

CT
may see dilation of bile ducts

MRCP
limited by resolution capabilities and artifacts
same key findings as ERCP

3.21 WILSON'S DISEASE

DEFINITION

disease of copper overload in liver and cerebral deep gray matter with hepatitis and neurological deterioration (hepatolenticular degeneration)

CLINICAL

autosomal recessive 1/200 000
normal copper uptake and transport to liver via albumin
no ceruloplasmin, no biliary copper excretion, low serum copper/ceruloplasmin
copper buildup in hepatocytes, chronic hepatitis and cirrhosis

Copper spillover, neural toxicity

putamen, lenticular degeneration
adolescent 'Parkinsonism'
Kayser-Fleischer rings (LATE clinical
    finding)

IMAGING

see Ch 11 for CNS
see cirrhosis

4. TRAUMA AND VASCULAR CONDITIONS

4.1 BUDD–CHIARI SYNDROME

DEFINITION

acute or subacute thrombosis of hepatic
    vein/veins or intrahepatic IVC

ETIOLOGY

Focal disease
WEBS
HEPATOCELLULAR CARCINOMA WITH
    TUMOR INVASION

Coagulopathy
ESTROGENIC
ORAL CONTRACEPTIVE PILL
PREGNANCY
HIGH ESTROGEN STATES

PARANEOPLASTIC
ABDOMINAL MALIGNANCY
POLYCYTHEMIA

IMAGING

US
intravenous thrombus

Angio
occlusion of hepatic veins

CT
hepatomegaly, ascites, later caudate
    hypertrophy

lack of hepatic vein and IVC enhancement
    (differential is severe right heart failure with
        backwards congestion)
patchy parenchymal enhancement

NUC MED

SULFUR COLLOID
bright caudate uptake, reduced uptake
    elsewhere

4.2 HYPOVOLEMIA COMPLEX (manifestations)

IMAGING

CT
intestinal dilation and third space
    accumulation of fluid (i.e. intraluminal)
collapse of great veins and 'contrast linger'
non washout (intense stain) of adrenals, gut
    wall, renal cortex
vasoconstriction with patchy enhancement
    of spleen, liver, kidneys

4.3 LIVER INFARCTS

4.3.1 ARTERIAL INFARCT

occurs in transplant liver only or following
    embolization

4.3.2 INFARCT OF ZAHN

occluded portal supply
marked sinusoid stasis and atrophy, no
    necrosis (therefore, not a true infarct)

4.3.3 HYPOVOLEMIC INJURY

zone 3/centrilobular coagulative necrosis

4.3.4 CARDIAC CONGESTION

IMAGING

in general, infarcts manifest as areas of
    altered vascular enhancement
in portal thrombosis, affected segments
    enhance in arterial phase
heterogeneous defects on CT arterial
    portography may mimic tumor, but are
    usually wedge shaped with apex towards
    blocked vessel

CARDIAC CONGESTION has delayed liver
    portal enhancement and delayed hepatic
    vein and IVC enhancement with dilated
    IVC

4.4 LIVER TRAUMA

CLASSIFICATION

4.4.1 Intracapsular rupture

4.4.2 Subcapsular hematoma

4.4.3 Laceration

4.4.4 Extracapsular rupture

4.4.5 Periportal tracking
see periportal tracking gamut

4.4.6 Traumatic/postoperative biloma

IMAGING

AXR
hemoperitoneum, right flank stripe
organ displacement: kidney, colon

US
hypoechoic or mixed irregular
    intraparenchymal collection with mass
    effect
subcapsular crescentic or lens-shaped
    collection
may be difficult to outline well on US
biloma (intraparenchymal or subcapsular) is
    a hypoechoic collection

CT
precontrast fresh hematoma hypodense;
    hematomas may resorb or transform to
    fluid collections
contrast required to definitively outline
    margins of collection and to diagnose
    rapid extravasation
if liver capsule torn, cut or punctured,
    intraperitoneal blood accumulates
    around liver and in dependent portions of
    cavity
bilomas are low density; often post
    operative; perihepatic or subcapsular;
    rarely intraparenchymal (usually
    posttraumatic)

IDA

bile extravasations show as extraanatomic non bowel collections of radiotracer that accumulate with time

usually postoperative or after penetrating trauma

?POSTOP BILE LEAK: continue imaging until leak confirmed or all tracer has passed into small bowel

4.5 PELIOSIS HEPATIS

DEFINITION

primary dilation of hepatic sinusoids to form lakes 1 mm to 1 cm

associated with steroids, oral contraceptives, danazol

IMAGING

CT

hypodense focal area precontrast (follows blood pool)

rapid enhancement post contrast, then follows blood pool

4.6 SPLENIC TRAUMA

beware of splenic trauma when left sided rib fractures are present!

CLASSIFICATION

4.6.1 Intracapsular rupture

4.6.2 Extracapsular rupture

4.6.3 Laceration

4.6.4 Fracture

4.6.5 Sentinel clot

high density clot adjacent to inapparent laceration

IMAGING

AXR

hemoperitoneum, left flank stripe

large splenic shadow

organ displacement: kidney, stomach, diaphragm, colon

CT

precontrast may show hypodense fracture line with fluid or subcapsular hematoma; often isodense and invisible

with contrast, subcapsular collections and fracture planes do not enhance; beware of vascular injury

intraperitoneal free blood or fluid

4.7 VASCULAR ANOMALIES AND VARIANTS

4.7.1 HEPATIC ARTERY VARIANTS

Conventional pattern

both right and left hepatic arteries arise from the proper hepatic artery and lie anterior to the portal veins

Common variants

right hepatic artery lies posterior to the right portal vein

right hepatic artery arises from the inferior pancreaticoduodenal artery (off superior mesenteric artery) in ~10%

left hepatic artery arises from the left gastric artery (off celiac axis) in ~10%

4.7.2 PORTAL VEIN VARIANTS

4.7.2.1 Prepyloric portal vein

4.7.2.2 Cavernous transformation

4.7.3 IVC WEBS AND BUDD–CHIARI SEQUELAE

4.8 VENOOCCLUSIVE DISEASE

DEFINITION

fibrosis around small hepatic vein radicles with eventual fibrous obliteration

ETIOLOGY

liver transplant

graft vs host disease

pyrrolizidine alkaloids

IMAGING FINDINGS (late)

obliteration of hepatic veins

5. LIVER MASSES

5.1 ABSCESS

ETIOLOGY

5.1.1 Amebic

5.1.2 Bacterial

PORTAL SPREAD
(E coli and other gut organisms)

appendicitis

diverticular disease

Crohn's disease

septic portal thrombosis

ARTERIAL SPREAD

Staphylococcal septicemia

immunosuppressed (particularly Candida)

ASCENDING CHOLANGITIS

IMAGING

US

EARLY

discrete hypoechoic area

progressive central cavitation

ESTABLISHED

usually hypoechoic collection with mass effect

thick ill defined wall

amebic abscess: tends to be at the dome under diaphragm

FUNGAL

multiple hypoechoic nodules with central echogenic dot (vascular core)

CT

EARLY

discrete hypodense area with mild contrast enhancement

progressive central hypodensity

ESTABLISHED

discrete hypodense area with mass effect

may have gas (pathognomonic)

thin or thicker ring contrast enhancement

5.2 CAVERNOUS HEMANGIOMA

DEFINITION

non malignant hamartomatous vascular
mass

CLINICAL

7% of population;female: male 5:1; most
commonly asymptomatic, rarely bleeds

commonest cause of mass after metastases
in imaging studies

90% <4 cm; 2% grow on followup

dilated vascular spaces with flat endothelial
lining, may thrombose and scar

IMAGING

US

TYPICAL (80%)

hyperechoic mass, no Doppler flow

small proportion may show power Doppler
flow

ATYPICAL (20%)

bright rim, isoechoic center

US guided biopsy

FNA: blood only

core cutting needle: may lead to catastrophic
bleeding

CT

precontrast: low density

arterial phase: peripheral blobs of contrast
(strongly suggestive)

portal venous phase and delayed: slow
edges-in enhancement (minutes);
eventually shows increased density
compared to liver parenchyma

atypical appearance includes arterial phase
enhancing mass (arterialized
hemangioma)

MR

FOLLOWS BLOOD ON ALL
SEQUENCES

T1W: low

T2W: signal as for fluid (including dual echo
T2W sequences [long TE and even longer
TE])

may have a central scar

Gd contrast: enhances edges in (peripheral
nodular enhancement, with peripheral
puddling 95% specific; delayed fill-in on
late images)

T2 constant of lesion >125 ms is 100%
specific for benign etiology

DIFFERENTIAL DIAGNOSIS

cystic tumor or simple cyst

Angio

blood lakes

NUC MED

SULFUR COLLOID

cold defect

RED BLOOD CELL SCAN

hot focus, similar to blood pool

usually fills in late on flow study and may
have cold focus on early blood pool
image ('flip-flop sign')

use SPECT for anything other than a gross
mass

sensitivity drops with small size, but ~95%
at >2 cm

5.3 CHOLANGIO-CARCINOMA (intrahepatic)

DEFINITION

uncommon intrahepatic adenocarcinoma of
biliary epithelium

CLINICAL

ASSOCIATIONS: sclerosing cholangitis,
clonorchiasis

unifocal or multifocal mass

adenocarcinoma with glandular or tubular
structures

often scirrhous, NOT BILE STAINED

invasion of veins rare (cf. hepatocellular
carcinoma)

Location

PERIPHERAL

HILAR (see biliary section)

Spread

LYMPHATIC 50%: local, paraaortic

HEMATOGENOUS 50%: lungs, vertebrae,
adrenals, brain

IMAGING

US

non specific mass of any echotexture, often
with segmental or lobar dilation of bile
ducts

CT

hypodense mass precontrast

often close to porta (may obstruct portal
veins)

often with segmental or lobar bile duct
dilation

mild or no enhancement

MR

non specific mass, low on T1W, high on T2W

mild or heterogeneous enhancement with
Gd

NUC MED

IDA

cold

SULFUR COLLOID

cold

PET

FDG avid

5.4 CIRRHOTIC NODULES

see under CIRRHOSIS (nodule – hepatocellular carcinoma progression and also CIRRHOSIS – imaging)

5.5 CYST

IMAGING

AXR

no findings

US

classic cyst

hypodense fluid echogenicity

pencil sharp margins

mass effect

increased through transmission

CT

problem if partial volume artifact and hard to diagnose if small
fluid density (e.g. <20 HU)
no enhancement
imperceptible wall

MR

classic cyst
low T1W, high T2W signal
no enhancement
imperceptible wall
follows CSF on all sequences (if spinal canal is in field of view)
T2W appearance remains bright with extra long TE (see cavernous hemangioma)

5.6 FOCAL NODULAR HYPERPLASIA

DEFINITION

hyperplastic (non neoplastic by definition) nodule with arterial supply and characteristic architecture

MORPHOLOGY

female > male, young adults, 20% multiple
mass with central fibrous spoke wheel scar; may be subcapsular
scar and septa contain arterial branches with fibromuscular hypoplasia, proliferating bile ducts and no normal hepatic veins
interspersed parenchyma consists of: normal hepatocytes and sinusoids, and possibly piecemeal necrosis

IMAGING

US

isoechoic solid
spoke wheel vascular architecture

CT

precontrast: homogenous hypodense to liver
arterial phase: strong enhancement
portal venous phase and delayed: isodense mass but with hypodense scar

MR

T1W: parenchyma and scar are isointense to liver
T2W: parenchyma is isointense, scar hyperintense

dynamic Gd: parenchymal arterial phase enhancement, with scar showing delayed enhancement

NUC MED

SULFUR COLLOID

10% intensely increased uptake (helpful)
30% increased uptake (helpful)
30% same as surrounding liver
30% reduced uptake

IDA

similar to liver (functioning hepatocytes present, no photopenia)
may be hot (impaired washout)

Differential diagnosis

GIANT HEMANGIOMA WITH SCAR (WRONG ENHANCEMENT)
FIBROLAMELLAR HEPATOCELLULAR CARCINOMA
HYPERVASCULAR METASTASIS WITH SCAR

5.7 HEPATOCELLULAR ADENOMA

DEFINITION

benign neoplasm of hepatocyte origin, with malignant transformation exceedingly rare, but a tendency to hemorrhage

CLINICAL

young female, oral contraceptives, may regress on cessation; in males consider anabolic steroid use
sheets and cords of near normal hepatocytes; may contain lipid
no portal tracts, no Kupffer cells, no bile ducts, arterial neovascularity

IMAGING

US/CT/MR

non specific solid mass; hemorrhage into tumor
arterial phase enhancing mass
T1W: high or low (depends on fat content and hemorrhage)
T2W: high

NUC MED

SULFUR COLLOID

majority cold (usually no Kupffer cells)

IDA

same uptake as liver (functioning hepatocytes)
may be increased compared to liver (accumulation with lack of biliary drainage)

5.8 HEPATOCELLULAR CARCINOMA (HCC)

DEFINITION

malignant tumor of hepatocytes with strong association with hepatitis B virus and cirrhosis

ETIOLOGY, EPIDEMIOLOGY

prevalence reflects hepatitis B virus (HBV) prevalence

Low HBV incidence areas

older patient, male:female 2:1
cirrhosis 90% (of any cause); alcohol is major, but hemochromatosis has highest incidence of HCC
most likely regenerative nodule – dysplastic nodule – HCC sequence
exact role of HCV?

High HBV incidence areas

high vertical transmission and carrier rates
younger patients, male:female 8:1
overall incidence 50 times higher
HBV main etiology; DNA integration, dysplasia

Fibrolamellar HCC

non cirrhotic liver
non HBV?
20–40 year olds; better prognosis especially if resectable

CLINICAL

mass, pain, malaise, jaundice, weight loss, intratumoral hemorrhage, decompensation of cirrhosis
elevated alpha fetoprotein (major serum marker of HCC)

Spread

invades hepatic and portal veins, may cause thrombosis (! metastases do not do this)
local lymph nodes
invasion in continuity (adrenal, kidney)
hematogenous late

MACRO

5.8.1 Unifocal (solitary)
yellow or hemorrhagic bile stained nodule

5.8.2 Multifocal
multiple masses and nodules

5.8.3 Diffuse
merges into cirrhotic background

5.8.4 Fibrolamellar HCC
single large scirrhous mass with fibrous bands

MICRO

Well differentiated HCC
trabecular or acinar architecture
hepatocytes, possibly bile canaliculi
variable amount of fatty change

Moderately differentiated

Anaplastic
pleomorphic cells, giant cells

Mixed HCC and cholangiocarcinoma

Fibrolamellar HCC
well differentiated polygonal cells in cords and nests, septa of dense collagen

IMAGING

Venous invasion on all modalities!

May contain hemorrhage on all modalities!

AXR
possible hepatomegaly

US
usually hypodense, may be bright (fatty change in tumor)
Doppler: AV shunting in 50% (hard if there is surrounding cirrhosis)

CT
precontrast: iso/hypodense mass with contour deformity
arterial phase: vivid enhancement (no normal portal venous supply)
portal venous phase: iso/hypodense, may become invisible

Lipiodol CT
retains lipiodol compared to normal hepatic parenchyma (no Kupffer cells)
(10 ml lipiodol injection into hepatic artery, scan at 1 week)

MR
T1W: usually low, may be high (fatty change inside tumor)
T2W: high
Gd: arterial phase enhancement analogous to CT
SCAR OF FIBROLAMELLAR HCC: T1W signal low, T2W signal also low and does not enhance after Gd (cf. focal nodular hyperplasia)

Angio
supplied by neovascular branches of the hepatic artery, and not by the portal vein
usually vascular with an arterial blush from hepatic artery
angiography may show the bleeding point in an acutely hemorrhaging HCC

NUC MED
IDA
usually photopenic with delayed accumulation of IDA compared to normal liver (tumor hepatocytes still take up IDA, but there is no drainage)
occasionally isointense to normal liver

SULFUR COLLOID
photopenic defect

GALLIUM
2/3 hot compared to surrounding parenchyma, rest isointense or cold

PET
FDG avid, variably hot
may be invisible in background of metabolically active liver

5.9 HYDATID DISEASE
(manifestations)

also see Ch 13

IMAGING

AXR
rounded calcification
mass effect if large

US
cystic or mixed mass with internal debris, daughter cysts peripherally, calcification, infrequently floating membranes

CT
hypodense cystic mass, daughter cysts
internal septa, areas of higher densities
may show ring enhancement (host capsule)
thin rim calcification (Echinococcus granulosus)
clumpy calcification and more irregular mass (Echinococcus alveolaris)

5.10 LIVER TUMORS WORKUP

see isolated liver mass gamut

IMAGING MODALITIES USED IN WORKUP

Ultrasound
color, Doppler

CT
precontrast, arterial phase, venous phase

CT arterial portography

Delayed (6 hour) CT
normal parenchyma still mildly enhanced (but not HCC etc)

Lipiodol CT
10 ml lipiodol injected into hepatic artery, scan at 10 days
tumors retain lipiodol (no Kupffer cells)

Sulfur colloid scintigraphy
cold focus = no perfusion or no Kupffer
normal = likely normal parenchyma (especially in focal fatty change)
elevated = probably focal nodular hyperplasia

Red blood cell (RBC) scintigraphy
hot focus = vessel or vascular space (i.e. hemangioma)

IDA scintigraphy
marker of hepatocyte function

Gallium scintigraphy

2/3 of HCC are gallium avid
lymphoma is gallium avid

MRI

T1W, T2W, dynamic Gd, chemical shift

MRI ferrumoxides (Resovist)

bright = no perfusion or no Kupffer cells

Biopsy (FNA or core)

5.11 METASTASIS

commonest cause of single solid liver mass
at imaging
commonest cause of multiple liver masses at
imaging

ETIOLOGY

colorectal carcinoma, other GIT
malignancies (including carcinoid)
lung carcinoma, breast carcinoma
pancreatic carcinoma
lymphomas
cervix and prostate carcinomas
uterine carcinoma
sarcomas
CHILD: neuroblastoma, nephroblastoma,
rhabdomyosarcoma

IMAGING

AXR

no findings unless hepatomegaly or
calcification

US

ECHOGENIC
GIT/vascular/urogenital

HYPOECHOIC
breast/lung/lymphoma/melanoma

BULLSEYE
breast/lung/colon

CALCIFIED
mucinous adenocarcinoma
chondrosarcoma/osteosarcoma

CYSTIC
neuroendocrine

CT

HYPERVASCULAR
carcinoid and other paragangliomas

pheochromocytoma and other
neuroendocrine
renal
thyroid
vascular sarcomas

HYPOVASCULAR, RING
ENHANCEMENT
generally all else

CT arterial portography (CTAP)

sensitivity equal to MR, but can not tell cysts
from metastases

Delayed CT at 6 hours

normal parenchyma still slightly high density
metastases low density

MR

generally, low T1W signal, high T2W signal,
Gd enhancement analogous to CT
can tell from cysts (on long TE)
melanoma and mucin high on T1W
sequences
lymphoma low on T1W sequences, iso to low
on T2W sequences, mild if any
enhancement

FERRUMOXIDES MR
example of trade name: Resovist
most sensitive MR sequence
normal liver parenchyma loses signal
(Kupffer cells take up ferrumoxides
leading to signal loss)
all foreign non hepatocyte containing masses
stand out (use T2W sequences)
detects but does not characterize masses

Angio

main use is intraarterial chemotherapy
hypervascular tumors: mass with
neoangiogenesis
hypovascular tumors: mass with ring
staining

NUC MED

cold defect on all tracers
(except for MIBG, iodine and octreotide in
relevant tumors)

PET

reflects metabolism of primary tumor
beware of low metabolic metastases in high
metabolic liver

HOT
lung
sarcoma
lymphoma

LESS HOT
breast
colon

OFTEN NOT
treated tumor

DEFINITION

acute gallbladder inflammation most
commonly precipitated by stones

ETIOPATHOGENESIS

6.1.1 90% Calculous

physical obstruction (stone impaction in
gallbladder neck)
increased intraluminal pressure, chemical
wall inflammation, venous ischemia

6.1.2 10% Acalculous

possibly obstruction by sludge, or
combination of chemical damage to wall
and ischemia
TRAUMA
BURNS
PARENTERAL NUTRITION
POSTPARTUM
SEPSIS, BACTERIAL CHOLECYSTITIS

CLINICAL

Classical presentation

biliary colic (RUQ pain, vomiting)
RUQ tenderness (Murphy's sign)
fever, signs of inflammation, elevated white
cell count, failure to settle
no jaundice by definition

Variants

especially pyrexia of unknown origin in
critically ill, hospitalized or debilitated
patient
relatively silent gangrenous cholecystitis in
the elderly (often perforates)

Complications

acalculous cholecystitis is more prone to
complications

GALLBLADDER

6.1.3 PERFORATION, BILE PERITONITIS

6.1.4 EMPYEMA, BACTERIAL SUPERINFECTION

6.1.5 EMPHYSEMATOUS CHOLECYSTITIS (rare; diabetics)

6.1.6 GANGRENOUS CHOLECYSTITIS, FOCAL ABSCESS, PERITONITIS

6.1.7 GALLSTONE ILEUS

CBD

OBSTRUCTION BY PASSING STONE
MIRIZZI'S SYNDROME
PANCREATITIS
ASCENDING CHOLANGITIS

IMAGING

AXR

~10% of gallstones are calcified

US

gallstones (one or many, generally mobile cleanly shadowing curved surfaces) +/– gallstone impacted in gallbladder neck (fixed stone at gallbladder neck) and
thickened (edematous) wall (commonly >2–3 mm)
pericholecystic free fluid and
sonographic Murphy's sign (direct tenderness)

CT

stones may be isodense to bile
thickened edematous gallbladder wall
ring enhancement of inner aspect of thickened gallbladder wall
gallbladder fossa enhancement

IDA

cardinal sign is non opacification of gallbladder implying cystic duct obstruction
demonstration of gallbladder by 30 min rules out cholecystitis with a high degree of certainty
demonstration between 30 min and 1 hour nominally still normal, but less reliable in ruling out acute cholecystitis (may be present with partial duct obstruction)
failure to demonstrate gallbladder indicates acute cholecystitis with high degree of certainty
acute acalculous cholecystitis usually has non demonstration of gallbladder due to high intraluminal pressure
demonstration of gallbladder between 30 min and 4 hours or with morphine is best regarded as abnormal but not specific

ANCILLARY SIGNS

rim sign: hypervascularity around gallbladder fossa implying inflammation with secondarily increased hepatic parenchymal uptake and/or blocked clearance by small bile ducts directly to gallbladder
nubbin sign: lower cystic duct fills retrogradely, but not gallbladder

PITFALLS

FALSE POSITIVE

patient fasted <4 hours (gallbladder contracted) or >24 hours (filled to capacity – use cholecystokinin (CCK) to empty)
liver failure (delayed and poor uptake by liver parenchyma, delayed and faint biliary tree demonstration) – no useful information about state of gallbladder; includes hyperalimentation in sick patients

FALSE NEGATIVE

sometimes acute acalculous cholecystitis
sometimes partial cystic duct obstruction (usually has delayed gallbladder filling)
attempts at further maneuvers

FURTHER MANEUVERS

aim to reduce false positives caused by chronic cholecystitis

delayed imaging to 4 hours

morphine to contract ampullary sphincter not recommended, as high risk of missing true positives!!
may demonstrate patency of cystic duct by increasing backflow to gallbladder
failure to see gallbladder within 30 min of morphine indicates cystic duct obstruction

6.2 ADENOMYOSIS

DEFINITION

totally benign focal or multifocal gallbladder mucosal diverticula with muscular hypertrophy

ALTERNATIVE NAMES

adenomyomatosis
diverticular disease of gallbladder
cholecystitis glandularis proliferans

CLINICAL

usually asymptomatic incidental finding
ASSOCIATIONS: stones, acute or chronic cholecystitis
solitary = adenomyoma (often fundal); multiple = adenomyosis
mucosal outpouching extending under serosa, often stone in lumen, complex mucosal folding, marked muscular hypertrophy

IMAGING

US

wall thickening or mass centered on wall; may have associated reverberation artifact; may have a stricture or focal narrowing

CT

gallbladder wall thickening or mass centered on wall and of same density
preserved smooth gallbladder outline, no evidence of direct invasion
preserved surrounding structures and fat planes

6.3 ASCENDING CHOLANGITIS

DEFINITION

ascending infection of biliary tree with secondary parenchymal abscess formation and high mortality

ETIOLOGY

Obstruction
stone
tumor
stricture
parasite
(choledochal cyst)

Manipulation
surgical
endoscopic

Foreign body
intraductal stones (strong association)
stent

Microorganisms

E coli, Gram negative aerobes and anaerobes, Enterococci

immunosuppressed – different pattern of cholangitis (see AIDS abdomen) or multifocal candidal liver abscesses

CLINICAL

elderly, debilitated, intraductal gallstones, preexisting biliary abnormalities, immune suppression

RUQ pain, sepsis and pyrexia, jaundice (Charcot's triad) +/– cardiovascular collapse

progresses to multifocal liver abscesses; high mortality

IMAGING

US

may show causative agent (intraductal stones, gallstones, dilated biliary tree, etc)

dilated biliary tree, thickened wall

intrabiliary debris

intraparenchymal abscesses

CT

usually shows causative agent

diffusely dilated biliary tree

focal dilations of biliary tree

edema of extrahepatic ducts and edema surrounding intrahepatic ducts

irregular low density spaces with mass effect centered on biliary tree with ring enhancement (developing abscesses)

MR

analogous to CT

dilation of biliary tree and wall thickening

PTC (percutaneous transhepatic cholangiography)

used to drain infected biliary tree

may demonstrate obstruction or intraductal filling defects

6.4 BILIARY CARCINOMAS

GROUP DEFINITION

adenocarcinomas of biliary epithelial origin

6.4.1 INTRAHEPATIC CHOLANGIOCARCINOMA

small duct origin

see separate entry in the liver masses section

6.4.2 GALLBLADDER CARCINOMA

CLINICAL

female > male, >70 years old

very strong association with gallstones (60 –90%)

usually present late; mass, pain, weight loss and jaundice

MACRO

90% unresectable; direct invasion of liver and metastases to portal nodes

95% adenocarcinoma

6.4.2.1 Scirrhous infiltrating

gritty pale mass centered on gallbladder with direct liver invasion

6.4.2.2 Fungating (less common)

IMAGING

US

gallbladder irregular mass

evidence of direct invasion of liver or adjacent structures

gallstones may be present

CT

relatively inhomogeneous or multilobulated avascular mass centered on the gallbladder or gallbladder wall

may obliterate the gallbladder or extend into the lumen; wall thickening of >1 cm suggestive

loss of surrounding fat planes with direct invasion; direct invasion of liver

may cause biliary obstruction if invades porta hepatis

portal, celiac, peripancreatic lymph nodes

may ring enhance; may have intrahepatic metastases

MR

analogous to CT

T2W sequence shows margin with bile in gallbladder and edge to liver

T1W sequence shows edge to liver and pancreas

6.4.3 BILE DUCT CARCINOMA

CLINICAL

male > female, >70 years old

adenocarcinoma, usually with marked scirrhous reaction

position critical in determining timing of presentation and so resectability

Associations

ulcerative colitis, sclerosing cholangitis (strong association), choledochal cyst, gallstones (30%), infestation

CLASSIFICATION BY LOCATION

6.4.3.1 High (Klatzkin tumor) – most common

located at hilum, commonly at confluence of lobar hepatic ducts

sclerosing much more than nodular or papillary

slow growing, extends along ducts

presents with jaundice, mass relatively uncommon

usually unresectable

6.4.3.2 Mid

nodular form (mass centered on duct wall) more common than sclerosing or papillary

presents with jaundice

6.4.3.3 Low (ampullary)

papillary form (intraluminal mass) more common than nodular

presents early – possible Whipple's procedure

differential is NON BILIARY AMPULLARY CARCINOMA (PANCREATIC or DUODENAL)

IMAGING

PTC/ERCP/MRCP

dominant or irregular or shouldered stricture

progressive stricture

US

biliary dilation, mass

CT

mass may or may not be present

mass relatively avascular and may be differentiated from the normally enhancing pancreas (20–30 s) or liver (portal venous phase)

dilation of biliary tree upstream from mass

irregular narrowing of biliary tree and wall thickening at site of tumor (may have no mass)

regional lymphadenopathy

intrahepatic metastases

MR

good problem solving modality especially for sclerosing form with little mass effect

abnormal thickening of biliary wall

mass

high peribiliary T2W signal

diffuse peribiliary enhancement with Gd

intrapancreatic tumors low signal on fat sat T1W sequence (pancreatic tissue high signal)

PET

moderately FDG avid

identification in metabolically active liver may be difficult

6.5 CHOLESTEROLOSIS and CHOLESTEROL POLYPS

DEFINITION

abnormal accumulation of cholesterol in gallbladder mucosa

CLINICAL

25% of surgical specimens

asymptomatic in itself but associated with other conditions

PATHOLOGY

strawberry gallbladder, lamina propria full of foamy macrophages containing cholesterol

focal protrusions of mucosa form polypoid masses ('cholesterol polyp')

IMAGING

cholesterolosis itself is invisible

US/CT (cholesterol polyp)

murally based polyp, echogenic but without shadowing, does not move with position change, usually not visible on CT without biliary contrast because similar density to bile

DIFFERENTIAL

adherent stone (casts shadow); mobile stone (casts shadow, moves); sludge ball (moves)

6.6 CHRONIC CHOLECYSTITIS

DEFINITION

chronic inflammation of gallbladder wall, usually related to stones or supersaturated bile, with a number of morphological appearances

ETIOLOGY

CHRONIC ON ACUTE

CHRONIC AB INITIO (90% gallstones, 10% acalculous)

BACTERIAL SUPERINFECTION

CLINICAL

chronic RUQ pain, flatulent dyspepsia

intermittent attacks of biliary colic or acute cholecystitis/exacerbation

MACRO

6.6.1 Chronic cholecystitis NOS

may have stones or no stones

contracted fibrotic gallbladder

mucosa preserved vs mucosa atrophic

prominent Rokitansky–Aschoff sinuses (subserosal outpouchings of mucosa)

6.6.2 Porcelain gallbladder

dystrophic wall calcification with markedly increased carcinoma risk (10% go on to carcinoma)

6.6.3 Mucocele

obstructed gallbladder containing mucus from mucosal secretions (benign mucocele)

6.6.4 Xanthogranulomatous cholecystitis

chronic inflammation with granulomatous (giant cells, activated macrophages) infiltrate and foam filled macrophages

macroscopically a mass with possible blood product staining

(analogous to xanthogranulomatous pyelonephritis)

6.6.5 Sphincter of Oddi dysfunction

postulated cause of post cholecystectomy syndrome

may cause physiological obstruction where no anatomical obstruction is evident at ERCP

IMAGING

AXR

porcelain gallbladder may be visible (pear shaped or curvilinear calcification in RUQ)

US/CT

gallstones

contracted gallbladder around gallstones

thickened gallbladder wall

xanthogranulomatous cholecystitis may mimic a gallbladder carcinoma

IDA

abnormal gallbladder ejection fraction (EF) does not automatically equal chronic acalculous cholecystitis!

abnormal EF in appropriately selected patients highly predictive of acalculous cholecystitis

PROTOCOL

fasting (between 4 and 24 hours)

definitely not pregnant

IDA, wait for gallbladder to fill

re-image after fatty meal – milk (normal is EF > 50%)

re-image after fatty meal – Ensure (R) (normal is EF of 60% ± 20%)

cholecystokinin 0.02 microgram per kilogram

A) over 3 min (abnormal is EF <35%; larger number of false positives – mechanism ?spasm of gallbladder neck)

B) over 30–40 min (reliable, but more tedious; abnormal is EF <50%; fewer false positives)

FALSE POSITIVES

diabetes
achalasia
malabsorption
drugs (morphine, atropine, octreotide, nifedipine, progesterone)
achalasia

6.7 GALLBLADDER POLYPS (overview)

Non neoplastic

HAMARTOMATOUS – RETENTION

CHOLESTEROL POLYPS

Neoplastic

TUBULAR ADENOMA
PAPILLARY ADENOMA
DIFFUSE DUCT PAPILLOMATOSIS

6.8 GALLSTONES

DEFINITION

largely asymptomatic cholesterol, pigment or mixed bile concretions and the commonest pathology underlying biliary symptoms

ETIOPATHOGENESIS

(80%) Cholesterol

supersaturated bile AND gallbladder stasis or dyskinesis AND nucleation nidus

STONES
solitary, multiple, soft or hard

LIMY BILE
small particles suspended in bile associated with stasis

SLUDGE BALLS
loose masses of small particles

RISK FACTORS
pregnancy, oral contraceptives
obesity, hyperlipidemia
gallbladder stasis
family history of gallstones

(20%) Pigment

BLACK (STERILE) – NIDUS AND ACCRETION

unconjugated calcium bilirubinate
small, soft, multiple, spiculated

RISK FACTORS
hemolytic disease
pancreatic insufficiency
biliary infestation
ileal disease (due to oxalate retention): Crohn's disease, intestinal bypass, resection

BROWN – INFECTION STONES

laminated greasy, radiolucent
tend to form in bile ducts with infection

CLINICAL

5% of all <40 year olds, female > male
25% of all >80 year olds, female > male
90% asymptomatic, convert at 1–3% per year
biliary colic, acute cholecystitis (gallbladder neck stone), jaundice (CBD stone or Mirizzi's syndrome)
COMPLICATIONS: ascending cholangitis, gallstone pancreatitis

IMAGING

AXR

small percent only calcified
may have 'Mercedes Benz' sign of internal low density clefts

US

rounded echogenic mobile or fixed masses with posterior shadowing
less dense stones and sludge balls may not completely shadow

CT

variable density rounded or facetted stones; may have rings of calcification; may have central low density clefts or clumpy calcification (cholesterol stones low density, pigment stones high density)
intraductal stones often are higher density than unopacified bile and may be visible in CBD

MRCP/CT IVC (CT intravenous cholangiogram)

rounded or irregular mobile filling defect
duct may be dilated
acute angles with duct walls

ERCP

as for MRCP, but beware air bubbles as differential
complete block to contrast flow

6.9 INFESTATIONS (overview)

ETIOLOGY

Flukes

FASCIOLA HEPATICA
OPISTHORCHIS SINENSIS, CLONORCHIS SINENSIS

Ascaris lumbricoides

Ova

FASCIOLA HEPATICA
SCHISTOSOMA

COMPLICATIONS

eosinophilic chronic cholangitis with fibrosis
'pipe stem' portal fibrosis with schistosoma
secondary bacterial superinfection leading to ascending cholangitis
brown (infection) gallstones
LATE: secondary biliary cirrhosis and cholangiocarcinoma

6.10 MIRIZZI'S SYNDROME

DEFINITION

extrinsic right sided compression of the common bile duct by a gallstone impacted in the lower end of the cystic duct (with jaundice)

IMAGING

extrinsic mid common bile duct compression with isocenter outside the wall
COMPLICATION: gallbladder to common hepatic duct fistulas

7. PANCREATIC CONDITIONS

7.1 ACUTE PANCREATITIS

DEFINITION

acute inflammation of pancreatic parenchyma characterized by autodigestion, necrosis, hemorrhage and extensive secondary systemic complications

ETIOLOGY

Gallstones

Alcohol

Rare

TRAUMA
ERCP/BLUNT

INFECTION
MUMPS, COXSACKIE VIRUSES

CLONORCHIS

MALFORMATION
PANCREAS DIVISUM

pancreatitis occurs in dorsal pancreas only
probably related to relative obstruction at
the accessory ampulla

VASCULAR
ISCHEMIC INJURY

VASCULITIS

METABOLIC
HYPERPARATHYROIDISM, HYPERCALCEMIA

DRUGS (DIURETICS)

PATHOGENESIS

interstitial release and activation of
pancreatic enzymes
protein autodigestion
fat autodigestion, calcium salt precipitation
acute neutrophilic inflammation

CLINICAL

acute abdomen with constant central and
epigastric pain radiating to back
increased serum pancreatic amylase and
lipase levels; white cell count may be
elevated

Acute interstitial pancreatitis
(acute pancreatitis NOS)
edema of pancreas and surrounding fat
planes
patchy or diffuse fat necrosis, globules of
calcium deposition

Acute hemorrhagic pancreatitis
hemorrhage predominant feature
severe end of pancreatitis spectrum

Complications

ACUTE

LOCAL
superinfection, abscess
calcium sequestration, hypocalcemia
endocrine pancreas dysfunction, acute
hyperglycemia
splenic and portal vein thrombosis
splenic artery aneurysm
acute bowel necrosis

SYSTEMIC
?secondary to pancreatic enzymes in
circulation
disseminated intravascular coagulation
acute adult respiratory distress syndrome
acute renal failure
fat embolism, microinfarcts
consumption coagulopathy

CHRONIC
pseudocyst formation
pancreatic insufficiency
bile duct obstruction

IMAGING

AXR
may have no findings
sentinel duodenal loop
evidence of prior pancreatitis: pancreatic
area calcification

US
usually inaccessible because of bowel gas
and pain
swollen hypoechoic pancreas
may see pseudocysts
ascites (greater and lesser sac)
portal and splenic vein thromboses
may show gallstones

CT
main modality
diffuse or more focal swelling of pancreas,
may be massive
edema and masking of peripancreatic fat
planes
increased and patchily inhomogeneous
pancreatic density (balance of prior
pancreatic fatty replacement/atrophy and
current edema and hemorrhage)
intrapancreatic collections, lesser and
greater sac fluid (may be dense – blood
or protein); peripancreatic collections;
these eventually develop rim
enhancement
exudate may permeate retroperitoneum –
anterior pararenal space, posterior
pararenal space, transverse mesocolon,
mesentery root, rarely perirenal space
after contrast, homogeneous (less severe
pancreatitis) or patchy (more severe
pancreatitis) enhancement; areas of non
enhancement indicate necrosis

BALTHAZAR CT SEVERITY INDEX
MORPHOLOGY CHANGES
normal 0
swelling, abnormal texture 1
peripancreatic inflammation, infiltrated fat 2
single fluid collection 3
many fluid collections 4
NB can not tell sterile pseudocyst from
abscess (but gas suggestive of abscess)

EXTENT OF NECROSIS
nil   0
<30%   2
30–50%   4
>50%   6

PROGNOSIS
prognosis worse the higher the score
score of 7 to 10 confers mortality 20%

MR
not a major modality
normal or edematous pancreas retains
signal characteristics
edema and collections low on T1W and high
on T2W sequences (depends on protein
content) and analogous to CT
hemorrhagic collections well shown (high on
T1W sequences)
non enhancement (T1W with Gd) carries
same significance as for CT

7.2 CHRONIC PANCREATITIS

DEFINITION

chronic pancreatic inflammation and
progressive atrophy usually presenting as
relapsing attacks (chronic relapsing
pancreatitis)

ETIOLOGY

Alcoholism

Gallstones (less common)

Pancreas divisum
pancreatitis occurs in dorsal pancreas
probably related to relative obstruction at
the accessory ampulla

Idiopathic ~40%

includes familial chronic pancreatitis

newer evidence suggests cystic fibrosis carriers are at higher risk for chronic pancreatitis

Familial

does not automatically follow simple duct obstruction

RISK OF CARCINOMA HIGHER IN FAMILIAL FORM

PATHOGENESIS

presence of inflammation differentiates from simple chronic duct obstruction ('chronic obstructive pancreatitis')

overlap with acute pancreatitis

calcification, stone formation, fibrosis are all major features

?repeated focal necrosis responsible for eventual fibrosis

CLINICAL

pain

pancreatic insufficiency (exocrine, endocrine)

pseudocysts

biliary obstruction, splenic vein thrombosis

MORPHOLOGY

shrunken hard fibrotic gland

patchy loss of acini, irregular fibrosis, chronic inflammatory infiltrate

duct dilations, stenoses, abnormal side branches, stones, mucus plugs, calcifications, pseudocysts

IMAGING

US, CT

CALCIFICATION is the cardinal sign

small atrophic gland with irregular contours BUT may be enlarged if imaged during a recurrent acute episode

less commonly swollen pancreas (chronic inflammatory swelling)

diffuse or patchy reduction in gland density

intrapancreatic clumpy or more diffuse calcification

dilation and tortuosity of main pancreatic duct

focal duct stenoses

intraductal filling defects (mucus plugs, stones)

---

pancreatic parenchymal cysts

peripancreatic pseudocysts, lesser sac collections

splenic vein thrombosis, splenic artery aneurysm/pseudoaneurysm

no changes of acute inflammation (see acute pancreatitis entry) unless imaged during a recurrent episode

ERCP/MRCP

duct dilation with focal stenoses

abnormal side branches

filling defects (mucus plugs, stones)

7.3 CYSTIC FIBROSIS (manifestations)

see Ch 06, Ch 13

IMAGING

CT

pancreatic parenchymal atrophy and fatty replacement

parenchymal pancreatic calcification and cysts

duct stenoses, mucus plugging

7.4 CYSTIC MASSES IN PANCREAS (overview)

Non tumor

PSEUDOCYST

LIQUEFACTIVE NECROSIS

RETENTION CYST

ABSCESS

CONGENITAL

POLYCYSTIC KIDNEY DISEASE (~5%)

VON HIPPEL–LINDAU SIMPLE CYSTS

associated with microcystic adenoma

Tumor (5% of all pancreatic tumors)

see pancreatic neoplasms

MICROCYSTIC SEROUS ADENOMA (SEROUS CYSTADENOMA)

PAPILLARY CYSTIC TUMOR (SOLID-CYSTIC TUMOR)

MUCINOUS CYSTADENOMA (MACROCYSTIC ADENOMA)

MUCINOUS CYSTADENOCARCINOMA

INTRADUCTAL PAPILLARY MUCINOUS NEOPLASM

7.5 DIABETES MELLITUS

GROUP DEFINITION

state of chronic hyperglycemia, associated metabolic abnormalities and their sequelae

CLASSIFICATION IS BY TYPE

10% IDDM (insulin dependent diabetes mellitus)

90% NIDDM (non insulin dependent diabetes mellitus)

Secondary diabetes

pancreatitis

post surgical

hemochromatosis

CLASSIFICATION OF COMPLICATIONS

Acute

METABOLIC

DIABETIC KETOACIDOSIS

HYPEROSMOLAR NON KETOTIC STATE

HYPOGLYCEMIA

INFECTIONS

Chronic

MACROVASCULAR

MICROVASCULAR

NEPHROPATHY

RETINOPATHY

NEUROPATHY

MONONEURITIS

PERIPHERAL

AUTONOMIC

7.5.1 IDDM (insulin dependent diabetes mellitus)

DEFINITION

absolute insulin deficiency from autoimmune beta cell destruction

EPIDEMIOLOGY

prepubertal onset, seasonal incidence
(?environmental ??viral trigger)
wide geographic variation
familial/genetic predisposition

Risk factors

family history (partial RF)
monozygotic concordance 50%
certain HLA haplotypes (some susceptible,
others protective)
autoimmune disease (10% have other
thyrogastric cluster diseases)

CLINICAL

lymphocytic insulitis, antibeta antibodies,
antibeta CD4 lymphocytes (all precede
IDDM; found in 90% of IDDM); eventual
beta cell destruction following a silent
window
hyperglycemia, hypoinsulinemia
glycemic hyperosmolality – glycosuria,
polyuria, thirst
hypercatabolic state, weight loss, hunger
ketosis = metabolic ketotic acidosis,
ketonuria, dehydration, coma
diabetic ketoacidosis (DKA) may be
precipitated by intercurrent infection
survival is dependent on exogenous insulin

7.5.2 NIDDM (non insulin dependent diabetes mellitus)

DEFINITION

combination of peripheral insulin resistance
and relative insulin deficiency

EPIDEMIOLOGY

usual onset >40 years
prevalence is 10% of >70 year olds, ~3% of
total population
associated with sedentary lifestyle, and has
wide geographic variation
very prevalent in Aborigines and
Polynesians

Risk factors

family history
genetic predisposition (90% monozygotic
concordance)
obesity

CLINICAL

Hyperglycemia

glycosuria, polyuria, thirst
hyperosmolar non-ketotic state (usually
coma) – HONK
usually no diabetic ketoacidosis (DKA)

Infections

fungal skin infections
other

Constitutional

lethargy
malaise

Associated metabolic abnormalities

hyperlipidemia, dyslipidemia

7.5.3 DIABETES COMMON PATHWAY

NATURAL HISTORY – ACUTE COMPLICATIONS

Diabetic ketoacidosis (DKA)

occurs in IDDM
hyperglycemia, dehydration, ketoacidosis,
respiratory compensation, glycosuria,
ketonuria
potassium derangement (secondary to
treatment or even without it)
eventual coma, neurological deficit

Hyperosmolar non-ketosis (HONK)

occurs in NIDDM
hyperglycemia, dehydration, glycosuria
eventual coma
Na derangement

Hypoglycemia (with treatment)

GLYCOPENIC NEUROLOGICAL
DEFICITS
visual disturbance, mood alteration, acute
deterioration in higher mental function,
obtundation, coma

SYMPATHETIC ADRENERGIC
SYMPTOMS AND SIGNS
shaking, tachycardia, sweating, anxiety

Infections

FUNGAL
cutaneous
mucormycosis (orbital, sinonasal)

GAS FORMING
emphysematous cholecystitis
emphysematous pyelonephritis
gangrene

BACTERIAL INFECTIONS
pyelonephritis and osteomyelitis in
particular

NATURAL HISTORY – CHRONIC COMPLICATIONS

Macrovascular

*see entry on atherosclerosis in Ch 15
vascular*
accelerated atherosclerosis (depends on
duration of disease)
synergism with smoking and hypertension in
accelerating morbidity
coronary, cerebral, renal, aortoiliac
atherosclerosis in particular
LARGE VESSEL OCCLUSIVE DISEASE
LARGE VESSEL ANEURYSMAL DISEASE
THROMBOEMBOLISM

Microvascular

HYALINE ARTERIOLOSCLEROSIS
homogenous or layered, PAS + hyaline small
vessel deposits around basement
membrane; abnormally thickened,
abnormally permeable basement
membrane

MICROVASCULAR OCCLUSIVE
DISEASE
small vessel trophic disease
ischemia
infection
glomerular disease

Nephropathy

*see entry on diabetic nephropathy in Ch 08
renal*

MACROVASCULAR RENAL DISEASE

MICROVASCULAR RENAL DISEASE
HYALINE ARTERIOLOSCLEROSIS

GLOMERULAR DISEASE
capillary deposits
mesangial deposits
Bowman's space deposits

CLINICAL PRESENTATION
microalbuminuria, proteinuria, chronic
renal failure
progression relentless but rate varies
major cause of renal failure
recurs in renal transplants

Retinopathy

diabetic retinopathy is the third leading cause of blindness worldwide

BACKGROUND RETINOPATHY

DOTS

microaneurysms from pericyte loss

BLOTS

hard exudate

COTTON WOOL SPOTS

infarcts

and RETINAL HEMORRHAGES

PROLIFERATIVE RETINOPATHY

neovascularization (?secondary to hypoxic drive) with vitreous and retinal hemorrhages and subsequent scarring

Neuropathy

MONONEURITIS

thrombosis of vascular supply (microvascular complication)

e.g. femoral mononeuritis

PERIPHERAL

symmetrical glove and stocking polyneuropathy

sensory > motor

infections, neuropathic joints

Schwann cell loss ?secondary to sorbitol formation

AUTONOMIC

postural hypotension

erectile dysfunction

7.6 PANCREATIC ANATOMICAL VARIANTS

7.6.1 DUCT VARIANTS

CONVENTIONAL ANATOMY ~70%

SEPARATE BILIARY PAPILLA 2%

PANCREAS DIVISUM

main pancreatic duct to minor papilla, CBD and accessory pancreatic duct to minor papilla

7.6.2 ECTOPIC PANCREAS

STOMACH, DUODENUM, MECKEL'S DIVERTICULUM, ILEUM

7.6.3 ANNULAR PANCREAS

DEFINITION

congenital malrotation of the ventral pancreatic bud producing a ring of pancreatic tissue which encircles descending duodenum and may cause obstruction

CLINICAL

neonate: duodenal obstruction (including duodenal atresia)

adult: chronic pain, perhaps chronic pancreatitis

IMAGING

Fluoro

rounded extraluminal narrowing of duodenum at level of ampulla

ERCP/MRCP

circular course of accessory pancreatic duct around duodenum

US/CT/MR

ring of pancreatic tissue (texture, density and signal follow rest of pancreas) surrounding duodenum

7.7 PANCREATIC CARCINOMA NOS

DEFINITION

malignant pancreatic ductal epithelial neoplasm presenting late and usually unresectable

EPIDEMIOLOGY

male > female, >60 years old

Risk factors

Western diet

diabetes

smoking

partial gastrectomy

FAMILIAL CHRONIC PANCREATITIS

chronic pancreatitis NOS

CLINICAL

late presentation unless the carcinoma's location causes early biliary obstruction

60% in head of pancreas, 20% in body or tail, 20% diffuse infiltrating

jaundice; pain (from involvement of celiac plexus nerves or invasion of adjacent structures)

most carcinomas advanced at diagnosis, and unresectable

Spread

IN CONTINUITY

PERINEURAL

celiac plexus derived pain

LYMPHATIC

peripancreatic, celiac, superior mesenteric and portal nodes

commonest site of recurrence after resection

VASCULAR

SMV tumor thrombosis

occludes splenic vein, superior mesenteric vein

liver metastases

systemic metastases late

TRANSCELOMIC

Staging

TNM

T1	intrapancreatic, <2 cm
T2	intrapancreatic, >2 cm
T3	direct invasion of duodenum, bile duct, peripancreatic fat
T4	direct invasion of stomach, spleen, colon, or portal vein and celiac artery; and superior mesenteric vessels

STAGE I	T1 or T2, N0 M0
STAGE II	T3, N0 M0
STAGE III	T up to T3, N1 M0
STAGE IV	any N T4 or any T any N M1

MORPHOLOGY

scirrhous hypovascular mass replacing normal pancreatic parenchyma

virtually never calcify (but may engulf existing calcium)

90% adenocarcinoma (most anaplastic), 10% adenosquamous

IMAGING

AXR

no findings unless there is duodenal obstruction

Fluoro

pancreatic mass indirectly shown by enlarged duodenal loop

may show fixed narrowed or obstructed duodenum

may show direct invasion of duodenum

US

hypoechoic pancreatic mass

obliteration of splenic vein, may involve superior mesenteric vein, portal vein; intravenous thrombus

may have distal duct dilation

CT

mass isodense to pancreatic tissue precontrast

strand extension into peripancreatic fat indicates invasion

in pancreatic phase of contrast (20–30s scans) carcinoma enhances poorly compared to normal parenchyma, allowing margin estimation

mass often blocks CBD and pancreatic duct (double duct sign)

may encase superior mesenteric artery and superior mesenteric vein (fat plane around artery is normally present; vein directly contacts pancreatic tissue)

may have tumor or bland thrombus in splenic, superior mesenteric or portal veins

liver metastases hypovascular with ring enhancement

lymphadenopathy (peripancreatic, gastric, celiac, superior mesenteric, portal)

UNRESECTABLE IF

local invasion into adjacent organs or vessels (encases SMA and SMV or tumor thrombus)

distant metastases or ascites

MR

low or iso T1W signal, high T2W signal compared to parenchyma

Gd enhancement differential analogous to CT

PET

FDG avid (moderate)

particularly useful for nodal staging

useful for recurrence detection

differentials: stomach physiological uptake; renal pelves; early postoperative change

---

7.8 PANCREATIC ISLET TUMORS

GROUP DEFINITION

proliferative pancreatic islet cell neoplasms of variable malignant potential and hormonal expression

INSULINOMA

commonest islet cell tumor

80% clinically manifest, 20% silent

hyperinsulinemia, documentable hypoglycemic attacks (precipitated by fasting, exercise)

70% solitary adenoma, 10% multiple adenomas, 10% carcinoma (proven by metastases), 10% hyperplasia

GASTRINOMA

presents with Zollinger–Ellison syndrome: hypergastrinemia, hypersecretion, diarrhea

severe peptic ulceration: multifocal, ectopic, distal; recurrent or refractory

90% pancreatic, 10% duodenal

60% carcinoma (only proof is metastases), 40% adenoma (solitary or multiple)

GLUCAGONOMA

mild diabetes mellitus, migratory necrotizing skin erythema, anemia

SOMATOSTATINOMA

diabetes mellitus, cholelithiasis, steatorrhea

VIPOMA

watery diarrhea, achlorhydria, hypokalemia

IMAGING (group)

in general, difficult to locate and excise

US

usually unhelpful if mass is small

larger tumor presents with mass

may show liver metastases

CT

calcification frequent (~20%), may be clumpy

small tumor: hypervascular pancreatic mass with arterial phase contrast enhancement (i.e. different kinetics from surrounding normal pancreas)

large tumor: hypervascular mass, may contain calcification

MR

fat saturated precontrast T1W sequence: low intensity mass

T2W sequence: isointense or hyperintense signal

fat saturated dynamic contrast sequence: hypervascular arterial phase enhancing mass (same kinetics as CT)

Angio

arterial blush

venous sampling: hepatic vein sampling with intraarterial calcium or secretin; TIPS with direct portal venous sampling

NUC MED

many are octreotide (In-111 octreotide) avid

sensitivity in gastrinoma best (~95%), in insulinoma least (~50%)

may be the only means of localizing the tumor (more successful in extrapancreatic locations)

metastases have same avidity as parent tumor

PET (FDG)

variable FDG avidity

7.9 PANCREATIC NEOPLASMS – CYSTIC
(minority: ~5%)

GROUP DEFINITION

pathologic definition refers to cyst formation on histology

imaging definition requires macroscopically visible cysts

7.9.1 MICROCYSTIC SEROUS ADENOMA (= serous cystadenoma)

CLINICAL

ASSOCIATED WITH VON HIPPEL–LINDAU SYNDROME

rare, nearly always benign, elderly females (sporadic form)

large mass composed of multiple cysts lined by cuboidal epithelium

may have a central scar, 20% calcify (characteristic)

IMAGING

CT

solid or honeycomb appearance (cysts may be too small to resolve)

prominent contrast enhancement, outlining septa between cysts

central radial scar, calcification

MR

analogous to CT

7.9.2 PAPILLARY CYSTIC TUMOR (solid-cystic tumor)

CLINICAL

female >> male, <35 years old, uncommon

well circumscribed large mass with cystic and solid areas, usually benign

uniform eosinophilic cells forming papillae or sheets, estrogen, progesterone receptors

areas of tumor breakdown form cystic spaces and pseudopapillary projections

areas of hemorrhage

IMAGING

MR

foci of hemorrhage

7.9.3 MUCINOUS CYSTADENOMA (= macrocystic adenoma)

CLINICAL

40–60 years old

presents as an incidental finding or as an abdominal mass

MORPHOLOGY

unilocular or multiloculated septated collection of mucus surrounded by a fibrous capsule

mucus produced by neoplastic cells either lining the cavity or forming papillary projections

usually in body and tail of pancreas

no communication with the ductal system

undergoes malignant transformation

IMAGING

US

complex cystic mass with posterior acoustic enhancement and variable amount of internal debris

CT

large (6–10 cm) multiloculated cyst or conglomerate of few cysts in body or tail of pancreas

thick septa with vivid enhancement and possible calcification

DIFFERENTIAL: PSEUDOCYST

mucinous cystadenoma has no surrounding inflammatory change and no regression with time

MR

analogous to CT

cyst content has variable MR signal depending on protein content

septa may be shown better than with CT, they contrast with mucus

Fine needle aspiration

amylase: pseudocyst

mucin: mucinous cystic tumor

carcinoembryonic antigen: serous cystic tumor

7.9.4 MUCINOUS CYSTADENOCARCINOMA

malignant equivalent of mucinous cystadenoma

7.9.5 INTRADUCTAL PAPILLARY MUCINOUS NEOPLASM

CLINICAL

presents with symptoms of chronic pancreatitis, biliary obstruction, or pain

prognosis better than for solid ductal adenocarcinoma NOS, but variable depending on aggressivity of neoplastic epithelial component

MORPHOLOGY

neoplastic flat or papillary epithelium of branch pancreatic duct or main duct producing excessive mucus

mucus distends the ductal system; if tumor of a side branch, develops into a complex cystic mass; if of main duct, develops gross dilation of main duct with mucus extruding through the ampulla, and with variable distal atrophy

IMAGING

CT

side branch neoplasm: complex cystic mass composed of tubular low density components in uncinate process or head of pancreas with enhancing septa (ductal walls)

main duct neoplasm: dilation of main duct with atrophy of pancreatic parenchyma distally

DIFFERENTIAL IS CHRONIC PANCREATITIS

usually evolves over time, and has signs of inflammation

MR/MRCP

analogous to CT; may show mass of dilated branch ducts better than CT (signal contrast)

ERCP

shows communication between main duct and dilated mucus filled ducts (side branch tumor)

demonstrates dilated main duct filled with mucus (main duct tumor); dilation can be massive

once mucus cleared, shows filling defects (tumor; mucus concretions)

7.10 PANCREATIC NEOPLASMS – SOLID (majority)

PAPILLARY DUCTAL ADENOMA

CLINICAL

men = women, 50–70 years old

presents with biliary or pancreatic duct obstruction

PATHOLOGY

soft friable intraductal mass
tubulovillous architecture with variable
degree of intraepithelial dysplasia

DUCTAL ADENOCARCINOMA

see pancreatic carcinoma NOS

ACINAR ADENOCARCINOMA (1%)

ISLET CELL TUMORS

see separate entry

METASTASES

LYMPHOMA

see Ch 16

7.11 PANCREAS TRAUMA (grading)

IMAGING

CT
I   CONTUSION/INTRACAPSULAR HEMATOMA
II LACERATION, DUCT SYSTEM INTACT
III FRACTURE >50% WIDTH
IV CRUSH INJURY, SHATTERED PANCREAS

can not confirm intact duct with injury grades I or II on CT alone
infer duct injury with injury grades III or IV
LATE COMPLICATION: TRAUMATIC PSEUDOCYST (days–weeks)

7.12 PSEUDOCYST

DEFINITION

focal walled off collection of exudate or pancreatic secretions

ETIOLOGY

acute pancreatitis; chronic pancreatitis; pancreatic trauma

MORPHOLOGY

often solitary
non epithelialized wall of variable thickness with chronic inflammatory exudate and variable fibrotic reaction
proteinaceous contents; may contain old blood or cholesterol crystals from prior hemorrhage

Location

7.12.1 INTRAPANCREATIC

7.12.2 RETROPERITONEAL PERIPANCREATIC

7.12.3 LESSER SAC

7.12.4 DISTANT (presumed dissection along tissue planes by exudate)

IMAGING

US
fluid collection within/around pancreas or in lesser sac
hypoechoic, or with internal debris
hyperechoic if it has been bled into
irregular wall
superimposed signs of acute or chronic pancreatitis

CT
hypodense rounded cystic mass; hyperdense if recent bleeding
thick or thin wall with contrast enhancement; no enhancement of cyst contents
signs of pancreatitis

MR
analogous to CT
T1W signal of cyst content variable depending on blood products; T2W signal usually high

8. PEDIATRIC CONDITIONS

see Ch 18

9. AIDS ABDOMEN

see Ch 06

8 Adrenal, renal and urinary tract

1. NORMAL

1.1 ADRENAL NUCLEAR MEDICINE

Adrenal cortex

NP59 = I-123 or I-131 6-beta
    iodomethyl 19-norcholesterol
(alternative: selenocholesterol)
cold I thyroid blockade
image at 3 days post injection
may add dexamethasone suppression
    (4 mg daily for 7 days)

NORMAL UPTAKE
liver, gallbladder
stomach and colon
faint normal adrenal

CUSHING'S SYNDROME
bilateral uptake = hyperplasia
unilateral uptake = functional adenoma,
    carcinoma
no uptake = dexamethasone suppressed
    normal adrenals or carcinoma

CONN'S SYNDROME
use dexamethasone suppression
early unilateral breakthrough = adenoma
early bilateral breakthrough = hyperplasia
late bilateral breakthrough (>5 days) =
    normal

MASS
non functional adenoma is cold
functional adenoma is hot
carcinoma (~10% are functional) is usually
    cold
metastasis, lymphoma are cold
hemorrhage is cold

Adrenal medulla

MIBG = I-123 or I-131
    metaiodobenzylguanidine
cold I thyroid blockade
image at 24 and 48 hours post injection

NORMAL UPTAKE
salivary glands and nasal mucosa
myocardium
spleen, liver
bowel (myenteric plexus)
kidneys, bladder, urinary (and
    contamination)
faintly normal adrenal medulla
(thyroid if not blocked)

ADRENAL UPTAKE
faint bilateral uptake = normal medulla
focally increased uptake =
    pheochromocytoma or paraganglioma
focally increased uptake (pediatric mass) =
    neuroblastoma

1.2 NUC MED DYNAMIC RENAL SCANNING

ROI: region of interest

Renogram phases
(20 minute renogram)

PERFUSION PHASE
30s to 60s
reference to abdominal aorta
kidney parenchyma evident within 5s
upstroke of curves similar

CORTICAL UPTAKE PHASE
60s to 3 min
whole kidney ROI (background corrected) is
    used for:
differential renal function (normal not less
    than 45:55)
GFR estimation with DTPA (need to know
    injected dose, assumes normal anatomy)

EXCRETORY PHASE
excretion of tracer into collecting system
merges into drainage phase

DRAINAGE PHASE
drainage of tracer from collecting system to
    bladder
relevant in dilated collecting systems and in
    obstruction
whole kidney ROI used with diuretic
    washout studies

Renogram derived indices

TIME TO PEAK
normally <5 min

20 MINUTE RETENTION
ratio of 20 min ROI to peak ROI
normal is <0.3 or 0.4 in the absence of
    collecting system pooling or obstruction

PARENCHYMAL TRANSIT TIME (PTT)
measure of cortical function independent of
    drainage
2 pixel cortical ROI (corrected for
    background) used to generate PTT by
    curve deconvolution; requires compact
    bolus and normal cardiac function
usually <200–240s

RENOGRAM GRADE OR TYPE

GRADE 0 (normal)
rapid upstroke, normal time to peak, rapid
    two phase fall-off, normal 20 min
    retention

GRADE I
rapid upstroke, delayed time to peak, two
    phase fall-off, increased 20 min retention

GRADE II
slow upstroke, delayed single phase fall-off
beware of collecting system accumulation

GRADE III
continually rising renogram
beware of collecting system accumulation

GRADE IV
'renal failure pattern'
washin and washout with measurable renal
    uptake

GRADE V
'blood background curve'
ROI curve same as background – no
    measurable renal uptake

Commonly used tracers

DTPA
MNEMONIC: D-TP-A; TP: TOTALLY PASSIVE
low protein binding, first pass clearance
    ~20%, approximates GFR
normal GFR range is wide but at least
    >120 ml/min for adults

MAG3
~50% protein binding, small volume of
    distribution, all free MAG3 actively
    secreted by tubules, approximates
    estimated renal plasma flow (ERPF)
normal ERPF approx 600 ml/min; should be
    at least >400 ml/min

DMSA
MNEMONIC: D-MS-A: MS: MOSTLY STUCK
excreted by tubules, but ~50% is bound to
    normal cortex
cortex: background intensity highest at 3–6
    hours post injection

CHROMIUM DTPA
not an imaging isotope
requires serial blood samples
most accurate nuclear medicine GFR
    calculation

Captopril scanning

RATIONALE
internally generated angiotensin constricts
    efferent arterioles, maintaining filtration
    pressure and GFR in face of reduced
    afferent arteriole perfusion pressure
ACE inhibitor blocks this action leading to
    efferent arteriole dilation and a drop in
    tracer excretion

PROTOCOL
withhold ACE inhibitors or angiotensin
    receptor blockers
withhold diuretics (increased incidence of
    symptomatic hypotension)
prehydrate

25 mg or 50 mg of captopril orally, continue hydration

monitor BP: asymptomatic 10 mmHg drop indicates effect

significant hypotension needs treatment and may produce false positives

use MAG3 (no difference in accuracy to DTPA, better images) or DTPA

post captopril vs baseline study

SIGNS OF RENAL ARTERY STENOSIS

detects functionally significant stenosis, i.e. down to ~70%

increase in 20 min retention fraction (by >0.2)

deterioration in renogram grade (by two grades)

increase in parenchymal transit time beyond normal

visual findings (delayed uptake and excretion compared to baseline)

CAVEAT: preexisting poor renal function invalidates results (e.g. grade III renogram, GFR <20 ml/min)

DIFFERENTIAL

obstruction with backpressure

renal vein thrombosis

hypotension, dehydration

1.3 FUNCTIONAL ASSESSMENT OF OBSTRUCTION

IVU Lasix washout

qualitative delay in washout

may require an upright film as well

reproduction of symptoms suggestive

NUC MED diuretic renogram

(Lasix washout)

PARTICULAR USE IN PEDIATRICS

furosemide (Lasix) 1 mg/kg or 20 mg at 20 min

imaging for 20 min, washout curve T1/2 calculated

NORMAL: T1/2 <10 min

INTERMEDIATE: 10 min < T1/2 <20 min

OBSTRUCTED: T1/2 >20 min

Whitaker test

urinary catheter

22G percutaneous needle to renal collecting system

saline or dilute contrast infused via needle

collecting system pressure measured intermittently

at 10 ml/min flow rate normal is <10 cm H2O

equivocal 12–22 cm H2O

moderate obstruction 22–40 cm H2O

severe obstruction >40 cm H2O

1.4 RENAL ARTERY DOPPLER

Renal artery stenosis criteria – native artery

after Thomas Stavros

DIRECT INDICES

require a good renal artery trace at an angle that allows reasonable measurement of peak velocities

peak systolic velocity >180 cm/s

distal velocity : proximal velocity >2.0

renal to aortic peak velocity ratio >3.5 (>3.0 suggestive)

post stenotic turbulence

stenosis visible in cross section and >70%

INDIRECT INDICES

assessment of interlobar arteries without demonstration of renal artery

controversial, as have given different results in different hands

decreased color flow

acceleration time >(0.07 to 0.1) second

acceleration <3 m/s2

loss of early systolic peak and tardus parvus waveform

decreased resistive index

CAVEATS

GENERAL

beware aliasing (go to lower frequency transducer)

beware of side to side asymmetry

similar approach to both kidneys (usually posterior)

resistive index distal to a renal artery stenosis DROPS

IF RESISTIVE INDEX IS ABNORMALLY ELEVATED

accuracy of indirect indices (loss of early systolic peak and drop in acceleration) is reduced

blood pressure will probably not respond to dilation of stenosis if a stenosis is present

Renal artery stenosis criteria – transplant

assess renal–iliac ratio and resistive index

localized substantial elevation in renal Vpeak indicates stenosis

Resistive index

normal adult <0.7

normal infant 0.7–0.8

transplant <0.7

technically demanding, sensitive and completely non specific

1.5 MR DYNAMIC RENAL SCANNING

Gd-DTPA has IDENTICAL kinetics to Tc-99m DTPA

see notes under DTPA in nuc med dynamic scanning

2. GAMUTS

2.1 GENERIC (all modalities)

2.1.1 ADRENAL BILATERAL ENLARGEMENT

METASTASES

LYMPHOMA

HYPERPLASIA

INFECTION

especially TB and fungal

UNILATERAL MASS OCCURRING BILATERALLY

2.1.2 ADRENAL INSUFFICIENCY

Pituitary cause

HYPOPITUITARISM

ADENOMA

POST SURGICAL

SHEEHAN'S SYNDROME = post partum pituitary apoplexy

INFILTRATION: SARCOIDOSIS, LYMPHOMA, HISTIOCYTOSIS, HYPOPHYSITIS

Adrenal cause

AUTOIMMUNE – ADDISON'S DISEASE

see its own entry

OTHER ADRENAL CAUSE – ADDISON'S SYNDROME

see its own entry

Iatrogenic

rapid steroid withdrawal following steroid suppression

2.1.3 ADRENAL MASS

Gamut

MASS OF ADRENOCORTICAL ORIGIN

ADRENOCORTICAL HYPERPLASIA

NON FUNCTIONING ADENOMA/NODULE

FUNCTIONING ADRENOCORTICAL
ADENOMA

ADRENOCORTICAL CARCINOMA

CONGENITAL ADRENAL HYPERPLASIA
(bilateral)

MASS OF ADRENAL MEDULLARY ORIGIN

NEUROBLASTOMA

PHEOCHROMOCYTOMA

MYELOLIPOMA

MASS OF OTHER ORIGIN

MOST: METASTASIS, LYMPHOMA

HEMORRHAGE

special clinical circumstances (neonate,
overwhelming sepsis, disseminated
intravascular coagulation)

blood products on MR; no contrast
enhancement

shrinks with time, calcifies

ADRENALITIS, ADRENAL TB

special clinical circumstances: Gram
negative sepsis, overwhelming sepsis,
meningococcus, TB

COMPLEX CYST

differential is usually resolving hemorrhage
vs cystic tumor

2.1.4 BIG SMOOTH KIDNEY
(one or both)

Normal = 3.5 vertebrae + disks

Unilateral
HYDRONEPHROSIS
RENAL MASS
PYELONEPHRITIS
RENAL INFARCT
RENAL VEIN THROMBOSIS
TRAUMATIC HEMATOMA
DUPLICATION OR CROSSED FUSED RENAL
ECTOPIA
COMPENSATORY HYPERTROPHY OR
SOLITARY KIDNEY

Bilateral

BILATERAL ONLY CAUSES
ACUTE TUBULAR NECROSIS

EARLY GLOMERULONEPHRITIS
EARLY DIABETES MELLITUS
MEDULLARY SPONGE KIDNEY
AUTOSOMAL DOMINANT POLYCYSTIC
KIDNEY DISEASE
LEUKEMIA, LYMPHOMA, BILATERAL
TUMOR INFILTRATION
STORAGE DISEASES
AMYLOIDOSIS

UNILATERAL CAUSE PRESENT BILATERALLY
BILATERAL HYDRONEPHROSIS
BILATERAL PYELONEPHRITIS
BILATERAL RENAL VEIN THROMBOSIS
BILATERAL RENAL MASSES

2.1.5 BLADDER GAMUTS

2.1.5.1 Small volume bladder
FIBROSIS
SURGERY, RADIOTHERAPY,
CHEMOTHERAPY
TB, SCHISTOSOMIASIS (bladder wall
calcification)

2.1.5.2 Pear shaped bladder
PERIVESICAL FLUID
BILATERAL LYMPHADENOPATHY
PELVIC LIPOMATOSIS
NEUROFIBROMATOSIS

2.1.5.3 Thick walled bladder

EDEMA
CYSTITIS

INFILTRATION
NEOPLASTIC
SCHISTOSOMIASIS (ACTIVE)

HYPERTROPHY

2.1.5.4 Bladder outflow obstruction

LOOSE BODY (stone, clot)

ANATOMICAL – MALE
BENIGN PROSTATIC HYPERTROPHY
URETEROCELE (OBSTRUCTING)
TUMOR
POLYP
TRANSITIONAL CELL CARCINOMA
PROSTATE CARCINOMA
RHABDOMYOSARCOMA (child)
STRICTURE
usually posterior or anterior urethra
usually post infective, post traumatic or post
operative
URETHRAL VALVES

MEATAL STENOSIS

ANATOMICAL – FEMALE
UTERINE PROLAPSE
URETHRAL DIVERTICULUM
TUMOR
POLYP
TRANSITIONAL CELL CARCINOMA
CERVICAL CARCINOMA
RHABDOMYOSARCOMA (child)

FUNCTIONAL
DETRUSOR/SPHINCTER DYSSYNERGIA

2.1.5.5 Calcified bladder wall
TB
SCHISTOSOMIASIS
RADIOTHERAPY

2.1.6 CALCIFICATION

see Ch 06

2.1.7 DILATED COLLECTING SYSTEM, NO OBSTRUCTION

REFLUX

PREVIOUS OBSTRUCTION NOW
RELIEVED

MEGACALYCOSIS

2.1.8 FOCAL KIDNEY DEFECTS

Scarring
POST INFECTIVE
POST OPERATIVE/POST TRAUMATIC

Post infarct fibrosis

Papillary necrosis

(Fetal lobulation)
normal variant that simulates cortical
defects
uniform, multifocal, anatomical
no reduction in parenchymal thickness

2.1.9 FREE INTRAPERITONEAL FLUID

see Ch 06

2.1.10 LARGE URETER

OBSTRUCTION (ureter or bladder)

REFLUX

PREGNANCY

INFECTION

ECTOPIA, URETEROCELE

POLYURIA

PRIMARY MEGAURETER

2.1.11 PAPILLARY NECROSIS

MNEMONIC: ADIPOSE

A-NALGESIC NEPHROPATHY

D-IABETES
ESPECIALLY WITH PYELONEPHRITIS

I-NFANTS
SICK, IN INTENSIVE CARE, ETC

P-YELONEPHRITIS

O-BSTRUCTION

S-ICKLE CELL DISEASE

E-THANOL
uncommonly, E-THYLENE GLYCOL

2.1.12 RENAL CYST OR CYST-LIKE STRUCTURE

Simple

CYST

PARAPELVIC CYST

CALYCEAL DIVERTICULUM

Complex

BENIGN

HEMORRHAGIC CYST

INFECTED CYST

SEPTATED CYST

HYDATID

TB, ABSCESS, HYDROCALYX

AV MALFORMATION, ANEURYSM

MALIGNANT

CYSTIC NEPHROMA

CYSTIC RENAL CELL CARCINOMA

CYSTIC WILMS' TUMOR

LYMPHOMA WITH CYSTIC CHANGE

PEDIATRIC DYSPLASIAS WITH CYSTS

MULTICYSTIC DYSPLASTIC KIDNEY

CYSTIC RENAL DYSPLASIA

2.1.13 RENAL HEMATOMA

Traumatic

Spontaneous

TUMOR
ANGIOMYOLIPOMA
RENAL CELL CARCINOMA

AV MALFORMATION

HEMORRHAGIC CYST

INFARCT

INFECTION

ARTERITIS

2.1.14 RENAL MASS
(space occupying lesion – SOL)

CYST (simple or complex)

CALYCEAL DIVERTICULUM

BLOCKED CALYX

BLOCKED DUPLEX

TUMOR
RENAL CELL CARCINOMA
TRANSITIONAL CELL CARCINOMA
ANGIOMYOLIPOMA
LYMPHOMA
METASTASIS

PSEUDOTUMOR
PROMINENT PARENCHYMA

ABSCESS, TB

XANTHOGRANULOMATOUS
  PYELONEPHRITIS

HYDATID CYST

RENAL HEMATOMA

2.1.15 RETROPERITONEAL FIBROSIS

INFLAMMATORY ANEURYSM,
  INFLAMMATORY
  ATHEROSCLEROSIS

METHYSERGIDE

RADIATION FIBROSIS

DIFFERENTIAL: SCIRRHOUS
  NEOPLASM

2.1.16 SMALL BUMPY KIDNEY

REFLUX SCARS

INFARCTS

TRAUMA

TB

DYSPLASIA

2.1.17 SMALL SMOOTH KIDNEY

Unilateral

OBSTRUCTIVE ATROPHY

INFARCTED KIDNEY

RENAL ARTERY STENOSIS

LATE SEQUELAE OF RENAL VEIN
  THROMBOSIS

WHOLE KIDNEY HYPOPLASIA OR
  APLASIA

Bilateral
LATE GLOMERULONEPHRITIS AND
  VARIANTS

LATE DIABETIC NEPHROPATHY

PAPILLARY NECROSIS

VASCULITIS

UNILATERAL CAUSE OCCURRING
  BILATERALLY

2.1.18 URETERIC OBSTRUCTION

Luminal

MOBILE

STONE

CLOT

PAPILLA

FUNGUS BALL

FIXED

TUMOR

Mural

EDEMA

STRICTURE

STONE, SURGERY, TB, INFECTION

External (from above down)

ARTERY

CLASSICALLY UPPER MOIETY RENAL ARTERY CROSSING PELVIS

PANCREATITIS

RETROPERITONEAL FIBROSIS

TUMOR OR LYMPH NODE METASTASES

INCLUDES ENDOMETRIOSIS

PREGNANCY

UTERINE PROLAPSE (female)

PROSTATE HYPERTROPHY (male)

ACCIDENTAL LIGATION

2.1.19 VOIDING DYSFUNCTION

Failure to store

BLADDER

DETRUSOR HYPERACTIVITY

FIBROTIC BLADDER

SENSORY URGENCY

usually inflammatory or neurological

OUTLET

STRESS INCONTINENCE

INCOMPETENT BLADDER NECK

URETHRAL INSTABILITY

Failure to empty

BLADDER

NEUROLOGICAL

MYOGENIC

PSYCHOGENIC

OUTLET

see bladder outflow obstruction gamut

2.2 IVU (intravenous urogram)

2.2.1 AMPUTATED CALYX

TB

TRANSITIONAL CELL CARCINOMA OR OTHER TUMOR

POST INFECTIVE STRICTURE

OBSTRUCTION BY CALYCEAL STONE

2.2.2 DELAYED EXCRETION

Obstruction

dense delayed nephrogram

faint delayed pyelogram
(may have crescent sign)

Acute hypotension

bilateral persistent corticogram
differential: acute prerenal renal failure

Renal artery stenosis

small delayed nephrogram
dense delayed pyelogram
(may have collateral notching)
see NUC MED gamuts

Renal vein thrombosis

large faint delayed nephrogram
spidery faint delayed pyelogram

Differential: pyelonephritis

(nephrogram and pyelogram appear on time)

large streaky faint nephrogram
spidery faint pyelogram

2.2.3 FILLING DEFECT

LUCENT STONE

CLOT

SLOUGHED PAPILLA

TRANSITIONAL CELL CARCINOMA

AV MALFORMATION, VARICES

FUNGUS BALL

2.2.4 MISSING KIDNEY

Kidney is hiding

PELVIC KIDNEY

CROSSED RENAL ECTOPIA

Kidney is absent

NEPHRECTOMY

DYSPLASIA (ESPECIALLY MULTICYSTIC DYSPLASTIC KIDNEY)

AGENESIS

Kidney does not enhance

2.2.5 NON-ENHANCING KIDNEY

HIGH GRADE OBSTRUCTION

RENAL ARTERY OCCLUSION OR VERY HIGH GRADE STENOSIS

RENAL VEIN OCCLUSION (complete, sudden)

Total replacement by tumor

EXPECT AN ABNORMALLY SHAPED RENAL BED MASS

TOTAL REPLACEMENT BY XANTHOGRANULOMATOUS PYELONEPHRITIS

RARE

ABSENT KIDNEY

2.2.6 PERSISTENT NEPHROGRAM

Unilateral

OBSTRUCTION

RENAL VEIN THROMBOSIS (GRADUAL)

RENAL ARTERY STENOSIS (RARE, USUALLY HAS A PYELOGRAM)

Bilateral

ACUTE HYPOTENSION/ACUTE TUBULAR NECROSIS

MULTIPLE MYELOMA/RENAL AMYLOIDOSIS

2.3 US

2.3.1 ACUTELY EDEMATOUS KIDNEY

MNEMONIC: PRANG

P-YELONEPHRITIS

R-ENAL VEIN THROMBOSIS

A-TN OR TRANSPLANT REJECTION

GN: G-LOMERULO-N-EPHRITIS

2.3.2 INCREASED PYRAMIDAL ECHOGENICITY

NEPHROCALCINOSIS

MEDULLARY SPONGE KIDNEY, TUBULAR ECTASIA

GOUT

MEDULLARY MICROCYSTIC DISEASE

2.4 NUC MED

2.4.1 COLD PARENCHYMAL DEFECT

TRUE RENAL MASS

INFARCT OR SCAR

FOCAL PYELONEPHRITIS (LOBAR NEPHRONIA)

RADIATION NEPHRITIS

2.4.2 CONTINUALLY RISING RENOGRAM

HIGH GRADE OBSTRUCTION

ACUTE TUBULAR NECROSIS (MAG3)

RENAL ARTERY STENOSIS

TRANSPLANT: SEE ITS OWN ENTRY

2.4.3 EXTRARENAL DTPA/DMSA ACCUMULATION

TAMPON

EXTRAVASATION

TUMOR
UNPREDICTABLE

ABSCESS
UNPREDICTABLE

2.4.4 ONE KIDNEY NOT DEMONSTRATED

Absent kidney

NEPHRECTOMY

DYSPLASIA (ESPECIALLY MULTICYSTIC DYSPLASTIC KIDNEY)

AGENESIS

Non functioning kidney

VERY HIGH GRADE OBSTRUCTION

RENAL ARTERY OCCLUSION OR VERY HIGH GRADE STENOSIS

REPLACEMENT BY TUMOR

REPLACEMENT BY XANTHOGRANULOMATOUS PYELONEPHRITIS

2.4.5 RENOGRAM: INCREASED TRANSIT TIME AND CORTICAL RETENTION

DIABETES MELLITUS (CHRONIC)

GLOMERULONEPHRITIS (CHRONIC)

OTHER CHRONIC PARENCHYMAL DISEASE

RENAL ARTERY STENOSIS

TRANSPLANT: SEE ITS OWN ENTRY

RENAL, URINARY TRACT AND ADRENAL CONDITIONS

3. ACQUIRED RENAL AND URINARY TRACT CONDITIONS

3.1 ACUTE CORTICAL NECROSIS

DEFINITION

rare selective death of renal cortical parenchyma with preservation of pyramids and medulla

ETIOLOGY

Adults
placental abruption, placenta previa hemorrhage
severe hypotension, septic shock
envenomation
hyperacute transplant rejection

Children
severe dehydration
hemolytic uremic syndrome
transfusion reaction

IMAGING

XR/CT (late)
cortical calcification

CT/MR (early)
non enhancing cortex with normally enhancing medulla

3.2 ACUTE TUBULAR NECROSIS (ATN)

DEFINITION

acute tubular epithelial death or dysfunction with preservation of reticulin skeleton and capacity for full regeneration

ETIOLOGY

Ischemic
cardiogenic shock, hypovolemic shock, septic shock

Toxic
heme, myoglobin, hemoglobin
immunoglobulin light chains
aminoglycosides, diuretics, heavy metals
contrast media
animal venom

CLINICAL

presents with acute renal failure resolving in 2–3 weeks on dialysis
common with cadaveric transplants (evident on day 1)
tubular epithelial necrosis, tubular casts

IMAGING

US
size normal or increased, resistive index >0.75

NUC MED (DTPA)
washin–washout curve
degree of excreted DTPA reflects amount of preserved function

NUC MED (MAG3)
dense cortical nephrogram proportional to surviving cell mass; no excretion in severe ATN
amount of excreted MAG3 reflects returning function
renograms deteriorate and recover reflecting progress of ATN (see renogram grades)

IVU, CT
contrast contraindicated, but if given inadvertently: dense very prolonged nephrogram

3.3 AMYLOIDOSIS

DEFINITION

progressive intercellular deposition of insoluble protein ('amyloid', with characteristic light microscopic appearance) leading to cellular atrophy and loss

ETIOLOGY

Systemic amyloidosis

AL (75% of cases)
immunoglobulin light chain ('Bence Jones protein')
multiple myeloma patients, patients with monoclonal gammopathy of other types
'primary amyloidosis' in the older classification

AA
SAA protein (liver synthesized protein, acute phase reactant, need levels of x10 to x1000 normal to lead to amyloid formation)
'secondary amyloidosis' in the older classification
CHRONIC AUTOIMMUNE DISEASE
RHEUMATOID ARTHRITIS
SCLERODERMA
SYSTEMIC LUPUS ERYTHEMATOSUS
INFLAMMATORY BOWEL DISEASE
CHRONIC INFECTION
TB
OSTEOMYELITIS
MALIGNANCY
HODGKIN'S DISEASE
RENAL CELL CARCINOMA
FAMILIAL MEDITERRANEAN FEVER

Localized amyloidosis

CEREBRAL
made of A beta protein (also called beta 2 amyloid protein) – associated with Alzheimer's disease

SKIN, LARYNX, UROGENITAL MUCOSA ('amyloidoma')
AL type amyloid, ?localized plasmacytoma

PATHOGENESIS

presence of elevated SAA protein or light chains in itself is insufficient to cause amyloidosis

failure of SAA or light chain breakdown is possibly causative
likely sequence is deposition of soluble precursor protein, precursor cleavage, formation of insoluble fibrils: indefinite length paired fibrils composed of beta pleated sheets made of the principal amyloid protein (which varies with amyloid type) and invariable minor P component
eventual cellular pressure atrophy, with clinical manifestations from cellular depletion or mass effect

MACRO

waxy pale large organs (amyloid deposition) vs small shrunken organs (cellular atrophy)
stain blue with iodine and sulfuric acid (hence 'amyloid')

MICRO

H+E: acellular pink hyaline deposits, cell loss
Congo red: pink/orange, and birefringent green with polarized light

CLINICAL

SYSTEMIC AMYLOIDOSIS MANIFESTATIONS: renal > cardiac > GIT > skin
renal involvement most common and most significant manifestation of amyloidosis
renal failure most important cause of amyloid related death
poor prognosis overall, particularly poor in multiple myleoma

Kidney
glomerular deposits > tubular deposits, small vessel deposits with angiopathy
nephrotic syndrome, chronic renal failure, renal vein thrombosis

Liver
interstitial deposits with hepatocyte pressure atrophy
hepatomegaly, liver failure occurs late

Spleen
geographic deposits or sago deposits (central follicular dot-like deposits) with splenomegaly

Lungs
interstitial deposits

GIT mucosa and tongue
tongue masses; focal GIT masses
mucosal thickening, malabsorption, bleeding

Thyroid and pancreas
infiltration with pseudogoitre

Heart
subendocardial deposits and deposits between muscle fibers

Skin, respiratory, urogenital mucosa
interstitial deposits, submucosal masses, cutaneous masses
laryngeal, bronchial focal masses

Joints, synovium, muscle
see Ch 03
soft tissue, synovial deposits, carpal tunnel syndrome
associated with dialysis amyloidosis

Cerebral amyloid
amyloid angiopathy with bleeding
Alzheimer's disease

IMAGING (renal manifestations)

US/non contrast CT
smooth large kidneys (early)
may have hypoechoic parenchyma
renal vein thrombosis a frequent complication

IVU
IV contrast contraindicated in multiple myeloma and renal amyloidosis (accelerates renal failure)
normal or fainter nephrogram
collecting system may be compressed by renal parenchymal enlargement

3.4 ANALGESIC NEPHROPATHY

DEFINITION

papillary necrosis and progressive renal failure from (non opiate) analgesic abuse

ETIOLOGY

tends to present in older females
prolonged ingestion of phenacetin, acetaminophen/paracetamol, aspirin, NSAIDs; analgesic mixtures (component effect is synergistic)

CLINICAL

proteinuria, hematuria, loss of concentrating
   ability, nocturia
papillary sloughing, obstruction leading to
   renal colic
inevitable renal failure
increased incidence of transitional cell
   carcinoma

IMAGING

see entries on:
PAPILLARY NECROSIS
OBSTRUCTION
TRANSITIONAL CELL CARCINOMA

3.5 ANGIOMYOLIPOMA

DEFINITION

benign renal hamartoma with tendency to
   spontaneous hemorrhage and a strong
   association with tuberous sclerosis

CLINICAL

incidental imaging finding – often a
   diagnostic problem
0.1% of general population, 80% of tuberous
   sclerosis (TS)
50% of patients with angiomyolipomas have
   TS; 100% if multiple
composed of fat, thick walled blood vessels,
   irregular smooth muscle; bleeds

IMAGING

in the absence of identifiable fat,
   unequivocal distinction from renal cell
   carcinoma is impossible

US

rounded hyperechoic mass without
   shadowing
if in patient with TS – very likely
if multiple – very likely

DIFFERENTIAL

atypical (hyperechoic) renal cell carcinoma
renal sinus fat in unusual position
milk of calcium cyst

CT

well circumscribed parenchymal mass
   containing fat and soft tissue components
neovascular enhancement (different from
   renal parenchyma)

MR

fat and soft tissue components
vascular flow voids

Angio

hypervascular mass with abnormal blood
   vessels

NUC MED (DMSA)

cold mass

3.6 CYSTITIS (overview)

ACUTE INFECTIVE

ACUTE BACTERIAL

EMPHYSEMATOUS

TUBERCULOUS

ACUTE NON INFECTIVE

DRUG INDUCED

RADIATION CYSTITIS

CATHETER INDUCED

CHRONIC INFECTIVE

STONE RELATED

FOLLICULAR

CYSTITIS CYSTICA
see ureteropyelitis cystica

MALAKOPLAKIA
friable yellow brown ulcerating plaques,
   fibrosis, increased malignant potential

CHRONIC NON INFECTIVE

INTERSTITIAL
chronic symptoms but culture negative;
   scars and ulcers on cystoscopy
diffuse chronic inflammation, eventual
   fibrosis

PAPILLARY POLYPOID
inflammatory polyps reacting to mechanical
   irritation

RELATED PHENOMENA

BLADDER ENDOMETRIOSIS

SQUAMOUS METAPLASIA

GLANDULAR METAPLASIA

3.7 DIABETIC NEPHROPATHY

DEFINITION

renal parenchymal changes of chronic
   diabetes
by definition different from renal
   atherosclerosis in diabetes

CLINICAL

very common cause of endstage renal
   failure, dialysis and renal transplantation
progression from proteinuria to nephrotic
   syndrome to endstage renal failure
develops years after onset of diabetes and
   progresses over years; progression more
   severe in IDDM (type I diabetes) than
   NIDDM

MICRO

DIABETIC GLOMERULOSCLEROSIS

ARTERIOLAR SCLEROSIS

PAPILLARY NECROSIS

IMAGING

non specific deterioration in renal function
   and GFR
kidneys may be enlarged early, atrophic later
no change in parenchymal appearance, or
   non specific bilateral alteration of texture
papillary necrosis may occur

US

normal or
early mild bilateral enlargement or
increased resistive index or
increased parenchymal echogenicity or
mild parenchymal width atrophy

NUC MED (DTPA/MAG3)

bilateral non specific deterioration in
   renogram grade and numeric indices
no evidence of obstruction to drainage

3.8 GLOMERULO-NEPHRITIS (GN)

DEFINITION

glomerular malfunction with a wide range of etiology and assumed immune pathogenesis presenting with several histological patterns and leading to acute or chronic renal failure

EPIDEMIOLOGY

heterogeneous group; children, young and older adults
associations with autoimmune disease
associations with viral infections (hepatitis B virus, hepatitis C virus, HIV)

ETIOLOGY

Idiopathic (most common)

Minimal change disease

children, post viral respiratory or bacterial infection
nephrotic syndrome resolving with treatment

Post bacterial acute GN

children and adults post bacterial sore throat
(Streptococcus pyogenes Lancefield group A >> others)
acute nephritic syndrome, acute renal failure
usually good outcome with treatment

IgA (Berger's) disease

children and young adults with intermittent bouts of hematuria
first episode may be precipitated by infection
slowly progressive with variable course
circulating polymeric IgA deposited in GBM

Lupus (SLE) GN

young adults, female > male
progressive slow proteinuria and chronic renal failure
variable histology, variable course

Polyarteritis nodosa (PAN) GN and Wegener's GN

rapidly progressive GN is the cardinal presenting feature in both diseases

Henoch–Schönlein purpura

children with hematuria; good outcome with treatment

Goodpasture's syndrome

uncommon, young male > female
antiGBM antibodies
presents with nephritic syndrome, acute renal failure and massive pulmonary alveolar hemorrhage
may have a good response to therapy

Drug induced

penicillamine, gold

Bacterial endocarditis

chronic GBM deposition of circulating antigen–immunoglobulin complexes
cured if endocarditis cured

HBV, HCV, HIV

?altered immunity, ?circulating complexes

Alport's syndrome

?X-linked hereditary chronic GN of young adults
sensorineural deafness, lens dislocation

PATHOGENESIS

deposition or formation of immune complexes on glomerular basement membrane (GBM), rarely direct antiGBM attack
inflammatory and proliferative reactions; glomerular collapse, vascular occlusion, fibrosis
classification of GN is by histologic appearance, and any one etiology can have different histological patterns each with its own prognosis

CLINICAL PRESENTATION

NEPHROTIC SYNDROME
NEPHRITIC SYNDROME
ACUTE RENAL FAILURE
CHRONIC RENAL FAILURE
(see renal failure entry for definitions)
ASYMPTOMATIC HEMATURIA/PROTEINURIA
SYMPTOMS OF PRIMARY AUTOIMMUNE DISEASE

NATURAL HISTORY

very variable and depends on clinical presentation and biopsy findings

treatment: steroids, immune suppression, plasmapheresis

IMAGING

see renal failure

3.9 HYPERTENSIVE RENAL DISEASE

CLINICAL

Chronic benign hypertension

granular small kidneys
'plasmatic vasculosis', occlusion of afferent arterioles, glomerular sclerosis

Malignant (accelerated) hypertension

enlarged kidneys with 'fleabite' hemorrhages
arteriolar fibrinoid necrosis, hemorrhages

IMAGING

see chronic renal failure

3.10 INTERSTITIAL NEPHRITIS (tubulointerstitial nephritis – TIN)

GROUP DEFINITION

histologically defined group of diverse conditions characterized by inflammatory cellular infiltrate in renal parenchymal interstitium and tubular damage

3.10.1 ACUTE TIN

ETIOLOGY

DRUG REACTION (sulfonamides, diuretics, NSAIDs, other)
IN BONE MARROW TRANSPLANTS (graft vs host disease)
(infective pyelonephritis is classified separately)

CLINICAL

fever, hematuria, proteinuria, eosinophilia, skin rash
acute renal failure in 50%

IMAGING

US

kidneys normal size or slightly swollen (acutely)
may have altered parenchymal echogenicity (non specific)

3.10.2 CHRONIC TIN

includes: reflux nephropathy, obstructive nephropathy, radiation nephropathy, analgesic nephropathy, medullary cystic disease

3.11 MULTIPLE MYELOMA
(renal manifestations)

see Ch 05

CLINICAL

renal failure a major cause of death in multiple myeloma
Bence Jones proteinuria (light chains)
acute renal failure may be precipitated by dehydration, infection or drugs

PATHOGENESIS

TUBULAR OBSTRUCTION

Bence Jones proteins (light chains) combine with urinary glycoprotein (Tamm–Horsfall protein) forming obstructive tubular casts
Bence Jones proteins also appear to be directly toxic to tubular cells

HYPERCALCEMIA

AMYLOIDOSIS

IMAGING

kidneys normal size or enlarged
see renal failure entry

3.12 NEUROGENIC BLADDER

3.12.1 REFLEX NEUROPATHIC BLADDER

CLINICAL

commonest form of neurogenic bladder
spinal cord injuries, multiple sclerosis, cerebrovascular accidents
loss of upper motor neuron detrusor and sphincter innervation
detrusor–sphincter dyssynergia (failure of sphincter to relax during detrusor contraction)
involuntary inappropriate contractions against resistance lead to detrusor hypertrophy and large residual volumes

IMAGING

Fluoro (cystogram)

reduced bladder volume
heavy trabeculation, multiple diverticula ('Christmas tree' bladder)
moderate post void residual

US/CT

thickened bladder wall, trabeculations, diverticula

3.12.2 AREFLEXIC BLADDER

CLINICAL

lower motor neuron or sensory neuron damage or both
diabetes, cauda compression, trauma, multiple sclerosis, tabes dorsalis
usually large atonic bladder with overflow incontinence and absence of sensation of fullness
if sensory innervation preserved, sensation of fullness without ability to empty
if some motor innervation preserved, some degree of tone may be present

IMAGING

Fluoro/CT/US

large dilated bladder, large post void residual

3.13 OBSTRUCTION

CLASSIFICATION

ACUTE VS CHRONIC (slow)

LOW GRADE VS HIGH GRADE VS COMPLETE

UNILATERAL VS BILATERAL

LEVEL OF OBSTRUCTION (high vs low)

THESE FACTORS WILL DETERMINE CLINICAL PRESENTATION AND IMAGING FINDINGS

ETIOLOGY

see ureteric obstruction gamut

PATHOGENESIS

early rise in pressure to 50–70 mmHg
increased renal lymph flow, decreased renal blood flow, increased resistive index
hyperperistalsis and colic
eventual aperistalsis, dilation, atony

CLINICAL

3.13.1 Acute bilateral obstruction

uremia and death
relief of obstruction restores normal function

3.13.2 Acute unilateral obstruction

renal colic on that side
total obstruction may cause irreversible deterioration in renal function by 1 week
with lesser degrees of obstruction deteriorating renal function reversible for a number of weeks
(complete obstruction may produce a shell nephrogram by 3 months)
eventual irreversible functional deterioration, parenchymal atrophy

3.13.3 Chronic unilateral obstruction

silent hydronephrosis
may be completely compensated by hypertrophy of the opposite kidney
degree of recoverable renal function depends on volume of remaining renal parenchyma, degree of obstruction and its duration

3.13.4 Chronic bilateral obstruction

silent bilateral hydronephrosis with slowly progressive renal failure

relief of obstruction usually prevents deterioration but less likely to restore lost functional capacity

3.13.5 Complications

FORNICEAL RUPTURE, PERIRENAL URINOMA

SUPERIMPOSED INFECTION

IMAGING (acute obstruction)

XR

calcified stone along the expected course of the ureter very suggestive

US

50% normal
50% mild dilation
may have increased resistive index
serial ultrasound much more accurate
DILATION DOES NOT EQUAL OBSTRUCTION
NO DILATION DOES NOT EQUAL NO OBSTRUCTION

IVU (high grade obstruction)

dense delayed nephrogram
faint delayed pyelogram
mild dilation to level of obstruction
forniceal rupture causes collecting system to decompress
pyelosinus backflow produces streaks of contrast overlying collecting system and extending into peritoneum

IVU (low grade obstruction)

delayed pyelogram
mild dilation
holdup at level of obstruction ('standing column')

NUC MED (DTPA/MAG3)

delay in drainage in proportion to degree of holdup
normal perfusion
delay in tracer uptake and excretion comparatively mild and determined by degree and duration of obstruction
abnormal whole renogram curve with delayed time to peak, or accumulation curve (no drainage at all)
cortical only curve less abnormal than whole kidney curve

CT (targeted at stone)

non contrast thin section volumetric CT

DIRECT FINDINGS

virtually all stones are high density on CT, including urate, but excluding rare low density matrix only stones
stone within ureter (full cuff of ureteric wall) or at vesicoureteric junction (may be a considerable distance into apparent bladder wall in a partly empty bladder)
ureter can be traced above and below stone (unequivocal identification)

DIFFERENTIAL: phlebolith
no cuff of ureteric soft tissue
may have a low density core
not in the expected position of the ureter

INDIRECT FINDINGS

ipsilateral renal pelvis stones
dilated ureter or collecting system above
peri-renal stranding (edema), slightly swollen kidney
extravasation, urinoma

CT (general)

dilated renal collecting system and ureter
may show a transition zone
perirenal stranding (edema), slightly swollen kidney
extravasation, urinoma
may show cause of obstruction: stone, tumor, surgical clip, etc
after contrast administration, contrast kinetics analogous to IVU with delay in excretion in proportion to degree of obstruction
retroperitoneal extravasated contrast demonstrated unambiguously

MR (general)

dilated collecting system and ureter (low T1W, high T2W signal)
may show a transition zone
no signal from stones (can only be induced from a filling defect)
Gd-DTPA kinetics identical to Tc-99m DTPA

IMAGING (chronic obstruction)

XR

may show an enlarged kidney contour in severe hydronephrosis

US

variable degree of dilation depending on degree of obstruction and duration of obstruction

hydronephrosis may be gross particularly in PELVIURETERIC JUNCTION OBSTRUCTION
increased resistive index
parenchymal thinning and atrophy (papillae atrophy first)
eventual thin shell of parenchyma around a bag of urine

IVU/CT (high grade or complete)

shell nephrogram (thin cortical stripe of remaining enhancing cortex) around a dilated bag of urine

IVU (low grade)

delayed nephrogram, negative pyelogram
dilated delayed pyelogram

SPECIFIC SIGN

crescent sign: dilated calyces elevate collecting ducts into a near-horizontal position, flattening the papilla
opacified horizontal ducts form a peripheral crescent overlying non enhanced calyx

CT (low grade)

similar to IVU; collecting system wall may be thickened and may enhance
may demonstrate the cause of obstruction (stone, tumor, compression by extrinsic mass, prostate, surgical clip, etc)

NUC MED (DTPA, MAG3)

minimal or no perfusion abnormality
delay in tracer uptake and excretion
more marked delay in drainage, dilated collecting system
reduced split renal function (may recover with relief of obstruction)
abnormal whole kidney renogram, either with delayed peak or with a continually accumulating curve

MR (general)

dilated collecting system and ureter, ureter often tortuous
may show cause of obstruction (but no signal from stone – induced from a filling defect)
Gd-DTPA kinetics identical to Tc-99m DTPA

Functional assessment of obstruction

see its own entry under normal

3.14 ONCOCYTOMA

DEFINITION

epithelial tumor of low malignant potential

CLINICAL

female > male
develops from teens on, commoner in older
  adults
5% multiple

MORPHOLOGY

homogenous tan colored encapsulated renal
  cortical mass of variable size
30% have a central scar (suggestive)
can only differentiate from renal cell
  carcinoma on full specimen histology
uniformly packed bland eosinophilic
  oncocytes (pink cells packed with
  mitochondria)
few mitoses, no necrosis, low malignant
  potential
metastases rare

IMAGING

IVU/US/CT/MR

homogenous renal cortical mass
central stellate scar (hypoenhancing)
  suggestive but not diagnostic

Angio

hypervascular with spoke wheel pattern of
  tumor blood vessels

3.15 PAPILLARY NECROSIS

DEFINITION

selective necrosis of renal papillae (and,
  therefore, long loop nephrons) from a
  variety of causes leading to deteriorating
  renal function and collecting system loose
  bodies

ETIOLOGY

see papillary necrosis gamut

PATHOGENESIS

final common pathway of multiple
  processes, including: vascular occlusion,
  toxic destruction (increased
  concentration in papillae), infection

MORPHOLOGY

Unilateral versus bilateral

most often bilateral involving multiple
  calyces

unilateral papillary necrosis does
  occur, and the differential is:
infection with secondary papillary necrosis
obstruction with secondary papillary
  necrosis
renal vein thrombosis with papillary
  necrosis

focal papillary necrosis may occur, and
  the differential is:
RENAL TB
hematogenous focal abscess (e.g. IV drug
  use)
renal Brucellosis

Medullary type

enlarging necrotic cavity in center of papilla
'egg in cup' appearance

Papillary type

circumferential necrosis from fornices
  inward
sloughed calcified papilla that becomes a
  filling defect and a nidus

In situ type

slow flattening, resorption, calcification

Calyceal changes

early normal cortical thickness, clubbed
  calyx
late scarred endstage calyx, thin cortex
  (differentiation from reflux nephropathy
  difficult)

IMAGING

XR

usually normal
bilateral papillary calcification (differential:
  medullary sponge kidney)

IVU

IV contrast usually contraindicated because
  of renal dysfunction present in papillary
  necrosis

therefore, if papillary necrosis is shown on
  IVU, this is likely to be previously
  unknown disease manifesting for the first
  time

EARLY

no abnormalities

LATE

see morphology

sloughed papilla may cause
  obstruction

Fluoro (retrograde/antegrade pyelogram)

same findings as at IVU, but study not
  contraindicated if renal function
  impaired

US

increased papillary echogenicity
  (calcification)
missing papillae, clubbed calyces

CT/MR

missing papillae, flattened papillae, clubbed
  calyces, sloughed papillae in renal pelvis

NUC MED (DTPA/MAG3)

impaired renal function with no holdup of
  drainage

3.16 PSEUDOTUMOR

see renal mass gamut

GROUP DEFINITION

a radiological entity: renal parenchyma
  presenting as a tumoral mass on imaging

IMAGING (generic)

identification of pseudotumor consists of
  proving the pseudotumor behaves exactly
  the same as normal renal parenchyma in
  rest of kidney
infarct and lobar nephronia are two
  common entities that do not follow this
  rule

US

possibility of tumor usually raised on US
  because of mass effect
pseudotumor has same echotexture as rest
  of parenchyma and normal vascular
  architecture (unless a dysmorphic lobe)

CT

pseudotumor isodense with normal
parenchyma

on dynamic multiphase CT pseudotumor
faithfully follows normal parenchyma

MR

pseudotumor isointense to normal
parenchyma

on dynamic MR pseudotumor faithfully
follows normal parenchyma (same
time–intensity curve)

NUC MED (DMSA)

SPECT usually required

same uptake of DMSA as normal renal
parenchyma

BUT infarct and lobar nephronia produce
DMSA defects

3.16.1 JUNCTIONAL PARENCHYMA

prominent deep reaching parenchyma
where the two renunculi (the posterior
division and the anterior division) join

may have a surface groove (junctional
groove)

location embryologically determined and
characteristic

3.16.2 PROMINENT COLUMN OF BERTIN

3.16.3 DROMEDARY HUMP

triangular outer contour of left kidney,
perhaps from a splenic impression

3.16.4 RENAL INFARCT

also see its entry under renal ischemia

Acute infarct

acutely swollen edematous parenchyma with
poor enhancement

DIFFERENTIATION FROM NEOPLASM

pyramid shaped with apex at site of
occlusion

subcapsular cortical enhancement on CT
and MR

segmental non perfusion on angio

Chronic infarct

volume loss with eventual segmental
atrophy

3.16.5 HYPERTROPHY OF NORMAL PARENCHYMA NEXT TO SCAR

3.16.6 LOBAR DYSMORPHISM

abnormally positioned and oriented renal
lobe between upper and lower pole
calyces

typically drains into a small posterior calyx

because of AP orientation, parenchyma of
the lobe produces an enhancing 'donut'
on IVU or angio around the calyx

3.16.7 PYELONEPHRITIS/ LOBAR NEPHRONIA

see its own entry

mild segmental or global edema, perirenal
edema and stranding

reduced contrast enhancement, streaky
enhancement

!defect on DMSA imaging

3.17 PYELONEPHRITIS (PN)

DEFINITION

PN: renal parenchymal bacterial infection
(acute, chronic, recurrent)

REFLUX NEPHROPATHY: scarring following
recurrent episodes of ascending infection

EPIDEMIOLOGY

YOUNG (usually associated with reflux)

ELDERLY (usually associated with debility,
lower urinary infections, urinary
obstruction)

PREGNANT (usually asymptomatic
bacteriuria)

DIABETIC

ETIOLOGY

Ascending pyelonephritis

E coli, Proteus, Streptococcus (usually fecal),
Gram negative rods, Staphylococcus,
Candida

Hematogenous pyelonephritis

Staphylococcus, TB pyelonephritis, Candida

Predisposing states

VESICOURETERIC REFLUX AND INTRARENAL REFLUX

vesicoureteric reflux delivers lower urinary
tract organisms to renal pelvis

intrarenal reflux delivers organisms into
renal parenchyma

excretory duct openings on compound
papillae are not squeezed shut with high
intrarenal pressure, and reflux

lobar nephronia from reflux tends to upper
and lower poles (sites of compound
papillae)

OBSTRUCTION

STRUCTURAL

FUNCTIONAL (pregnancy, neuropathic
bladder)

NIDUS

STONE OR SLOUGHED PAPILLA

CATHETER OR TUBE

IMMUNOSUPPRESSION

DIABETES

emphysematous pyelonephritis in particular

MACRO SPECTRUM

3.17.1 Acute lobar nephronia

3.17.2 Renal abscess

3.17.3 Perirenal abscess

3.17.4 Pyonephrosis

3.17.5 Emphysematous pyelonephritis

associations: diabetics, stones, high
mortality

gas producing infection of (often) obstructed
kidney

rapidly progressive, with high mortality

3.17.6 Xanthogranulomatous pyelonephritis (XGP)

chronic low grade infection with fibrosis

FOCAL XGP (female > male) behaves as
abscess

DIFFUSE XGP (male > female) has
superimposed vasculitis

heterogeneous mass of abscesses, dilation,
fibrosis, calcification

staghorn stone in 75%

inflammatory infiltrate with fat laden
macrophages

3.17.7 Renal candidiasis

starts as acute PN but becomes chronic

ASSOCIATIONS

immunosuppressed, diabetics, neonates, transplant kidneys

ileal diversion, conduits, tubes, stents

COMPLICATIONS

dilation, obstruction, fungus ball

3.17.8 Reflux nephropathy

SCARRING results from ascending lobar nephronia (conventionally taken to occur under 5 years)

irregular cortical scarring centered on compound calyces (i.e. upper and lower poles), loss of papillae and calyceal dilation

intervening segmental hypertrophy

IMAGING (PN)

XR

may show cause: stent, nephrostomy tube, stone

emphysematous pyelonephritis: gas within renal pelvis, perirenal gas

IVU/CT

(non contrast: same comments as for XR)

focal or global renal enlargement, hypodense on CT

spidery compressed calyces

decreased contrast enhancement (segmental or global)

tubular striations on CT (blocked segments)

hazy outline

perirenal stranding

US

big kidney, focal hypoechoic area

loss of corticomedullary and parenchymosinus junctions

decreased vascularity on color/power Doppler

DMSA

no uptake in affected segments (80% sensitivity)

most sensitive imaging test available

absent uptake does not differentiate acute lobar nephronia from infarct from scar

with successful treatment defects of lobar nephronia resolve on followup DMSA

Xanthogranulomatous pyelonephritis

see under macro

Renal/perirenal abscess

heterogeneous usually hypodense mass with poor enhancement or no central enhancement

as abscess matures, thick enhancing wall develops

may contain gas

perirenal abscess usually crescentic as confined by fascia

3.18 RADIATION NEPHRITIS (manifestations)

IMAGING

NUC MED (DTPA/MAG3)

area of reduced function with straight margins corresponding to radiotherapy portal

may have increased uptake of MDP in the same area

may eventually resolve

3.19 RARE BLADDER TUMORS (overview)

3.19.1 HEMANGIOMA

3.19.2 NEUROFIBROMA

3.19.3 PHEOCHROMOCYTOMA

3.19.4 URACHAL ADENOCARCINOMA

3.19.5 LEIOMYOMA, LEIOMYOSARCOMA

3.19.6 RHABDOMYOSARCOMA

3.19.7 ENDOMETRIOSIS

3.20 RENAL ARTERY ANOMALIES

3.20.1 AV MALFORMATION (AVM)

CLINICAL

female > male

vascular steal

renovascular hypertension

hematuria

IMAGING

IVU

non specific space occupying lesion

US

may demonstrate cluster of vessels or arterialized renal vein Doppler signal if shunt sufficiently large

Angio

early venous drainage with cluster of small vessels or vascular spaces

CT

may show arterial phase enhancing mass or cluster of vessels

3.20.2 AV FISTULA (AVF)

CLINICAL

post renal biopsy

renal cell carcinoma (5% have arteriovenous shunt)

presents with recurrent hematuria, vascular steal

IMAGING

see entry on renal cell carcinoma and renal transplants

3.20.3 RENAL ARTERY ANEURYSM

CLINICAL

most often an incidental finding
may be multiple or bilateral

ETIOLOGY

atherosclerotic
post traumatic, post surgical, post
    intervention
polyarteritis nodosa (small, multiple,
    bilateral)
mycotic
following renal artery dissection
secondary to fibromuscular dysplasia

IMAGING

XR

rarely, has a calcified wall producing non
    specific ring calcification

IVU

non specific mass (arterial phase usually not
    filmed)

US

diagnostic (unless thrombosed)

CT

arterial phase enhancing mass (unless
    thrombosed)

Angio

diagnostic

3.21 RENAL ARTERY STENOSIS

DEFINITION

as loosely defined by common clinical use,
    stenosis of sufficient severity to be
    hemodynamically significant and produce
    renovascular hypertension

ETIOLOGY

Children

NEUROFIBROMATOSIS

HYPOPLASTIC AORTA AND
    BRANCHES

Adults

ATHEROSCLEROSIS
main cause overall
predominant cause in the over 50 year olds

FIBROMUSCULAR HYPERPLASIA
common cause in younger patients,
    especially female

ARTERITIS
TAKAYASU'S ARTERITIS
POLYARTERITIS NODOSA
RADIATION

SPONTANEOUS DISSECTION

EXTERNAL COMPRESSION

TRANSPLANT ANASTOMOTIC
STENOSIS

CLINICAL

usual clinical context is of difficult to control
    hypertension
may present with a renal bruit
may have progressively worsening renal
    function

IMAGING

IVU

classic (and rare) findings of delayed small
    nephrogram, delayed dense pyelogram

US

*see renal Doppler ultrasound entry under
normal*
subject to patient anatomy, difficulty with
    overlying gas and breath holding, and
    operator skill

CT (general)

renal artery calcification suggests renal
    atherosclerosis

CT (CT angio)

accuracy approaches catheter angio
large contrast load required
subject to metal, movement, flow artifacts
findings as for angio
limited accuracy in small branch vessels or
    small accessory arteries

MR (MR angio)

white blood techniques or contrast enhanced
    techniques
approaching accuracy of CT
has difficulty with metallic stents
findings as for angio

MR (MR captopril renography)

rationale, technique and findings analogous
    to nuclear medicine captopril renography
not widespread at present

Angio

consider using carbon dioxide as contrast
focal narrowing or multifocal narrowing,
    beading or dissection flap
atherosclerosis: irregular narrowing, plaque
    may be calcified; often ostial
fibromuscular dysplasia: beading of artery,
    commonly mid-artery
dissection: 'rat-tail' appearance; may have
    associated fibromuscular dysplasia;
    intimal flap
prelude to stenting

NUC MED

see captopril renography entry under normal

3.22 RENAL CELL CARCINOMA

DEFINITION

malignant neoplasm of renal tubular cell
    origin
other name: hypernephroma
renal adenoma: a small renal cell carcinoma

EPIDEMIOLOGY

most common malignant renal tumor (85%)
45–60 years old, male > female
1 in 13000, 13% multicentric, 13% calcify,
    13% cystic

Risk factors

von Hippel–Lindau syndrome
smoking, analgesic abuse
polycystic kidney disease
endstage renal failure/hemodialysis (not
    firmly proven because adult polycystic
    kidney disease is a common cause of
    endstage renal failure)

CLINICAL

Presentation

PREDICTABLE
flank pain, mass, hematuria
venous obstruction, varices, edema
with metastases

PARANEOPLASTIC

ENDOCRINE

erythropoietin, polycythemia

parathyroid hormone related protein,
    hyperparathyroidism

renin, renal hypertension

high ESR, high ferritin

CONSTITUTIONAL

weight loss, malaise, anemia

Spread

DIRECT INVASION

VENOUS INVASION

LYMPHATIC

HEMATOGENOUS

liver, lung, brain, adrenal

bone (typically highly lytic)

soft tissues

Staging – TNM

T STAGING

T1   limited to kidney, <7 cm diameter

T2   limited to kidney, >7 cm diameter

T3a   into adrenal gland or perinephric fat

T3b   into renal vein or IVC

T3c   extends along IVC above diaphragm

T4   invades outside Gerota's fascia

N STAGING

N1   single regional node

N2   more than one regional node

GROUPING

STAGE I	T1, N0, M0
STAGE II	T2, N0, M0
STAGE III	up to T3, up to N1, M0
STAGE IV	T4 or N2 or M1

Staging (Robson)

I	IN	intracapsular
II	OUT	through capsule or to adrenal
III	NEAR	(a) veins (b) nodes (c) both
IV	FAR	(a) organs in continuity
		(b) metastases

MACRO

round lobulated gray-white-yellow mass
    with invasive edge compressing and
    replacing kidney

lipid content determines amount of yellow
    color

hemorrhage, necrosis, cystic change

hypervascular with tumor neoangiogenesis

Cystic renal carcinoma

MULTILOCULAR CYSTIC CARCINOMA

UNILOCULAR CYSTADENOCARCINOMA

CYSTIC NECROSIS IN CARCINOMA

CARCINOMA DEVELOPING IN CYST

MICRO

CLEAR CELL (70%) (with glycogen and lipid)

GRANULAR CELL (packed with
    mitochondria)

SPINDLE CELL (sarcomatoid, aggressive)

tubuloacinar architecture, cystic spaces with
    papillary projections, highly vascular

prognosis relates to cytology not histology

IMAGING (primary)

XR

normal or

enlarged kidney with obvious mass
    with/without calcification

US

hypoechoic (no through transmission) or less
    commonly hyperechoic renal mass with
    distortion of renal contour and disruption
    of normal vascular architecture

patches of cystic change, calcification

may be an intracystic mass

IVU

space occupying lesion, possibly with some
    vascular phase contrast enhancement

CT

isodense or hyperdense renal mass

cystic change, necrosis (lower density),
    hematoma (higher density)

diffuse or patchy calcification

may be predominantly cystic or arise in a
    cyst (see macro)

by definition does not contain macroscopic
    fat but may entrap renal sinus or
    perirenal fat

DYNAMIC CONTRAST CT (multiphase)

does not follow normal renal parenchyma in
    all phases

may enhance similarly to contrast in early
    phases

less vivid than normal parenchyma in later
    interstitial phase

enhancement often heterogeneous

SMALL RENAL CARCINOMA

practical differentiation on CT is from cyst

precontrast density is in the soft tissue range

post contrast there is a rise in Hounsfield
    number indicating solid vascularized
    mass

RENAL VEIN INVASION

non enhancement

expansion

varices/varicocele

DIRECT INVASION

may need multiplanar reformats

unequivocal when perirenal fat is lost

MR

heterogeneous mass (depending on
    hemorrhage)

small masses isointense on T1W and
    isointense on T2W sequences to renal
    parenchyma

does not follow normal renal parenchyma
    with contrast

does enhance (differentiation from simple
    cyst)

typically, ring enhancement on early images,
    with poor enhancement compared to
    normal parenchyma in later interstitial
    phase

excellent demonstration of renal vein, IVC
    and right atrial invasion

SMALL RENAL CARCINOMA

dynamic post gadolinium MR with ROI
    curves on mass and normal parenchyma
    shows some enhancement (i.e. not a cyst)
    but slower and less intense enhancement
    than normal parenchyma

NUC MED (DTPA/MAG3/DMSA)

space occupying mass

Angio

abnormal arterial vascularity with tumor
    blush

AV shunts common

prelude to embolization

PET (FDG)

very FDG avid

however, difficult to differentiate from FDG
    excreted into calyces even with Lasix
    washout; small renal cell carcinomas
    may therefore be obscured

metastases are FDG avid

IMAGING (METASTASES)

XR

classically lytic or very expansile skeletal
    metastases

cannon ball lung metastases

CT

hypervascular liver metastases (enhance in arterial phase)

NUC MED (MDP)

hypervascular metastases
skeletal metastases often photopenic or 'donut'

3.23 RENAL CYSTS

GROUP DEFINITION

simple cysts fulfil rigid imaging criteria and can be left alone as totally benign
complex cysts require differentiation of cystic carcinoma from simple cysts with superimposed complications

3.23.1 SIMPLE CYST

CLINICAL

at least one half of the population over 50 years
unusual in childhood or adolescence; multiple cysts suggest cystic renal syndromes
commonest presentation is as an incidental finding on imaging performed for another reason
may present with mass effect, compression or obstruction (if strategically positioned)

IMAGING

must fulfill simple cyst criteria

US

hypoechoic fluid echogenicity rounded structure
posterior acoustic enhancement (proportional to size)
pencil thin regular wall that may have an edge shadow
no internal texture
no internal flow (color/power/wave Doppler)

CT

rounded fluid density structure
density is between 0 and 20 Hounsfield units (but beware partial volume effect if small)
pencil thin wall, may have a 'claw' of renal cortex if exophytic

allowed small specks of pencil thin calcification in wall
no contrast enhancement (i.e. no rise in Hounsfield number)

MR

rounded fluid signal mass
low on T1W, high on T2W sequences, gets brighter with longer TE (compare to collecting system urine and CSF)
morphology as for CT
no contrast enhancement

3.23.2 PARAPELVIC CYST

CLINICAL

may cause collecting system compression
more commonly an incidental finding
differentiating parapelvic cyst from hydrocalyx may be difficult

IMAGING

same criteria as for simple cyst
may be deformed to conform to renal sinus
BY DEFINITION, does not communicate with collecting system
contrast filled collecting system adjacent to or displaced or deformed by the cyst

3.23.3 COMPLEX CYST

CLINICAL

most often an incidental imaging finding (same as a simple cyst)
a specific problem in adult polycystic kidney disease (APCKD), as cysts hemorrhage, rupture or become infected and present with pain, hematuria or fever

IMAGING

Generic features of a complex cyst

thick wall or irregular wall (circumferential or focal)
many septations (unless walls of two adjacent simple cysts form a 'septum')
nodule arising from wall or within septation
irregularity at base
heavy calcification
high Hounsfield number or altered MR signal
enhancement

BOSNIAK CLASSIFICATION OF RENAL CYSTS

I SIMPLE CYST

II COMPLEX HOMOGENOUS HYPERDENSE

non suspicious septations
non suspicious calcification
hyperdense

III INDETERMINATE WITH SUSPICIOUS FEATURES

thickened septations
heavy calcification
mural/septal nodule

IV CLEARLY MALIGNANT

3.23.4 HEMORRHAGIC CYST

CLINICAL

by definition, a simple cyst with internal hemorrhage
particularly common in APCKD
if no other suspicious signs present, can be watched (or aspirated if large and of concern)
any other findings of a complex cyst (especially wall or base nodularity or soft tissue) suggest malignancy

IMAGING

US

internal mobile debris
all other criteria of simple cyst

CT

high Hounsfield number
no enhancement

MR

altered MR signal
signal is that of blood products and depends on age
(commonest is high T1W and high T2W)
may have fluid-fluid level!
no enhancement

3.23.5 MILK OF CALCIUM CYST

CLINICAL

not a cyst but a calyceal diverticulum lined by transitional epithelium

can be 'turned into' a calyceal diverticulum if communication with collecting system can be proven

IMAGING

US
internal echogenic debris, may shadow
debris may layer or move with posture
(diagnostic)

CT
high Hounsfield number
no enhancement
shifting of calcification with posture
diagnostic

3.23.6 URINE PSEUDOCYST
(urinoma)

CLINICAL

associated with obstruction, manipulation,
trauma

IMAGING

US/CT/MR
shape usually conforms to anatomical
spaces (e.g. renal sinus or perirenal
fascia) and is not rounded
may show slow accumulation of contrast in
urinoma

NUC MED (DTPA/MAG3)
activity outside the collecting system
indicative

3.23.7 CYSTIC DISEASE IN ENDSTAGE FAILURE

CLINICAL

40% of endstage renal failure patients
1% develop renal cell carcinoma
multiple cysts up to 3 cm with clear fluid
low cuboidal epithelium, hyperplasia,
dysplasia

IMAGING

same criteria of simple or complex as above

3.24 RENAL FAILURE

DEFINITIONS

Proteinuria
>0.3 g protein per 24 hours

Hematuria
any RBC (glomerular or non) on microscopy

Nephrotic syndrome
proteinuria >3.5 g over 24 hours,
hypoalbuminemia and edema,
hypercholesterolemia

MECHANISM
glomerular loss of protein exceeds tubular
resorption and liver synthetic capacity
producing hypoalbuminemia and
hypercholesterolemia
low oncotic pressure leads to salt and water
retention with edema

Nephritic syndrome
proteinuria, hematuria, oliguria,
hypertension, edema

Acute renal failure (ARF)
oliguria <400 ml output over 24 hours,
edema

Chronic renal failure (CRF)
insufficient renal function to maintain
internal homeostasis
generally a slow progression and the end
manifestation of chronic renal disease
symptoms and signs develop as CRF
progresses, and correlate with
decreasing glomerular filtration rate

ETIOLOGY

ARF
PRERENAL
HYPOVOLEMIA
ACUTE TUBULAR NECROSIS (ATN)

RENAL
ATN
ACUTE GLOMERULONEPHRITIS (GN)
ACUTE TUBULOINTERSTITIAL NEPHRITIS (TIN)

POSTRENAL
ACUTE BILATERAL OBSTRUCTION

CRF
PRERENAL
CHRONIC ISCHEMIA

RENAL
CHRONIC GLOMERULONEPHRITIS (GN)
DIABETIC NEPHROPATHY
BILATERAL REFLUX NEPHROPATHY
ANALGESIC NEPHROPATHY
CONGENITAL RENAL DISEASES

POST RENAL
BILATERAL CHRONIC OBSTRUCTION

CLINICAL MANIFESTATIONS

Acute
FLUID OVERLOAD
oliguria and anuria
hypertension, pulmonary edema

METABOLIC
malaise and weakness
uremia, seizures
hyperkalemia, arrhythmias

Chronic
FLUID IMBALANCE
polyuria and dehydration
oliguria and edema
hypertension, fluid overload

METABOLIC/ELECTROLYTE
hyperkalemia
metabolic acidosis
azotemia

CALCIUM/BONE
hypocalcemia
hyperphosphatemia
secondary hyperparathyroidism
renal osteodystrophy

HEMATOLOGIC
anemia
coagulopathy
superinfections

COMPLICATIONS OF UREMIA
myopathy
peripheral neuropathy
encephalopathy
dermatitis, pigmentation, pruritus
esophagitis, gastritis, ulcers

ACCELERATED ATHEROSCLEROSIS

GROWTH DISTURBANCE IN CHILDREN

IMAGING (CRF – general)

may demonstrate cause of renal failure, e.g. obstruction, polycystic kidneys, renal artery stenosis, reflux

description below is of findings in non specific renal parenchymal dysfunction in renal failure

XR

usually no findings

US

small kidneys, reduced parenchymal bulk
lost corticomedullary differentiation
increased parenchymal echogenicity
multiple small cysts may be present
elevated resistive index

IVU

CONTRAST CONTRAINDICATED

CT (non contrast)

small kidneys with parenchymal atrophy
multiple small cysts possible

MR

loss of corticomedullary differentiation on T1W sequences
!low T1W and T2W signal suggests iron deposition and sickle cell disease or thalassemia underlying renal failure

NUC MED (DTPA/MAG3)

perfusion deteriorates more slowly than uptake and excretion
reduced tracer uptake, delayed excretion
progression of renal curve grades
delayed time to peak
delayed time to bladder
increased cortical transit time
increased retention index
increased background tissue activity (including 'white spine')
no evidence of holdup of drainage BUT
with progressively deteriorating renal function too little tracer is excreted into collecting system and obstruction can no longer be excluded
eventual progression to washin–washout pattern, and ultimately no renal uptake

3.25 RENAL HYPERTENSION

DEFINITION

hypertension caused by renal disease

NOT equivalent to RENOVASCULAR HYPERTENSION, which is in turn NOT equivalent to RENAL ARTERY STENOSIS

CLASSIFICATION

Non vascular hyperreninemia

PRIMARY TUMORAL (reninoma)

SECONDARY
CHRONIC GLOMERULONEPHRITIS
REFLUX NEPHROPATHY
DIABETIC NEPHROPATHY
ANALGESIC NEPHROPATHY
POLYCYSTIC KIDNEY DISEASE

Fluid and salt retention hypertension

a variable contributor in all renal diseases
classic mechanism of hypertension in renal insufficiency and chronic renal failure, but unlikely to be the only one

Renovascular hypertension

LARGE VESSEL DISEASE (renal artery stenosis)
by definition, renal artery stenosis is the culprit of hypertension if treatment of the stenosis cures or improves the hypertension
differential is: essential hypertension, incidental renal artery narrowing
see its own entry

SMALL VESSEL DISEASE AND OTHER
NEPHROSCLEROSIS
DIABETIC NEPHROPATHY
VASCULITIS (MEDIUM AND SMALL VESSEL)
TRANSPLANT REJECTION
RENAL STEAL SYNDROME
AV MALFORMATION, AV FISTULA, TUMOR SHUNT

3.26 RENAL INFARCTION AND ISCHEMIA

DEFINITION

renal arterial ischemia, sudden or gradual
see renal vein thrombosis and renal artery stenosis under separate entries

ETIOLOGY

Acute occlusion (infarct)

TRAUMA, THROMBOEMBOLISM, DISSECTION

thin rim of subcapsular cortex is additionally supplied by the capsular arteries

Chronic ischemia

RENAL ARTERY STENOSIS (see its own entry)
SMALL VESSEL DISEASE AND OTHER (see renal hypertension)
gradual nephrosclerosis, glomerular loss, dropping GFR, renovascular HT

IMAGING (renal infarct)

XR

no findings

IVU

non opacified wedge in nephrogram, base to kidney contour, apex centrally

US

may be normal
absent color/power/wave Doppler flow in infarcted segment
(early) hypoechoic mildly swollen segment
(late) segmental atrophy and scarring

CT/MR

non contrast: mild segmental edema (wedge shaped)
(cause of a pseudotumor)
dynamic with contrast: wedge of non perfused tissue
cortical subcapsular rim sign (1–3 mm of subcapsular enhancing tissue) – may not be present
whole kidney infarction – no perfusion to entire kidney
amount of swelling and perirenal edema depends on timing and size of infarct
late segmental scar

Angio

definitive demonstration of cause
non flow in renal artery, branch, segmental artery
sharply geographically demarcated wedge shaped non perfused area

NUC MED (DMSA, DTPA, MAG3)

photopenic wedge shaped defect
best shown on DMSA SPECT

3.27 RENAL LEUKEMIA, LYMPHOMA, METASTASES

see Ch 16

metastases: lung, GIT, breast, melanoma
fundamentally, metastatic or lymphomatous
    mass is indistinguishable from renal cell
    carcinoma

3.28 RENAL TUBULAR ACIDOSIS

DISTAL RENAL TUBULAR ACIDOSIS (TYPE 1)
principal imaging manifestation is calcified
    stones (usually calcium oxalate)

PROXIMAL TUBULAR ACIDOSIS (TYPE 2)
no imaging findings

3.29 RENAL TUMOR OVERVIEW

Adults

BENIGN (5%)

ANGIOMYOLIPOMA
see its own entry

ONCOCYTOMA
see its own entry

RENINOMA

RENAL PHEOCHROMOCYTOMA

HEMANGIOMA

FIBROMA

MALIGNANT (vast majority)

RENAL CELL CARCINOMA (85%)
see its own entry

TRANSITIONAL CELL CARCINOMA (10%)
see its own entry

LEUKEMIA, LYMPHOMA
see its own entry

SARCOMA

    LEIOMYOSARCOMA

    RHABDOMYOSARCOMA

    LIPOSARCOMA

HEMANGIOPERICYTOMA

METASTASES

Children
see Ch 19

BENIGN

CONGENITAL MESOBLASTIC NEPHROMA

MULTILOCULAR CYSTIC NEPHROMA

MALIGNANT

NEPHROBLASTOMATOSIS

NEPHROBLASTOMA

CLEAR CELL SARCOMA

RHABDOID TUMOR

RENAL CELL CARCINOMA

3.30 RENAL VEIN ANOMALIES

3.30.1 NORMAL VARIANTS

Left inferior vena cava

Double inferior vena cava

Retroaortic left renal vein

3.30.2 RENAL VEIN VARICES

Left >> right

Secondary to AV malformation or fistula

Occlusive

Idiopathic

Portal varices with splenorenal varices
(IVU differential is ureteropyelitis cystica)

3.30.3 NUTCRACKER SUPERIOR MESENTERIC ARTERY SYNDROME

CLINICAL

thin young females with left flank pain and
    hematuria

IMAGING (CT/angio)

vertically positioned superior mesenteric
    artery compresses left renal vein
>5 cm H2O gradient across compression

3.31 RENAL VEIN THROMBOSIS

ETIOLOGY

Secondary to tumoral invasion along vein
RENAL CELL CARCINOMA
TRANSITIONAL CELL CARCINOMA
NEPHROBLASTOMA
RENAL SARCOMA
ADRENAL CARCINOMA
HEPATOCELLULAR CARCINOMA

Bland
CHILDREN
DEHYDRATION
SEPSIS
INFANT OF DIABETIC MOTHER
COAGULOPATHY
POLYCYTHEMIA
LYMPHOMA, LEUKEMIA

ADULT
NEPHROTIC SYNDROME
GLOMERULONEPHRITIS
COAGULOPATHY, POLYCYTHEMIA
POST PARTUM
AMYLOIDOSIS
TRAUMATIC

Clinical
ACUTE
large congested painful kidney, hematuria
    and proteinuria

CHRONIC
silent hematuria, proteinuria, nephrotic
    syndrome

LATE
if thrombosis does not resolve or is not
    treated, the kidney atrophies

IMAGING (acute/subacute renal vein thrombosis)

XR
no findings

IVU
large delayed faint nephrogram
spidery delayed faint pyelogram

US

direct demonstration of soft tissue within renal vein

may show thin peripheral flowing crescent on color/power Doppler

intrathrombus vascularity indicates tumor

CT

renal parenchymal findings similar to IVU: swollen kidney with delay in enhancement

perirenal haze and edema

non opacification of renal vein (differential: flow phenomenon)

expanded renal vein containing soft tissue collateral channels

MR

BLAND

thrombus unequivocal (as opposed to flow) if it has blood product signal on multiple sequences

TUMOR

expanded renal vein containing soft tissue

diffuse enhancement of thrombus indicates tumor thrombus

MR is the modality of choice to image extent of renal cell carcinoma tumor propagation

NUC MED (DTPA/MAG3)

poor renal function pattern

perfusion usually normal

can not differentiate from other causes of poor renal function

Angio

renal venogram: direct demonstration of fixed filling defect

prelude to thrombolysis

renal arteriogram: shows fixed filling defect in venous phase

PET (FDG)

if all else fails, PET may differentiate bland from tumor thrombus as tumor thrombus is FDG avid

3.32 SICKLE CELL DISEASE

see Ch 16

3.33 STONES

also see obstruction

DEFINITION

solid intraurinary crystalline precipitated mass (renal, ureteric, bladder)

EPIDEMIOLOGY/CLINICAL

5% of population

50% of asymptomatic stones become symptomatic in 5 years

1/5 of symptomatic stones need intervention

50% recur

outcome very variable and depends on co-pathology

obstruction and infection account for most of the morbidity

CLASSIFICATION BY COMPOSITION AND BY ETIOLOGY

Calcium oxalate (70%), calcium phosphate (5%)

METABOLISM NORMAL, NO IDENTIFIABLE CAUSE (MOST!)

URINARY TRACT CAUSE

STASIS AND OBSTRUCTION

DIVERTICULA

MEDULLARY SPONGE KIDNEY

PAPILLARY NECROSIS NIDUS

FOREIGN BODY NIDUS

METABOLIC CAUSE – CALCIUM METABOLISM

HYPERPARATHYROIDISM

OTHER HYPERCALCEMIA

IDIOPATHIC

SARCOIDOSIS

CUSHING'S SYNDROME

PARATHYROID HORMONE RELATED PROTEIN

RENAL TUBULAR ACIDOSIS (distal or type 1)

VITAMIN D RESISTANT RICKETS

IDIOPATHIC HYPERCALCIURIA

METABOLIC CAUSE – OXALATE METABOLISM

PRIMARY OXALURIA IN OXALOSIS

SECONDARY OXALURIA

SHORT GUT SYNDROME

CROHN'S DISEASE

BILIARY DISEASE

reduced enteric bile salt retention of oxalate, increased oxalate absorption

VITAMIN C INTOXICATION (precursor of oxalate)

Calcium magnesium ammonium phosphate (15%)

occurs in infection: 'TRIPLE STONE', 'INFECTION STONE' OR 'STRUVITE'

urea split by bacterial enzymes with increase in ammonium levels and urine pH

Urate (9%) – radiolucent on plain film or IVU

urate precipitates out of solution at low pH

GOUT

HYPERURICOSURIA

HEMOLYTIC ANEMIA

MYELOPROLIFERATIVE DISORDERS

HEMATOLOGICAL MALIGNANCY ON CHEMOTHERAPY

IDIOPATHIC

Cystine and xanthine (1%) – radiolucent on plain film and IVU

CYSTINURIA, XANTHINURIA

PATHOGENESIS

supersaturated solution of stone-forming electrolyte first precipitates as crystals around a nidus, with the stone then growing by progressive crystal precipitation

urine contains natural crystal inhibitors, and their relative lack contributes

IMAGING

also see obstruction

AXR

RADIOOPAQUE STONE

elongated, angular, moves on serial imaging

BEWARE

presacral stone, lucent stone

DIFFERENTIAL: PHLEBOLITH

laminated, rounded, below ischial spine

DIFFERENTIAL: other causes of intraabdominal calcification

US

echogenic shadowing renal focus

US usually sees only very proximal ureter and not beyond

reliable with large stones, less reliable with small (e.g. <3 mm) stones

Fluoro

nephrostomy, stone extraction, antegrade stent insertion

IVU

radioopaque stones usually become completely invisible when surrounded by contrast

ureteric column pointing at a density in two projections confirms it is a stone, and estimates degree of obstruction

radiolucent stone in renal pelvis manifests as (potentially mobile) filling defect (see filling defect gamut)

radiolucent ureteric stone is suggested by lower end of the ureteric contrast column filling 'corners' between ureteric wall and stone

CT (targeted at stone)
see obstruction entry

3.34 TRANSITIONAL CELL CARCINOMA (TCC)/ UROTHELIAL TUMORS

EPIDEMIOLOGY AND ETIOLOGY

male > female (approximately 3:1); >50 years old

smoking (accounts for ? of all TCC)

analgesic abuse

arylamines (rubber, dye, leather industries – latent period 15 to 40 years)

cylcophosphamide

Stasis and infection

stasis (especially diverticula)

stones

schistosomiasis (mostly SCC)

chronic cystitis

malakoplakia

PATHOGENESIS

final common pathway: multifocal synchronous and metachronous tumors (tend to be similar grade) – field change theory

bladder >> upper tract (64:1)

renal/ureteric TCC carries a 40–80% risk of TCC elsewhere

bladder TCC has a 30% risk of upper tract TCC

CLINICAL

low grades have good long term survival with treatment, despite multiple recurrences

high grades are progressive with poor survival

adenocarcinoma, squamous cell carcinoma, undifferentiated carcinoma all carry poor prognosis

RECURRENCE IS TYPICAL (SURVEILLANCE IS ESSENTIAL)

Staging (TNM)

bilateral synchronous upper tract 1% or less

T STAGE

Tis	in situ
Ta	non invasive mucosal papillary carcinoma only
T1	lamina propria
T2	invasion into muscularis
T2a	(bladder) inner half of muscle
T2b	(bladder) outer half of muscle
T3	peripelvic/periureteric fat or renal parenchyma
T3a	(bladder) microscopic perivesical invasion
T3b	(bladder) macroscopic perivesical extension
T4	invades adjacent organs (or beyond kidney)
T4a	(bladder) prostate/uterus/vagina
T4b	(bladder) pelvic or abdominal wall

N STAGE

N1	single lymph node <2 cm
N2	node or nodes <5 cm
N3	node or nodes >5 cm

STAGE GROUPING (renal pelvis/ureter)

STAGE I	T1 N0 M0
STAGE II	T2 N0 M0
STAGE III	T3 N0 M0
STAGE IV	T4 or N >0 or M1

STAGE GROUPING (bladder)

STAGE I	T1 N0 M0
STAGE II	T2 N0 M0
STAGE III	T3 or T4a N0 M0
STAGE IV	T4b or N >0 or M1

MORPHOLOGY

INVERTED PAPILLOMA (rare, usually benign)

TRANSITIONAL CELL PAPILLOMA (2–3%)

frond like delicate pedunculated outgrowth (bladder trigone > dome)

---

differentiation from grade I TCC not absolute

TRANSITIONAL CELL CARCINOMA (90%)

MACRO

PAPILLARY TYPE (exophytic polypoid mass, may invade at the base)

FLAT TYPE plaque like thickening of mucosa, tends to be anaplastic and invasive)

MICRO

IN SITU, GRADE I (well differentiated) to GRADE III (anaplastic)

GLANDULAR METAPLASIA AND ADENOCARCINOMA (1%)

SQUAMOUS METAPLASIA AND CARCINOMA (3%)

IMAGING (upper tract)

US

renal sinus mass

invasion into renal parenchyma

IVU

immobile filling defect

amputated calyx, hydrocalyx

murally based mass protruding into lumen

intraluminal mass, variable degree of obstruction

mucosal nodularity or focal irregularity

CT

filling defect (post contrast)

expanded collecting system

non calcified invasive mass centered on renal sinus

non enhancing or poorly enhancing with contrast

eventual obliteration of renal sinus fat and invasion of renal parenchyma

(renal vein invasion rare)

nodal metastases (commonly enhance)

distant metastases

IMAGING (bladder)

normal imaging does not exclude bladder TCC

primary diagnostic modality is cystoscopy

MR best for local staging of deep invasive tumors

CT/MR/PET locoregional staging

US

full bladder required

sessile or papillary mass

IVU

murally based mass

occasionally, pseudoureterocele or ureteric
obstruction

CT

bladder wall thickening or murally based
mass

(need a fully distended bladder)

gross mass extension into adjacent organs
or perivesical fat

nodal staging (lymph nodes often enhance
with contrast)

MR

normal bladder wall intermediate signal on
T1W and dark on T2W

tumor is higher signal than bladder wall

multiplanar, FSE thin section T2W
sequences (with full bladder)
with/without post Gd sequences used for
assessment of local invasion

tumor: higher T2W mass protruding into
bladder and extending into bladder wall
for a variable depth

stranding of perivesical fat suggests invasion

unequivocal invasion if nodular extension or
involvement of adjacent organs

tumor enhances with Gd at the same time as
mucosa and enhances more than muscle

PET (FDG)

generally of no use in T staging as tumor not
distinguishable from urinary activity

useful for regional lymph node assessment
for planning of resection or radiation
therapy

3.35 TRANSPLANT COMPLICATIONS OVERVIEW

SURGICAL COMPLICATIONS – IMAGING

3.35.1 URINOMA, HEMATOMA, LYMPHOCELE, ABSCESS

Fluoro (cystogram)

demonstrates any bladder wall defect

US

collection

needle aspiration differentiates type of
collection

NUC MED (DTPA/MAG3)

extravasation of urine into urinoma

3.35.2 ACUTE ARTERIAL THROMBOSIS

US

thrombosed artery with no color/Doppler
signal

no arterial perfusion in kidney

NUC MED (DTPA/MAG3)

no uptake – at all

3.35.3 ACUTE VENOUS THROMBOSIS

US

absent venous flow in transplant vein

swollen kidney

increased resistive index

3.35.4 CHRONIC ARTERIAL STENOSIS

US

may show anastomotic stenosis

post stenotic jet

renal artery to aortic ratio >3.5

3.35.5 ARTERIAL ANEURYSM, PSEUDOANEURYSM

3.35.6 AV FISTULA

usually intraparenchymal following biopsy

US

arterialized venous flow

Angio

shows location and extent; prelude to
embolization

3.35.7 CHRONIC URINARY OBSTRUCTION

US

progressive hydronephrosis

may show ureteric dilation to a transition
zone

3.35.8 STONES

MEDICAL COMPLICATIONS – IMAGING

3.35.9 REJECTION

Types of rejection

HYPERACUTE

preformed antibodies from previously
sensitized host

occurs within minutes (i.e. intraoperative),
irreversible

ACUTE

occurs between ~1 week and ~3 months

reversible cell mediated rejection

acute renal failure, fever, swelling, pain

CHRONIC

takes years to manifest

irreversible, immunoglobulin mediated

subendothelial arteriolar hyaline
immunoglobulin deposits with
thrombosis, focal and segmental
hyalinosis and sclerosis

slowly deteriorating function, GFR, and
ERPF

CYCLOSPORIN TOXICITY

US – acute rejection

swollen kidney with lost corticomedullary
junction

patent arteries and veins, no ischemia

increased resistive index

NUC MED (MAG3) – acute rejection

reduced perfusion

poor overall function

delayed uptake and excretion

usually not enough excretion to show
drainage (but if tracer reaches collecting
system, no obstruction)

accumulation renogram (grade III)

can not definitively differentiate from ATN
on a single study

serial imaging differentiates from ATN

time course: usually very good or good renal
function on day 1

progressive deterioration in the absence of
vascular obstruction

reverses with immunosuppression

3.35.10 ACUTE TUBULAR NECROSIS (ATN)

cadaveric donor

poor renal function evident within hours

patchy cell necrosis, tubules blocked by casts

resolves spontaneously over weeks with
supportive treatment

NUC MED (DTPA)
normal or mildly reduced perfusion
'washin–washout' pattern
poor uptake and excretion

NUC MED (MAG3)
normal or mildly reduced perfusion
reasonable uptake, but no excretion
MAG3 is taken up by residual tubular cells
and is retained as tubules are filled with
casts
intensity of uptake reflects volume of
residual viable cells
classically the renogram is grade III
(accumulation)
can not definitively differentiate from acute
rejection on a single study
serial imaging differentiates: time course is
of poor function on day 1 followed by
improvement over weeks

3.35.11 PYELONEPHRITIS

3.35.12 RECURRENCE OF PRIMARY DISEASE

3.35.13 SYSTEMIC COMPLICATIONS OF IMMUNOSUPPRESSION

3.36 TRAUMA OVERVIEW

3.36.1 RENAL TRAUMA

IMAGING

CT
CONTUSION
mild to moderate edema
patchy contrast enhancement
perinephric hematoma or edema
blood clot in renal pelvis

PERINEPHRIC HEMATOMA
crescentic non enhancing collection of
variable density

SUBCAPSULAR HEMATOMA
crescentic collection contained within renal
contour; may compress adjacent kidney

LACERATION/FRACTURE
separation of enhancing fragments with
intervening hematoma

LACERATION INTO COLLECTING
SYSTEM

RENAL PELVIS TEAR, URINOMA
nephrogram normal or abnormal
contrast pooling outside kidney
clot within collecting system
non opacification of distal ureter

RENAL ARTERY LACERATION,
DISSECTION, THROMBOSIS
CT: non enhancement of either whole kidney
or lobe supplied by injured artery, often
with a capsular rim (supplied by
collaterals)
ANGIO: dissection or abrupt cut-off; contrast
linger in no-flow vessel

TRAUMATIC RENAL VEIN
THROMBOSIS
non opacification of renal vein, swollen
kidney, other injuries

SHATTERED KIDNEY

3.36.2 URETERIC TRAUMA

SHARP

LIGATION

3.36.3 BLADDER TRAUMA

IN UP TO 10% OF PELVIC FRACTURES

PERIVESICAL HEMATOMA

EXTRAPERITONEAL RUPTURE

INTRAPERITONEAL RUPTURE

IMAGING

CT
clot within bladder (filling defects)
extraperitoneal hematoma, often related to
fracture
bladder displaced or compressed
free intraperitoneal blood

Cystogram
if urethral injury suspected, do retrograde
urethrogram first
extraperitoneal extravasation: usually
anterior streaky contrast that does not
migrate
intraperitoneal extravasation: contrast
outlines loops of bowel

3.36.4 URETHRAL TRAUMA

10% of male, 5% of female pelvic fractures

Male urethra
see Ch 09

Female urethra
DISRUPTION, LACERATION

URETHROVAGINAL FISTULA

3.36.5 HYPOVOLEMIA COMPLEX

see Ch 07

3.37 URETERIC PSEUDODIVERTICULOSIS

CLINICAL

reactive urothelial hyperplasia with
extension into lamina propria secondary
to inflammation (with eventually
developing atypia)
50% eventually develop transitional cell
carcinoma

IMAGING

IVU/retrograde
multiple ureteric outpouches
bilateral in 70%
may contain transitional cell carcinoma

3.38 URETERIC TUMOR OVERVIEW

CLASSIFICATION

Urothelial (field change)
SEE TRANSITIONAL CELL CARCINOMA

Mesodermal
FIBROMA

LEIOMYOMA

IMAGING

IVU/retrograde

fixed intraluminal filling defect
cupping above AND below (if stone has
    cupping, it is usually only above)
differential: any other filling defect

CT

soft tissue density intraluminal mass with
    expansion of ureter
contrast outlines mass above +/– below
mass may extend into/through ureteric wall
non specific thickening of ureteric wall
    (differential: edema, inflammatory
    thickening)

3.39 URETEROPYELITIS CYSTICA, CYSTITIS CYSTICA

DEFINITION

reactive urothelial proliferation probably
    related to recurrent urinary tract
    infections

CLINICAL

female > male, history of recurrent
    infections
downward proliferating urothelium,
    glandular von Brunn nest metaplasia
    with goblet proliferation

IMAGING

IVU/retrograde

small smooth multiple defects in contrast
    column or along wall
differential: varices

3.40 URETHRAL TUMOR OVERVIEW

3.40.1 FIBROEPITHELIAL POLYP

presents in a young child
benign fibroepithelial polyp with transitional
    epithelium covering
attached near the verumontanum

3.40.2 ADENOMATOUS POLYP

young male
polyp adjacent to verumontanum
lined by prostatic columnar epithelium

3.40.3 TRANSITIONAL CELL PAPILLOMA

older male
prostatic or bulbomembranous urethra
often associated with bladder papillomas

3.40.4 TRANSITIONAL CELL CARCINOMA

majority of urethral tumors are TCCs
60% are at bulbomembranous urethra, 30%
    in penile urethra, 10% in prostatic
    urethra

3.41 URINARY SCHISTOSOMIASIS

also see Ch 07 hepatic schistosomiasis

DEFINITION

parasitic infection of bladder and distal
    ureters with secondary chronic
    inflammation producing a fibrosed
    contracted bladder and increased risk of
    metaplastic squamous cell carcinoma

CLINICAL

Schistosoma hematobium (African helminth)
    larvae develop in freshwater snails,
    penetrate intact human skin and
    eventually reach pelvic venous plexus
live adults in pelvic veins provoke little
    inflammation
eggs deposited preferentially in the wall of
    bladder and ureters, cause intense
    granulomatous inflammation, hematuria,
    fibrosis and squamous metaplasia (late
    SCC)

IMAGING

XR/IVU

small volume bladder with linear wall
    calcification
calcified distal ureters produce a 'tram
    track' appearance (parallel linear
    calcification)

IVU/CT

early: mural based masses (acute
    inflammatory masses) indistinguishable
    from tumor
late: contracted small volume bladder,
    ureteric strictures, vesicoureteric reflux

3.42 URINARY TB

also see Ch 02, Ch 09, Ch 11, Ch 13, Ch 23

CLINICAL

10% of lung TB; 50% of patients give history
    of previous lung TB
may reactivate independently of lung disease
    (e.g. with immunosuppression)

MACRO

TB hematogenous foci in renal cortex
    (bilateral) either heal with a small scar or
    progress
progression usually focal and therefore
    unilateral
TB bacilluria, caseating necrosis,
    breakthrough to medulla and pelvis

Ulcerocavernous TB

tissue destruction and cavitation
    predominate, with relatively little
    scarring and stricture formation

Fibrocavernous TB

intense fibrotic response, with scarring and
    stricturing superimposed on tissue loss

Associated involvement

ADRENAL TB
GENITAL TB
PERINEPHRIC ABSCESS
SPINAL TB
PSOAS ABSCESS
PERITONEAL TB with/without ascites ('wet'
    or 'dry')

IMAGING

IVU

disease progression characteristically
    unilateral

EARLY
moth eaten fuzzy calyx
papillary necrosis
irregular cavity (drained caseation)

LATE

cavitation (ulcerocavernous TB)
infundibular stenosis
amputated calyx
purse string renal pelvis
autonephrectomy (caseocavernous)
variable clumpy calcification

URETER

distal ulcers
serrations (multiple ulcers)
vesicoureteric junction stricture
fibrosis, strictures, beading
CALCIFICATION DIAGNOSTIC

BLADDER

initially mucosal irregularity
late: contracted irregular indistensible
    bladder

US

may be near normal, but kidney non
    excretory
papillary destruction, hydrocalyx
scarred pelvis, purse string hydronephrosis
small echogenic focal mass
focal ring with hypoechoic core
large, heterogeneous, calcified mass
irregular mass similar to
    xanthogranulomatous pyelonephritis
    (25%)

CT

detects gross rather than mucosal disease
healed tuberculous focus: small calcified
    scar (differential: stone)
parenchymal TB: unilateral unipapillary or
    multipapillary area of low density with
    variable ring enhancement
density depends on amount of caseation
    versus amount of drainage
collecting system has mucosal enhancement
    in active inflammation
ulcerocavernous TB: papillary and calyceal
    destruction with cavitation – affects one
    or several calyces
fibrocavernous TB: with stricture formation,
    dilated calyces with scarred overlying
    parenchyma form a 'cloverleaf' pattern
may have involvement of all calyces with
    massive destruction and residual
    peripherally enhancing sac (tuberculous
    pyonephrosis)
may have ureteric stricture with collecting
    system dilation
calcification varies from none to heavy and
    from punctate to ring calcification

ASSOCIATED FINDINGS

perinephric collection
paraspinal mass
adrenal mass
vertebral body irregular destruction
psoas abscesses: low density masses
    with/without ring enhancement and with
    possible tracking into femoral triangle
paraaortic lymphadenopathy (normal or low
    density, with or without ring
    enhancement; low density with ring
    enhancement suggestive)

'WET' PERITONEAL TB

relatively high density ascites
thickened infiltrated omentum
celiac, superior mesenteric low density
    lymphadenopathy with possible ring
    enhancement

3.43 UROGENITAL BRUCELLOSIS

DEFINITION

bacterial granulomatous infection with
    hematogenous seeding of multiple organs
    by Brucella species (Gram negative
    coccobacillus from infected milk or
    abbatoirs)

IMAGING

testis is most commonly involved; kidneys
    and bladder rarely; ureter almost never
    indistinguishable from urogenital TB

4. CONGENITAL CONDITIONS AND MALFORMATIONS

4.1 ADULT POLYCYSTIC KIDNEY DISEASE

DEFINITION

autosomal dominant disease with inexorable
    multiple cyst formation (kidneys, liver,
    other), progressive renal parenchymal
    loss and inevitable chronic renal failure

CLINICAL

autosomal dominant, 100% penetrance,
    variable expressivity
1/1000, male = female

Kidneys

renal cysts evident by 30 years, polyuric
    chronic renal failure by 50 years
massive renal enlargement, complex
    hemorrhagic and superinfected cysts,
    urolithiasis
risk of renal carcinoma increased by x10

Other

liver cysts (30–50%)
pancreatic cysts (10%)
splenic, gonadal cysts
hypertension
aortic valve disease
CEREBRAL ARTERIAL ANEURYSMS 10–30%

IMAGING

XR

bilateral massively enlarged kidneys with
    displacement of all other organs

IVU (contrast contraindicated in worsening renal function)

no normal nephrogram, or 'Swiss cheese'
    nephrogram
massively enlarged kidneys
spidery elongated distorted collecting
    systems
usual IVU signs of obstruction if obstruction
    is present

US

EARLY: abnormal number of simple cysts
progressive increase in cyst number
eventually massively enlarged kidneys
    composed of multiple simple and
    complex cysts
complex cysts contain variably echogenic
    debris (new or old hemorrhage) possibly
    with layering
calyx or collecting system dilation difficult to
    identify among cysts

CT/MR

massively enlarged kidneys with multiple
    simple and complex cysts (hemorrhage
    particularly common)
streaky contrast enhancement
compressed and elongated collecting system

cyst signal on MR reflects presence of blood products and their age
stones and patchy areas of calcification difficult to differentiate
may need contrast to diagnose obstruction

NUC MED (DTPA/MAG3)

enlarged kidneys with multiple photopenic defects
reduced renal function, no obstruction

NUC MED (white cell scan)

may identify an infected cyst

4.2 BLADDER AND URETHRA MALFORMATIONS

see Ch 19

4.3 CALYCEAL DIVERTICULUM

usually silent congenital diverticulum arising from a fornix, more rarely from the renal pelvis
may become sealed off (differentiation from cyst impossible)

IMAGING

US

appearance similar to renal cyst or parapelvic cyst – differentiation very difficult

IVU

rounded opacifying smooth walled cavity opacifying from a fornix

CT

fluid density cyst, opacifies from renal collecting system
may contain position dependent stones

4.4 CONGENITAL CYSTIC RENAL MASSES

see Ch 19

4.5 INFANTILE AND JUVENILE POLYCYSTIC KIDNEY DISEASE

see Ch 19

4.6 MEDULLARY SPONGE KIDNEY (MSK)

DEFINITION

congenital dilation of collecting ducts, most commonly asymptomatic but occasionally presenting with urolithiasis and obstruction

CLINICAL

0.5% of population, male > female
bilateral in 75%, stones in 50%
ASSOCIATIONS: Caroli's disease, parathyroid adenoma, Ehlers–Danlos syndrome

IMAGING

AXR

thin elongated stones in clusters

IVU

collecting duct stones in about 50%
dilated collecting ducts in papillae
papillary blush (no individual ducts seen)
large papillae

differential is nephrocalcinosis

in nephrocalcinosis calcification is interstitial
in MSK, calcification is in collecting ducts
differentiation depends on demonstrating normal renal function with dilated collecting ducts
if calcification is heavy, differentiation from nephrocalcinosis is impossible

CT

thin stones clustered in papillae

NUC MED (DTPA)

prolonged transit time, with possibly asymmetrical function

4.7 PELVIURETERIC JUNCTION OBSTRUCTION AND VARIANTS

see Ch 19

4.8 URETERIC MALFORMATIONS

see Ch 19

4.9 VASCULAR MALFORMATIONS

4.9.1 CONGENITAL ARTERIOVENOUS MALFORMATIONS (AVM)

Cirsoid AVM

younger, female > male, vascular steal, hypertension, hematuria
early venous drainage with cluster of small vessels or vascular spaces

Aneurysmal AVM

older, female > male, vascular steal, hypertension, hematuria

4.9.2 ACQUIRED AV FISTULA

BIOPSY
TUMOR (5% of renal cell carcinomas contain shunts)
vascular steal, recurrent hematuria

4.9.3 RENAL ARTERIAL ANEURYSM

20% bilateral, 30% multiple

4.10 VESICOURETERIC REFLUX (VUR)

see Ch 19

4.11 VON HIPPEL–LINDAU SYNDROME (vHL)

EPIDEMIOLOGY

1/40 000, autosomal dominant, incomplete penetrance, variable expression, 3% new mutation; tumor suppressor gene on chromosome 3p25 (VHL gene)

20's: retinal angiomas, 30's: hemangioblastomas, 40's: renal cell carcinomas, young adult: pheochromocytomas

requires 2 tumors (one in CNS) or 1 tumor and 1 relative

ABDOMEN

renal cysts
renal carcinomas (50% bilateral multifocal)
pheochromocytomas (40%)
liver cysts
liver adenomas
pancreatic cysts, microcystic adenoma, islet cell tumors

CNS

Hemangioblastomas (50%, multiple)
see Ch 11
90% cerebellum, 10% spinal cord
80% cystic
may secrete erythropoietin

EYE

RETINAL ANGIOMAS (50%, half bilateral)
histologically identical to hemangioblastoma (hemangioblastoma of retina)
hemorrhages and retinal detachment

EAR

tumor of the endolymphatic sac

DIAGNOSTIC CRITERIA

1. hemangioblastoma of CNS or retina and a typical vHL tumor; OR
2. hemangioblastoma of CNS or retina and a positive family history

4.12 WHOLE KIDNEY MALFORMATIONS

see Ch 19

5. ADRENAL CONDITIONS

5.1 ADDISON'S DISEASE

DEFINITION

autoimmune adrenalitis (with autoantibodies and lymphocytic infiltrate) leading to chronic hypoadrenalism +/– acute hypoadrenal crises

CLINICAL

female > male, 30–60 years old
HLA DR3 associated
ASSOCIATIONS: autoimmune thyroiditis, pernicious anemia, autoimmune gastritis, vitiligo ('thyrogastric cluster')
high ACTH and K, low cortisol, Na, glucose
failure of mineralocorticoid function (salt wasting hyperkalemia) and glucocorticoid function (impaired stress response, hypoglycemia, hypotension)

Addison's syndrome (see below)

Acute hypoadrenal (Addisonian) crisis
malaise and fever
cardiovascular collapse and overwhelming sepsis

IMAGING

Generic
normal or small or non–identifiable adrenal glands
exclusion of other causes of hypoadrenalism: e.g. adrenal TB (calcification), adrenal infiltration (bilateral masses)

5.2 ADDISON'S SYNDROME

DEFINITION

syndrome of chronic adrenal insufficiency (of any non–iatrogenic cause), not part of a panhypopituitarism

ETIOLOGY

AUTOIMMUNE ADRENALITIS (ADDISON'S DISEASE)

BILATERAL ADRENAL LYMPHOMA

BILATERAL ADRENAL TB

BILATERAL ADRENAL TUMORS (RARE!)

RELATED CONDITION: CONGENITAL ADRENAL HYPERPLASIA (MIXED HORMONAL STATE)

RELATED CONDITION: ACUTE SEPTICEMIC ADRENAL HEMORRHAGE AND FAILURE (WATERHOUSE–FRIDERICHSEN SYNDROME)

CLINICAL MANIFESTATIONS

Suntanned and floppy
weakness
weight loss
hyperpigmentation (ACTH fragments acting on melanocyte stimulating hormone (MSH) receptors; also elevated MSH levels)

Cardiovascular
hypotension
salt wasting
hyperkalemic arrhythmias
hypoglycemia

Metabolic
hypoglycemia, hyperkalemia
nausea, vomiting, abdominal pain
diarrhea or constipation

5.3 ADRENAL HYPERPLASIA

DEFINITION

diffuse benign adrenal enlargement
secondary to high adrenocorticotrophic
hormone (ACTH) levels with or without a
block in adrenal hormonal synthesis

ETIOLOGY

Primary elevation of ACTH

female > male, 20–40 years old
PITUITARY ADENOMA (CUSHING'S
DISEASE)
HIGH HYPOTHALAMIC CORTICOTROPHIN
RELEASING FACTOR LEVELS

Ectopic ACTH

male > female, older patient
BRONCHOGENIC SQUAMOUS CELL
CARCINOMA

Congenital adrenal hyperplasia

blocks at every step of sex steroid,
mineralocorticoid and glucocorticoid
synthesis have been documented;
associated with sex phenotype disorders

MACRO

DIFFUSE: both glands smoothly enlarged,
minimal nodularity
NODULAR: diffuse form with superimposed
nodules
CEREBRIFORM: markedly enlarged
convoluted glands in congenital adrenal
hyperplasia

IMAGING

CT/MR

bilateral uniformly enlarged adrenal glands
(see macro)
medulla and cortex may be distinguishable
on MR

NUC MED

NP59 positive (bilateral), suppresses with
dexamethasone

5.4 ADRENAL NON FUNCTIONING ADENOMA

(adrenocortical nodule)

DEFINITION

common nodular overgrowth of normal
adrenal tissue with no adrenal
dysfunction

CLINICAL

asymptomatic and incidental
2% bilateral
yellow nodule containing normal
adrenocortical cells
in presence of known primary malignancy
elsewhere, there is ~50% probability of a
small adrenal mass being a non
functioning adenoma

IMAGING

CT

fat density small (<3 cm) discrete nodule
density <10 HU on non contrast CT implies
benignity (cutoff is arbitrary; lower
density carries higher probability of
benign nodule)
can do equivalent of non contrast CT 1 hour
after contrast administration if nodule
first detected at time of contrast CT

MR

phase shift (in-phase and out-of-phase) MR
shows lipid content (lipid has low signal
on out of phase images)

5.5 ADRENOCORTICAL ADENOMA (functioning)

DEFINITION

benign hormonally active adrenocortical
neoplasm

CLINICAL

30–50 years old, female > male
CUSHING'S SYNDROME (most)
CONN'S SYNDROME (few)
(VIRILIZING ADENOMA – RARE)

(NON HORMONAL PRODUCT ADENOMA –
EXCLUDED BY DEFINITION)
discrete yellow mass up to 3–4 cm
regular lipid laden fasciculata like cells,
fibrovascular core

IMAGING

CT/MR

adrenal soft tissue or lower density mass
well defined margin, regular
mild if any contrast enhancement
may have atrophy of rest of ipsilateral gland
and of contralateral gland (in contrast to
a non functioning adenoma)

NUC MED (NP59)

NP59 = I-123 or I-131 6-beta iodomethyl
19-norcholesterol
in Cushing's syndrome, unilateral increased
uptake (differential is very well
differentiated functioning carcinoma)
in Conn's syndrome, early unilateral
breakthrough with dexamethasone
suppression when scanned

5.6 ADRENOCORTICAL CARCINOMA

DEFINITION

malignant adrenal cortical neoplasm –
usually not hormonally active

CLINICAL

female >> male; bimodal age peaks:
childhood and adult
NON FUNCTIONAL (most), poor prognosis as
presents late
~10% PRODUCE CUSHING'S SYNDROME
NON HORMONAL PRODUCTS (uncommon,
male > female)
(VIRILIZING RARE)

Spread

VASCULAR INVASION DIAGNOSTIC
LYMPH NODES AND LYMPHATIC SPREAD
HEMATOGENOUS: other adrenal, lungs,
bones

MORPHOLOGY

not yellow (little lipid)
cords, nests, sheets of lipid sparse large
malignant cells

VASCULAR INVASION DIAGNOSTIC

IMAGING

CT/MR

often large (e.g. >5 cm) irregular adrenal
mass
areas of hemorrhage, cystic change, necrosis
may contain dystrophic calcification
variable contrast enhancement – patchy,
vivid, ring, may show delayed washout
irregular edge, invasion of surrounding
structures
vascular (especially renal vein and IVC)
invasion
nodal or distant metastases prove
malignancy

NUC MED (NP59)

NP59 = I-123 or I-131 6-beta iodomethyl
19-norcholesterol
usually no uptake (differential is any other
aggressive adrenal mass)
~10% are hormonally active, and may show
uptake (differential is adenoma)

5.7 CUSHING'S SYNDROME

DEFINITION

manifestations produced by excess
glucocorticoid levels (of any cause)

ETIOLOGY

Iatrogenic (exogenous steroid)

Non iatrogenic
70% pituitary ACTH adenoma
20% adrenal functional adenoma
10% ectopic ACTH

CLINICAL MANIFESTATIONS

Obese and weak
central obesity
osteoporosis
myopathy
moon face, skin striae, 'buffalo hump' of
dorsal fat

Cardiovascular
hypertension
plethora

Metabolic
diabetes
hirsutism, acne
menstrual changes

5.8 MULTIPLE ENDOCRINE NEOPLASIA (MEN) SYNDROMES

GROUP DEFINITION

well defined clusters of endocrine
neoplastic/hyperplastic tumors occurring
together

MEN I (Wermer syndrome)

CLINICAL

mnemonic: PPP
male = female, usually silent for many years

(15–50%)   P-ITUITARY ADENOMA
(no products or prolactin)

(30–80%)   P-ANCREATIC ISLET CELL
TUMOR
ADENOMA >> CARCINOMA
gastrin, insulin, serotonin, VIP

(95%)   P-ARATHYROID
HYPERPLASIA
multicentric

MEN II (Sipple syndrome)

CLINICAL

mnemonic: PMP
variable age, male > female, has ret
protooncogene

(10%) P-arathyroid hyperplasia

(100%) M-edullary carcinoma thyroid
significant cause of mortality/morbidity

(50%) P-heochromocytoma
often extraadrenal

MEN III

CLINICAL

mnemonic: MPM
male > female
Marfanoid appearance (100%)
presents early with mucosal neuromas

(100%) M-EDULLARY CARCINOMA
THYROID

(50%) P-HEOCHROMOCYTOMA
indolent malignant, often extraadrenal

(100%) M-UCOSAL NEUROMAS

5.9 MYELOLIPOMA

CLINICAL

uncommon benign adrenal medullary tumor,
hormonally inactive
composed of mature fat and hematopoietic
cells

IMAGING

CT/MR

adrenal fat density/fat signal mass,
frequently with calcification
may have contrast enhancement
may be quite large
no invasion of neighboring structures

5.10 PARAGANGLIOMAS

see Ch 12

5.11 PHEOCHROMO-CYTOMA (PHEO)

*also see mutliple endocrine neoplasia, Ch 11
von Hippel–Lindau syndrome and
neurofibromatosis, Ch 12 paragangliomas*

DEFINITION

benign or malignant tumor of adrenal
medulla or neural crest paraganglial cells
associated with paroxysmal hypertension
intraadrenal tumor (vast majority functional)
= pheochromocytoma
functional extraadrenal tumor =
extraadrenal pheo

non functional extraadrenal tumor = paraganglioma (includes specific names for specific locations)

EPIDEMIOLOGY

ADULTS: 30–50 years old, female > male, usually adrenal
CHILDREN (~5% of pheo): male > female, extraadrenal > adrenal

Rule of 10's
neural crest paraganglial tumor (chromosome 10 abnormalities)
10% bilateral, 10% extraadrenal, 10% malignant (only proof of malignancy is distant metastases), 10% familial (pheo alone; MEN II; MEN III, von Hippel–Lindau, NF1)

CLINICAL

1/3 have sustained hypertension (0.1% or less of all hypertensives)
2/3 have paroxysmal hypertension
24 hour urine collection: elevated vanillylmandelic acid (VMA), homovanillic acid (HMA) and metnoradrenalin (all catecholamine metabolism end products)

Extraadrenal locations

RETROPERITONEUM
the organ of origin is the legendary organ of Zuckerkandl which in fetal life was located at the origin of the inferior mesenteric artery

BLADDER WALL

MEDIASTINUM

Complications
COMPLICATIONS OF HYPERTENSION
CEREBRAL HEMORRHAGE
MYOCARDIAL FIBROSIS
DISTANT METASTASES
10% RECUR LOCALLY

MICRO

cords, clumps, diffuse collections of large cells in fibrovascular stroma
only proof of malignancy is distal metastases (vascular invasion not a criterion)

IMAGING

CT
3–5 cm on average, may be larger
mixed heterogeneous adrenal mass, calcifies (may form a ring of calcification)
cystic, necrotic, hemorrhagic change
vivid contrast enhancement
theoretically, contrast may release catecholamines – non contrast CT preferable (or use beta blockade)

MR
morphology of mass same as CT
very high T2W signal, simulating fluid (but also contains areas of hemorrhage)
vivid contrast enhancement

NUC MED
see entry on adrenal nuclear medicine

MOST ARE MIBG (I-123 OR I-131 METAIODOBENZYLGUANIDINE) AVID
MIBG is overall 80–90% sensitive and ~90% specific
useful particularly to locate extraadrenal pheo
(block thyroid with cold iodine prior to scanning)

MANY ARE OCTREOTIDE (In-111 OCTREOTIDE) AVID
octreotide sensitivity is comparable to MIBG, but specificity is lower

MANY ARE MDP AVID

9 Male reproductive system

1. NORMAL

1.1 NORMAL TESTIS

volume 15–20 ml, dimensions $2 \times 3 \times 4$ cm approximately

homogeneous echotexture, mediastinum testis slightly hyperechoic, vertical and posterior

CT: density similar to muscle

MR: intermediate (higher than fluid) T1W signal, high T2W signal (mediastinum testis darker on T2W, tunica albuginea dark)

epididymal head approximately 1 cm in diameter, slightly more heterogeneous than testis

arterial and venous color and Doppler traces present in testis parenchyma symmetrically right to left

1.2 NORMAL PROSTATE

non hypertrophied size: approximately $2 \times 3 \times 4$ cm in younger male (15 ml); $3 \times 4 \times 5$ cm in older male (25 ml)

apex of gland is inferiorly, base superiorly

urethra forms major landmark, urethral angle 135 degrees

Zonal anatomy

TRANSITIONAL ZONE (TZ)
upper periurethral
5% of gland volume
hypoechoic, moderate T1W, low T2W signal
gives rise to benign prostatic hypertrophy

CENTRAL ZONE (CZ)
upper periurethral, surrounds TZ, enlarges towards base, shrinks towards apex; extends approximately from base to urethral angle (junction of ejaculatory ducts)
25% of gland volume
intermediate echogenicity, moderate T1W, low T2W signal
10% of carcinoma arises in CZ

PERIPHERAL ZONE (PZ)
lies posterolaterally at base (external to CZ), periurethral towards apex where CZ is smaller/absent
70% of gland volume, hyperechoic or intermediate (margin with CZ then by contour), moderate T1W, high T2W signal
70% of carcinoma arises in PZ

ANTERIOR FIBROMUSCULAR STROMA (AFS)
non glandular wedge anterior to urethra

hypoechoic
low T1W, low T2W signal

PERIPROSTATIC VENOUS PLEXUS
low T1W, high T2W signal

transitional and central zones not distinguishable from each other on US or MR

prostate capsule low on T1W and low on T2W

neurovascular bundles enter capsule at 5 and 7 o'clock

2. GAMUTS

2.1 GENERIC (all modalities)

2.1.1 CYSTIC STRUCTURE IN PROSTATE

ABSCESS

SEMINAL VESICLE CYST

EJACULATORY DUCT CYST

PROSTATIC CYST
CYSTIC CHANGE IN BENIGN PROSTATIC HYPERTROPHY
CYSTIC CHANGE IN PROSTATITIS
RETENTION CYST

MULLERIAN REMNANT CYST

2.1.2 DIFFUSE CHANGE IN TESTIS TEXTURE

ORCHITIS
INCREASED VASCULARITY, TENDER, EPIDIDYMITIS

ISCHEMIA, INFARCTION, TORSION
HYPOECHOIC EDEMATOUS AVASCULAR
BEWARE incomplete or intermittent torsion; hyperemia post reversal; venous obstruction producing poor diastolic flow

LYMPHOMA, LEUKEMIA, OTHER INFILTRATING TUMOR
PAINLESS DIFFUSE INFILTRATION OR MASS

2.1.3 EPIDIDYMAL/SCROTAL CYST

SIMPLE CYST

SPERMATIC CYST

VARICOCELE

2.1.4 FOCAL EPIDIDYMAL NODULE

EPIDIDYMITIS

SPERMATIC GRANULOMA

ADENOMATOID TUMOR
benign and rare

2.1.5 FOCAL TESTICULAR CYST

TUNICA ALBUGINEA CYST

RETE CYST, TUBULAR ECTASIA OF RETE TESTIS

SUBSTANCE CYST
rare, beware of cystic neoplasm simulating simple cyst

CYSTIC CHANGE IN SOLID NODULE

2.1.6 FOCAL TESTICULAR MASS

HEMATOMA
INHOMOGENEOUS, POST TRAUMA

FOCAL ORCHITIS, ABSCESS
POORLY MARGINATED, TENDER, HYPERVASCULAR

SEMINOMA
SOLID HOMOGENEOUS

NON SEMINOMATOUS TUMOR
MIXED, CYSTIC, CALCIUM, FAT

LYMPHOMA, LEUKEMIA
DIFFUSE INFILTRATION OR MASS

EPIDERMOID
CALCIFIED WALL

Leydig/Sertoli tumors
NO SPECIFIC APPEARANCE

3. CONDITIONS OF THE MALE REPRODUCTIVE SYSTEM

3.1 BENIGN PROSTATIC HYPERPLASIA (BPH)

DEFINITION

benign idiopathic fibroadenomyomatous proliferation of transitional zone glands

CLINICAL

silent: 20% of 40 year olds, 90% of 70 year olds

symptomatic: 50% at >60 years; 20% need treatment

bladder outflow obstruction, urinary infections, neuropathic bladder, obstructive nephropathy

MORPHOLOGY

hormonally driven hyperplasia

irregular pale gray firm nodules (stromal hypertrophy) with microcystic spaces (dilated glands)

foci of squamous metaplasia and infarction (may calcify)

IMAGING

XR

prostatic calcification

IVU

prostatic indentation at bladder base, 'fishhook' ureters

outflow obstruction: significant residual volume and bladder trabeculation/diverticula

US (abdominal and rectal)

overall gland enlargement

volume increase from 25 ml to 50 ml or more

indentation of bladder base by median lobe

enlargement of transitional/central zone ('inner gland') with compression of peripheral zone +/– displacement of seminal vesicles

nodular texture, hypoechoic and hyperechoic inner gland nodules

focal or curvilinear calcification (reflectors), cystic change

urethra distorted, stretched or obscured

change of BPH may hide focal carcinomatous nodule

CT

prostate enlargement, bladder base indentation

MR

enlargement of inner gland

heterogeneous nodular echotexture

nodules low or intermediate signal on T1W, and low, intermediate or high signal on T2W with a low intensity peripheral pseudocapsule

peripheral zone retains low T1W high T2W signal but may be stretched or compressed

prostatic capsule and periprostatic fat planes remain intact

7 o'clock and 5 o'clock nerve bundle entry points remain normal

3.2 INGUINAL HERNIA

CLASSIFICATION

Direct

weakened conjoint tendon of abdominal oblique muscles with direct bulging

Indirect

hernial contents enter internal ring and travel along inguinal canal

Sliding

contains extraperitoneal structure (usually colon) with a pocket of peritoneum

Reducible vs incarcerated

Obstructed vs strangulated vs infarcted

CLINICAL (adult)

much more common in males

intermittent, small indirect inguinal hernias are often difficult to demonstrate and may progress to ultrasound or herniography

CONTENTS: extraperitoneal fat, pocket of peritoneum, small bowel, colon, corner of bladder

IMAGING (adult)

XR

gas extending into scrotum or beyond hernial orifice

CT

demonstrates contents (if present at the time)

US

real time imaging for small inguinal hernias

STRUCTURES TO IDENTIFY

external ring (anatomical landmarks)

cord and coverings (tubular structure running diagonally through inguinal canal, with testicular artery as component)

internal ring (midpoint of inguinal ligament; cord 'dives' deep into retroperitoneum out of field of view)

inferior epigastric artery medial to deep ring

MANEUVERS

two plane supine and/or erect observation of external ring, canal, internal ring with coughing or straining

comparison with normal side

FINDINGS

protrusion of abnormal contents through internal ring along canal

abnormal widening of internal ring

commonest early finding is a small tongue of extraperitoneal fat moving down inguinal canal

small bowel entering internal ring or inguinal canal is an unequivocal finding

3.3 ORCHITIS/ EPIDIDYMITIS

ETIOLOGY

Non specific epididymoorchitis

younger male – usually sexually transmitted

older male – urinary tract infections secondary to bladder outlet obstruction

other associations: prostatitis, urogenital malformations, urological procedures

presents with red, hot, tender swollen scrotum

Mumps orchitis

TB epididymoorchitis

secondary to renal and bladder TB

distended fluctuant epididymis, bead like cord, sinuses to skin, calcifies

TB orchitis late

HIV orchitis

IMAGING (group)

US – epididymitis

small to moderate hydrocele, may contain debris or pus

hypervascular epididymis, may be swollen and hypoechoic

testicular parenchymal echogenicity normal, vascularity present or increased

CALCIFICATION suggests TB

US – orchitis

usually occurs with epididymitis (unless viral orchitis, e.g. mumps)

swollen testis with diffusely hypoechoic echotexture

markedly hyperemic on color and pulsed Doppler

(principal differential of acute scrotum is torsion with ischemia, where no flow is present, but beware reactive hyperemia post spontaneous detortion)

focal orchitis: only part of testis is hypoechoic and swollen, and may mimic a tumor mass (principal differentiator is acute painful presentation in orchitis)

abscess: focal irregular hypoechoic mass with central necrosis

3.4 PROSTATIC CARCINOMA

DEFINITION

prostatic glandular epithelial neoplasm with a wide range of biological behavior, aggressivity and clinical significance

EPIDEMIOLOGY

most common male cancer, true incidence not known (?8%) because of large incidence of latent tumor

3% of males die of prostate carcinoma

CLINICAL

wide range of presentations

Incidental asymptomatic finding at TURP

Found at screening

Overt disease

LOCAL SYMPTOMS

urinary obstruction

pain, hematuria, rectal invasion

DISTANT SYMPTOMS

bony metastases (migratory deep bony pain), lung metastases, lymphangitis, brain metastases

weight loss, systemic symptoms

paraaortic nodal masses, etc

Prostate specific antigen (PSA)

glycoprotein specific to prostate epithelium; normal is <4

>10 is diagnostic of cancer; >20 indicates systemic metastases

FALSE POSITIVES: recent manipulation, biopsy or surgery; benign prostatic hypertrophy

FALSE NEGATIVES: microscopic foci; dedifferentiated anaplastic carcinoma

Spread

DIRECT

perineural (neurovascular bundles at 5 and 7 o'clock)

along seminal vesicles

to bladder and rectum

LYMPHATIC

to pelvic then paraaortic nodes

HEMATOGENOUS

(historically accepted) lumbar venous plexus retrogradely

systemic hematogenous

bones, lungs, liver, brain

Staging

AMERICAN UROLOGICAL ASSOCIATION STAGING (adapted)

A1   microscopic focal
A2   microscopic diffuse
B1   palpable <1.5 cm one lobe
B2   palpable, >1.5 cm or multifocal
C1   extracapsular (not seminal vesicles)
C2   extracapsular (seminal vesicles)
D1   <4 lymph nodes involved
D2   >3 lymph nodes or distant metastases
(i.e. A and B potentially curable)

TNM STAGING

T1   not palpable or visible
T2   confined to prostate
T3a through prostatic capsule
T3b involving seminal vesicles
T4   fixed or invading adjacent structures
N1   regional nodes
M1   non regional nodes or distant metastases

MACRO

70% arise in peripheral zone, 20% in transitional zone, 10% in central zone

firm desmoplastic focus or multiple foci

may be obscured by benign prostatic hypertrophy

MICRO

Well differentiated

papillary adenocarcinoma or cribriform adenocarcinoma, back to back glands

Poorly differentiated

cords, sheets, nests of anaplastic cells

Grading by Gleason score

overcomes histological variability – single best correlation with prognosis

most prevalent and second most prevalent histological patterns each scored 1 to 5 (1 is most differentiated, 5 is least differentiated); total is 2 to 10

IMAGING

XR – bones

sclerotic bony metastases

commonly pelvis, lumbar vertebrae, upper femora

more advanced: other vertebrae, skull, ribs, distal femora, shoulder girdles

infrequent pathological vertebral fractures, rarely pathological fractures elsewhere

very rarely, lytic metastases

CXR

multiple nodules or lymphangitis carcinomatosa pattern, or both (advanced disease)

US (TRUS)

transrectal US

hypoechoic nodule 70%; hyperechoic or mixed nodule 30%

commonest in peripheral zone (70% of carcinoma)

capsule irregularity, bulge, invasion

color or power Doppler may identify a nodule where it is not apparent with gray scale

carcinoma may be lost in changes of benign prostatic hypertrophy

frank extension through capsule into other structures (e.g. rectum)

US (TRUS) guided biopsy

core biopsy of any suspicious nodules

non targeted quadrant or sextant biopsy

antibiotic coverage essential (protocols vary)

potential complications: hemorrhage, infection, urinary retention

CT

paraaortic lymphadenopathy, iliac lymphadenopathy, pelvic side wall lymphadenopathy

hypodense peripherally enhancing liver metastases

sclerotic vertebral metastases

not accurate at local staging of early prostate carcinoma: only gross invasion visible

not useful in detecting response to radiation therapy

MR – prostate

body coil or (in preference) endorectal coil

peripheral zone carcinoma low T1W and low T2W signal mass within peripheral zone (visible on T2W, not on T1W)

stellate or lobulated

contrast is not helpful

central or transitional zone carcinoma difficult to distinguish from normal prostate or benign prostatic hypertrophy

invasion of capsule (extends to capsule, capsule deformed or thickened)

invasion through capsule (spiculated extension into periprostatic fat)

invasion of neurovascular bundles (5 and 7 o'clock) particularly common (thickening or extension of tumor along bundle)

invasion of surrounding structures (seminal vesicles, rectum, bladder)

regional lymphadenopathy (pelvic sidewall, presacral)

possibly bony metastases (low T1W, low or high T2W signal) within the field of view

NUC MED (MDP)

prostate metastases have intense MDP uptake (blastic metastases)

pelvis, lumbar spine, upper femora

multiple random foci first in axial, then in appendicular skeleton

superscan: diffuse massively increased uptake throughout the skeleton (kidneys not visible or extremely faint)

NUC MED (Sr-89)

effective palliation of metastatic pain

potential side effects: platelet and white cell count drop

PET (F-)

same findings as for MDP

PET (FDG)

prostate carcinoma moderately FDG avid, but not all tumors are visible (i.e.

sensitivity not as good as for other tumors)

proximity to bladder makes identification of primary potentially difficult (need catheter)

used for problem solving particularly nodal staging if considering radical surgery or radiotherapy or in restaging

3.5 SPERMATIC GRANULOMA

nodule of extravasated sperm phagocytosed by reactive macrophages; particularly common post vasectomy

IMAGING

US

extratesticular spermatic mass of variable echogenicity, usually <1 cm

3.6 TESTICULAR CYSTS

3.6.1 TUNICA ALBUGINEA CYST

simple cyst centered on margin of testis, immediately subcapsular

can be left alone

3.6.2 SIMPLE PARENCHYMAL CYST

simple cyst on strict ultrasound criteria

very low risk of neoplasia if no solid component, especially if cyst small

3.6.3 TUBULAR ECTASIA OF RETE TESTIS

multiple cysts and fluid filled tubules within the mediastinum testis, following its expected position

benign, can be left alone

3.7 TESTICULAR EPIDERMOID

rare developmental non neoplastic inclusion mass containing keratin debris

IMAGING

US

well marginated intratesticular mass

calcified regular rim (suggestive)

no internal vascularity

NO DISTINGUISHING CHARACTERISTICS FROM GERM CELL TUMORS

3.8 TESTICULAR GERM CELL TUMORS

DEFINITION

malignant testicular germ cell tumor with capacity for pluripotent differentiation and high malignant potential

EPIDEMIOLOGY

1/100 000, but commonest carcinoma in 15–35 year old males

geographic variation (Europe > Japan)

seminoma: older male than other germ cell tumor types, cryptorchidism

yolk sac tumor: 40% of all childhood testicular tumors

Associations

cryptorchidism (risk of undescended testis > post orchidopexy > contralateral descended testis > normal controls)

testicular dysgenesis

ETIOPATHOGENESIS

starts as intratubular germ cell neoplasia (found in undescended testes and around invasive carcinoma)

CLINICAL

testicular pain, mass

presents with metastases (paraaortic, mediastinal, lung) in approximately 15%

alphafetoprotein (alphaFP) elevated: embryonal carcinoma, yolk sac tumor, choriocarcinoma

beta human chorionic gonadotrophin (beta hCG) elevated: choriocarcinoma, seminoma with syncytiotrophoblastic component

Staging

NON TNM STAGING

STAGE I   confined to testis and spermatic cord

STAGE II   nodal metastases below diaphragm (IIa nodes not palpable, IIb bulky nodes)

STAGE III   nodal metastases beyond diaphragm or extranodal metastases

TNM STAGING

T1   testis/epididymis, no lymphatic/vascular invasion

T2   testis/epididymis, vascular/lymphatic invasion OR invasion of tunica vaginalis

T3   spermatic cord

T4   scrotal wall

N1   node or nodes <2 cm

N2   node or nodes >2 cm, <5 cm

N3   node or nodes >5 cm

MORPHOLOGY

3.8.1 Seminoma

SEMINOMA NOS
sheets of undifferentiated germ cells
fibrous bands with reactive lymphocytes

SPERMATOCYTIC (5%)
early sperm line differentiation, indolent tumor

ANAPLASTIC (10%)
less differentiated

3.8.2 Choriocarcinoma
hemorrhagic necrotic mass
bilaminar (syncytiotrophoblast, cytotrophoblast) angioinvasive architecture

3.8.3 Yolk sac tumor
fetal yolk sac cells, glomeruloid bodies, alphaFP positive
pure yolk sac tumor in children, mixed in adults

3.8.4 Embryonal carcinoma
irregular mass with necrosis and hemorrhage
sheets and tubules of anaplastic cells (dark nuclei, clear cytoplasm)

3.8.5 Teratoma
CHILDREN: mature form (but has malignant potential)

ADULTS: immature (polycystic necrotic and hemorrhagic mass)

IMAGING

US
testicular intraparenchymal mass
usually non tender
may replace most or entire testis
seminoma more likely to be uniform homogeneous hypoechoic
non seminomatous germ cell tumor more likely to be heterogeneous hypoechoic, or complex cystic
may contain areas of necrosis, calcification, hemorrhage (more likely to be high grade)

CT (staging)
nodal metastases to paraaortic nodes (drainage pattern of testis), then thoracic nodes
metastases may be of low density or have central low density
may form lymph node conglomerates
with treatment, develop central necrosis or calcification
residual tissue common

PET (FDG)
differentiates inactive residual fibrotic tissue from metabolically active residual nodal metastases
immature germ cell tumor is very FDG avid
mature teratoma has low grade FDG uptake

3.9 TESTICULAR LYMPHOMA/LEUKEMIA

see Ch 16
painless enlargement of testis in patient with lymphoma or leukemia

3.10 TESTICULAR MICROLITHIASIS

DEFINITION

formation of microliths from degenerating cells in seminiferous tubules

CLINICAL

uncommon; associations are:
    cryptorchidism, Klinefelter's syndrome, Down's syndrome, male pseudohermaphroditism, alveolar microlithiasis
associated with subfertility and 20 fold increased risk of testicular malignancy
asymptomatic but up to 40% develop germ cell tumors; usual followup is yearly ultrasound once discovered

IMAGING

US
multiple small non shadowing intraparenchymal reflectors

3.11 TESTICULAR TORSION

CLINICAL

narrow pedicle predisposes ('bell-clapper testis')
commoner in adolescents and young males
less common in children (before testicular growth)
presents with acute scrotum

IMAGING

US
(use other side for comparison)
echotexture may be normal early or diffusely hypoechoic and swollen later
CARDINAL SIGN: absent normal intraparenchymal color flow and Doppler signal
scrotal wall flow may be increased
BEWARE intermittent torsion and reactive hyperemia following spontaneous reduction

NUC MED
'scrotal scan' for acute torsion no longer justifiable on radiation protection grounds because of widespread availability of US
cardinal sign is absent perfusion to testis (central photopenia inside perfused scrotum)

3.12 TESTICULAR TRAUMA

CLINICAL

spectrum from patchy edema or hemorrhage to major rupture
fracture or rupture usually requires surgical decompression but has a good salvage rate early
traumatic infarction may also occur

IMAGING

US

hematocele: contains variable amount of echogenic debris
patchy hemorrhage is mixed on US
focal hematoma is hypoechoic initially, then mixed echogenicity
infarction: see testicular torsion
major rupture: usually not a diagnostic problem!

Differential

focal hematoma has no special distinguishing characteristics (see gamuts for testicular mass)
diagnosis is made on history
if in doubt, followup US shows resolution appropriate to the timecourse

3.13 VARICOCELE

CLINICAL

varicose dilation of the pampiniform plexus presents with pain, 'dragging' sensation, mass or a 'bag of worms'
left earlier or larger than right

IMAGING

US

multiple extratesticular tortuous thin walled venous channels with color flow; usually around epididymal head

3.14 URETHRAL INJURY

CLINICAL

hematuria
acute traumatic urinary retention
physical signs of injury to perineum
pelvic fractures

IMAGING (retrograde urethrogram)

Cardinal safety rule
DO NOT PASS URINARY CATHETER IF IN DOUBT

DO RETROGRADE URETHROGRAM FIRST
alternative to urethral urinary catheter (short or medium term) is a suprapubic catheter

Posterior urethra

3.14.1 GRADE I   URETHRA INTACT, PERIURETHRAL HEMATOMA
displaced, stretched or thin urethra
no extravasation by definition

3.14.2 GRADE II   INJURY OR TRANSSECTION ABOVE UROGENITAL DIAPHRAGM
usual location is just distal to the prostate
also bladder neck, prostatic urethra
partial or complete transsection with contrast extravasation into pelvis (retroperitoneum or peritoneum)

3.14.4 GRADE III   INJURY OR TRANSSECTION BELOW UROGENITAL DIAPHRAGM
usual location is just below urogenital sphincter
partial or complete transsection with contrast extravasation into perineum

Anterior urethra

3.14.5 COMPLETE LACERATION

3.14.6 INCOMPLETE LACERATION

CNS, head and neck

10 CNS normal and gamuts

1. NORMAL

1.1 ANASTOMOSES BETWEEN EXTERNAL AND INTERNAL CAROTID CIRCULATIONS

facial artery – ophthalmic artery
maxillary artery (deep) – inferolateral trunk of internal carotid artery
occipital artery – muscular branches of vertebral artery
middle meningeal artery – recurrent meningeal artery

1.2 CAROTID DOPPLER

Carotid artery stenosis on doppler criteria

INTERNAL CAROTID ARTERY

0–15%   systolic Vp <125 cm/s and no other findings
15–50%   systolic Vp <125 cm/s spectral broadening
50–80%   systolic Vp >125 cm/s diastolic velocity <40 cm/s 2< IC/CC <4
80–100%   systolic Vp >125 cm/s diastolic velocity >140 cm/s IC/CC >4

IC/CC: ratio of peak systolic velocities internal carotid artery:common carotid artery; Vp: peak velocity

EXTERNAL CAROTID ARTERY

<50%   spectral broadening
>50%   systolic Vp >125 cm/s

Plaque description

SMOOTH VS ROUGH

CALCIFIED VS SOFT

SOFT PLAQUE
INTIMAL THICKENING
HOMOGENEOUS
HETEROGENEOUS/COMPLEX
(FOCAL ANECHOIC = HEMORRHAGE)

1.3 ELOQUENT CORTEX

cortex that directly controls function, and damage to eloquent cortex usually produces major focal neurological deficits

includes: primary motor cortex, primary somatosensory cortex, primary visual cortex, Broca's area and Wernicke's area therefore, either not resectable or resectable but with deliberate sacrifice of function
may need mapping using anatomical knowledge or functional MR techniques

1.4 GLASGOW COMA SCORE

Eyes open in response to:

NONE = 1, TO PAIN = 2, TO SPEECH = 3, SPONTANEOUS = 4

Best verbal response

NONE = 1, NOISE = 2, INAPPROPRIATE = 3, CONFUSED = 4, ORIENTED = 5

Best motor response

NONE = 1, EXTENDS LIMBS = 2, FLEXES LIMBS = 3, WITHDRAWS FROM PAIN = 4, LOCALIZES PAIN = 5, CARRIES OUT INSTRUCTION = 6

Add the scores together for a total score 3–15/15

1.5 MR SPECTROSCOPY (MRS) SURVIVAL BASICS

MR spectroscopic imaging = chemical shift imaging

Generation of spectra

different molecules with unmatched protons precess at slightly different frequencies that depend on the main magnetic field strength
ratios of the frequency differences between different molecules remains the same at different main field strengths
tetramethylsilane is used as a reference, and frequency shift relative to it is expressed as a difference in parts per million (ppm), taken from the frequency ratio
by convention, zero point (tetramethylsilane) is on the right of plot of signal intensity vs shift in ppm ('spectrum'), and molecules with progressively higher frequency shift are displayed further to the left

Common sequences

MRS can be performed after gadolinium contrast
water is suppressed out of spectrum, and baseline adjusted to be stable; if water suppression fails, dominant water peak (4.7 ppm) makes spectrum difficult to interpret

STEAM (Stimulated Echo Acquisition Mode)

similar to gradient echo sequences
shorter TE (e.g. 30–40 ms)
signal to noise ratio lower
allows resolution of short TE metabolites (e.g. myo-inositol/glutamine and glutamate)

PRESS (point resolved spectroscopy)

similar to spin echo sequences
longer TE (e.g. 135–144 ms or longer)
signal to noise ratio higher
unable to resolve short TE metabolites
more commonly used sequence
preferred for longer TE work (e.g. tumor spectroscopy: good resolution of choline, creatine, NAA)

Common metabolites

unsuppressed water: 4.7 ppm, dominates entire spectrum
fat: 1.3 ppm (mixture of species)

CLINICALLY RELEVANT METABOLITES (shift in ppm)

LIPID (FAT, OTHER LIPID SPECIES) 1.3
lipid fragments present in necrosis
external (scalp) fat is a source of contamination
broad lipid peak overlaps lactate peak and may obscure it

LACTATE (DOUBLET) 1.33
inverted peak at intermediate TE, e.g. 135–144 ms
marker of anaerobic metabolism or necrosis

ALANINE (DOUBLET) 1.48
present in some meningiomas, not present in normal brain

N-ACETYL ASPARTATE (NAA) 2.02 (FIRST PEAK)
marker of neuronal density

GLUTAMATE/GLUTAMINE 2.05–2.5

CREATINE/PHOSPHOCREATINE 3.03
marker of cell metabolism
commonly used as an internal reference

CHOLINE 3.22
marker of cell membrane proliferation/ density and turnover

MYO-INOSITOL 3.56
marker of gliosis and an osmolyte
elevated in Alzheimer's disease
reduced in hepatic encephalopathy

GLUTAMINE/GLUTAMATE 3.65–3.8
elevated in hepatic encephalopathy

NORMAL RATIOS
easiest ratios are peak heights
areas under curve ratios are more accurate
    and preferred for semi-quantitation of
    metabolites
ratios are used to differentiate tumor from
    radiation necrosis, follow evolution of
    disease and progression of tumor
ratios below are peak area ratios; values are
    based on a PRESS sequence with TE 135
    or 144 ms, (NYU Medical Center/Siemens
    Spectroscopy at 1.5T)
choline:creatine 0.75 (SD 0.14)
NAA:creatine 1.45 (SD 0.22)
choline:NAA 0.54 (SD 0.13)

Single voxel vs multivoxel spectroscopy

SINGLE VOXEL SPECTROSCOPY
1 cm cube, 1.5 cm cube, 2 cm cube
larger voxel gives higher signal to noise
    ratio but more volume averaging
smaller voxel requires longer acquisition
    time for good signal to noise ratio
problems: sampling error, positioning error,
    volume averaging

MULTIVOXEL SPECTROSCOPY
commonly 2D array of adjacent voxels
overcomes sampling error (provided entire
    mass is in the slab)
current software allows multivoxel
    acquisitions in similar time to single
    voxel spectroscopy
problems: voxel 'bleeding' and
    contamination from adjacent voxels over
    scalp/fat/CSF
particularly useful in large heterogeneous
    masses
not relevant to masses smaller than one
    voxel
3D multislice whole brain spectroscopy is
    the focus of current research

1.6 MYELINATION

see Ch 20

1.7 NORMAL LEPTOMENINGEAL ENHANCEMENT

thin <1 mm, smooth and linear
focal and discontinuous
mild (less intense than cavernous sinus)

1.8 NORMAL PINEAL

4 × 4 × 8 mm; does not calcify <10 years of
    age

1.9 NORMAL PITUITARY

Fossa size
16 mm AP 11 mm SI

Gland size
MALE up to 8 mm high
FEMALE up to 10 mm high
INFUNDIBULUM thickness 2–3 mm

Incidentalomas 15%
incidental poorly enhancing lesions: cysts,
    microadenomas

1.10 NORMAL SKULL MR

see Ch 01

1.11 VENTRICLES AND SULCI

also see normal values in Ch 20

White matter
volume stable from 20 years on
increasing perivascular spaces with age

White matter focal T2W hyperintensity
white matter UBOs commonly occur on T2W
    sequences in patients over 50 years old
    (UBO: unidentified bright object)
perivascular space (normal)
perivascular vacuolated myelin (essentially
    normal)
focal areas of demyelination
spongy degeneration, deep focal ischemia
lacunar infarction

Gray matter
slow linear decline in volume from 20 years
    on

Ventricles and sulci
large range of normal sizes
size increases from 50–60 years on

Brain iron
not detectable at birth, then normal
    accumulation in:
globus pallidus
substantia nigra and red nucleus
dentate nucleus of cerebellum
putamen (late)

2. GAMUTS

2.1 GENERIC (all modalities)

2.1.1 ABSCESS SOURCES

Hematogenous
SEPTICEMIA

BACTERIAL ENDOCARDITIS

RIGHT TO LEFT VASCULAR SHUNT
(HEART OR LUNGS)

IV DRUG ABUSE

Direct
MIDDLE EAR INFECTION

MASTOID INFECTION

PARANASAL INFECTION

PENETRATING TRAUMA OR
SURGERY

(CONGENITAL SINUS)

2.1.2 AIDS IN THE CNS

see Ch 11 for condition entries

Meningitis
HIV CONVERSION

FUNGAL

TB AND MAC

LYMPHOMA

Parenchymal diffuse processes
HIV ENCEPHALOPATHY

PROGRESSIVE MULTIFOCAL LEUKOENCEPHALOPATHY

CMV CEREBRITIS

Parenchymal focal processes

TOXOPLASMOSIS

TB OR FUNGAL ABSCESS

SYPHILITIC GUMMA

LYMPHOMA

KAPOSI'S SARCOMA

GLIOBLASTOMA

Myelopathy

VZV (VARICELLA ZOSTER VIRUS)

CMV (CYTOMEGALOVIRUS)

TOXOPLASMOSIS

LYMPHOMA

2.1.3 BACK PAIN IN CHILDREN

see Ch 17

2.1.4 CEREBRAL HEMORRHAGE GAMUTS

2.1.4.1 Hemorrhage classification by location

SUBARACHNOID

DEEP INTRAPARENCHYMAL

LOBAR

2.1.4.2 Hypertensive hemorrhage locations

PUTAMEN

THALAMUS

PONS

CEREBELLUM
(~10% due to aneurysm)

2.1.4.3 Differential diagnoses of hypertensive hemorrhage

HEMORRHAGE WITHOUT AN UNDERLYING MASS

HYPERTENSIVE HEMORRHAGE

AMYLOID ANGIOPATHY

INFARCT WITH SUBSEQUENT HEMORRHAGE

VENOUS INFARCT

COAGULOPATHY

HEMORRHAGE INTO AN UNDERLYING MASS

ANEURYSM

AV MALFORMATION

HEMANGIOMA

TUMOR

METASTASES THAT BLEED

MELANOMA

CHORIOCARCINOMA

RENAL CELL CARCINOMA

LUNG CARCINOMA

BREAST CARCINOMA

2.1.4.4 Characteristics of a benign hemorrhage

WELL DEFINED HEMOSIDERIN RIM

ORDERLY EVOLUTION

2.1.4.5 Characteristics of hemorrhage into malignancy

INCOMPLETE HEMOSIDERIN RIM

ENHANCEMENT UNRELATED TO BLEED

BIZARRE

DISORDERED EVOLUTION

GROWS

2.1.5 CEREBRAL EDEMA, INTRAAXIAL EDEMA

Diffuse neuraxial edema

TRAUMA

HYPOXIA

INFECTION

Focal neuraxial edema

TRAUMA

INFARCT

INFECTION

TUMOR

2.1.6 DISK DISEASE DIFFERENTIALS

Focal lumbar intraspinal mass

DISK FRAGMENT

CONJOINED ROOT

INTRASPINAL CYST

NERVE SHEATH TUMOR

Ring enhancing focal mass

DISK FRAGMENT

SCHWANNOMA

CONJOINED ROOT

INTRASPINAL CYST

Solidly enhancing mass

SCAR

TUMOR NOS

SCHWANNOMA

2.1.7 INFARCT DIFFERENTIAL DIAGNOSES

differential causes for each cardinal finding in infarction

2.1.7.1 Edema (differential of edema: gliosis)

TRAUMA

INFECTION

TUMOR

INFARCT

2.1.7.2 Volume loss

ATROPHY

INFARCT

CONGENITAL LESION

2.1.7.3 Ring enhancement
see gamut for ring enhancement (MAGIC DR AL)

2.1.7.4 Leptomeningeal enhancement

POSTOPERATIVE

UNDERLYING INFARCT

AV MALFORMATION

METASTASIS, LYMPHOMA, LANGERHANS CELL HISTIOCYTOSIS

SARCOIDOSIS, TB, FUNGI

MENINGIOMA

2.1.7.5 Hemorrhage
see cerebral hemorrhage gamuts

2.1.8 INFARCTS – UNUSUAL

Mnemonic: 3H 4VM

H-eart

R TO L SHUNTS

CONGENITAL HEART DISEASE

PROSTHETIC VALVES

CARDIOMYOPATHY, ATRIAL FLUTTER

ENDOCARDITIS, IV DRUG ABUSE

H-ypertension

MALIGNANT HYPERTENSION

ECLAMPSIA

H-ypercoagulability

ANTIPHOSPHOLIPID ANTIBODIES
see Ch 15

ANTITHROMBIN III DEFICIENCY

PROTEIN C DEFICIENCY

PROTEIN S DEFICIENCY

ORAL CONTRACEPTIVE PILL

PUERPERIUM

HEMOLYTIC UREMIC SYNDROME +
   THROMBOTIC
   THROMBOCYTOPENIC PURPURA
see Ch 16

V-enous

INFECTION WITH DURAL SINUS
   THROMBOSIS

FOCAL VASCULAR ANOMALY

HYPERCOAGULABLE STATE

V-asospasm

SUBARACHNOID HEMORRHAGE

ECLAMPSIA

IV DRUG ABUSE

MIGRAINE

V-asculitis

INFECTIVE

TB, FUNGI

PSEUDOINFECTIVE

SARCOID AND SYPHILIS

AUTOIMMUNE

GIANT CELL ARTERITIS

TAKAYASU'S ARTERITIS

POLYARTERITIS NODOSA

PRIMARY CNS VASCULITIS

V-asculopathy

FIBROMUSCULAR DYSPLASIA,
   DISSECTION

MARFAN'S, EHLERS–DANLOS
   SYNDROMES

MOYA MOYA SYNDROME

M-itochondrial encephalopathy

MELAS

M-yopathy, E-ncephalopathy, L-actic
   A-cidosis, S-troke like episodes

MERRF

M-yoclonic E-pilepsy, R-agged R-ed F-ibers

LEIGH DISEASE

2.1.9 METASTASES

2.1.9.1 Metastases that bleed

MELANOMA

CHORIOCARCINOMA

RENAL CELL CARCINOMA

LUNG CARCINOMA

BREAST CARCINOMA

2.1.9.2 Metastases that calcify

OSTEOSARCOMA

COLON CARCINOMA

MUCINOUS TUMORS NOS

PANCREATIC CARCINOMA

2.1.10 PARKINSON'S DISEASE DIFFERENTIALS

IDIOPATHIC PARKINSON'S DISEASE

PROGRESSIVE SUPRANUCLEAR
   PALSY

SHY–DRAGER SYNDROME

STRIATONIGRAL DEGENERATION

TOXIC PARKINSONISM

2.1.11 PITUITARY GAMUTS

2.1.11.1 Abnormal stalk enhancement

SARCOIDOSIS, TB, SYPHILIS

HISTIOCYTOSIS

LYMPHOMA, LEUKEMIA

HYPOPHYSITIS

2.1.11.2 J shaped sella

CHIASMATIC GLIOMA

ACHONDROPLASIA

NEUROFIBROMATOSIS

MUCOPOLYSACCHARIDOSES

PYKNODYSOSTOSIS

2.1.11.3 Short list of causes of high T1W intrasellar signal

HEMORRHAGE INTO PITUITARY
   ADENOMA

RATHKE'S CLEFT CYST

(CRANIOPHARYNGIOMA)

THROMBOSED ANEURYSM

2.1.12 RING ENHANCEMENT

Mnemonic: MAGIC DR AL

M-ETASTASIS

A-BSCESS

G-LIOMA

I-NFARCT

C-ONTUSIONS

D-EMYELINATION

R-ADIOTHERAPY

A-NEURYSM

L-YMPHOMA

2.1.13 TEMPORAL BONE DISEASE GOING TO CEREBELLOPONTINE ANGLE

CHOLESTEROL GRANULOMA

PETROUS APICITIS (GRADENIGO
   SYNDROME)

GLOMUS TUMOR

FRACTURE

NOT CHOLESTEATOMA!

2.1.14 TUMOR BY LOCATION – INTRACRANIAL

2.1.14.1 Intraaxial hemispheric

MNEMONIC: I'M PONG

I-NFECTION

M-ETASTASIS, LYMPHOMA

P-NET LINE TUMORS

MNEMONIC FOR PNET LINE TUMORS: PNETEM

P-INEOBLASTOMA

N-EUROBLASTOMA – RHABDOID VARIANT

E-PENDYMOBLASTOMA

RE-T-INOBLASTOMA

MEDULLO-E-PITHELIOMA

M-EDULLOBLASTOMA

O-LIGODENDROGLIOMA

N-EURAL LINE

NEUROCYTOMA, DYSEMBRYOPLASTIC NEUROEPITHELIAL TUMOR, GANGLIOCYTOMA, GANGLIOGLIOMA

G-LIAL LINE (astrocytic)

CIRCUMSCRIBED ASTROCYTOMAS

SUBEPENDYMAL GIANT CELL ASTROCYTOMA

PILOCYTIC ASTROCYTOMA

PLEOMORPHIC XANTHOASTROCYTOMA

DIFFUSE ASTROCYTOMAS

PROTOPLASMIC ASTROCYTOMA, FIBRILLARY ASTROCYTOMA, GEMISTOCYTIC ASTROCYTOMA

ANAPLASTIC ASTROCYTOMA

GLIOBLASTOMA MULTIFORME

2.1.14.2 Parasellar, sellar (intra and extraaxial)

MNEMONIC: CAT GAME

C-RANIOPHARYNGIOMA, RATHKE'S CLEFT CYST

A-DENOMA (pituitary adenoma)

T-ERATOMA, OTHER GERM CELL TUMORS

G-LIOMA (optic or hypophyseal)

A-NEURYSM, ARACHNOID CYST

M-ENINGIOMA

E-PIDERMOID, DERMOID, EOSINOPHILIC GRANULOMA

2.1.14.3 Pineal

MNEMONIC: PIG

P-INEAL CYST, PINEOCYTOMA, PINEOBLASTOMA

I-NCLUSION 'TUMOR'

G-ERM CELL TUMOR

2.1.14.4 Ventricles (intraaxial by definition)

GENERAL

MNEMONIC: METC

M-ENINGIOMA

E-PENDYMOMA, SUBEPENDYMOMA

T-ERATOMA, DERMOID

C-HOROID PLEXUS TUMORS

AT FORAMEN OF MONRO

COLLOID CYST

NEUROCYTOMA

GIANT CELL ASTROCYTOMA

2.1.14.5 Posterior fossa (intra and extraaxial)

MNEMONIC: I'M MADE SAME

I-NFECTION

M-ETASTASIS

MIDLINE OR CLOSE TO MIDLINE (MADE)

M-EDULLOBLASTOMA

A-STROCYTOMA (PONTINE OR CEREBELLAR)

D-ERMOID

E-PENDYMOMA

LATERAL OR CEREBELLOPONTINE ANGLE (SAME)

S-CHWANNOMA

A-RACHNOID CYST

M-ENINGIOMA

E-PIDERMOID

2.1.14.6 Extraaxial

MENINGIOMA

HEMANGIOPERICYTOMA

METASTASIS, LYMPHOMA

SARCOMA

FIBROUS DYSPLASIA

2.1.15 TUMOR BY LOCATION – SPINAL

2.1.15.1 Spinal intramedullary

FINDINGS

mass within cord substance expanding cord in two projections

isocenter of mass in cord

CSF tapers around expanded cord in all projections

may expand canal if indolent

virtually all enhance with gadolinium

may have a secondary syrinx

60% ependymoma, 35% astrocytoma

DIFFERENTIAL

MNEMONIC: I'M SALTED

I-NFECTION

M-ETASTASIS

S-YRINX

A-STROCYTOMA

L-IPOMA

T-ERATOMA, GERM CELL TUMOR

E-PENDYMOMA

D-ERMOID, EPIDERMOID

2.1.15.2 Intradural extramedullary

FINDINGS

mass that lies between dura and cord

cord not expanded

cord deviated from one wall of canal in at least one projection

CSF widened around mass and may 'cup' the mass, forming acute angles with dura and with cord

DIFFERENTIAL

MNEMONIC: SAME DAME

S-CHWANNOMA

A-RACHNOID CYST

M-ENINGIOMA

E-PIDERMOID

D-ERMOID

A-V MALFORMATION

M-ETASTASIS

E-PENDYMOMA

BUT NOTE INTRADURAL EXTRAMEDULLARY NON TUMORS

CONJOINED NERVE ROOT

DIFFUSE BENIGN ROOT ENLARGEMENT

2.1.15.3 Extradural

FINDINGS

isocenter of mass falls outside the canal

mass lifts a smooth curve of dura with it

cord may be compressed by mass, with dural
   sac dimensions abnormally reduced first

CSF tapers around cord in narrowed
   subarachnoid space

MNEMONIC: DAMDENONG

D-ISK

A-BSCESS

M-ETASTASIS (LYMPHOMA)

D-ERMOID

E-PIDERMOID

N-EUROFIBROMA

O-SSEOUS PRIMARY

N-EUROBLASTOMA

G-ANGLIONEUROMA

2.1.16 TUMOR BY CHARACTER

2.1.16.1 Dense tumors (high density on CT, possibly low-low on MR)

CONSIDER HEMORRHAGE

MENINGIOMA

EPENDYMOMA

MEDULLOBLASTOMA

LYMPHOMA

DENSE METASTASIS

2.1.16.2 Enhancing tumors which are biologically low grade

EPENDYMOMA, CHOROID PLEXUS TUMORS

MENINGIOMA

GIANT CELL ASTROCYTOMA

PILOCYTIC ASTROCYTOMA

PLEOMORPHIC XANTHOASTROCYTOMA

HEMANGIOMA, HEMANGIOBLASTOMA

SCHWANNOMA

2.1.16.3 Calcifying tumors which are biologically low grade

NEUROCYTOMA

MENINGIOMA

EPENDYMOMA, CHOROID PLEXUS TUMORS

PINEOCYTOMA

OLIGODENDROGLIOMA

2.1.16.4 Cyst with mural nodule

PILOCYTIC ASTROCYTOMA (CHILD)

HEMANGIOBLASTOMA (ADULT)

GANGLIOGLIOMA

PLEOMORPHIC XANTHOASTROCYTOMA (RARE)

DIFFERENTIAL: CYSTIC NECROSIS IN HIGH GRADE TUMOR

2.1.17 TUMORS BY LINEAGE

2.1.17.1 Ependymoneuroglial

EPENDYMAL, SUBEPENDYMAL, CHOROID

NEURAL, NEUROGLIAL

NEUROCYTOMA

DYSEMBRYOPLASTIC NEUROEPITHELIAL TUMOR ('NEUROGLIOMA')

GANGLIOCYTOMA

GANGLIOGLIOMA

ASTROGLIAL, OLIGODENDROGLIAL, UNDIFFERENTIATED

ASTROGLIAL

   CIRCUMSCRIBED (WHO GRADE I)
      SUBEPENDYMAL GIANT CELL
      PILOCYTIC

   PLEOMORPHIC XANTHOASTROCYTOMA (WHO GRADE II)

   DIFFUSE ASTROCYTOMA (WHO GRADE II)
      PROTOPLASMIC
      FIBRILLARY
      GEMISTOCYTIC

ANAPLASTIC ASTROCYTOMA (WHO GRADE III)

GLIOBLASTOMA (WHO GRADE IV)

OLIGODENDROGLIOMA

PNETs

PRIMITIVE NEUROECTODERMAL TUMORS

MNEMONIC: PNETEM

P-INEOBLASTOMA

N-EUROBLASTOMA, RHABDOID TUMOR

E-PENDYMOBLASTOMA

RE-T-INOBLASTOMA

MEDULLO-E-PITHELIOMA

M-EDULLOBLASTOMA

2.1.17.2 Specialized endocrine

PITUITARY

PINEAL

2.1.17.3 Neuraxis coverings

MENINGOTHELIAL

NERVE SHEATH

2.1.17.4 Vascular

HEMANGIOMA

HEMANGIOBLASTOMA

HEMANGIOPERICYTOMA

2.1.17.5 Lymphoid

LYMPHOMA

2.1.17.6 Embryonal

GERM CELL TUMORS

DYSGERMINOMA

YOLK SAC TUMOR

CHORIOCARCINOMA

EMBRYONAL CELL CARCINOMA

IMMATURE TERATOMA

MATURE TERATOMA

CRANIOPHARYNGIOMA

RATHKE'S CLEFT CYST

CHORDOMA

COLLOID CYST

2.1.17.7 Non neoplastic masses

INCLUSION 'TUMORS'

LIPOMA

ARACHNOID CYST

2.1.18 TUMOR DESCRIPTORS

LOCATION is the most important differentiator (EXTRAAXIAL versus INTRAAXIAL; specific location of ISOCENTER for each)

characterization descriptors below allow further classification

MNEMONIC: MEDECHE

M-ORPHOLOGY

E-DGE

D-ENSITY OR SIGNAL

E-NHANCEMENT

C-ALCIFICATION

H-EMORRHAGE

E-DEMA

2.2 CT (and XR)

2.2.1 INTRACRANIAL CALCIFICATION

Mnemonic: STIVENS

S-yndromic

STURGE–WEBER (>2 years old)

TUBEROUS SCLEROSIS (>1 year old)

NEUROFIBROMATOSIS (choroid plexus)

T-umor

MENINGIOMA

CRANIOPHARYNGIOMA

PINEAL TUMORS

CHOROID TUMORS

OLIGODENDROGLIOMA

POST RADIATION THERAPY – ANY TUMOR

I-nfection [TB LATCH]

TB

L-ISTERIA

A-BSCESS

T-ORCH INFECTIONS

C-YSTICERCOSIS

(H-YDATID)

V-ascular

ANEURYSM

HEMANGIOMA

AV MALFORMATION

E-ndocrine

HYPERPARATHYROIDISM

HYPOPARATHYROIDISM (basal ganglia)

HYPERVITAMINOSIS D

LEAD POISONING

N-ormal

DURA

PINEAL

CHOROID (>10 years old)

S-ubdural hematoma

2.2.2 SKULL GAMUTS

see Ch 01

2.3 MR

2.3.1 BONE MARROW CHANGES ON MR

see Ch 01

2.3.2 DURAL ABNORMAL ENHANCEMENT

Carcinomatous

BREAST

PROSTATE

LYMPHOMA, LEUKEMIA

Benign

INTRACRANIAL HYPOTENSION

MUCOPOLYSACCHARIDOSES

IDIOPATHIC HYPERTROPHIC PACHYMENINGITIS

2.3.3 DYSMYELINATING DISEASES

see condition entries in Ch 11

division into white vs gray, deep vs superficial is a simplified conceptual framework, allows straightforward grouping, but is approximate

White matter

MNEMONIC: GAMP CAMP

DEEP [GAMP]

G-LOBOID (KRABBE) LEUKODYSTROPHY

A-DRENOLEUKODYSTROPHY/ A-DRENOMYELONEUROPATHY

M-ETACHROMATIC LEUKODYSTROPHY

P-HENYLKETONURIA

SUBCORTICAL [CAMP]

C-ANAVAN DISEASE

A-LEXANDER DISEASE

M-ERLZBACHER–P-ELIZAEUS (or PELIZAEUS–MERLZBACHER) DISEASE

Gray matter

MNEMONIC: LEWISH MUCEG HUNTS

DEEP [LEWISH]

LE-IGH DISEASE

WI-LSONs DISEASE

S-PATZ–H-ALLERVORDEN DISEASE (or HALLERVORDEN–SPATZ DISEASE)

CORTICAL [MUCEG]

MU-COLIPIDOSES (NIEMANN–PICK disease in particular)

CE-ROID LIPOFUSCINOSIS

G-LYCOGEN STORAGE DISEASE (POMPE DISEASE in particular)

BOTH [HUNTS]

HUNT-INGTON'S DISEASE

TAY–S-ACHS DISEASE (and GM2 GANGLIOSIDOSIS)

Both white and gray

MNEMONIC: MMMZ

M-ELAS

Myopathy, Encephalopathy, Lactic Acidosis, Stroke like episodes

M-ERRF

Myoclonic Epilepsy, Ragged Red Fibers (in skeletal muscle)

M-UCOPOLYSACCHARIDOSES

Z-ELLWEGER SYNDROME

2.3.4 HEMORRHAGE ON MR

see Ch 11

2.3.5 INCIDENTAL FOCI OF HIGH T2W SIGNAL

for dominant multiple foci of high T2W signal, see white matter multiple foci of high T2W signal gamut

Findings
by definition, not the dominant finding
one or few
in keeping with patient's age
not relevant to presenting problem

Differential
PERIVASCULAR SPACES

VACUOLATED MYELIN

DEEP FOCAL ISCHEMIA (PERFORATORS)

FRANK LACUNAR INFARCTION

OLD FOCI OF HEMORRHAGE

SMALL EMBOLI (ESP AT GRAY-WHITE JUNCTION)

2.3.6 LEPTOMENINGEAL ABNORMAL ENHANCEMENT

see normal leptomeningeal enhancement entry under normal
abnormal enhancement is anything in excess of that

2.3.6.1 Diffuse
MENINGITIS (INFECTIVE OR CHEMICAL)

LEPTOMENINGEAL CARCINOMATOSIS (METASTASES OR LYMPHOMA)

POSTOPERATIVE

SARCOIDOSIS

DURAL VENOUS SINUS THROMBOSIS

2.3.6.2 Focal
POSTOPERATIVE

OVER AN UNDERLYING INFARCT

AVM

METASTASIS, LYMPHOMA, HISTIOCYTOMA

2.3.6.3 Basal cisterns
SARCOIDOSIS, TB, FUNGI, SYPHILIS

MENINGIOMA

2.3.7 SPINAL CYSTS

see Ch 01

2.3.8 SPINAL NERVE ROOT THICKENING (diffuse)

LEUKEMIA, LYMPHOMA, CARCINOMATOSIS

SARCOIDOSIS, HISTIOCYTOSIS

CONGENITAL HYPERTROPHIC NEUROPATHIES

2.3.9 SUBARACHNOID METASTASES

Drop metastases
GLIOBLASTOMA

EPENDYMOMA

MEDULLOBLASTOMA

PNET TUMORS

CHOROID PLEXUS TUMORS

Hematogenous metastases
LUNG CARCINOMA

BREAST CARCINOMA

MELANOMA

LYMPHOMA, LEUKEMIA

Findings
ALL ENHANCE

NODULAR DEPOSITS OR FOCAL MASSES

DIFFUSE THICKENING OR CLUMPING

ROOT SLEEVE OBLITERATION

2.3.10 T1W HIGH SIGNAL MATERIAL

BLOOD

FAT

THICK PROTEIN

MELANIN

CALCIUM (DIFFUSE RATHER THAN CLUMPY)

GADOLINIUM

SLOW FLOW

2.3.11 T2W LOW SIGNAL MATERIAL

BLOOD

DENSE TISSUE (FIBROUS, CELLULAR, PROTEINACEOUS)

IRON

CALCIUM (CLUMPY RATHER THAN DIFFUSE)

AIR

METAL (NON IRON)

FLOW VOID

2.3.12 WHITE MATTER MS LIKE PATTERN

MNEMONIC: MAPS

M-ULTIPLE SCLEROSIS

A-CUTE DISSEMINATED ENCEPHALOMYELITIS

P-ROGRESSIVE MULTIFOCAL LEUKOENCEPHALOPATHY

S-UBACUTE SCLEROSING PANENCEPHALITIS

2.3.13 WHITE MATTER MULTIPLE FOCI OF HIGH T2W SIGNAL

this is the gamut where the white matter high T2W foci are the principal or dominant finding

MNEMONIC: MAVIS MAVIS

M-ULTIPLE SCLEROSIS AND M-ETASTASES

A-GING AND A-BNORMAL MYELIN (DYSMYELINATION)

V-IRAL ENCEPHALITIS AND V-ASCULITIS

I-NFARCTS (SMALL VESSEL ISCHEMIA) AND I-NFECTION (VIRAL, LYME DISEASE, ETC)

S-HEAR INJURY AND S-ARCOIDOSIS

2.4 PET

see Ch 25

SECTION 3

3. GENERAL PRINCIPLES AND CONDITIONS

3.1 ASTROGLIAL CYTOPATHOLOGY

Gliosis

CNS equivalent of granulation and scar tissue

astrocytes proliferate+ in area of damage to form gliotic tissue and eventually restore the blood–brain barrier

proliferation, gemistocytic astrocytes (pink and stubby), eventual shrinkage

Astrocyte lineage markers

glial fibrillary acidic protein, intermediate cytofilaments

Inclusion bodies occurring in astrocytes

ROSENTHAL FIBERS

CORPORA AMYLACEA

Alzheimer II astrocyte

occurs in hepatic encephalopathy, not Alzheimer's disease!

3.2 BLOOD–BRAIN BARRIER (BBB)

DEFINITION

histological/biochemical interface between the intravascular compartment and the subarachnoid space which limits passage of charged species and macromolecules into the CSF

endothelial tight junctions, continuous basement membrane, astrocyte foot processes

FUNCTION

Freely permeable to

water

ions that pass by facilitated diffusion (Na, K, Cl, HCO3)

glucose (and FDG)

lipophilic non charged molecules (and anesthetics)

gases (including Xe)

Impermeable to

proteins unless active transport mechanism is present

large charged molecules (e.g. Tl, DTPA, Gd)

large non charged hydrophilic molecules (e.g. iodinated contrast material)

CNS AREAS NORMALLY WITHOUT BLOOD–BRAIN BARRIER

lower hypothalamus (tuber cinereum) and anterior pituitary

area postrema

pineal gland

choroid plexus (but a choroid–CSF barrier is present)

DISRUPTION OF BBB

Necrosis (non-neoplastic, BBB eventually restored by gliosis)

Tumor

tumoral neoangiogenesis

no BBB in high grade tumors

no BBB in metastatic tumors (capillaries same as in tissue of origin)

no BBB in extraaxial tumors

CONTRAST ENHANCEMENT IN DISRUPTED BBB

spectrum of enhancement from none to vivid

does not delineate tumor from surrounding edema

tumor (especially gliomas) can be expected to infiltrate beyond the area of enhancement

Non-structural disruption

altered vascular permeability

altitude sickness

peritumoral vasogenic edema

encephalitis/cerebritis

IMAGING

Commonly used agents that pass through the BBB

HMPAO (CERETEC)

ECD (NEUROLITE)

FDG

Xe GAS

Commonly used agents that do not pass through the BBB

X-RAY/CT CONTRAST

MR CONTRAST

THALLIUM

MIBI (taken up in choroid)

3.3 EDEMA TYPES

GROUP DEFINITION

focal or diffuse abnormal increase in intra axial extracellular or intracellular fluid volume

3.3.1 VASOGENIC

MECHANISM

increased capillary permeability with reversible disruption of tight junctions

increased interstitial water content affecting white matter (loose) more than gray matter (compact)

associated with tumor, abscess, demyelination, less so hematoma

IMAGING

decreased density and T1W signal and increased T2W/PD/FLAIR signal with mass effect (usually already occurring around a mass)

predominantly white matter affected, with fingers of edema following white matter tracts subcortically

3.3.2 CYTOTOXIC

MECHANISM

cell death with accumulation of intracellular and interstitial water

affects both gray and white matter

associated with infarcts and other causes of necrosis

IMAGING

decreased density and T1W signal and increased T2W/PD/FLAIR signal with mild mass effect

affects gray and white matter equally, with gray/white matter interface lost

3.3.3 TRANSEPENDYMAL
(interstitial)

MECHANISM

increased CSF pressure with transependymal CSF transudation occurs with hydrocephalus

IMAGING

decreased density and T1W signal and increased T2W/PD/FLAIR signal surrounding the lateral ventricles

3.4 HEMORRHAGE ON CT/MR (imaging findings)

Species	Timing	CT	T1W	T2W
oxyhemoglobin	0 to 6 hours	dense	isointense	high
deoxyhemoglobin	6 hours to 3 days	dense	isointense	low
intracellular methemoglobin	3 days to 1 week	dense	high	low
extracellular methemoglobin	1 to 4 weeks	iso or hypodense	high	high
chronic ferritin	late	hypodense	low	low

all species have low or very low GRE signal

3.5 HYDROCEPHALUS

see Ch 20

3.6 LAMINAR NECROSIS

AREAS OF VULNERABILITY

NEOCORTEX LAYERS 3, 5, 6
HIPPOCAMPUS SECTORS CA 1, 3, 4
CEREBELLUM Purkinje cells > stellate cells > other
STRIATUM small cells > large cells

IMAGING

MR

gyriform cortical contrast enhancement subacutely, gyriform increased cortical T1W signal (probably laminar hemorrhage)
eventual atrophy

3.7 MESIAL TEMPORAL SCLEROSIS

CONDITIONS UNDERLYING COMPLEX PARTIAL SEIZURES

MESIAL TEMPORAL SCLEROSIS (70%)

MIGRATION ANOMALIES

TUMOR (USUALLY NEUROGLIAL LOW GRADE)

GLIOSIS (PERINATAL HYPOXIA, TRAUMA)

POSTENCEPHALITIC

HAMARTOMAS

CLINICAL

variable range of ages from children to young adults
presents with complex partial seizures of variable severity and frequency
often refractory to medication

IMAGING

MR

hippocampal atrophy
decreased hippocampal volume
decreased outflow structures volume (fornix, mamillary body)
low T1W, high T2W hippocampal signal
loss of internal structure
change in temporal white matter signal

PET (interictal FDG)

hypometabolic area mesial or lateral temporal cortex or temporal pole
comparison with other side (15% difference is significant) or rest of cortex
seizures during FDG uptake may render scan non diagnostic

NUC MED (HMPAO or ECD)

INTERICTAL: reduced perfusion to mesial temporal cortex, lateral temporal cortex or temporal pole
seizures during radiotracer uptake may render scan non diagnostic
ICTAL: increased perfusion of the ictal focus (injection must be truly ictal)
POSTICTAL: unpredictable pattern of reducing perfusion at focus with a frequent ring of increased perfusion as seizure propagates

4. TRAUMA

4.1 ARTERIAL INJURY

CLASSIFICATION

Type of injury

DIRECT INJURY: TRANSSECTION, LACERATION (PENETRATING INJURY OR FRACTURE EDGE)

INDIRECT INJURY: SUBINTIMAL HEMATOMA, DISSECTION, LACERATION

Complications

CAROTID SHEATH HEMATOMA, EXSANGUINATION

THROMBOSIS

FALSE ANEURYSM

TRAUMATIC AV FISTULA

4.1.1 TRAUMATIC DISSECTION

direct injury (skull base fractures, vertebral fractures)
indirect injury (sports injuries, car accidents, spinal manipulation)
ICA location: distal cervical ICA, ICA at skull base (at entry to and through carotid canal), cavernous portion of ICA
VA location: between C2 and foramen magnum, or related to vertebral fractures

IMAGING

see Ch 15

4.1.2 TRAUMATIC FALSE ANEURYSM

ICA at skull base; cavernous ICA
distal ACA (usually cortical branches passing under falx)
distal arterial branches related to skull fractures

IMAGING

CT/MR/CTA/MRA

abnormal expansion of lumen or abnormal mass adjacent to vessel with a flow void; may contain laminated thrombus of various ages

Angio

saccular broad based or narrow based aneurysm

4.1.3 TRAUMATIC AV FISTULA

ICA to internal jugular vein
middle meningeal vessels
caroticocavernous fistula (CC fistula): presents with engorged superior ophthalmic vein branches, pain, reduced vision, proptosis (may be pulsatile); clinical differential is cavernous sinus thrombosis

IMAGING (CC fistula)

CT

skull base fractures commonly involving petrous apex, sphenoid and carotid canal
engorged superior ophthalmic vein, swollen extraocular muscles, orbital edema, proptosis

MR

swollen superior ophthalmic vein, orbital and conal edema
high velocity flow void in superior ophthalmic vein
patent cavernous sinus (may have different flow signal from other side)
no cavernous sinus thrombosis by definition, but thrombosis of superior ophthalmic vein and cavernous sinus may occur as a secondary complication

Angio

passage of carotid contrast into cavernous sinus too early to be venous return
may demonstrate fistula directly
possibly contrast reflux into orbit
may be a prelude to balloon occlusion

4.2 DIFFUSE BRAIN INJURY

DEFINITION

neuronal and axonal injury produced primarily by shearing forces from indirect trauma

CLASSIFICATION (simplified)

Concussion

by definition, no structural damage detectable

Cortical contusions

Diffuse axonal injury

Diffuse cerebral edema

4.2.1 CORTICAL CONTUSIONS

MORPHOLOGY

Contusions

cortical surfaces in contact with irregular surfaces or dural edges (inferior frontal lobes and frontal poles, temporal poles, midbrain at tentorial notch)
direct injury to cortex, petechial or larger hemorrhages
old contusion: hemosiderin stained gliosis, hemosiderosis

IMAGING

CT

usually normal or intracortical hematomas

MR

superficial cortical location or brainstem at tentorial notch

ACUTE

petechial or intralobar hemorrhages, foci of edema

superficial foci of high T2W, PD and FLAIR signal
blood products may be evident

SUBACUTE/CHRONIC

petechial hemorrhages with hemosiderosis
foci of hemosiderin related low signal best seen on GRE sequences
gliosis and atrophy

4.2.2 DIFFUSE AXONAL INJURY

MORPHOLOGY

produced by differential movement in shearing injury
gray-white matter interface, deep white matter long tracts, corpus callosum (especially splenium), internal capsule, dorsal midbrain
axonal retraction balls, swollen axons
injury is usually severe despite relatively minor imaging abnormalities

IMAGING

CT

usually normal

MR

deep white matter and white-gray matter interface location

ACUTE

multiple foci of edema, petechial hemorrhages not as obvious
deep foci of high T2W, PD and FLAIR signal
PD and FLAIR more sensitive than T2W
foci ovoid, oriented along axonal tracts
MRS appears promising

SUBACUTE/CHRONIC

petechial hemorrhages with hemosiderosis
foci of hemosiderin related low signal best seen on GRE sequences

4.2.3 DIFFUSE CEREBRAL EDEMA

CLINICAL

massive shearing injury, hypoxia or ischemia
50% acute mortality

IMAGING

CT/MR

diffuse global edema

may have small multifocal petechial hemorrhages

4.3 HERNIATIONS

4.3.1 SUBFALCINE

MORPHOLOGY

caused by supratentorial unilateral mass

midline shift (ventricles, corpus callosum, third ventricle, cingulate gyrus)

corpus callosum, cingulate gyrus herniate under falx

trapped contralateral ventricle (by occlusion at foramen of Monro) with dilation, rarely occluded distal anterior cerebral artery under falx (with eventual infarction)

4.3.2 TRANSTENTORIAL DOWN

MORPHOLOGY

caused by supratentorial mass and usually unilateral

occasionally caused by gross hemispheric edema and then bilateral

uncus and parahippocampal gyrus displaced medially into suprasellar cistern and then through tentorial notch into the perimesencephalic cistern

ipsilateral midbrain compressed, shortened and displaced

contralateral dorsal midbrain compressed against tentorial free edge ('Kernohan notch')

stretching of brainstem perforating arteries (occlusion, avulsion) produces central tegmental petechial hemorrhages (Duret hemorrhage)

ipsilateral oculomotor (CNIII) palsy

trapped contralateral ventricle

occluded ipsilateral posterior cerebral artery with distal infarction

4.3.3 TRANSTENTORIAL UP

MORPHOLOGY

caused by posterior fossa mass (usually slowly enlarging)

vermis pushed up through tentorial notch with tectal compression, aqueduct obstruction, hydrocephalus

4.3.4 TONSILLAR

MORPHOLOGY

caused by either supratentorial mass with transtentorial herniation occurring first, or by posterior fossa mass

cerebellar tonsils pushed through foramen magnum compressing inferior medulla (and tonsils and cerebellum also fill cisterna magna)

'coning': compression of medulla in tonsillar herniation with inhibition of respiratory centers

IMAGING

plane of foramen magnum is defined by a line from tip of clivus (basion) to posterior lip of foramen magnum (opisthion), best shown on sagittal MR

tonsillar herniation is protrusion of tonsils >5 mm below foramen magnum (less in elderly)

compressed medulla, lost cisterna magna

imaging differential is Chiari I

4.4 SKULL FRACTURES

4.4.1 VAULT

Linear

Diastatic (runs into suture, continues along it)

4.4.2 BASE OF SKULL

Sphenoid

Petrous pyramids/temporal bone

Orbital roofs

Basiocciput/foramen magnum

4.4.3 TEMPORAL BONE FRACTURES

see Ch 12

4.5 TRAUMATIC CSF LEAKS

CLINICAL

occurs following significant head injury (commonly car accidents)

presents acutely or after a delay with CSF rhinorrhea, CSF otorrhea, headache

may complicate transsphenoidal hypophysectomies, craniofacial resections with dural flaps, or sinus surgery

may progress to meningitis if untreated

IMAGING

XR

brow up skull x-ray: intracranial gas (specific; very insensitive)

CT

intracranial air (acutely)

fluid in facial bone paranasal sinuses (non specific; differential is blood, retained secretions and incidental sinusitis)

BASE OF SKULL FRACTURES

cribriform plate and ethmoid bone

frontal bone/orbital roof into frontal sinus

orbital roof and medial orbital wall

sphenoid bone with extension to sphenoid sinus

middle cranial fossa into lateral extension of sphenoid sinus

temporal bone into middle ear cavity or external ear canal

CT with subarachnoid contrast

usually imaged for cribriform plate fractures, prone, direct coronal slices

contrast leaks into superior nasal meatus

NUC MED (radionuclide ventriculogram)

lumbar injection of radiotracer (e.g. TcDTPA)

patient flat or head down

4, 24 hour imaging of facial bones looking for evidence of extravasation

nasal pledgets (or ear pledgets) inserted during imaging, removed at a set time and counted; blood counted for background control several fold elevation of pledget count relative to blood indicates CSF leak (exact number depends on departmental protocol)

4.6 TRAUMATIC HEMORRHAGE AND COLLECTIONS

4.6.1 EXTRADURAL (EPIDURAL) HEMATOMA

CLINICAL

vast majority are arterial injury with hemorrhage between dura and calvarium (dural venous sinus lacerations rare cause)
fracture in 90%, lucid interval in 50%
nearly all supratentorial, unilateral
typically middle meningeal artery tear
temporoparietal, frontal, posterior fossa
cross dural attachments not sutures, biconvex

IMAGING

CT
dense unilateral collection
classically biconvex
majority have an associated fracture
mass effect

MR
collection of blood products
MR signal characteristics depend on age of hematoma
biconvex
elevates dura (thin black line) away from calvarium
mass effect

Angio
mass effect, deformity and displacement of cortical capillary blush

4.6.2 SUBDURAL HEMATOMA

CLINICAL

tearing of bridging cortical veins running to dural venous sinuses

associated with child abuse, old age, alcoholism, anticoagulation
variable clinical presentation depending on size of collection and speed of its enlargement
present at variable hematoma ages
95% supratentorial, 15% bilateral
cross sutures but not dural attachments, concavoconvex, extend along dural reflections (falx and tentorium)
interhemispheric subdurals particularly associated with child abuse
ACUTE, SUBACUTE, CHRONIC

IMAGING

CT
variable density concavoconvex collection
15% bilateral
pitfall if bilateral isodense to cortex (need contrast or MR)
acute subdurals dense
subacute subdurals isodense to cortex or hypodense
chronically form subdural hygromas
may rebleed with a blood-fluid level
mass effect

MR
collection containing fluid (hygroma) and blood products of variable age
may contain blood-fluid levels
may contain multiple membranes and compartments (multiple bleeds of different ages)
mass effect

4.6.3 SUBDURAL HYGROMA

Resorbing subdural hematoma

Tear in arachnoid producing subdural CSF collection

4.6.4 TRAUMATIC INTRAPARENCHYMAL HEMATOMA

IMAGING

associated with other evidence of injury
frontal, temporal, deep gray
mass effect, herniations

4.6.5 SUBARACHNOID HEMORRHAGE (traumatic)

IMAGING

MR is relatively insensitive compared to CT

5. TUMORS

5.1 ARACHNOID CYST

DEFINITION

non neoplastic developmental CSF-containing cyst with walls of arachnoid mater

CLINICAL

male:female 3:1
middle cranial fossa/Sylvian fissure, suprasellar, quadrigeminal cistern, cerebellopontine angle, cisterna magna; rarely intraventricular
occasional hemorrhage into cyst

IMAGING

CT
extraaxial mass isodense to CSF, classically at temporal pole tip
often little mass effect for size of cyst, possibly expansion or erosion of surrounding bone and underdevelopment or compression of adjacent brain
sometimes no mass as such but subtle to gross expansion of a CSF cistern
definitive diagnosis is by CT cisternography (with intrathecal contrast and possibly delayed imaging)

MR
extraaxial mass that follows CSF on all sequences and has same morphology as for CT
non vascular (and has no vessels) but vessels can invaginate into it
definitive diagnosis is by diffusion weighted sequences (cyst follows CSF exactly; epidermoid cyst (the principal differential diagnosis) does not)

5.2 ASTROCYTOMAS

DEFINITION

heterogeneous group of neoplastic tumors of astrocytes, with the majority demonstrating diffuse infiltration of normal brain and tendency to dedifferentiate and to recur

CLASSIFICATION (WHO 2000)

Circumscribed gliomas (grade I)

PILOCYTIC ASTROCYTOMA

SUBEPENDYMAL GIANT CELL ASTROCYTOMA

Pleomorphic xanthoastrocytoma (grade II)

generally benign behavior but can have malignant degeneration

Diffuse astrocytomas (grade II)

FIBRILLARY ASTROCYTOMA

PROTOPLASMIC ASTROCYTOMA

GEMISTOCYTIC ASTROCYTOMA

Anaplastic astrocytoma (grade III)

Glioblastoma multiforme (grade IV)

EPIDEMIOLOGY
(Astrocytomas as a group)

commonest intracranial tumor
60% of all primary brain tumors
increased incidence following brain irradiation, in immune suppression, in AIDS, as well as familial clusters

Syndromes with astrocytomas

Li–Fraumeni
Turcot
Neurofibromatosis 1
Tuberous sclerosis

PATHOGENESIS
(Astrocytomas as a group)

diffuse and higher grade astrocytomas infiltrate into surrounding brain

blood–brain barrier breakdown in higher grade tumors
microscopic infiltration extends beyond visible tumor edge
surrounding vasogenic edema usually extends beyond infiltration
tumor may produce focal neurological deficit or new seizures
mass effect from tumor, hemorrhage and edema usually exceed local effects of tumor on adjacent cortex
diffuse involvement or eloquent structures makes tumor not fully resectable
cell type is usually mixed, making typing and grading difficult and subject to sampling error

Prognostic factors

tumor biology
geographic position

Survival with treatment

long term for pilocytic astrocytoma
5 years for diffuse astrocytomas (WHO grade II)
2–5 years for anaplastic astrocytoma
<1 year for glioblastoma

5.2.1 PILOCYTIC ASTROCYTOMA (circumscribed astrocytoma, grade I)

CLINICAL

generally presents <20 years, male = female
commonest childhood glioma ('juvenile pilocytic astrocytoma')
mass effect or hydrocephalus; rarely seizures
bipolar cells in bundles, Rosenthal fibers
full resection (if possible) is curative

IMAGING

cerebellar hemispheres, rest of brainstem, hypothalamus, thalamus
intraaxial cystic mass with tumoral mural nodule (but usually completely solid if in optic nerve/chiasm) with uniform strong enhancement

CT

hypodense cyst with enhancing mural nodule
mass effect, but little edema

MR

fluid containing cyst (may not follow CSF exactly)

mural nodule or part solid tumor (iso or low signal on T1W, high on T2W) with uniform contrast enhancement of solid component and cyst wall
sometimes fully solid
little surrounding edema
no calcification, no hemorrhage, no necrosis
leptomeningeal invasion with enhancing leptomeningeal nodules

5.2.2 SUBEPENDYMAL GIANT CELL ASTROCYTOMA
(circumscribed astrocytoma, grade I)

CLINICAL

occurs in patients with tuberous sclerosis
slow growing mass at foramen of Monro, large fusiform cells

IMAGING

calcifying heterogeneous mass at the foramen of Monro
iso to low T1W signal, heterogeneous or low T2W signal
no hemorrhage, no necrosis, enhances with contrast

5.2.3 PLEOMORPHIC XANTHOASTROCYTOMA (grade II)

CLINICAL

rare slow growing astrocytoma of young adults presenting with seizures
superficial mass in cerebral hemisphere, involving cortex and meninges, with a cyst and mural nodules morphology and pleomorphic histology

IMAGING

intraaxial superficial mass with enhancing nodule and deeper fluid containing cyst
no calcification, bleed or necrosis
enhances with contrast

5.2.4 DIFFUSE ASTROCYTOMAS (grade II)

CLINICAL

20–40 years, male > female, overall ~10% of all astrocytomas

seizures, subtle focal neurological deficits, personality and higher mental function changes, mass effect

FIBRILLARY (fusiform astrocytes)

PROTOPLASMIC (large protoplasmic astrocytes)

GEMISTOCYTIC (eosinophilic polygonal astrocytes)

IMAGING

intraaxial mass with isocenter on white matter or gray-white junction and relatively little vasogenic edema

in adults, cerebral hemispheric > other locations

in children, pons and brainstem > cerebellum

CT

hypodense mass

25% calcify

no hemorrhage or necrosis by definition

no contrast enhancement

MR

mass low on T1W, high on T2W and PD sequences

TUMOR EXTENDS BEYOND ABNORMAL SIGNAL

no hemorrhage or necrosis by definition

overlying cortex may be preserved or diffusely expanded

may have cystic areas

usually no contrast enhancement

NUC MED (TI)

no thallium staining unless blood–brain barrier disrupted

PET (FDG)

variable amount of FDG uptake relative to surrounding normal cortex

may be contrasted by low FDG uptake if a ring of edema is present

5.2.5 ANAPLASTIC ASTROCYTOMA (grade III)

CLINICAL

40–60 year olds, male > female, ~1/3 of astrocytomas overall

seizures, focal neurological deficits, higher mental function changes, mass effect

nuclear atypia, definite tendency to progress to glioblastoma

may have drop metastases

IMAGING

intraaxial mass with isocenter on white matter or gray-white junction and variable amount of vasogenic edema

CT

hypodense mass

no calcification

may have cystic areas

variable amount of contrast enhancement

MR

mass low on T1W, high on T2W and PD sequences

no necrosis by definition

hemorrhage on MR still allows diagnosis of anaplastic astrocytoma

contrast enhancement present, of variable degree

BEWARE OF DROP METASTASES

NUC MED (TI)

generally show thallium uptake and retention (unless treated)

PET (FDG)

FDG avid, often with a ring of low FDG uptake in surrounding vasogenic edema

5.2.6 GLIOBLASTOMA MULTIFORME (grade IV)

CLINICAL

>50 years, male > female

most common primary brain tumor

60% of all astrocytomas

short duration of presentation with seizures, rapidly increasing intracranial pressure and mass effect, acute brain syndrome, non specific neurological symptoms and personality changes, stroke-like episodes (intratumoral bleeds)

pseudopalisading bizarre cells with pleomorphism, mitoses, necrosis, neovascularity

IMAGING

intraaxial mass with isocenter on white matter with extensive vasogenic edema and prominent mass effect

cerebral hemispheres: frontal, temporal and parietal > occipital

infiltrative and destructive extension along white matter tracts (particularly across corpus callosum: 'butterfly glioma') and into overlying cortex

CT

hypodense mass (unless with hematoma)

extensive vasogenic edema

edema +/– mass extend across corpus callosum

hemorrhages common

strong ring enhancement

MR

variable signal mass on T1W depending on blood products and age; generally low signal on T1W, high on T2W but heterogeneous

hematomas and areas of necrosis present (cystic necrosis: higher on T2W and lower on T1W; hemorrhage has blood products signal)

frequently irregularly shaped with masses connected by infiltrated white matter tracts producing several related areas of ring enhancement

satellite nodules

LOOK FOR DROP METASTASES

neovascularity flow voids

vivid ring enhancement after contrast

TUMOR INFILTRATES BEYOND ENHANCEMENT

extensive vasogenic edema well beyond the area of enhancement and often into other hemisphere

mass effect with herniations, trapping of ventricles, cisternal effacement

NUC MED (TI)

strong Tl uptake and retention

PET (FDG)

strongly FDG avid (unless massively necrotic) in a ring of low FDG avid edema

IMAGING – ASTROCYTOMAS AS A GROUP

MR SPECTROSCOPY

creatine used as internal control/reference, and choline:creatine and NAA:creatine ratios can be used to grade tumor

choline:creatine ratio elevated (high cellularity)

NAA:creatine reduced (neuronal replacement by tumor)

LOW GRADE GLIOMAS
choline:creatine <2.0
variably reduced NAA:creatine
beware of heterogeneity (need to sample entire tumor)

HIGH GRADE GLIOMAS
choline:creatine >2.0
NAA markedly reduced
necrotic areas have lactate/lipid signal (beware of artifactually low choline:creatine secondary to necrosis)
tumor infiltration into surrounding brain produces increased peritumoral choline:creatine ratio (not increased in metastases)

GLIOMA RECURRENCE
decreased NAA:creatine
choline:creatine >2.0 may indicate recurrence
choline:creatine <2.0 equivocal (major differential is radiation encephalitis, see below)
heterogeneity leads to sampling errors (ideally, need to cover entire tumor bed)

DIFFERENTIAL DIAGNOSIS
radiation necrosis (dead tissue)
radiation encephalitis
(see radiation necrosis entry)

5.2.7 GLIOMATOSIS CEREBRI

DEFINITION

diffuse glial neoplastic infiltration of brain and spinal cord without destruction of underlying anatomical structures

CLINICAL

20–40 year olds
presents late with higher mental function and personality changes

IMAGING

MR
abnormal T2W signal particularly in white matter
symmetrical gray and white matter expansion with sulcal effacement, involving one or both hemispheres
no contrast enhancement
no mass

DIFFERENTIAL
HERPES SIMPLEX ENCEPHALITIS
WHITE MATTER DISEASE
HEMIMEGALENCEPHALY

5.3 CHORDOMA

see Ch 05

5.4 CHOROID PLEXUS TUMORS

DEFINITION

intraventricular papillary tumors of choroid plexus epithelium

CLINICAL

80% in children (majority <2 years), rare in adults, male > female
10–20% malignant
usual location is in atrium of lateral ventricle in children, and fourth ventricle in children and adults
presents with hydrocephalus (obstructive, overproduction)
DROP METASTASES OCCUR
papillomas cured by total resection; carcinomas have poorer prognosis

IMAGING

CT
calcified intraventricular lobulated mass with ventricle expansion
asymmetrical hydrocephalus secondary to obstruction (e.g. at foramen of Monro)
symmetrical hydrocephalus from ? CSF overproduction
vivid contrast enhancement
gross brain invasion indicates carcinoma

MR
intraventricular lobulated mass (as for CT)
iso to low on T1W, heterogeneous low on T2W and heterogeneous increased on PD
cystic change and hemosiderin staining may occur
flow voids and clumpy calcium voids
vivid contrast enhancement

5.5 COLLOID CYST OF THIRD VENTRICLE

DEFINITION

rare epithelial lined simple cyst within superior anterior third ventricle

IMAGING

CT
midline rounded mass in anterior third ventricle
2/3 hyperdense, 1/3 isodense
no calcification
no contrast enhancement

MR
intraventricular (superior aspect of anterior third ventricle) rounded mass
high on T1W, isointense to gray on T2W but signal characteristics variable
no contrast enhancement (thin rim of enhancement may occur)

5.6 CRANIO-PHARYNGIOMA

DEFINITION

benign locally aggressive squamous epithelial (?Rathke's cleft origin) suprasellar/sellar tumor

CLINICAL

3% of CNS primaries, 1/2 in 5–15 year olds, rest in adults
50% of pediatric suprasellar masses
origin from squamous epithelial rests of Rathke's cleft (junction of pituitary stalk and hypophysis): squamous nests and cords, squamous lined cysts with keratin
visual loss, endocrinopathies, raised intracranial pressure and altered higher mental function
prognosis good if complete resection can be achieved

Adamantinomatous type

nodular solid mass with variable cystic component filled with viscous dark cholesterol laden fluid ('motor oil')
frequently calcifies

Papillary type

usually occurs in adults
tends to be solid without cystic components or calcification

IMAGING

extraaxial midline basal mass, 75% suprasellar with sellar extension, 20% suprasellar only, 5% intrasellar only

XR

skull plain film may show clinoid erosion, sellar expansion and suprasellar calcification

CT

mixed solid/cystic lobulated dense sellar/suprasellar mass
clumpy calcification (90%)
vivid contrast enhancement
displaces or encloses surrounding structures (see MR)
pressure erosion of clinoids and pituitary fossa

MR

ADAMANTINOMATOUS TYPE

mixed solid and cystic lobulated mass
cystic component has high T1W and T2W signal
solid component has heterogeneous signal but generally low on T1W, high on T2W
areas of hemorrhage (blood products) and signal void in clumpy calcification
vividly contrast enhancing

PAPILLARY TYPE

solid mass often low on T1W and high on T2W
vividly contrast enhancing

EITHER

direct invasion into sella, cisterns; displaces, stretches and elevates chiasm or surrounds it (need to identify relationship to chiasm)
displaces, compresses or surrounds pituitary (need to identify)
surrounds adjacent vessels (need to identify)
may invade cavernous sinuses or enclose carotid arteries

carotid artery flow voids usually maintained
if sufficiently large may cause hydrocephalus

5.7 DERMOID

DEFINITION

developmental ectodermal inclusion mass containing both epithelium and epidermal appendages; not a neoplasm; uncommon compared to epidermoid

IMAGING

Location

brain: midline subarachnoid (tends to basal cisterns)
spine: lumbar
orbit/sphenoid: through skull tables at sutures
subcutaneous (especially scalp)

CT

fat density non enhancing extraaxial mass
often follows a fissure (interhemispheric, suprasellar, Sylvian)
wall may have thin calcification
beware of free fat globules in CSF

MR

extraaxial circumscribed mass
high T1W signal, intermediate T2W signal
saturates with fat sat sequences
if ruptured, free globules and deposits of fat scattered through the subarachnoid space
no contrast enhancement

5.8 EPENDYMOMA

DEFINITION

ependymal neoplasm of variable aggressivity with tendency to obstruct CSF flow

CLINICAL

children > adults (10% of childhood CNS tumors), male > female
fourth ventricle (hydrocephalus), spinal (pain, neural deficit), less commonly cerebrum and lateral ventricles (non specific)

presents with hydrocephalus, raised intracranial pressure, focal neurological deficits
CSF SPREAD WITH DROP METASTASES
bipolar ependymal cells forming rosettes
subtypes: CELLULAR, CLEAR CELL, TANYCYTIC (spinal variant), ANAPLASTIC (aggressive), MYXOPAPILLARY (indolent, cauda and conus)

IMAGING

CT

dense intraventricular or intramedullary or spinal subarachnoid mass
vivid contrast enhancement with areas of cystic change
50% calcify

MR

intraventricular or spinal intramedullary mass
fills fourth ventricle and exits through CSF foramina
hydrocephalus above
expands spinal canal, compresses adjacent cord (often over a few levels); often associated syrinx
low T1W, intermediate T2W signal
vivid heterogeneous contrast enhancement
areas of cystic change, necrosis, hemorrhage
IMAGE ENTIRE NEURAXIS LOOKING FOR DROP METASTASES

5.9 EPIDERMOID

DEFINITION

developmental ectodermal inclusion mass containing only epithelium; not a neoplasm

CLINICAL

20–60 year olds
very rarely secondary to traumatic implantation of epithelium (spinal)
presents with mass effect and compression of adjacent structures
mid ear cholesteatoma is a special category (see head and neck chapter)

IMAGING

Location

not restricted to midline; cerebellopontine angle (commonest), parasellar, intraventricular

CT

low density (or CSF density) non enhancing extraaxial lobulated mass

MR

extraaxial mass with extension into cisterns and sulci and later compression of adjacent structures

T1W and T2W signal often close to CSF; PD signal may also be close to CSF

differentiation of epidermoid and arachnoid cyst best done on diffusion weighted imaging (no diffusion restriction in CSF or arachnoid cyst; diffusion restriction (= high DWI signal) in epidermoid)

no contrast enhancement (thin rim of peripheral enhancement may occur)

5.10 GERM CELL TUMOR (CNS)

DEFINITION

pediatric neoplasm of pluripotent germ cells with tendency to pineal and suprasellar regions

CLINICAL

childhood tumor; commonest pineal tumor

male:female 10:1 pineal, 1:1 suprasellar

60% pineal, 30% suprasellar, 10% thalamic, fourth ventricle

presents with focal neurological symptoms depending on location

CSF SPREAD, SUBEPENDYMAL SPREAD

germinoma: soft yellow-white mass with cystic change, regular cell sheets

other types: gelatinous myxoid stroma (yolk sac tumor); hemorrhage and necrosis (particularly choriocarcinoma); mesodermal and ectodermal elements (teratomas)

IMAGING

midline mass in pineal, suprasellar or occasionally other location

CT

dense mass with calcification and contrast enhancement

mature teratoma may contain cystic and fatty components

MR

germinoma: low T1W and low T2W signal mass (pineal, suprasellar, other) with vivid contrast enhancement

homogenous uniform, but hemorrhagic foci may occur

teratoma: markedly heterogeneous with cystic change, fat and hemorrhage; strong but variable contrast enhancement

CSF SPREAD OCCURS

5.11 HEMANGIO-BLASTOMA

DEFINITION

vascular benign tumor strongly associated with von Hippel–Lindau disease (vHL)

CLINICAL

90% sporadic (solitary, cerebellar): 30–60 year old adults

10% vHL (multiple tumors – cerebellar, spinal, younger adults)

present with mass effect and obstruction to CSF flow

neoplastic stroma, extensive vascular channels

produce erythropoietin and may cause secondary polycythemia

benign but 25% recur

IMAGING

80% cerebellar, 15% spinal cord (often with syrinx)

CT

hypodense cyst with mural nodule; nodule has vivid contrast enhancement

MR

intraaxial well circumscribed mass (nearly always infratentorial) with relatively little edema

60% cyst with peripheral nodule, 40% solid

tumor iso on T1W, high on T2W with vivid uniform contrast enhancement

large flow voids associated with mass

necrosis, calcification and hemorrhage rare

cyst is fluid filled (may not follow CSF exactly) and may have a thin enhancing wall (gliosis not tumor)

Angio

mural nodule has a vivid vascular blush with prolonged contrast staining

5.12 HEMANGIO-PERICYTOMA

see Ch 05

5.13 HYPOTHALAMIC HAMARTOMA

see Ch 20

5.14 LANGERHANS CELL HISTIOCYTOSIS
(CNS manifestations)

also see Ch 05

CLINICAL

CNS involved classically in multifocal histiocytosis (Hand–Schuller–Christian disease)

pituitary dysfunction, hypothalamic dysfunction, cranial nerve palsies, raised intracranial pressure

Hand–Schuller–Christian triad: diabetes insipidus, exophthalmos, lytic bone lesions

IMAGING

XR/CT

calvarium and skull base lytic defects

MR/CT

hypothalamus, pituitary masses in Hand–Schuller–Christian disease

isodense or hyperdense on CT

isointense on T1W, isointense on T2W, vivid contrast enhancement

leptomeningeal deposits/enhancement in Letterer–Siwe disease

5.15 LIPOMA

DEFINITION

benign lipoma indistinguishable from
lipomas elsewhere

ASSOCIATIONS

corpus callosum agenesis
integral part of myelolipomeningocele and
tethered cord spectrum

IMAGING

CT

fat density mass in characteristic location
(pericallosal, filum terminale)
no enhancement

MR

typical mature lipoma located in the midline
around or adjacent to corpus callosum or
at the conus/filum terminale
wraps around arteries and nerves
fat content can be proven by fat sat
sequences

5.16 MEDULLO-BLASTOMA

see Ch 20

5.17 MENINGIOMA

DEFINITION

benign (uncommonly malignant)
meningothelial neoplasm with a wide
range of histological variants

EPIDEMIOLOGY

commonest non glial CNS primary
20% of all CNS primaries, 30% of all spinal
primaries
adults 40–60 years, female:male 2:1;
particular female predominance in spinal
meningiomas
~2% have malignant behavior, ~1% have
metastases

ETIOLOGY

arachnoid cap cell origin
association with neurofibromatosis 2 (NF2) –
50% of multifocal meningiomas is NF2
if occurs in a child – suspect NF2

CLINICAL

seizures; focal neurological deficit; headache
occasionally there is enough reactive edema
for mass effect
NF2 meningiomas can present with cranial
nerve palsies

MACRO

Location

SUPRATENTORIAL
PARASAGITTAL, CONVEXITY, SPHENOID
RIDGE, OLFACTORY GROOVE,
PARASELLAR

INFRATENTORIAL (10%)
CEREBELLOPONTINE ANGLE, CLIVAL

EXTRACRANIAL
SKULL BASE, PERIPHERAL NERVES (OPTIC
NERVE SHEATH)

UNUSUAL
INTRAVENTRICULAR, PINEAL, OPTIC
NERVE SHEATH

INTRASPINAL (common)
strong female predominance
association with NF2
90% intradural extramedullary
5% dumbbell with extradural component
thoracic > cervical > lumbar

Gross morphology

GLOBULAR
commonest form
fleshy or firm whitish mass with a firm dural
attachment or invasion

EN PLAQUE (uncommon)
flat meningioma growing along dural
surfaces

Commoner histological types

MENINGOTHELIAL (neoplastic lobules, thin
collagenous septa)
FIBROBLASTIC
TRANSITIONAL (whorls and mixture of
above two)
PSAMMOMATOUS (usually SPINAL) –
mineralized psammoma bodies

PAPILLARY (aggressive behavior)
ANAPLASTIC (aggressive behavior)

IMAGING

CT

dense or isodense well circumscribed
extraaxial durally based mass
compresses underlying brain (variable
amount of reactive edema)
25% calcify
vivid contrast enhancement with 'dural tail'
hyperostosis of overlying skull characteristic
for calvarial invasion
no hyperostosis in spinal meningiomas

MR

well circumscribed durally based extraaxial
mass

TYPICAL
iso or low T1W signal, isointense but
heterogeneous T2W signal, high or
isointense PD signal
homogenous, no necrosis or hemorrhage
vivid but heterogeneous contrast
enhancement
DURAL TAIL (thickened enhancement along
dura): suggestive and typical of
meningioma but not exclusive to
meningioma; both direct tumor invasion
along dura and reactive fibrosis
contribute to the tail
thin CSF cleft separating tumor from
underlying brain
brain compressed with minimal edema
prominent flow voids within tumor
major imaging differential of spinal
meningioma is nerve sheath tumor
MR spectroscopy: high choline (cellularity),
absent NAA (no neurons), may have lipid
and lactate; alanine (doublet at 1.48
ppm) relatively specific, but not always
present

ATYPICAL
clumpy calcification voids, high T2W signal,
poor or patchy contrast enhancement,
invasion of underlying brain;
extensive reactive vasogenic edema
10% form cysts

Angio

hypervascular tumor supplied by meningeal
arteries
may parasitize pial arteries
'sunburst' appearance

5.18 METASTASES

EPIDEMIOLOGY

25% of all tumors
40% of all adult CNS tumors, rare in children

ETIOLOGY

Parenchymal

HEMATOGENOUS

LUNG CARCINOMA

BREAST CARCINOMA

COLON CARCINOMA

MELANOMA

RENAL CELL CARCINOMA

OTHER

Leptomeningeal

HEMATOGENOUSLY SEEDED

LYMPHOMA

LEUKEMIA

BREAST CARCINOMA

LUNG CARCINOMA

COLON CARCINOMA

MELANOMA

CSF SPREAD

PRIMITIVE NEUROECTODERMAL TUMORS

GLIOBLASTOMA

CHOROID PLEXUS CARCINOMA

EPENDYMOMA

PRIMARY LYMPHOMA

Spread along nerve trunks

HEAD AND NECK CANCERS

NERVE SHEATH TUMORS

Direct transdural spread from bony metastases

IMAGING

multiple masses strongly suggest metastases; solitary nature of mass does not exclude

CT

classic intraaxial, contrast enhancing mass with surrounding vasogenic edema
gray-white matter interface, interfaces between arterial territories

cerebral hemispheres (80%) > cerebellum
ring enhancement with contrast
see GAMUTS for causes of metastases with unusual appearance

MR

classic intraaxial, contrast enhancing mass with surrounding vasogenic edema
location as for CT
low on T1W, high on T2W and PD sequences
ring or solid enhancement: thick, irregular wall of ring (as opposed to other causes of ring enhancement); nodular enhancement
central necrosis
hemorrhage (see GAMUTS)
MR spectroscopy: reduced NAA within metastasis itself; lactate and lipid may be present; elevated choline and reports of reduced creatine within the lesion; peritumoral T2W signal abnormality has no elevation of choline:creatine ratio (indicating a well circumscribed non infiltrating tumor)

DIFFERENTIAL: HIGH GRADE GLIOMA

relatively greater choline and lower lactate/lipid within tumor; peritumoral T2W signal abnormality infiltrated by glioma and has elevated choline:creatine ratio

5.19 NEURAL AND NEUROGLIAL TUMORS

GROUP DEFINITION

low grade benign tumors with neural differentiation and variable amount of glial differentiation
neural differentiation can be into ganglial cells or neural cells (prefix of name) and there may be a glial component (ending of name in 'glioma' vs 'cytoma')

5.19.1 GANGLIOCYTOMA/ GANGLIOGLIOMA

CLINICAL

rare (1% of brain tumors), mature ganglionic neurons
children, young adults, male > female
long history of headaches, seizures, associated with temporal lobe epilepsy
good prognosis or cure with resection

Dysplastic cerebellar gangliocytoma
see its own entry below

Desmoplastic infantile ganglioglioma

rare tumor of infants
massive cystic/solid contrast enhancing parietal mass

IMAGING

cortically or superficially located intraaxial supratentorial mass

CT

isodense or hyperdense solid mass without contrast enhancement (gangliocytoma)
cyst with mural nodule and variable enhancement (ganglioglioma)
may calcify

MR

similar to gray matter on T1W and T2W and high on PD (gangliocytoma); no enhancement
cyst with mural nodule (low T1W, high T2W signal) and variable enhancement (ganglioglioma)
little if any edema

5.19.2 NEUROCYTOMA

CLINICAL

rare benign tumor of young adults (foramen of Monro); small mature neurons

IMAGING

CT

isodense or hyperdense rounded intraventricular mass with contrast enhancement; may calcify

MR

iso or high T1W signal and iso or high T2W signal
mild contrast enhancement

5.19.3 DYSEMBRYOPLASTIC NEUROEPITHELIAL TUMOR (DNT)

(should have been called 'neuroglioma' judging by its components)

CLINICAL

young adults, male > female; columnar
   'specific glioneuronal elements'
presents with intractable complex partial
   seizures
surgery curative

IMAGING

MR

cortically located intraaxial well
   circumscribed mass
low T1W and high T2W signal
no surrounding edema
microcystic change possible
no contrast enhancement
mesial temporal sclerosis may coexist

5.19.4 DYSPLASTIC CEREBELLAR GANGLIOCYTOMA
(Lhermitte–Duclos syndrome)

CLINICAL

found as the principal CNS manifestation of
   Cowden syndrome (Ch 06)
presents with posterior fossa mass effect
   and cerebellar symptoms
?cortical dysplasia, ?true gangliocytoma

IMAGING

MR

expanded cerebellar folia with abnormally
   elevated T2W signal
no contrast enhancement

5.20 NEUROFIBROMA

DEFINITION

benign peripheral nerve tumor of Schwann
   cells, perineural cells and fibroblasts

CLINICAL

Sporadic

common, fusiform only, peripheral or
   cutaneous, male = female

SYNDROMIC (neurofibromatosis 1, NF1)

multiple neurofibromas, fusiform and
   plexiform

MORPHOLOGY

Fusiform

firm gray mass along nerve trunk;
   unecapsulated spindle cells permeating
   axons
CUTANEOUS (30% have NF1)
PERIPHERAL NERVES (not cranial nerves)
SPINAL NERVES

Plexiform (NF1)

diffuse mass extending along multiple
   nerves
CUTANEOUS
PERIPHERAL LARGE NERVES
SPINAL
ORBITAL

IMAGING

spinal neurofibroma: see spinal section

US

non specific solid fusiform well demarcated
   cutaneous or subcutaneous mass
may be related to a major identifiable nerve
   trunk

CT

solid soft tissue density fusiform mass

MR

iso T1W and mixed T2W signal
heterogeneous contrast enhancement
~50% have 'target' appearance
may be related to a major identifiable nerve
   or trunk
can not distinguish from schwannoma
complex mass involving multiple nerves if
   plexiform

5.21 OLIGO-DENDROGLIOMA

DEFINITION

uncommon tumor of oligodendrocytes (~5%
   of all primary CNS tumors)

CLINICAL

uncommon, 30–60 years old, male > female;
   uniform oligodendroglia ('fried egg' cells)
predominantly supratentorial
long history of headaches, seizures
prognosis better in pure oligodendroglioma
   with treatment (survival of years)
>50% mixed with astrocytoma elements
   (more aggressive)

IMAGING

intraaxial cerebral mass (frontal > other)
   with isocenter on subcortical white
   matter and often little edema

CT

hypodense or isodense
calcifies (characteristic)
superficial mass may scallop calvarium
contrast enhancing

MR

low T1W signal, high T2W signal
areas of hemorrhage and cystic change
calcification produces signal voids
involvement of overlying cortex with
   expansion or diffuse abnormal signal
contrast enhancing

5.22 PINEAL CELL TUMORS

5.22.1 PINEAL CYST

CLINICAL

extremely common and largely
   asymptomatic
true incidence not known
very rarely presents with intracystic
   hemorrhage

IMAGING

CT

enlarged regular pineal gland with low
   density regular core (if large enough to
   be seen)

MR

cystic replacement of some to most of the pineal, with cyst signal close (but usually not identical) to CSF

smooth margins, regular, but may contact or displace surrounding structures

peripheral enhancement is probably residual pineal tissue

5.22.2 PINEOCYTOMA

DEFINITION

low grade slow growing mature pineal cell tumor

CLINICAL

rare; 10% of all pineal masses; pineocytes in rosettes

young adults, male = female

presents with aqueduct obstruction, raised intracranial pressure and failure of upward gaze (Parinaud syndrome)

IMAGING

CT

dense pineal mass with calcification and vivid contrast enhancement

MR

relatively well circumscribed pineal mass usually without hemorrhage or necrosis

variable signal, in general low T1W high T2W signal

vivid contrast enhancement

little surrounding edema

5.22.3 PINEAL PARENCHYMAL TUMOR OF INTERMEDIATE DIFFERENTIATION

intermediate behavior between pineocytoma and pineoblastoma

5.22.4 PINEOBLASTOMA

DEFINITION

malignant embryonal pineal small round blue cell tumor (one of the PNETs)

CLINICAL

rare

young children, male = female; immature small blue pineal cells in rosettes

may occur with bilateral retinoblastoma ('trilateral retinoblastoma')

presents with aqueduct obstruction, raised intracranial pressure and failure of upward gaze (Parinaud syndrome)

CSF DROP METASTASES COMMON

poor prognosis

IMAGING

CT

dense pineal mass with calcification and contrast enhancement

MR

lobulated solid mass with hemorrhagic areas

iso or low T1W signal and iso or low T2W signal

vivid contrast enhancement

variable amount of vasogenic edema

LEPTOMENINGEAL DEPOSITS

5.23 PITUITARY ADENOMA

DEFINITION

benign tumor of anterior pituitary (adenohypophysis) origin with variable hormonal products and a tendency to recur after incomplete resection

CLINICAL

10% of all intracranial primaries, true incidence of non functioning microadenomas not known

commonest sellar/juxtasellar mass (50%)

90% occur in adults

variable cellularity, pleomorphism; variably regular endocrine cells in loose stroma

male predominance: GH type; female predominance: PRL, ACTH types

Presentations

ENDOCRINOPATHY (usually microadenoma)

amenorrhea, lactation (PRL)

acromegaly or pituitary gigantism (GH)

Cushing's syndrome (ACTH)

MASS (macroadenoma)

optic chiasm compression with slow bitemporal hemianopsia

pituitary compression with hypopituitarism

PITUITARY APOPLEXY

hemorrhage into adenoma with headache, sudden visual disturbance

IMAGING

XR (macroadenoma)

expansion of sella

pressure erosion of sellar bone

for acromegaly, see Ch 02

CT (macroadenoma)

isodense sellar/suprasellar mass

calcification rare; cystic change occurs

possibly hematoma

prominent contrast enhancement

surgical planning: which sphenoid sinus is dominant, where the optic nerve canals are in relation to the sphenoid sinuses, how extensive sphenoid/clival pneumatization is relative to tumor extent (consider direct coronal scanning)

MR

MACROADENOMA (>10 mm)

heterogeneous T1W and T2W signal; hemorrhage with blood products of various ages

adenoma itself usually has low T1W high T2W signal

enhances except for cystic, necrotic and hemorrhagic areas

variable invasion of cavernous sinuses and encasement of cavernous carotid arteries (usually no obstruction) – differentiation from venous enhancement in sinuses may be difficult

chiasm elevated and stretched (need to identify it)

pituitary stalk and floor of third ventricle elevated and deviated (need to identify extent)

MICROADENOMA (<10 mm)

no MR findings (isointense tumor)

minimal bulkiness of one lateral lobe with convex roof

stalk deviation to other side (unreliable)

low T1W, high T2W signal in tumor (precontrast)

DIRECT DEMONSTRATION: rounded mass with delayed enhancement compared to normal pituitary on dynamic contrast run

INCIDENTAL PITUITARY FINDINGS

small cysts or non functioning adenomas (usually 2–3 mm) are very common and are usually of no clinical significance

Angio

petrosal venous sampling used for confirmation and localization of ACTH secretion

5.24 PRIMARY LYMPHOMA

DEFINITION

primary intraaxial non Hodgkin's lymphoma without evidence of prior lymphoma elsewhere

CLINICAL

IMMUNOSUPPRESSED (AIDS/NON AIDS) – very poor prognosis
IMMUNOCOMPETENT (elderly, rare)

IMAGING

intraaxial solitary or multiple masses
deep cerebral white, basal ganglia, thalami, corpus callosum
leptomeningeal, subependymal, uveal tract
posterior fossa and spine uncommon

CT

isodense mass or masses with variable amount of edema
enhance with contrast

MR

ill-marginated mass or masses as above
signal intensity similar to gray matter, but may be high T2W signal
variable amount of edema (sometimes extensive in AIDS)
hemorrhage and necrosis uncommon
solid or ring contrast enhancement
perivascular infiltration
MR spectroscopy: markedly elevated choline:creatine ratio (very cellular tumor); lactate/lipid commonly present; decreased myo-inositol, NAA, creatine

DIFFERENTIAL: TOXOPLASMOSIS IN AIDS

usually low choline, creatine and NAA; high lactate/lipid levels

NUC MED (TI)

lymphoma takes up and retains Tl (unlike toxoplasmosis)

PET (FDG)

increased FDG uptake

5.25 RATHKE'S CLEFT CYST

DEFINITION

embryonal remnant cyst of Rathke's cleft epithelial origin containing cholesterol rich dark fluid ('motor oil')

IMAGING

CT

low density sellar mass without calcification
no contrast enhancement

MR

regular thin walled cyst with no contrast enhancement
high T1W signal; variable signal on T2W (depending on fluid composition)
no contrast enhancement (thin rim enhancement allowed)
DIFFERENTIAL: cystic craniopharyngioma; pituitary adenoma with dominant hemorrhage (neither of these has smooth and regular walls)

5.26 SCHWANNOMA

DEFINITION

usually benign tumor of Schwann cells involving peripheral, spinal and cranial sensory nerves

CLINICAL

40–60 years old, female:male 2:1, 95% sporadic
5% syndromic (neurofibromatosis 2)
CRANIAL NERVES – sensory change precedes motor deficit
SPINE – dorsal roots involved, usually lumbosacral; presents with pain and nerve root/conus/cauda compression symptoms

PERIPHERAL – presents as a mass attached to but not infiltrating nerve
BIPHASIC HISTOLOGY: Antoni A – dense bundles of spindle cells; Antoni B – loose matrix, few cells

Acoustic schwannoma

7% of all primary intracranial tumors
bilateral acoustic schwannomas is diagnostic of NF2
presents with tinnitus, vertigo and progressive hearing loss

IMAGING

spinal schwannoma: see spinal section

US

ovoid non specific solid well circumscribed subcutaneous mass

CT

isodense or soft tissue density mass, rarely may calcify
strong contrast enhancement
cerebellopontine angle: widening of bony internal auditory meatus (1 mm side to side symmetry)

MR

isointense T1W, high T2W signal; T2W signal may be similar to CSF; texture heterogeneous in larger tumors (cystic change)
vivid contrast enhancement
~50% have 'target' sign; indistinguishable from neurofibroma or peripheral nerve sheath tumor
cerebellopontine angle: strongly enhancing mass with a tail in internal auditory meatus ('ice cream cone' appearance)
small intracanalicular schwannoma: minimal widening of vestibular nerve; enhances with contrast (beware of normal fat within temporal bone)

6. VASCULAR

6.1 ANEURYSMS

DEFINITION

abnormal focal expansion of arterial lumen involving all wall layers (true aneurysm) or a defect (false aneurysm) that has local mass effect and a tendency to rupture

ETIOLOGY

Hemodynamic 'berry' aneurysm

2–8% of population, peak of rupture at 40–60 years of age

ASSOCIATIONS

family history; polycystic kidney disease; hypertension, aortic coarctation
fibromuscular dysplasia, Marfan's and Ehlers–Danlos syndromes
AVM (high focal flow)

Traumatic false aneurysm (1%)

distal ACA, cavernous ICA, cortical branches MCA

Mycotic aneurysm (2%)

distal vessels
IV drug abuse, bacterial endocarditis, R to L shunts

Atherosclerotic fusiform aneurysms (>60 years old)

PATHOGENESIS (hemodynamic aneurysms)

branchpoint fragmentation and loss of internal elastic lamina with progressive atrophy of media and bulging of wall at points of stress
wall of aneurysm made of intima + adventitia with layers of thrombus
aneurysm has inflow, vortex, outflow zones

CLINICAL

Unruptured – rupture rate

<7 mm ~1% per year
>7 mm ~25% per year

Focal cranial nerve palsy

CNIII: posterior communicating artery aneurysm
CNIII to CNVI: cavernous internal carotid artery aneurysm

Spontaneous subarachnoid hemorrhage

IMAGING (subarachnoid hemorrhage)

see subarachnoid hemorrhage

IMAGING (aneurysms)

80% solitary; 15% two; 5% three or more

Location

30% ACommA
30% distal ICA/PCommA
20% terminal M1 segment MCA
10% basilar tip
10% elsewhere: distal ACA, PICA, post traumatic
ASSOCIATED WITH AVM: 60% have aneurysm at nidus, 10% at pedicle
unusual locations for mycotic and vasculitic aneurysms
GIANT ANEURYSM (>2.5 cm): cavernous ICA, rarely basilar tip; presents with cranial nerve palsies and mass effect; contains laminated thrombus with a smaller patent lumen

CT

if large, a rounded or lobulated mass in characteristic location
wall may calcify
fusiform aneurysms commonly calcify

CT angio

ADVANTAGES

acceptable accuracy for screening purposes (e.g. family history)
non invasive, but requires a large contrast load

FUNDAMENTAL LIMITATIONS

differentiation of enhancing blood from bone ('extraction' of the vasculature)
thrombus filled aneurysms (with no flowing lumen) not demonstrated
differentiation of arterial from venous structures

MR

ROUNDED OR LOBULATED MASS IN TYPICAL LOCATION WITH VARIABLE SIGNAL
flow void
pulsation artifact
slow flow (usually bright on T1W images)
clot (blood products signal depending on age)
combination of above (e.g. flow void with cuff of thrombus)

BEWARE IF INTRASELLAR (differential is intrasellar solid mass, e.g. pituitary adenoma with hemorrhage)

MR angio

ADVANTAGES

usually 'bright blood' time of flight sequences without or with intravenous contrast
acceptable accuracy for screening purposes (e.g. family history)
non–invasive, but susceptible to motion artifact

FUNDAMENTAL LIMITATIONS

thrombus filled aneurysms not demonstrated
differentiation of slow flowing arterial from venous structures
spatial resolution of smaller flowing arteries

Angio

still the gold standard for detection and the prelude to coil embolization
two negative angiograms effectively rules out aneurysmal hemorrhage for practical purposes
demonstrates aneurysm lumen, pedicle, nipple (multiple projections)
4 vessel study shows all potential aneurysms
shows any coexistent AVMs (except capillary AVMs)
vasospasm: thin irregular narrowing of distal vessels

PITFALL

posterior communicating artery (PCommA) infundibulum
diameter <2 mm, smooth funnel with PCommA at apex

6.2 ARTERIAL DISSECTION

ETIOLOGY

SPONTANEOUS
TRAUMATIC
VASCULOPATHY (fibromuscular dysplasia, Marfan's syndrome, Ehlers–Danlos syndrome, cystic medial necrosis)

CLINICAL

ICA dissection

pain
infarcts in ICA territory
Horner's syndrome
secondary caroticocavernous fistula

VA dissection

infarcts in basivertebral territory

IMAGING

ICA: mid cervical to skull base
VA: C2 to skull base, C6

CT/MR/CTA/MRA

FINDINGS OF DISSECTION

ICA location: distal cervical ICA, ICA at skull base (at entry to and through carotid canal), cavernous portion of ICA
VA location: between C2 and foramen magnum, or related to vertebral fractures
may have findings of fibromuscular dysplasia (Ch 15)
may have fractures of foramina transversaria (vertebral dissection)
tapering true lumen (with arterial enhancement on CT and MR signal that follows the uninjured side – flow void or high T1W/GRE signal)
true lumen may spiral gently
thrombus under dissection flap (no enhancement on CT, blood product signal on MR which depends on age of dissection)

DISTAL FINDINGS

normal flow (either through remaining patent true lumen or via Circle of Willis or other collaterals)
sluggish flow (altered enhancement timing, altered MR signal)
thrombosis, absent flow (no CT enhancement, no MR flow void)
no infarct, or completed or patchy infarction in relevant arterial territory

Angio

location: distal cervical ICA, ICA at skull base (at entry and through carotid canal), cavernous portion of ICA; vertebral artery between C2 and foramen magnum
may have findings of fibromuscular dysplasia not evident on CTA/MRA
'rat-tail' tapering lumen either with no flow (contrast linger, slow washout) or variable amount of reduced flow (delayed contrast flow distally compared to normal side)
true lumen may outline course and location of subintimal hematoma under flap
angiography of external carotid and opposite ICA shows extent of collateral supply

NUC MED (HMPAO, ECD)

not a common indication
if used, unequivocally documents state of cortical perfusion from all sources

6.3 INTRAPARENCHYMAL HEMORRHAGE

also see cerebral hemorrhage gamuts (Ch 10) and hemorrhage on CT/MR (general principles section)

GROUP DEFINITION

non traumatic intraparenchymal hemorrhage

ETIOLOGY

HYPERTENSIVE
ANEURYSMAL
UNDERLYING MASS
HEMORRHAGIC INFARCT
AMYLOID ANGIOPATHY
COAGULOPATHY/OVER-ANTICOAGULATION

LOCATION

LOBAR: subcortical or cortical cerebral; association with amyloid angiopathy
DEEP INTRAPARENCHYMAL: deep white or gray, thalami, basal ganglia, cerebellum, pons; tends to be hypertensive (~10% are aneurysmal; need to exclude underlying mass)

6.3.1 HYPERTENSIVE HEMORRHAGE

PATHOGENESIS

LIPOHYALINOTIC DEGENERATION of arterial media, occasional Charcot–Bouchard microaneurysms in deep perforating arteries

IMAGING

CT/MR

intraparenchymal hematoma with variable amount of mass effect and variable appearance depending on time of imaging
see hemorrhage on CT/MR in general principles section
variable amount of secondary subarachnoid and intraventricular blood
may cause secondary hydrocephalus or herniation from mass effect

FOR DIFFERENTIAL DIAGNOSIS ON IMAGING, see gamuts (Ch 10)

6.3.2 ANEURYSMAL HEMORRHAGE

variable amount of parenchymal hematoma versus subarachnoid blood
an intraparenchymal hemorrhage often follows previous minor or subclinical subarachnoid hemorrhages with developing subarachnoid adhesions and fibrosis

6.3.3 HEMORRHAGE INTO A MASS

see entries on AV malformation and hemangioma

6.3.4 HEMORRHAGE SECONDARY TO AMYLOID ANGIOPATHY

PATHOGENESIS

cortical and pial vessel A beta protein amyloid deposition; Alzheimer's disease in 40%

IMAGING

CT/MR

usually lobar rather than deep parenchymal location of hematoma

6.4 ISCHEMIC STROKE

DEFINITION

acute ischemic loss of brain tissue

EPIDEMIOLOGY

third leading cause of death after AMI and cancer
80% ischemic, 10% intraparenchymal hemorrhage, 10% subarachnoid hemorrhage

Risk factors

CEREBRAL ATHEROSCLEROTIC RISK FACTORS

SMOKING, HYPERTENSION, DIABETES, DYSLIPIDEMIA

if asymptomatic carotid stenosis >75%, rate of stroke is 3% per year

if transient ischemic attacks, rate of stroke is 1/3 in 5 years

CARDIOEMBOLIC RISK FACTORS

ATRIAL FIBRILLATION
CONGENITAL HEART DISEASE
PROSTHETIC VALVES

ETIOLOGY

Embolic: cardioembolic, atheroembolic

Atherothrombotic: carotid or intracerebral

LARGE VESSEL

LACUNAR

UNUSUAL
see Ch 10 infarcts – unusual

Hypotensive: watershed, global

Venous
see its own entry

MORPHOLOGY

<6 hours: no visible changes

6–24 hours: pallor, early softening, loss of gray-white junction, reactive edema; red neurons, neutrophil influx

1 day to 1 week: friable gelatinous infarcted area sharply demarcated from normal brain; RESORPTION: macrophage influx, phagocytosis

1 week on: progressive liquefaction, gliosis lined cystic cavities, eventual encephalomalacia and volume loss; GLIOSIS: glial proliferation (gemistocytes), neovascular capillaries

blood–brain barrier reconstituted with a delay of weeks to months

TERRITORIES

80% supratentorial, 10% infratentorial, 10% with hemorrhagic transformation

Arterial

ANTERIOR
(80%) MCA: COMPLETE, INCOMPLETE, STRIATOCAPSULAR
ACA

POSTERIOR
PCA
TOP OF BASILAR SYNDROME
SCA
PICA (lateral medullary syndrome)
(AICA rare)

PERFORATORS
LENTICULOSTRIATE, THALAMIC, PONTINE
RECURRENT ARTERY OF HEUBNER
ANTERIOR CHOROIDAL ARTERY

Unusual arterial patterns

tend to occur with proximal occlusion and result from the completeness of the Circle of Willis and adequacy of collaterals

Watershed territories

PREMATURE NEONATES: DEEP WHITE (CENTRAL/CORTICAL)
CHILDREN, ADULTS: INTERARTERIAL WATERSHED INFARCTS or PSEUDOLAMINAR NECROSIS

Global ischemia

DEEP GRAY: BASAL GANGLIA, SUBSTANTIA NIGRA, THALAMI
CORTEX: MESIAL TEMPORAL especially

INFARCT TIME COURSE AND PROGRESSION OF IMAGING FINDINGS

infarcted area has to be large enough for the imaging modality's resolving power to be visible (i.e. CT and Nuc Med will not show acute lacunar infarction)

6.4.1 Immediate

CT
NO FINDINGS (rules out bleed)

MR
loss of flow voids, occlusion of vessel on MRA
intravascular stagnant enhancement
diffusion restriction onset (off at 2 weeks time) – latest time of onset unclear
perfusion – no findings or delayed parenchymal transit time
MR spectroscopy: beginning of evolution to abnormal spectrum ('infarct spectrum')

NUC MED (HMPAO, ECD)
no perfusion to infarcted area

6.4.2 Hyperacute 1–6 hours

CT
rules out bleed
50% no findings

50% hyperdense artery, subtle decreased density of deep gray

MR
T1W gyral swelling, sulcal effacement, loss of gray-white matter junction; area of diffusion restriction, intravascular stagnant enhancement

6.4.3 Acute 6–24 hours

CT
loss of gray-white junction
sulcal effacement
in classical middle cerebral artery infarction: hypodense insula (insular ribbon sign), basal ganglia

MR
T1W mass effect, T2W area of high signal, area of diffusion restriction, intravascular stagnant enhancement
MR spectroscopy: lactate peak up, N-acetyl aspartate peak down, no change in choline peak, elevation in glutamine and glutamate (hence combination of short and intermediate TE acquisitions are recommended to resolve glx/glu and lactate respectively)

6.4.4 Late acute 1–3 days

CT
discrete hypodense area, mild mass effect; possible patchy hemorrhage

MR
T1W mass effect, T2W area of very high signal, area of diffusion restriction, leptomeningeal enhancement
offset intravascular enhancement
onset parenchymal enhancement (gyriform) at approximately 3 days
MR spectroscopy: lactate peak up, N-acetyl aspartate peak further down, choline may become elevated with cell membrane breakdown; extent and degree of NAA loss inversely correlate with clinical outcome

6.4.5 Subacute 1 week to 2 months

CT
mass effect resolves
onset gyral enhancement

MR
T1W mass effect resolves; T2W fogging (loss of increased T2W signal in infarcted area)
offset diffusion restriction at approximately 2 weeks

parenchymal enhancement (gyriform) persists

MR spectroscopy: lactate peak decreases or persists, and extent and persistence inversely correlate with clinical outcome

6.4.6 Months–years

CT

atrophy, encephalomalacia

dilation ex vacuo

no enhancement

MR

atrophy, encephalomalacia, gliosis, Wallerian degeneration

parenchymal enhancement offset at approximately 3 months

MR spectroscopy: lactate peak decreasing and eventually absent, N -acetyl aspartate peak down, choline peak variable, or down (gliosis); myo-inositol may be elevated (gliosis)

NUC MED (HMPAO, ECD)

variably decreased perfusion in distribution of infarct depending on degree of residual or reestablished blood supply

usually markedly reduced or absent perfusion in infarcted area

6.5 SUBARACHNOID HEMORRHAGE (SAH)

DEFINITION

extravasation of blood into CSF (subarachnoid space proper, intraventricular)

ETIOLOGY (spontaneous SAH)

90% ANEURYSMAL

PERIMESENCEPHALIC: small volume probable venous self limiting

AVM

VARIABLE CAUSES: ANTICOAGULANTS, COAGULOPATHY, HEMORRHAGIC INFARCTS, VASCULITIS, LEUKEMIA

CLINICAL

classic: sudden onset very severe headache, often occipital

other: collapse with or without focal neurological signs

SPONTANEOUS SUBARACHNOID HEMORRHAGE (90% of all spontaneous SAH)

MORTALITY 1/3, MAJOR MORBIDITY 1/3

intraparenchymal hemorrhage

vasospasm

acute hydrocephalus

REBLEED RATE 50% IN 2 WEEKS

mortality of rebleed ~50%

COMPLICATIONS

acute pulmonary edema

vasospasm, ischemia

cranial nerve palsies

hydrocephalus

CNS SUPERFICIAL SIDEROSIS

deposition of hemosiderin on subarachnoid surfaces of the brain secondary to repeated small volume SAH; cranial nerve palsies

IMAGING

CT

95% sensitive in demonstrating subarachnoid blood in first 48 hours

lumbar puncture required beyond then

increased density clot in ventricles and basal cisterns

associated intraparenchymal hematoma in ? (differential is primary hypertensive hemorrhage)

hemorrhage origin is usually where the majority of blood is found

SUBARACHNOID BLOOD LOCATIONS

CLASSIC DEPENDENT LOCATIONS:

occipital horns, interpeduncular cistern, posterior third ventricle

CLASSIC PERIANEURYSMAL LOCATIONS:

interhemispheric fissure (ACommA), Sylvian fissure (M1 MCA), suprasellar and ambient cisterns (distal ICA, PCommA)

DIFFICULT LOCATIONS:

posterior fossa

spinal subarachnoid space

NON ANEURYSMAL SAH (10%)

THROMBOSED ANEURYSM

OCCULT AVM (??off external carotid circulation)

TUMOR

PERIMESENCEPHALIC VENOUS

MR

subarachnoid blood (insensitive!)

insensitive to acute hemorrhage AND CAN NOT EXCLUDE IT

may demonstrate clot as filling defects within CSF

acute intraparenchymal hematoma has signal characteristics dependent on age (usually low T1W, mid to high T2W)

may demonstrate superficial siderosis from previous episodes of hemorrhage

rim of low signal on all sequences, and blooming on GRE and other hemosiderin sensitive sequences

covers pial surfaces, particularly in posterior fossa (brainstem) and cranial nerves

Angio

see aneurysms – imaging

6.6 VASCULAR MALFORMATION SPECTRUM

GROUP DEFINITION

heterogeneous group of vascular malformations but with a common tendency to hemorrhage

6.6.1 ARTERIOVENOUS MALFORMATION (AVM)

DEFINITION

congenital network of abnormal arteriovenous shunts

EPIDEMIOLOGY

?1/1000

90% present under 50 years of age

98% solitary, 2% multiple: hereditary hemorrhagic telangiectasia (Osler–Weber–Rendu syndrome) and Wyburn–Mason syndrome (brain + ocular AVMs)

CLINICAL

Presentation

(50%) HEMORRHAGE

intraparenchymal (commonest),
   intraventricular, subarachnoid, mixed
risk is ~3% per year, mortality ~15%, major
   morbidity ~30% per episode

(25%) SEIZURES

usually cortical AVMs

FOCAL NEUROLOGICAL DEFICIT

?arterial steal
?venous hypertension
?direct pressure and repeated hemorrhage

HEADACHE, MASS EFFECT

Grading

SPETZLER–MARTIN (out of 5)

size <3 cm   1
size 3–6 cm   2
size >6 cm   3
eloquent cortex   1
deep venous drainage 1
grade 6 is assigned to extensive or diffuse
   inoperable AVMs

RISK OF BLEEDING HIGH IF:

deep location
associated aneurysm
deep venous drainage
venous stenosis (outflow stenosis)

MACRO

80% supratentorial
enlarged arterial feeders (pedicle aneurysm
   10%)
nidus: tangle of abnormal dilated AV vessels,
   aneurysm 60%, apex usually deep, base
   at cortex
venous outflow
adjacent brain: usually surrounding gliosis
   and no functioning tissue

IMAGING

CT

isodense mass
may bleed (hematoma), calcify
none to variable surrounding edema
   (depending on recent AVM
   activity/thrombosis/hemorrhage)
strong serpentine contrast enhancement
enhancement variable if thrombosed

MR

PATENT AVM

tightly packed flow voids
variable amount of surrounding hemosiderin
   and edema/gliosis
contrast enhancement of slowly flowing
   channels and often venous outflow

THROMBOSED AVM

variable blood products signal within AVM
vessel walls may enhance

HEMORRHAGE

surrounding blood products of different ages
   or frank hematoma with mass
also see superficial siderosis within the entry
   on SAH

CORTICAL LOCATION

need to identify relation to eloquent cortex

MRA

coil of flowing channels (demonstration
   depends on flow velocity)
may show pedicle aneurysms

Angio

nest of coiled abnormal channels with
   variable mass effect
no recognizable normal cortical branches off
   vessel leading to AVM, but take-off may
   be from a large cortical branch
may be supplied by multiple feeders from
   different vascular territories (including
   external carotid)
pedicle or intranidal aneurysm/aneurysms
venous drainage to enlarged cortical or deep
   veins (often dilated and may be very
   abnormal)
often a prelude to preoperative or
   preradiotherapy embolization

6.6.2 ARTERIOVENOUS FISTULA (AVF)

DEFINITION

probably acquired abnormal fistulous
   arteriovenous communication with
   secondary venous hypertension

CLINICAL

10–15% of all malformations
presents at 40–60 years
LOCATION: TRANSVERSE + SIGMOID +
   CAVERNOUS SINUSES; TENTORIUM;
   SPINAL

feeding arteries usually dural/
   leptomeningeal
subarachnoid and intraparenchymal
   hemorrhage relatively rare
venous infarcts (cerebral, spinal)
cranial nerve palsies, reduced conscious
   state (dural sinus thrombosis)
pulsatile proptosis, deteriorating vision
   (caroticocavernous fistula)
?chronic intracranial hypertension (dural
   venous sinus hypertension)

IMAGING

CT/MR

dilated veins or dural venous sinuses
venous/dural sinus thrombosis
reversed flow (phase contrast MRV)

Angio

direct arteriovenous drainage (from
   meningeal arteries)
dural sinus stenoses, thromboses, venous
   dilation and tortuosity
reversed venous flow direction

ANGIOGRAPHIC TYPES

I   dural sinus, antegrade flow (benign
    course)
II dural sinus, retrograde flow (venous
    hypertension)
III cortical vein, no ectasia
IV cortical vein, with ectasia (bleed more
    likely)
V   spinal dural AVF (50% progressive
    myelopathy)

6.6.3 VEIN OF GALEN ANEURYSM

DEFINITION

dilation of vein of Galen (VofG) secondary to
   increased flow and pressure from
   different causes

CLASSIFICATION

I   direct AVF (post choroidal artery,
    anterior cerebral artery, perforators)
II thalamic AVM draining to V of G
III mixture of I and II
IV AVM with venous drainage in V of G
    territory

CLINICAL

incidental imaging finding
high flow left ventricular failure (neonates)
bruit, hydrocephalus (children):
    hydrocephalus from ?direct pressure
    ?venous HT
focal mass effect (children, adults)

IMAGING

US

midline mass with complex vascular flow

CT

vascular enhancing midline mass below
    splenium, posterior to thalami and above
    midbrain
variable mass effect

MR

mixture of flow voids, slow flow high signal,
    thrombosis and variable vascular
    enhancement
MRA may show direct communication of
    arteries to aneurysm

Angio

demonstrates source of increased flow and
    classifies
may be a prelude to embolization

6.6.4 VENOUS ANGIOMA

CLINICAL

commonest single vascular CNS anomaly
usually an incidental totally asymptomatic
    angiographic or MR finding
minority associated with hemangioma
sometimes associated with hemorrhage
    (?causal relationship to venous angioma
    itself)

MACRO

medullary vein medusa head, transcortical
    draining vein
commonest location deep white near
    ventricle (infratentorial, supratentorial)

IMAGING

CT

often invisible
enhancing draining vein

MR

abnormal tributary veins and draining vein
    may be visible precontrast
vascular enhancement with contrast making
    veins obvious

Angio

diagnostic 'medusa head' tributaries with a
    draining vein
80% drain to surface, 20% drain deep

6.6.5 CAPILLARY TELANGIECTASIA

CLINICAL

second most common malformation after
    venous angioma
nests of racemose dilated capillaries with no
    muscular wall in normal brain
    parenchyma
usually multiple; brainstem, spinal cord
most asymptomatic; small minority bleed

IMAGING

CT

possible dystrophic calcification

MR

blood products

Angio

normal: ('angiographically cryptic' or
    'angiographically occult' malformation)

6.6.6 CAVERNOUS HEMANGIOMA

DEFINITION

abnormal dilated endovascular spaces with
    no intervening brain; analogous to
    cavernous hemangiomas elsewhere

EPIDEMIOLOGY

1/2000, male = female
SPORADIC: 90% solitary, 10% multiple
FAMILIAL (autosomal dominant): multiple in
    75%
overall 50% are multiple, other
    malformations common

CLINICAL

risk of bleed ?1% per year
seizures, focal neurological signs, or
    incidental
slow flow or thrombosed endothelial lined
    spaces with a ring of hemosiderin and
    gliosis

IMAGING

CT

hyper or isodense mass
may calcify
variable contrast enhancement

MR

'popcorn lesion with hemosiderin ring'
cluster of high T2W spaces with variable
    amount of blood products (i.e. variable
    T1W signal) and a rim of hemosiderin

Angio

USUALLY NORMAL ('angiographically
    cryptic' or 'angiographically occult'
    malformation)

6.7 VENOUS INFARCTION

DEFINITION

neurological deficit (irreversible, reversible)
    secondary to venous hypertension or
    thrombosis/obstruction

ETIOLOGY

Infection

SINUSITIS

MASTOIDITIS

Focal vascular anomaly

AVF

FLOW REVERSAL WITH VENOUS
    HYPERTENSION

STENOSIS

EXTRINSIC COMPRESSION

Hypercoagulable state

DEHYDRATED NEONATE

ANTIPHOSPHOLIPID ANTIBODIES
    (SLE)

ANTITHROMBIN III DEFICIENCY

PROTEIN C DEFICIENCY

PROTEIN S DEFICIENCY

ORAL CONTRACEPTIVE PILL

PUERPERIUM

HYPERVISCOSITY

POLYCYTHEMIA

ONCOLOGY PATIENTS

CLINICAL

headache, papilloedema, reduced conscious state, focal neurological deficits

classic adult presentation is neurological deficit with reduced conscious state in a young adult female post partum or on oral contraceptive pill

neonates and children (classically with dehydration)

Complications

RESIDUAL IDIOPATHIC INTRACRANIAL HYPERTENSION

CORTICAL INFARCTS

DEEP THALAMIC INFARCTS, DEATH

EDEMA, CONING, DEATH

MORPHOLOGY

venous hypertension in subtended VENOUS DRAINAGE area, edema, frank hemorrhagic infarction in non arterial territory

Main types

DURAL SINUS THROMBOSIS

superior sagittal sinus commonest

DEEP CEREBRAL VEIN THROMBOSIS

INTERNAL CEREBRAL VEIN, VEIN OF GALEN

usually child or neonate with severe neurological deficit

IMAGING

Angio

gold standard: non filling of normally expected veins

filling defects on venous phase of angiogram

delayed washout of patent upstream veins, collateral demonstration

associated anomalies (AVM, AVF)

prelude to venous thrombolysis

CT

thrombosed cortical vein (high density tubular structure running along cortex to dural venous sinus) or thrombosed vein of Galen (abnormally high density)

variable amount of (cytotoxic) edema

non arterial distribution of edema

patchy hemorrhage (non arterial distribution)

'empty delta' sign with contrast (filling defect within descending portion of superior sagittal sinus) – unreliable

bilateral thalamic and surrounding low density very suggestive of vein of Galen territory infarction

MR

loss of dural venous sinus flow void or direct clot visualization in multiple sequences and planes (signal depends on clot age): differential is slow flow

variable amount of edema (as for CT)

non arterial patchy hemorrhages (as for CT)

MR time of flight venography – flow defect

false negatives – subacute clot (high T1W signal)

false positives – apparent non flow depending on vein orientation

MR phase contrast venography – flow defect

7. INFECTION

7.1 ACUTE MENINGITIS

DEFINITION

rapidly evolving viral or bacterial infection of the meninges and CSF

EPIDEMIOLOGY

commonest CNS infection

viral meningitis very common as a complication of other viral infections

distinct patterns of infection in particular subgroups (neonates, immunocompromised)

Risk factors

skull base fractures/CSF leaks

adjacent infections (mastoiditis, ethmoiditis)

contact with other infected persons (meningococcus)

ETIOLOGY

Viral

enteroviruses

echoviruses

AIDS: HIV, cytomegalovirus, herpes viruses

Bacterial

NEONATE: Group B Streptococcus, Escherichia coli, Listeria, Staphylococcus, Gram negative organisms

CHILD: Hemophilus, meningococcus, pneumococcus

ADULT: meningococcus, pneumococcus

IMMUNOSUPPRESSED: Gram negatives

ENDOCARDITIS: Staphylococcus

CLINICAL

Route of access

HEMATOGENOUS access (most common)

IN CONTINUITY (ENT infections)

ENTRY TRACK, SKULL BASE FRACTURE, CSF LEAK

IMPLANTATION (e.g. surgical, ventriculoperitoneal shunt)

Presentation

prodromal viral illness (viral meningitis)

fever, headache, meningism, vomiting

meningococcus: rash, cardiovascular collapse

neonates: bulging fontanelle, decreasing conscious state, seizures

viral meningitis usually self limiting

Complications of bacterial meningitis

cerebritis/abscess (may be from seeding of infarct)

subdural empyema or hygroma

dural venous sinus thrombosis, venous infarcts

vasculitis, cranial nerve palsies

arterial thrombosis and infarcts

labyrinthitis, deafness

hydrocephalus (late)

IMAGING

US

often normal

echogenic material in sulci

variable echogenicity extraaxial fluid collections

cerebral hyperechoic foci (?cerebritis, ?infarct)

CT

viral meningitis: normal
bacterial meningitis: usually normal (excludes hemorrhage or intracranial mass)
abnormal meningeal enhancement
complications (subdural collections, abscesses)
may show dural sinus thrombosis
neonates/children: subdural empyemas/ hygromas, extraaxial sources (mastoid collections, sinonasal collections)

MR

viral meningitis: usually normal (rarely, meningeal enhancement)
bacterial meningitis: may have abnormal leptomeningeal enhancement/basal cistern enhancement; rarely, massive exudate may fill basal cisterns
allows detection of complications
SUBDURAL EMPYEMA: see its own entry

7.2 AIDS, AIDS DEMENTIA COMPLEX

DEFINITION

an overall clinical syndrome in AIDS patients with deteriorating cognitive function due to a number of possible causes

CLINICAL

Infective agents
HIV
TOXOPLASMOSIS
JC PAPOVAVIRUS (PROGRESSIVE MULTIFOCAL LEUKOENCEPHALOPATHY – PML)
CYTOMEGALOVIRUS (VENTRICULOENCEPHALITIS, VASCULITIS, CHORIORETINITIS)
FUNGAL (CRYPTOCOCCUS, OTHERS)
TB (TB >> MAC)

7.2.1 Meningitis
HIV CONVERSION
FUNGAL (CRYPTOCOCCUS > OTHERS)
TB
LYMPHOMATOUS MENINGITIS

7.2.2 Parenchymal diffuse disease
HIV ENCEPHALOPATHY
PROGRESSIVE MULTIFOCAL LEUKOENCEPHALOPATHY
CYTOMEGALOVIRUS (CMV) INFECTION

7.2.3 Parenchymal focal disease
TOXOPLASMOSIS
LYMPHOMA
TB OR FUNGAL ABSCESS
SYPHILITIC GUMMA
GLIOBLASTOMA MULTIFORME
KAPOSI'S SARCOMA

7.2.4 Myelopathy
VARICELLA ZOSTER VIRUS
CYTOMEGALOVIRUS
TOXOPLASMOSIS
LYMPHOMA

IMAGING (general features of CNS AIDS)

MR (CT)
cerebral and cerebellar atrophy out of keeping with age
abnormal foci of high T2W signal usually in white matter, without contrast enhancement
focal or multifocal intraaxial masses with or without contrast enhancement (see differential above, and gamuts)
meningitis: abnormal meningeal contrast enhancement

7.3 CEREBRITIS and BRAIN ABSCESS

DEFINITION

focal parenchymal infection of the brain (and spinal cord)

ETIOLOGY

also see acute meningitis

Organism
BACTERIAL (MOST): Streptococcus, Hemophilus, Staphylococcus (especially trauma), E coli, anaerobes
UNUSUAL (immune suppression, HIV): TB, cryptococcus, toxoplasmosis

Mode of spread

7.3.1 HEMATOGENOUS
endocarditis
IV drug abuse
pulmonary infection (abscess, bronchiectasis)
right to left cardiac shunts or pulmonary AVMs

7.3.2 SINUSITIS (frontal, ethmoidal, sphenoidal)

7.3.3 MASTOIDITIS, OTITIS MEDIA
usually accompanied by dural venous sinus thrombosis

7.3.4 TRAUMA, DIRECT INOCULATION, CSF LEAK

7.3.5 SECONDARY TO ACUTE BACTERIAL MENINGITIS

CLINICAL

mass effect and raised intracranial pressure
focal neurological signs or seizures
fever, sepsis

Location

AT SITE OF DIRECT ENTRY: USUALLY SOLITARY

HEMATOGENOUS
distribution reflects perfusion: frontal, parietal, temporal, occipital, cerebellum
frequently at gray-white interface
solitary or multifocal (especially in immune suppression)

Stages

EARLY CEREBRITIS 0–5 DAYS
focal edema and hyperemia
neutrophilic perivascular infiltrate, no capsule

LATE CEREBRITIS ~5 DAYS TO 2 WEEKS
coalescing patchy necrosis, surrounding cuff of inflammation and peripheral edema
neutrophil and macrophage infiltrate, early granulation tissue

EARLY ABSCESS ~2 WEEKS TO MONTHS
central liquefactive necrosis, debris, capsule of thin collagen and reticulin, surrounding edema

LATE ABSCESS – MONTHS
central liquefactive necrosis, fibrous capsule (granulation fibroblasts), neovascularization, reactive gliosis with gemistocytes, edema

IMAGING

CEREBRITIS

US

increased parenchymal echogenicity ('cotton wool')

DIFFERENTIAL: infarct

CT

ill marginated intraaxial area of reduced density with variable amount of mass effect and edema

early cerebritis: no contrast enhancement

enhancement develops progressively from mild, delayed, patchy to eventual ring enhancement as inflammation and granulation tissue develop

MR

ill marginated intraaxial area of mildly decreased T1W and high T2W signal with variable amount of mass effect and edema

contrast enhancement evident earlier than on CT; progresses from mild patchy to peripheral ring enhancement

center develops progressively higher T2W signal

ABSCESS

unifocal, multifocal

CT

subcortical rounded low density mass with variable amount of vasogenic edema

ring enhancement with contrast: thin (early); thick (late)

enhancing ring frequently thicker peripherally (?better blood supply from cortical vessels)

MR

subcortical rounded or ovoid mass, high on T2W/PD and low on T1W sequences

surrounded by capsule of low T1W and T2W signal (regular and smooth)

variable amount of vasogenic edema outside the capsule (high on T2W)

regular, thin (earlier) or thick (later) vivid contrast enhancement of capsule, classically thicker subcortically

may see communication with ventricles with ependymitis (abnormal enhancement)

may see focal or more diffuse meningeal abnormal enhancement

possible daughter abscesses (usually medially)

MR spectroscopy: usually reduced or no NAA, variably reduced choline and creatine; bacterial products: acetate (1.92 ppm), succinate (2.4 ppm), other amino acid peaks; lactate/lipid peak

DIFFERENTIAL DIAGNOSIS

see gamuts – ring enhancing lesion

high grade gliomas have elevated choline and choline:creatine ratio typically >2.0 (see astrocytomas)

7.4 CHRONIC MENINGITIS

DEFINITION

heterogeneous group of chronic conditions involving CSF spaces, infective, non infective, and of uncertain cause

ETIOLOGY

Infective

7.4.1 TB

7.4.2 FUNGAL (cryptococcus, coccidiomycosis)

Non infective

7.4.3 SARCOIDOSIS

7.4.4 WEGENER'S GRANULOMATOSIS

7.4.5 LANGERHANS CELL HISTIOCYTOSIS

MORPHOLOGY

tendency to involve basal cisterns

thick fibrinous exudate

eventual basal cistern fibrosis and hydrocephalus

CN palsies, vasculitis of arteries passing through basal cisterns

IMAGING (general features)

CT

normal

basal dural thickening with meningeal contrast enhancement

possibly patchy dural calcification, obliteration of basal cisterns

MR

normal

basal meningeal thick or nodular enhancement with variable extension further cranially

manifestations of complications (arterial occlusions, infarcts, hydrocephalus, cranial nerve enhancement)

7.5 FUNGAL CNS INFECTIONS

DEFINITION

heterogeneous group of CNS infections by fungi (and fungi-like bacteria) usually affecting the immunocompromised and producing a number of similar clinical and imaging patterns

ETIOLOGY

Fungi

ASPERGILLUS

diabetics and immunosuppressed

spores inhaled

hematogenous spread (from lung deposits)

direct spread from sinonasal or orbital infection (uncommon)

angiocentric, angioinvasive infection

abscess formation

MUCORMYCOSIS

diabetics, immunosuppressed

direct spread from sinonasal infection ('rhinocerebral mucormycosis')

frontal lobe and orbital infection, cavernous sinus thrombosis and infection

angiocentric, angioinvasive

cavernous sinus thrombosis in particular

also forms abscesses

CRYPTOCOCCUS

HIV population in particular

hematogenous spread

basal meningitis

perivascular space infection

CANDIDA

immunosuppressed, HIV, oncology patients

hematogenous spread

basal meningitis

abscess formation

COCCIDIOIDES

rare, endemic; spores inhaled

hematogenous spread

basal meningitis, occasional parenchymal granuloma formation

OTHERS (histoplasma, blastomyces)

Fungi–like bacteria

NOCARDIA
immunosuppressed and AIDS
hematogenous spread
multiple brain abscesses

ACTINOMYCES
rare
hematogenous spread from chronic focus of
    actinomycosis elsewhere
abscess formation

MORPHOLOGY

Patterns of involvement

7.5.1 PARENCHYMAL ABSCESS
Candida, Coccidioides, Aspergillus, others

7.5.2 ANGIOCENTRIC ANGIOINVASIVE INFECTION
Mucor and Aspergillus
thrombosis with local parenchymal
    infarction or distal cerebral infarction;
    secondary conversion of bland to fungal
    septic infarcts
devastating rapidly progressive infection

HEMATOGENOUS SPREAD

RHINOCEREBRAL SPREAD
inferior frontal lobe, anterior temporal lobe
    abscesses, cavernous sinus infective
    thrombosis

7.5.3 PERIVASCULAR INFECTION
Cryptococcus
gelatinous collections in perivascular spaces
    particularly affecting perforating arteries
    (basal ganglia, deep gray, brainstem)

CHRONIC MENINGITIS
see its own entry

IMAGING

FUNGAL ABSCESS

CT
low density mass with thick contrast
    enhancing rim or nodular enhancement
vasogenic edema

MR
low T1W signal and isointense T2W and PD
    signal mass
low T1W and T2W signal rim (?dense
    hyphae, ?manganese, ?blood products)
surrounding vasogenic edema
thick ring or nodular contrast enhancement

PERIVASCULAR INFECTION

CT
usually normal
small hypodense foci in basal ganglia

MR
small multiple foci of high T2W and low
    T1W signal along course of perforating
    arteries (deep gray, midbrain)
do not enhance with contrast

INFARCTS

same features as arterial or venous infarcts
    of other causes
location, number and distribution unusual
    and related to underlying fungal
    abscesses, angiitis or basal meningitis
superinfection evolves to cerebritis/fungal
    abscess

DIFFUSE FUNGAL MENINGOENCEPHALITIS

CT/MR
generalized or more focal cerebral edema

7.6 HSV ENCEPHALITIS

DEFINITION

cerebral parenchymal infection with the
    herpes simplex virus (HSV)

ETIOLOGY

adults (immunocompetent): HSV1
    reactivation
neonates: perinatal HSV2 infection

CLINICAL

Adults
retrograde ascent from trigeminal ganglion
rapidly progressive conscious state
    deterioration, mortality ~50%
hemorrhagic encephalitis in limbic areas:
    temporal, subfrontal, cingulate areas,
    insula; Cowdry inclusion bodies (HSV
    particles)
initially unilateral becoming bilateral

Neonates
diffuse meningoencephalitis, hemorrhage,
    necrosis, eventual porencephalic cysts,

parenchymal calcification and
    microcephaly
see entry on TORCH infections in Ch 20

IMAGING (adult form)

CT
normal till 3 to 5 days
ill defined low density in temporal lobe/lobes
eventual patchy or gyriform contrast
    enhancement

MR
abnormal at ~2 days
gyral edema on T1W sequences, diffusely
    increased T2W signal in affected cortex
    and underlying white matter
temporal cortex, subfrontal cortex, insula
    but not putamen
eventual gyriform enhancement

NUC MED (HMPAO, ECD)
abnormal by ~4 to 5 days
marked hyperemia in infected areas

7.7 HYDATID
(CNS manifestations)

see Ch 13 hydatid disease

CLINICAL

2% of all hydatids
presents with rising intracranial pressure

IMAGING

CT/MR
solitary, less often multiple thin-walled
    round CSF density cyst; wall may calcify;
    rarely enhances
cyst signal close to but not identical to CSF
may show daughter cysts

7.8 NEURO-CYSTICERCOSIS

DEFINITION

CNS infection by larva of Taenia solium (pig
    tapeworm) with several distinct
    presentation forms ('stages')

7.8.1 LIVE VESICULAR

IMAGING

CT/MR

CSF like intraparenchymal cyst, mural
    nodule (protoscolex)
mature cyst is 5–20 mm in size
no edema or mass effect

7.8.2 COLLOIDAL VESICULAR
(dead larva)

IMAGING

CT/MR

hyperdense/hyperintense (T1W and T2W)
    intraparenchymal cyst
ring contrast enhancement and marked
    edema

7.8.3 GRANULAR NODULAR
(central dead scolex)

IMAGING

CT/MR

isodense/isointense parenchymal mass with
    contrast enhancement
persisting edema

7.8.4 CALCIFIED GRANULAR
(at 1 to 10 years; 'healed')

IMAGING

CT/MR

small parenchymal calcified nodule
no edema

7.8.5 RACEMOSE FORM

IMAGING

CT/MR

intraventricular cysts
grape like clusters without scolices in basal
    cisterns
do not enhance
may cause hydrocephalus

7.9 NEUROSARCOIDOSIS

see Ch 13 sarcoidosis

CLINICAL

5% of all sarcoid
granulomatous leptomeningitis and
    vasculitis (basal cisterns)
CN II, VII, VIII palsies
pituitary: diabetes insipidus,
    hypopituitarism, visual disturbance
    (chiasm)
focal neurological deficits (vasculitic infarcts)
globe, conus, bulbar fat

IMAGING

MR

abnormally intense and thickened contrast
    enhancement variably present in: basal
    cisterns, meninges (cranial, spinal),
    cranial nerves, ependyma
abnormal focal areas of increased T2W
    signal with little or no mass effect in
    brain (perivascular distribution) and
    spinal cord; may enhance with contrast
abnormally expanded pituitary and stalk,
    with possible involvement of inferior
    hypothalamus and optic chiasm; uniform
    contrast enhancement

DIFFERENTIAL

lymphoma
histiocytosis
lymphocytic hypophysitis

7.10 NEUROSYPHILIS

CLINICAL

10% of untreated syphilis
MENINGEAL (10 years delay): chronic
    meningitis, obliterative endarteritis
PARETIC (20 years delay): parenchymal
    spirochetes, widespread atrophy, memory
    and personality disturbances (general
    paralysis of the insane)
TABES DORSALIS (30 years delay): sensory
    root damage with dorsal column atrophy,
    Charcot joints and absent deep tendon
    reflexes

IMAGING

MR (non specific)

multiple parenchymal foci of T2W
    hyperintensity

possible meningeal contrast enhancement
diffuse parenchymal atrophy

7.11 SUBDURAL EMPYEMA

IMAGING

CT

relative 'blind areas' adjacent to bone
    (orbital roof, tegmen tympani)
variable density extraaxial collection with a
    contrast enhancing delimiting membrane
usually parasagittal or related to ENT
    infection
frequently bilateral
differential: chronic subdural hematoma
    with organization
may see complications (dural venous sinus
    thrombosis, etc)

MR

SUBDURAL EMPYEMA
extraaxial collection as for CT
purulent collections higher on T1W and
    lower on T2W sequences (?due to
    proteinaceous components)
thick enhancing membrane with contrast
adjacent cerebral edema

SUBDURAL HYGROMA (differentiation
    not absolute)
by definition, extraaxial collection isointense
    with CSF and no evidence of other
    changes (enhancing membranes,
    adjacent edema)

SUBDURAL HEMATOMA (differentiation
    not absolute)
contains blood products
see under its own entry

7.12 TB (CNS)

EPIDEMIOLOGY

Endemic

Immunosuppressed: HIV, IV drug abuse, alcoholics

PATHOGENESIS

reactive type TB (specific immune response)
    produces characteristic tuberculous
    granulomas

unreactive TB (poor immune response) produces non granulomatous abscesses or perivascular miliary CNS TB

MORPHOLOGY

7.12.1 Chronic TB meningitis with vasculitis

basal cistern involvement, thick fibrinous exudate, may calcify

basal cistern vasculitis causes arterial infarcts

7.12.2 Fibrocaseous focus (tuberculoma)

usually small focus at gray-white junction, may be multiple

7.12.3 Non granulomatous abscess

7.12.4 Miliary CNS TB

IMAGING

CT/MR

TB MENINGITIS

possible basal cisterns and fissures obliteration

thick basal cistern meningeal contrast enhancement

dystrophic meningeal calcification

secondary infarcts, hydrocephalus

FIBROCASEOUS FOCUS (tuberculoma)

solitary or multiple small subcortical mass/masses at gray-white junction

isointense on T1W, low on T2W

nodular or ring contrast enhancement

healed or old foci calcify

NON GRANULOMATOUS ABSCESS

same imaging features as cerebral abscess (see its own entry)

MILIARY CNS TB

multiple small foci of high T2W signal with nodular contrast enhancement (gray-white junction; deep perforator territory)

7.13 TORCH INFECTIONS
(manifestations)

see Ch 20

7.14 TOXOPLASMOSIS
(adult)

DEFINITION

parenchymal CNS infection by Toxoplasma gondii in the immunocompromised (particularly AIDS)

CLINICAL

AIDS: commonest clinically overt CNS infection

non AIDS: oncology patients, immunosuppression (steroids)

headache, drowsiness, altered cognitive function, seizures, fever

antibiotic treatment (sulfa drugs, other) effective

Distribution

basal ganglia, gray-white junction, cerebrum and cerebellum

vast majority are multiple at diagnosis

Parenchymal toxoplasma lesion zones

(inner to outer)
CENTRAL NECROSIS
FREE TOXOPLASMA ORGANISMS
ENCYSTED TOXOPLASMA ORGANISMS
VASOGENIC EDEMA

IMAGING

CT

multiple intraparenchymal hypodense or isodense areas with ring or nodular contrast enhancement

enhancement maximal with double dose, delayed (1 hour) imaging

variable amount of mass effect and edema

treated toxoplasmosis may calcify

MR

multiple intraparenchymal masses, low T1W signal, variable T2W signal (hypointense to hyperintense)

ring or nodular contrast enhancement

surrounding vasogenic edema

treated toxoplasmosis has variable signal (low or high)

NUC MED (Tl)

no uptake or mild washin with no delayed retention

PET (FDG)

no increased uptake

TOXOPLASMOSIS vs LYMPHOMA

TOXOPLASMOSIS

multiple, small

hypodense

gray-white junction, basal ganglia

fluorodeoxyglucose, thallium cold

responds to antibiotics (follow through to resolution, as multiple pathologies coexist)

MR spectroscopy: high lactate/lipid, decreased/no choline; decreased myo-inositol, creatine, NAA

LYMPHOMA

few, large

hyperdense

periventricular, corpus callosum

fluorodeoxyglucose, thallium avid

no response to antibiotics

MR spectroscopy: markedly elevated choline:creatine ratio, lactate/lipid is also present

7.15 VIRAL/POST VIRAL NON HERPES ENCEPHALITIS

GROUP DEFINITION

immune mediated myelinolysis and neuronal destruction caused by either current viral CNS infection (encephalitis) or by a postulated post viral autoimmune response

GENERAL GROUP FEATURES
(imaging)

MR

foci of high T2W signal affecting white matter more than gray matter, and both subcortical or deep; low or isointense on T1W

7.15.1 ACUTE DISSEMINATED ENCEPHALOMYELITIS

autoimmune crossreaction post viral infection (measles, HZV), commoner in children

rarely, follows vaccination to viral diseases of childhood

perivascular demyelination

IMAGING

subcortical and deep white matter; also brainstem and cerebellum
deep gray (thalami, basal ganglia) may be involved
lesions may show contrast enhancement

7.15.2 SUBACUTE SCLEROSING PANENCEPHALITIS

very rare measles reactivation

IMAGING

lesions do not enhance with contrast

7.15.3 MURRAY VALLEY ENCEPHALITIS

arbovirus (mosquito borne)

7.15.4 RABIES

encephalitis and wound paresthesias
Negri inclusion bodies

7.15.5 PROGRESSIVE MULTIFOCAL LEUKOENCEPHALOPATHY

JC polyoma virus (70% of population seropositive) infection of immunocompromised
uncommon, but more prevalent with AIDS
infection and destruction of oligodendroglia

IMAGING

subcortical white matter and also deep white and gray matter, but usually not cortex or cerebellum
rarely, lesions enhance with contrast

7.15.6 CMV

immune suppression or AIDS
ventriculoependymitis, vasculitis, choroid plexitis, chorioretinitis

7.15.7 HIV

conversion meningitis
HIV subacute encephalitis

dorsal column vacuolar myelopathy
cranial and peripheral mononeuropathy

IMAGING

see AIDS dementia complex entry

8. DEGENERATIONS

8.1 ALCOHOL RELATED DISEASE

8.1.1 WERNICKE'S ENCEPHALOPATHY

vitamin B1 deficiency
ataxia and nystagmus, confusion and psychosis
petechial hemorrhages and necrosis in mamillary bodies, medial thalamus, deep periaqueductal gray, deep periventricular gray

8.1.2 CHRONIC ATROPHY
(alcohol related)

CEREBELLOVERMIAN
GENERALIZED
ALCOHOLIC DEMENTIA

8.1.3 SUBACUTE COMBINED DEGENERATION OF THE CORD

see acute/subacute transverse myelopathy

8.1.4 CENTRAL PONTINE MYELINOLYSIS

see its own entry

8.1.5 HEPATIC ENCEPHALOPATHY

CLINICAL

complication of alcoholic cirrhosis and liver failure
may be precipitated by gastrointestinal hemorrhage
asterixis, confusion, decreasing conscious state, coma
glia transform to Alzheimer II astrocytes

(large nuclei, glycogen inclusions) – not related to Alzheimer's disease!

IMAGING

MR

bilateral diffusely increased T1W signal in putamen and globus pallidus, normal T2W signal

8.2 ALZHEIMER'S DISEASE (AD)

DEFINITION

common progressive dementia with neuronal loss, cerebral amyloid, neuritic plaques and neurofibrillary tangles

EPIDEMIOLOGY

single commonest type of dementia (some 60–70% of all dementias)
20% of 75–85 year olds have dementia (mostly AD), 40% have cognitive impairment

Risk factors

old age (prevalence doubles every 5 years)
family history of AD (risk x3.5) (NB rare familial type also exists)
Down's syndrome (APP gene) – histological AD by 40 years of age; APP: amyloid precursor protein
ApoE gene (chromosome 19) epsilon4 allele

CLINICAL

progressive slow cognitive decline with memory deficits, loss of higher mental function, personality changes, and eventual motor apraxia (gross motor function preserved well)

MACRO

frontotemporoparietal atrophy (esp hippocampal CA1 sector, amygdala, endorhinal cortex)
general cortical atrophy with enlargement of sulci and ventricles; more pronounced than normal age related volume loss, but with extensive overlap in populations

MICRO

NO PATHOGNOMONIC FINDINGS (all can be seen in normals); prevalence of dementia rises with pathologic burden

Lesions with A beta amyloid
AMYLOID ANGIOPATHY
DIFFUSE PLAQUES
NEURITIC PLAQUES

Lesions without A beta amyloid
NEUROFIBRILLARY TANGLES
HIPPOCAMPAL DEGENERATION

IMAGING

CT
rules out surgical conditions
cortical atrophy (overlaps with normal)

MR
early atrophy: amygdala and hippocampi; (producing enlargement of temporal horns)
late atrophy: diffuse with large temporal horns and third ventricle
may show increased hippocampal T2W signal
white matter T2W hyperintense foci similar to normal aging or vascular disease, and do not discriminate

VOLUMETRICS
whole brain or temporal lobe volumetrics shows greater atrophy in AD than in age matched normals – and the separation of the two populations is not sufficiently specific

MR SPECTROSCOPY
hippocampus difficult to target because of adjacent temporal bone causing artifact; parietal white and occipital gray matter may show characteristic changes
decreased NAA, decreased NAA:creatine ratio
increased myo-inositol and myo-inositol:creatine ratio (may be related to gliosis, amyloid/neuritic plaques)
elevation of MI may distinguish Alzheimer's disease from dementias of other types (although recently elevation of MI has been reported in diseases other than AD including AIDS dementia and dementia of frontal type)

NUC MED (HMPAO, ECD)/PET (FDG)
cerebellum, visual cortex used as intensity controls
HMPAO or ECD show pattern of cerebral perfusion and hence PERFUSION DEFECTS
FDG correlates with cerebral glucose metabolism and hence shows HYPOMETABOLIC AREAS
classical pattern: reduced biparietal activity (parietal association cortex) with bitemporal extension (including hippocampi); this may be asymmetrical; relatively preserved activity elsewhere in cortex
more severe disease shows progressive involvement of frontal cortex from posterior to anterior
discrimination between differential diagnoses not perfect (see DIFFERENTIAL) but has utility in changing odds ratios
totally normal study has a high negative predictive value (i.e. utility in exclusion of AD)
CAVEATS: standardized injecting conditions required; need MR correlation to exclude old infarction, gliosis, etc as causes of reduced perfusion

DIFFERENTIAL

MULTIINFARCT DEMENTIA
distribution of defects asymmetrical and corresponds to vascular territories
DEMENTIA OF FRONTAL TYPE
frontal lobe defects (symmetrical, asymmetrical)
PARKINSON'S DISEASE WITH DEMENTIA
uncommon
differentiation of Lewy body disease from AD may progress to I-123 iodobenzamide (dopaminergic marker)
MITOCHONDRIAL ENCEPHALOPATHIES
rare
COMBINATION OF DIFFERENT TYPES OF DEMENTIA!

8.3 AMYOTROPHIC LATERAL SCLEROSIS

CLINICAL

male > female, 50–70 years
progressive loss of upper and lower motor neurons, corticospinal tract and anterior horn gliosis and atrophy

limb muscular atrophy and weakness (amyotrophy = denervation atrophy) with hyperreflexia

IMAGING

MR
high T2W/PD signal in position of corticospinal tracts
atrophy and volume loss involving lateral columns of spinal cord (i.e. lateral corticospinal tract) and possibly anterior horns

8.4 BIG DEMENTIAS
(overview and differentiating findings)

GROUP DEFINITION

slowly progressive neurodegenerative conditions with cognitive and higher mental function impairment in the presence of a clear sensorium and relatively preserved gross motor function

CLASSIFICATION

number in brackets indicates which diseases from the top of each list are numerically important

Idiopathic/familial dementias (5)

ALZHEIMER'S DISEASE (AD)

FRONTAL LOBE DEMENTIA SPECTRUM

LEWY BODY DISEASE (AD TO PD SPECTRUM)

PARKINSON'S DISEASE (PD) WITH DEMENTIA

PARKINSON'S VARIANTS

PROGRESSIVE SUPRANUCLEAR PALSY

OTHERS

HUNTINGTON'S DISEASE

CREUTZFELDT–JAKOB DISEASE (infective)

Secondary dementias (5)

ALCOHOLIC DEMENTIA

MULTIINFARCT DEMENTIA

DEMENTIA OF DIFFUSE
MICROVASCULAR DISEASE

HIV DEMENTIA (AIDS dementia complex)

MULTIPLE SCLEROSIS

MITOCHONDRIAL
ENCEPHALOPATHIES

ILLICIT DRUG ABUSE

DYSMYELINATING DISEASES

NEUROSYPHILIS

Mimickers of dementia (4)

TUMOR (primary, secondary)

CHRONIC SUBDURAL HEMATOMA

DEPRESSION

HYDROCEPHALUS (including normal
pressure)

SIDE EFFECTS OF MEDICATION (esp in
elderly)

HYPOTHYROIDISM

8.4.1 ALZHEIMER'S DISEASE (AD)

see its own entry

CLINICAL DIFFERENTIATORS

commonest type of dementia
slowly progressive course, absence of
features of MID or PD

IMAGING DIFFERENTIATORS

MR
hippocampal atrophy
decreased NAA/MI ratio

NUC MED/PET
symmetrical decreased parietotemporal
activity that does not fit vascular
territories

8.4.2 MULTIINFARCT DEMENTIA (MID)

CLINICAL DIFFERENTIATORS

multiple cortical and subcortical infarcts
evidence of vascular disease elsewhere
stepwise time course with identifiable
individual infarcts

IMAGING DIFFERENTIATORS

multiple infarcts or gliosis on MR with
multifocal perfusion defects that fit
vascular territories

8.4.3 ALCOHOLIC DEMENTIA

see alcohol related disease entry

CLINICAL DIFFERENTIATORS

history of longstanding alcohol abuse always
present, but may be concealed
findings of alcoholic liver disease, etc

IMAGING DIFFERENTIATORS

mammillary and thalamus and deep gray
atrophy; generalized cortical atrophy;
cerebellar atrophy

8.4.4 PARKINSON'S DISEASE AND RELATIVES

see its own entries

CLINICAL DIFFERENTIATORS

motor deficits and neurological findings of
Parkinson's disease; appropriate
response to medication
may coexist with other dementias

IMAGING

difficult; see its own entry

8.4.5 FRONTAL LOBE DEMENTIA (including Pick's disease)

see its own entry

IMAGING DIFFERENTIATORS

CT/MR
marked bifrontal atrophy

NUC MED/PET
symmetrical bifrontal reduced activity

8.4.6 AIDS DEMENTIA COMPLEX

see its own entry

CLINICAL

cognitive or conscious state deterioration in
an AIDS patient (many causes)

IMAGING (possible findings)

gray matter atrophy, foci of high T2W signal
in white matter, mass lesions

8.4.7 HUNTINGTONS DISEASE (HD)

*see its entry under gray matter
degenerations*

CLINICAL DIFFERENTIATORS

onset 40–60 years old, family history usually
present
choreoathetosis, dementia, personality
change

IMAGING DIFFERENTIATORS

progressive and eventually massive caudate
atrophy (with matching frontal horn
dilation)
putamen atrophy

8.4.8 CREUTZFELDT–JAKOB DISEASE (infective?)

CLINICAL

rare rapidly progressive dementia
postulated cause is a 'prion' infection
(infective protein particle with no DNA)
associations: human purified growth
hormone injection, cerebral electrode
implantation, corneal transplantation
animal analogues: scrapie (sheep), bovine
spongiform encephalopathy ('mad cow
disease') (?transmissivity to humans)
spongiform degeneration of neurons,
neuronal loss, gliosis, no inflammatory
change

IMAGING FINDINGS

CT

usually normal

MR

normal

diffuse atrophy

symmetric high T2W signal in basal ganglia, thalami, possibly cortex, little other early findings

late cortical atrophy

8.5 CARBON MONOXIDE (CO) POISONING

CLINICAL

necrosis of globi pallidi, selective cell death of large neurons (pseudolaminar necrosis)

IMAGING

CT

classically, bilateral symmetrical hypodensity of globi pallidi

if severe, diffuse loss of gray-white interface, cortical low density and diffuse cerebral edema

MR

symmetrical high T2W signal in anterior 2/3 of globi pallidi, possibly with spillover into surrounding structures

if severe, diffuse cortical high T2W signal, diffuse cerebral edema

8.6 CENTRAL PONTINE MYELINOLYSIS

(osmotic myelinolysis)

CLINICAL

alcoholic liver disease, burns, sepsis, diffuse malignancy

destruction of myelin

bulbar palsy and quadriparesis

probably caused by rapid correction of severe hyponatremia

IMAGING

MR

symmetrical central pontine high T2W triangular signal

other areas of myelinolysis: midbrain, deep gray nuclei and white matter

8.7 GRAY AND WHITE MATTER DEGENERATING CONDITIONS

MNEMONIC: MMMZ

8.7.1 M-ELAS

see mitochondrial encephalopathies entry

8.7.2 M-ERRF

see mitochondrial encephalopathies entry

8.7.3 M-UCOPOLY-SACCHARIDOSES

8.7.4 Z-ELLWEGER DISEASE

peroxisomal enzyme deficiency

IMAGING

MR/CT

pachymicrogyria, polymicrogyria, heterotopic gray matter, dysmyelination, cortical atrophy

8.8 GRAY MATTER DEGENERATING CONDITIONS

MNEMONIC: LEWISH MUCEG HUNTS

DEEP LEWISH

8.8.1 LE-IGH DISEASE

CLINICAL

lactic acidosis with mitochondrial encephalopathy (autosomal recessive or X-linked)

infantile form: hypotonia, extraocular palsies, seizures

juvenile, adult forms exist

IMAGING

MR

bilateral symmetric necrotizing foci in deep gray matter (basal ganglia, thalami, periaqueductal gray, cerebellum, medulla): low T1W and high T2W signal

8.8.2 WI-LSON'S DISEASE (CNS manifestations)

also see Ch 07

IMAGING

CT

symmetrical low density basal ganglia

MR

findings similar to hepatic encephalopathy

basal ganglia (especially globus pallidus and putamen) progressively high on both T1W and T2W

increased T2W signal in surrounding white matter

eventual fibrosis with decreasing T2W signal

8.8.3 S-PATZ-H-ALLERVORDEN (HALLERVORDEN–SPATZ) DISEASE

infantile onset

movement disorder with dystonia and mental retardation

IMAGING

degeneration and iron deposition in globi pallidi responsible for MR changes

globi pallidi low on T2W (iron) with high T2W foci ('eye of the tiger sign')

SUPERFICIAL [MUCEG]

8.8.4 MU-COLIPIDOSES

NIEMANN–PICK DISEASE

sphingomyelin accumulation
generalized brain atrophy, thin cortex
visceromegaly

OTHER MUCOLIPIDOSES

8.8.5 CE-ROID LIPOFUSCINOSIS

accumulation of ceroid and lipofuscin-like
    substances with neuronal loss and
    atrophy
cortical atrophy, abnormal gray matter
    signal

8.8.6 G-LYCOGEN STORAGE DISEASE

see Ch 07

IMAGING (CNS manifestations)

macrocephaly

CT
diffuse hypodensity
thick dura
dilated ventricles

MR
cortical atrophy
subcortical white matter radially oriented
    foci of high T2W signal
thickened low signal dura
possible spinal cord compression (especially
    at craniocervical junction)

BOTH [HUNTS]

8.8.7 HUN-TINGTON'S DISEASE

CLINICAL

autosomal dominant progressive
    striatocortical atrophy manifesting as
    choreoathetosis and progressive
    dementia
1/10 000, new mutations extremely rare
onset at 40–50 years, choreoathetosis, early
    and relentless dementia, bradykinesia,
    behavioral changes, death
massive caudate and putamen atrophy
massive basal ganglia fibrillary gliosis
frontal cortical atrophy

IMAGING

MR
marked atrophy of caudate nucleus (and
    expansion of frontal horn)
atrophy of putamen and frontal cortex
high T2W signal in striatum

8.8.8 T-AY–S-ACHS DISEASE

8.9 LEUKODYSTROPHIES

MNEMONIC: GAMP CAMP

DEEP [GAMP]

8.9.1 G-LOBOID (KRABBE) LEUKODYSTROPHY

autosomal recessive lysosomal enzyme
    deficiency

IMAGING

symmetric deep white matter
    dysmyelination (high T2W signal) with
    stippled thalamic calcification
atrophy

8.9.2 A-DRENO-LEUKODYSTROPHY (ALD)/ ADRENOMYELONEUROPATHY

CLINICAL

X-linked or autosomal recessive peroxisomal
    enzyme deficiency

accumulation of very long chain fatty acids
    in brain, adrenals, red blood cells

Classic ALD (50%, X-linked)
onset at 5–10 years old, rapid progression

Adrenomyeloneuropathy (25%)
corticospinal tract and spinal cord
    involvement

Addison's disease only (10%)

IMAGING

MR
parietooccipital deep dysmyelination,
    abnormally high white matter T2W
    signal (includes splenium of corpus
    callosum)
posterior white matter predominance
dysmyelination progresses central to
    peripheral, posterior to anterior

8.9.3 M-ETACHROMATIC LEUKODYSTROPHY

autosomal recessive lysosome enzyme
    deficiency
abnormal brain tissue has metachromatic
    histological staining

IMAGING

symmetrical deep white matter
    dysmyelination (high on T2W) with
    atrophy and cerebellar involvement

8.9.4 P-HENYLKETONURIA (PKU)

CLINICAL

autosomal recessive deficiency of enzyme
    catabolizing phenylalanine
incidence approximately 1/10 000, but
    manifestations are rare (screened at
    birth)
classic PKU: severe intellectual impairment
    with normal sensory and motor functions

IMAGING

non specific abnormal high T2W deep white
    matter signal

SUPERFICIAL [CAMP]

8.9.5 C-ANAVAN DISEASE

CLINICAL

autosomal recessive inheritance of aspartate catabolic enzyme with accumulation of N-acetyl aspartate in neurons
macrocephaly, hypotonia, motor abnormalities

IMAGING

CT
diffuse symmetric cerebral and cerebellar hypodensity

MR
diffuse subcortical white matter high T2W signal
macrocephaly
ELEVATED NAA PEAK ON MR SPECTROSCOPY

8.9.6 A-LEXANDER DISEASE

macrocephaly, spasticity, may have intellectual retardation (in infantile form)

IMAGING

dysmyelination of subcortical and deep white matter starting with frontal lobes
macrocephaly

8.9.7 M-ERZBACHER–P-ELIZAEUS DISEASE

rare X-linked deficiency of a component of myelin
pendular nystagmus

IMAGING

patchy white matter dysmyelination ('tigroid pattern') or total dysmyelination (high T2W signal)
diffuse atrophy

8.10 MITOCHONDRIAL ENCEPHALOPATHIES

8.10.1 LEIGH DISEASE

see under gray matter degenerations

8.10.2 MELAS

= M-ITOCHONDRIAL MYOPATHY, E-NCEPHALOPATHY, L-ACTIC A-CIDOSIS AND S-TROKE LIKE EPISODES

CLINICAL

progressive neuronal dysfunction and other systemic manifestations resulting from a mitochondrial enzyme defect leading to inadequate oxidative phosphorylation
presents in late childhood, adolescence, early adulthood

Myopathy

Encephalopathy
seizures
sensorineural deafness
cortical blindness
hemiparesis

Lactic acidosis

Stroke like episodes
step wise progression
complete infarcts, laminar cell death, reversible injury with full or partial recovery (present as herpes simplex virus encephalopathy)

IMAGING

CT
no findings or low density consistent with infarction but not corresponding to arterial vascular territories

MR
high T2W signal in cortical ribbon of affected cortex
cortical abnormalities come before deep white matter changes
occipital lobes > parietal lobes > other
deep gray (basal ganglia, thalami) involved with patchy infarcts

DOES NOT FOLLOW ARTERIAL TERRITORIES

8.10.3 MERRF

= M-YOCLONIC E-PILEPSY WITH R-AGGED R-ED F-IBERS
mitochondrial DNA mutation
multiple infarcts, dentate and olive body degeneration, dysmyelination

8.10.4 KEARNS–SAYRE DISEASE

autosomal dominant, high serum pyruvate, behaves like Leigh disease

8.11 MULTIPLE SCLEROSIS (MS)

DEFINITION

autoimmune demyelinating disease presenting with multiple focal neurological deficits and usually with a progressive relapsing–remitting natural history

EPIDEMIOLOGY

incidence in Europeans 1/1000; young adults; female:male 2:1; prevalence higher in cold climates
family history a risk factor (x15 for first degree relative; monozygotic twin concordance 25%)

PATHOGENESIS

initiation mechanism unclear; no viral agent isolated yet; no link to other autoimmune diseases
cell mediated immune destruction of myelin in patches (plaques) centered on venules
neurological deficit from conduction failure
quiescence mechanism unclear
healing by gliosis with some remyelination

CLINICAL

Clinical definition
multiple neurological deficits separated both in space and in time
visual disturbance, orbital pain; spastic paresis; ataxia; paresthesias, neuralgia; bladder or bowel spasticity or flaccidity; personality disturbance

neurological deficits may resolve fully or partly (on or off treatment)

in general, slowly progressive relapsing–remitting disease with considerable morbidity and disability burden

Subtypes

8.11.1 CLASSIC MS (relapsing–remitting)

8.11.2 CHRONIC PROGRESSIVE MS

8.11.3 OPTIC NEURITIS

single isolated episode
as a prequel to MS

8.11.4 DEVIC DISEASE (neuromyelitis optica)

Asians; 20% rapid progression; rest as for MS

spinal cord and bilateral optic neuritis

8.11.5 ACUTE MS

rapid progressive course

MACRO

Plaque

firm gray well defined area of abnormal white matter; size and number variable

follows venules and veins radially ('Dawson's fingers')

classically corpus callosum, centrum semiovale, deep white matter, pons, middle cerebellar peduncle, medulla, cervical cord

Shadow plaque

less well defined healing or healed plaque, with partial remyelination

IMAGING

CT

most commonly normal

rarely shows active large plaques as focal hypodense areas

occasionally shows tumefactive plaques as focal hypodense masses with contrast enhancement

MR

single best imaging modality BUT a false negative rate exists, and MR abnormalities are not perfectly specific to MS (see DIFFERENTIAL)

many MR lesions are CLINICALLY SILENT

CRANIAL MS

90% of MS patients have MR lesions

isointense signal on T1W, high signal on T2W, PD and FLAIR sequences

diffusion restriction is present in active plaques

mild mass effect may be present (active plaques)

active plaques may enhance with contrast: ring enhancement is typical, BUT patchy or targetoid enhancement may occur

giant plaques (tumefactive MS)

late atrophy and gliosis, loss of enhancement, possibly cystic malacia

LOCATION

typically white matter

callososeptal interface (93% sensitivity, 97% specificity)

subependymal periventricular white matter (90% of MS) – particularly angles of lateral ventricles

10% posterior fossa: middle cerebral peduncle, pons, cerebellar white matter

10% spinal cord only

medial longitudinal fasciculus (relatively specific)

HELPFUL FINDINGS

abnormal T2W foci >3 mm in diameter, at least one >6 mm

callososeptal interface, brainstem, post fossa, cord lesions

SPINAL CORD MS

cervical cord tends to be involved ahead of thoracic cord and conus

acutely, foci if intramedullary high T2W signal which may have mild mass effect or may enhance

'healed' plaques produce atrophy and volume loss; enhancement may resolve; gliosis may cause persistent high T2W signal

contrast enhancement tends to demonstrate active plaques

OPTIC NEURITIS

also see Ch 12 entry

sequences: T2W, T2W (fat sat) or STIR; T1W pre and post gadolinium; axial and coronal

abnormal high T2W or PD signal along course of optic nerve (one or both) with occasional extension to chiasm

mild swelling, loss of CSF cuff around nerve

may have patchy contrast enhancement

MR SPECTROSCOPY

findings common to demyelinating disease in general, and not specific to MS

acutely increased choline:creatine due to demyelination and increased cell turnover

lactate/lipid increased; NAA:creatine not reduced in acute stage

chronic stage has reduced choline, creatine and NAA and elevated myo-inositol (all indicating gliosis)

(tumor has markedly elevated choline and reduced NAA, whereas in MS, NAA usually not reduced in acute stage)

Imaging differential of foci of high T2W
see Ch 10

8.12 NORMAL PRESSURE HYDROCEPHALUS

DEFINITION

triad of ataxia, dementia, incontinence

intracranial pressure monitor: intermittent abnormal waves

IMAGING

MR (communicating hydrocephalus)

large ventricles out of proportion to both sulci and dementia; bowing of corpus callosum (on sagittal images); dilated temporal horns with hippocampi intact (perihippocampal fissures small); distension of optic and infundibular recesses of the third ventricle

CSF flow void in aqueduct; may have transependymal edema

NUC MED (radionuclide ventriculography)

reflux of tracer into ventricles without clearance by 24 hours

delayed radiotracer clearance at vertex (shunting of most value in this pattern)

clearance may be normal or via ependymal pathways

8.13 OLIVO-PONTOCEREBELLAR ATROPHY

CLINICAL

ataxia, cerebellar symptoms

IMAGING

MR

volume loss and flattening of pons and middle cerebellar peduncles; abnormal pontine T2W/PD signal

volume loss and gliosis of olives

cerebellar bilateral hemispheric atrophy
pyramidal tracts not involved

8.14 PARKINSON'S DISEASE (PD)

DEFINITION

idiopathic Parkinsonism with substantia nigra degeneration and loss of dopaminergic neurons

CLINICAL

relatively common (incidence 1/1000 over 50 years old)
bradykinesia, mask facies, festinating gait, classical tremor, unilateral onset, persistent asymmetry; response to levodopa

IMAGING

CT
normal (unless there is coexistent atrophy)

MR
pars compacta is sandwiched between hypointense pars reticulata and red nucleus (T2W and PD sequences)
pars compacta width decreases in Parkinson's disease and related conditions (there is overlap with normal aging)
pars compacta may contain abnormal high T2W signal
cerebral atrophy (non specific and overlaps with other dementias and with normal age related volume loss)

NUC MED (dopaminergic imaging)
reduced substantia nigra DA activity

8.15 PARKINSON'S DISEASE RELATED CONDITIONS

GROUP DEFINITION AND CLASSIFICATION

spectrum of conditions which have loss of dopaminergic neurons and Parkinsonism in common

conditions which have Parkinsonism and other manifestations informally known as the 'Parkinson plus' conditions

8.15.1 PROGRESSIVE SUPRANUCLEAR PALSY

= Richardson–Steele–Olszewski syndrome
Parkinsonism, loss of upgaze, trunkal disequilibrium; dementia may occur
atrophy of substantia nigra, colliculi, subthalamic nuclei, globi pallidi, dentate nuclei
imaging findings of Parkinson's disease with possible further atrophy as above

8.15.2 SHY–DRAGER SYNDROME

Parkinsonism and autonomic dysfunction
imaging findings of Parkinson's disease or of striatonigral degeneration (depending on which is dominant)

8.15.3 STRIATONIGRAL DEGENERATION

CLINICAL

Parkinsonism unresponsive to levodopa; striatum and substantia nigra atrophy
MR findings of Parkinson's disease AND abnormal putaminal T2W/PD signal: low signal (deposition of paramagnetic material) or high signal (underlying gliosis)

8.16 PICK'S DISEASE

CLINICAL

rare dementia with marked frontal lobe atrophy and neuronal Pick bodies
part of the frontal lobe dementia spectrum
may be difficult to differentiate from Alzheimer disease
frontal signs (abnormal behavior, motivational disturbances, hypersexuality)

IMAGING

CT/MR
frontal and temporal atrophy, caudate atrophy, large frontal horns of lateral ventricles

NUC MED (HMPAO, ECD)/PET (FDG)
symmetrical bifrontal decreased activity

8.17 RADIATION NECROSIS

CLINICAL

EARLY post radiotherapy edema is usually not a diagnostic problem
LATE radiation necrosis occurs at 6 months to several years post radiotherapy: gliotic response, obliterative endarteritis with necrosis, neoangiogenesis, disrupted blood–brain barrier; clinical presentation may be similar to tumor recurrence, or an asymptomatic imaging finding

IMAGING (late radiation necrosis)

MR
edema (vasogenic or mixed)
area of abnormal thick contrast enhancement in tumor bed
possible central cavitation (especially if debulking had occurred)
stable mass effect
conforms to radiation portal (this is of use if the mass and abnormal enhancement are away from the tumor bed in incidentally traversed normal brain)
morphologically on a single scan in time, radiation necrosis and tumor recurrence are difficult to distinguish

MR SPECTROSCOPY (MRS)

RADIATION NECROSIS (dead tissue)
reduced choline
reduced NAA
reduced creatine
lactate/lipid may be present

RADIATION ENCEPHALITIS
underlying process is demyelination and astrocytosis
increased choline:creatine
decreased NAA:creatine
increased myo-inositol:creatine
DO A FOLLOWUP MRS: TUMOR RECURRENCE WILL LEAD TO FURTHER INCREASES in choline:creatine ratio, AND RADIATION NECROSIS WILL REDUCE the choline:creatine ratio
heterogeneity leads to sampling errors (ideally, need to cover entire tumor bed)

DIFFERENTIAL: GLIOMA RECURRENCE
decreased NAA:creatine

choline:creatine >2.0 indicates recurrence

choline:creatine <2.0 equivocal (major differential is radiation encephalitis, see above)

heterogeneity leads to sampling errors (ideally, need to cover entire tumor bed)

NUC MED (TI)

thallium is taken up and retained in viable tumor, including recurrence, where blood–brain barrier is disrupted

in radiation necrosis there is no thallium uptake or early staining with significant washout

PET (FDG)

no FDG uptake in area of abnormal contrast enhancement indicates radiation necrosis not tumor recurrence

FDG uptake comparable to normal brain is equivocal

markedly increased FDG uptake suggests tumor recurrence

9. SPINAL CORD

9.1 ACUTE/SUBACUTE TRANSVERSE MYELOPATHY

DEFINITION

clinical syndrome of acute/subacute spinal cord dysfunction (usually with a demonstrable segmental level) in the absence of mechanical cord compression

DIFFERENTIAL DIAGNOSIS: COMPRESSIVE MYELOPATHY

ETIOLOGY

Idiopathic
diagnosis of exclusion
possibly autoimmune etiology

Infective

INFECTIVE MYELITIS

VIRAL

  HERPES SIMPLEX VIRUS

  POLIO VIRUS

  HIV

  COXSACKIE

BACTERIAL

TB

Vascular disease

HEMORRHAGE

ARTERIAL INFARCT, ISCHEMIA

VENOUS HYPERTENSION, VENOUS INFARCT

AVM, AVF, HEMANGIOMA

Tumor

Radiation myelopathy

Autoimmune

MULTIPLE SCLEROSIS

SYSTEMIC LUPUS ERYTHEMATOSUS (SLE)

POST VIRAL/ACUTE DISSEMINATED ENCEPHALOMYELITIS (ADEM)

Metabolic

B12 DEFICIENCY: SUBACUTE COMBINED DEGENERATION OF THE CORD

ALCOHOLIC

IMAGING (general features of group)

CT
usually unhelpful except to exclude bony compression

MR

normal OR

'TRANSVERSE MYELITIS'

single or multiple foci of intramedullary low T1W and high T2W signal with variably defined margin, and variable amount of mass effect

may or may not enhance with contrast

prominent mass effect suggests tumor (should enhance)

multiple lesions with intervening normal cord makes tumor very unlikely

VS 'SURGICAL LESION' (differential)

COMPRESSION

ABSCESS

TUMOR

HEMATOMA

AV MALFORMATION, HEMANGIOMA

AV FISTULA (indirect signs)

9.1.1 INFECTIVE MYELITIS

viral (herpes simplex, poliovirus, HIV, Coxsackie virus)

TB

bacterial

IMAGING

MR
may enhance with contrast
abscess has mass effect

9.1.2 SPINAL INFARCTION

see its own entry

9.1.3 SPINAL CORD TUMOR

ependymoma is commonest

astrocytoma (usually fibrillary) is second commonest

other: metastasis, lymphoma, other CNS primary tumors

9.1.4 RADIATION MYELOPATHY

CLINICAL

appropriate history: spinal irradiation
onset between 3 months and 3 years

IMAGING

MR

intramedullary focus of high T2W signal, low T1W signal with contrast enhancement and mass effect

CONTAINED WITHIN RADIATION PORTAL

evolves into atrophy with volume loss

9.1.5 MULTIPLE SCLEROSIS

see degenerations section

9.1.6 POST VIRAL/ADEM

see its own entry

9.1.7 SUBACUTE COMBINED DEGENERATION OF THE CORD

very rare

B12 deficiency, vacuolation of myelin

ataxia and paresthesias

classically, selective involvement of dorsal columns with abnormally high T2W signal

9.2 ASTROCYTOMA

CLINICAL

commonest spinal tumor in children
second commonest spinal tumor in adults
(female = male)
cervical > thoracic
usually low grade fibrillary astrocytoma

IMAGING

MR

long multisegment intramedullary mass
diffusely expanding cord with cystic
change
isointense on T1W, high T2W signal
all spinal astrocytomas enhance with
contrast (solid portion of tumor)
syrinx above and below
mass/syrinx may expand canal if
longstanding

9.3 DEGENERATIVE DISEASE

see Ch 04 disk degenerative disease

9.4 DISK PROTRUSIONS

see Ch 04 disk protrusions

9.5 EPENDYMOMA

(myxopapillary type)

female > male, ~30 year old, commonest
spinal tumor
fleshy sausage shaped moderately vascular
mass
involves conus medullaris and filum
terminale
slow growing, cystic change, hemorrhage
see tumors section

9.6 MENINGIOMA

second commonest intradural extramedullary
(primary) mass
see tumors section

9.7 MULTIPLE SCLEROSIS

also see degenerations section

9.8 NERVE SHEATH TUMORS

also see schwannoma and neurofibroma
under tumors

CLINICAL

most common intradural extramedullary
(primary) tumor
schwannoma or neurofibroma (associated
with NF1)
present with pain, radiculopathy, cord or
conus compression
15% extradural, 70% extradural
intramedullary, 15% dumbbell, 1%
intramedullary

IMAGING

XR

classically, smooth widening of neural exit
foramina at one or multiple levels
without cortical loss or destruction
(pressure expansion)
may have posterior scalloping of vertebral
bodies (dural ectasia)

Fluoro

mobile on myelography (meningiomas are
fixed to dura)

CT

classic intradural extramedullary rounded
mass
often not detectable on CT without
subarachnoid contrast

MR

frequently multiple (neurofibromatosis 1)
isointense or slightly high T1W signal, high
T2W signal (may be similar to CSF)
heterogeneous texture in larger tumors, may
have central areas of low T2W signal
('target sign')
vivid contrast enhancement
'dumbbell' tumors extend along nerve root
sleeves into neural exit foramina
(particularly so in neurofibromatosis)

9.9 SPINAL CANAL/CORD MALFORMATIONS

see Ch 20

9.10 SPINAL CANAL CYSTS AND MIMICKERS

see Ch 04

9.11 SPINAL CANAL STENOSIS

see Ch 04

9.12 SPINAL INFECTION

see Ch 02, Ch 03
for cord abscess, see cerebritis

9.13 SPINAL ISCHEMIA/ INFARCTION

ETIOLOGY

aortic dissection with occlusion of artery of
Adamkiewicz and other radicular feeders
aortic surgery with cross clamping
rare complication of spinal angiography
unusual causes of infarction (see infarcts –
unusual)

CLINICAL

9.13.1 Anterior spinal artery (ASA) infarct

commonest spinal infarct
cervical rare, thoracic and lumbar more
common
infarction of cord except posterior columns
produces flaccid paralysis with loss of
pain and temperature sensation, but
preserved touch and proprioception

9.13.2 Posterior spinal artery (PSA) infarct

very rare in isolation

9.13.3 ASA and PSA (full cord) infarct

IMAGING

MR

high T2W signal within gray or both gray and white matter either diffusely involving entire cross section or corresponding to a vascular territory (usually ASA)

mild swelling acutely, eventual gliosis and atrophy

infarct enhances after several days and persists for weeks to months

9.14 SPINAL VASCULAR MALFORMATIONS

also see vascular section

9.14.1 SPINAL DURAL ARTERIOVENOUS FISTULA (AVF)

CLINICAL

presumed acquired dural AVF of older adults involving a thoracolumbar nerve root sleeve

presents with chronic or 'stuttering' lumbar or thoracic myelopathy secondary to spinal venous hypertension

IMAGING

Angio

(direct catheter spinal angiography of segmental arteries)

demonstrates level and origin of the fistula

cardinal sign early abnormal contrast filling of dilated spinal veins

prelude to endovascular embolization

MR

occasionally may be totally normal

affected cord (not always directly related to the level of the AVF) has high T2W and low T1W signal

mild swelling may be present; cord infarcts may enhance

chronic atrophy eventually supervenes

dilated pial veins visible as serpiginous flow voids that show vascular contrast enhancement

9.14.2 SPINAL CORD ARTERIOVENOUS MALFORMATION (AVM)

CLINICAL

intraparenchymal AVM, usually presenting with acute hemorrhage in younger patients

associated with other AV malformations elsewhere

IMAGING

MR

nidus: a tight or more extensive mix of slow flows or flow voids; may extend outside the spinal cord

surrounding blood products of different ages, possibly with gliosis

Angio

(direct catheter spinal angiography of segmental arteries)

gold standard examination showing supply and drainage of the nidus and any associated aneurysms etc

prelude to endovascular embolization

9.14.3 SPINAL CORD ARTERIOVENOUS FISTULA

intradural AVF in the thoracolumbar area with fistula from spinal arteries to spinal veins

9.14.4 CAVERNOUS HEMANGIOMA

may present with acute hemorrhage, 'stuttering' neurological deficit or slow myelopathy

IMAGING

see vascular section, cavernous hemangioma may have an associated syrinx

9.15 SUBARACHNOID METASTASES

ETIOLOGY

Drop metastases

GLIOBLASTOMA

EPENDYMOMA

MEDULLOBLASTOMA

PRIMITIVE NEUROECTODERMAL TUMOR

CHOROID PLEXUS TUMORS

Hematogenous metastases

LUNG CARCINOMA

BREAST CARCINOMA

MELANOMA

LYMPHOMA, LEUKEMIA

IMAGING

MR

nodular deposits or focal masses

low signal on T1W sequences, and outlined by CSF as masses or thickening on T2W sequences

diffuse thickening or clumping without focal mass

all enhance with contrast

root sleeve obliteration

9.16 SYRINGO-HYDROMYELIA

DEFINITION

abnormal intraspinal accumulation of CSF or other fluid either in the central canal, in an intramedullary cleft, or both

ETIOLOGY

Non neoplastic

TRAUMA

50% of spinal cord injury patients presenting with new symptoms will have a syrinx

CHRONIC COMPRESSION

CONGENITAL
SYRINGOHYDROMYELIA

ISOLATED

PART OF CHIARI I

PART OF CHIARI II

POST SUBARACHNOID
HEMORRHAGE

Neoplastic

SPINAL CORD PRIMARY TUMOR

LEPTOMENINGEAL
CARCINOMATOSIS

PATHOGENESIS

spinal cord cystic myelomalacia in trauma
?altered CSF flow dynamics with CSF
pulsation probably responsible for syrinx
growth

CLINICAL

incidental finding vs progressive myelopathy
cervical syringohydromyelia: dissociated
sensory loss (loss of pain and
temperature sensation in upper limbs),
classically with neuropathic shoulder
joints

IMAGING

CT

expanded cord contour (may not be present
if there is simultaneous atrophy)
with myelography, late trapping of contrast
within syrinx

MR (non neoplastic syrinx)

well marginated cystic elongated spaces
within cord parenchyma
unicameral or multicompartmental, variable
length
usually slightly hyperintense to CSF on both
T1W and T2W (protein contents)
cord expanded or atrophied around syrinx,
or both

MR (neoplastic syrinx)

spinal cord tumor mass (contrast enhancing)
associated with syrinx

margins of syrinx may enhance as well,
often irregularly and incompletely (syrinx
may be secondary to tumor, but be
outside of it)

10. SYNDROMES

10.1 SYNDROME ENTRIES IN Ch 20

CEPHALOCELES

CHIARI MALFORMATIONS

CORPUS CALLOSUM AGENESIS

HOLOPROSENCEPHALY SPECTRUM

MIGRATION AND SULCATION
ANOMALIES

POSTERIOR FOSSA
MALFORMATIONS

10.2 ATAXIA TELANGIECTASIA

1/40 000, AR, chromosome 11q
cerebellar atrophy, ataxia
cutaneous telangiectasias
immunodeficiency, recurrent lung infections
progression to leukemia/lymphoma

10.3 BASAL CELL NEVUS SYNDROME (Gorlin–Goltz)

autosomal dominant, chromosome 9q31
mutations

CNS

lamellar dural calcification
falx calcification (100%)
callosal dysgenesis
may develop medulloblastoma

HEAD AND NECK

multiple odontogenic keratocysts
hypertelorism
multiple basal cell carcinomas
short fourth metacarpal

10.4 CADASIL

C-EREBRAL A-UTOSOMAL
D-OMINANT A-RTERIOPATHY,
S-UBCORTICAL
I-NFARCTS,
L-EUKOENCEPHALOPATHY
eosinophilic arteriolosclerosis of deep
perforating arteries
progressive multifocal deep white, gray
demyelination and stroke like episodes
leads to pseudobulbar palsy and multiinfarct
dementia at 40–60 years

10.5 NEURO-FIBROMATOSIS 1 (NF1)

EPIDEMIOLOGY

1/2000 to 1/4000 (50% new mutations), 90%
of all NF
autosomal dominant, neurofibromin (tumor
suppressor gene) mutation on
chromosome 17q11

CNS

10% OPTIC GLIOMA
variable contrast enhancement
10% aggressive

NON OPTIC GLIOMA
usually low grade brainstem astrocytoma

(>75%) BENIGN BRAIN HAMARTOMAS
glial proliferation, spongiosis
classic unidentified bright objects (high on
T2W), regress after 12 years
basal ganglia, internal capsule, cerebellar
peduncles

SPINAL CORD ASTROCYTOMA

PERIPHERAL NERVES/ NEUROENDOCRINE

SIMPLE NEUROFIBROMAS
central
cutaneous

30% PLEXIFORM NEUROFIBROMAS
orbit, scalp
spinal roots
plexi
10% sarcomatous change

MALIGNANT PERIPHERAL NERVE SHEATH TUMORS

PHEOCHROMOCYTOMAS

CARCINOID TUMORS

SKELETAL

30% SCOLIOSIS

DURAL ECTASIA

vertebral scalloping
meningoceles, large exit foramina

HYPOPLASTIC SPHENOID WING

temporoorbital herniation

FOCAL GIGANTISM

RIBBON RIBS, TIBIAL BOWING, PSEUDOJOINTS

OPHTHALMOCUTANEOUS

café-au-lait spots
inguinal and axillary freckles
Lisch nodules
buphthalmos
retinal phacomas
orbital plexiform neurofibromas

VASCULAR

intimal proliferation (fibromuscular dysplasia), arterial occlusions
cerebral arterial occlusions

DIAGNOSTIC CRITERIA: TWO OR MORE OF

1. 6 or more café-au-lait patches (>5 mm prepubertal, >15 mm adult)
2. 2 or more neurofibromas or 1 plexiform neurofibroma
3. axillary and/or inguinal freckling
4. optic nerve glioma
5. characteristic bony abnormality
6. first degree relative with NF1

10.6 NEUROFIBROMATOSIS (NF2)

EPIDEMIOLOGY

1/40 000 (50% are new mutations), 10% of all NF

autosomal dominant mutation of tumor suppressor gene (NF2 gene) on chromosome 22q12

BRAIN

vestibular schwannomas (bilateral)
other cranial nerve schwannomas
multiple meningiomas
choroid plexus calcification
glial hamartomas
cerebral parenchymal and choroid calcification

SPINE

spinal cord ependymomas
nerve root schwannomas
meningiomas/meningioangiomatosis
cutaneous nerve schwannomas

EYE

posterior lens opacities
retinal hamartomas

DIAGNOSTIC CRITERIA

1. bilateral vestibular schwannomas; or
2. patient has a first degree relative with NF2 and has:
a. one vestibular schwannoma or
b. two of: meningioma, schwannoma, glioma, lens opacity, cerebral calcification
OR
3. two of
a. vestibular schwannoma
b. multiple meningiomas
c. schwannoma, glioma, neurofibroma, lens opacity, cerebral calcification

10.7 OSLER–WEBER–RENDU (hereditary hemorrhagic telangiectasia)

see Ch 15

10.8 STURGE–WEBER SYNDROME

= ENCEPHALOTRIGEMINAL ANGIOMATOSIS

PATHOGENESIS

embryonal leptomeningeal angioma leading to deficient normal superficial cortical venous network
secondary cortical ischemic atrophy and calcification and prominent deep vein collaterals

BRAIN (parietooccipital cortex >other)

gyriform tramtrack calcification (visible on skull XR from 2 years on)
cortical and subcortical gliosis
small hemicranium, hypertrophic cortex
prominent deep veins
pial angioma (may enhance with contrast)

EYE

ocular choroid angioma

FACE

cranial nerve V1 port wine stain

10.9 TUBEROUS SCLEROSIS

EPIDEMIOLOGY

1/10 000, autosomal dominant, low penetrance; 2/3 have chromosome 9q34 abnormality (TSC1 gene), 1/3 have chromosome 16p13 abnormality (TSC2 gene)
(<50%) classic triad of mental retardation, seizures, adenoma sebaceum
abnormal radial glial-neuronal unit

CNS

SUBEPENDYMAL HAMARTOMAS (95%)
calcify from 1 year on, may contrast enhance

CORTICAL TUBERS (95%)
expanded elevated gliotic bumpy gyrus
associated with epilepsy
CT: hypodense white, 50% calcify
MR: IN NEONATES: high T1W, low T2W signal;
IN ADULTS: low T1W, high T2W signal

ABNORMAL RADIAL MYELIN (white matter hamartoma) (95%)

linear, curved, wedge shape high T2W signal white matter tracts

SUBEPENDYMAL GIANT CELL ASTROCYTOMA (10%)

slowly enlarging contrast enhancing nodule at foramen of Monro

see its own entry

VASCULAR DYSPLASIAS

CARDIAC

RHABDOMYOMA (50%)
see Ch 14

KIDNEYS

ANGIOMYOLIPOMAS (50%)
see Ch 08

LUNGS

LYMPHANGIOLEIOMYOMATOSIS LIKE CHANGE
see Ch 13

EYE

retinal hamartomas (50%)

VISCERAL HAMARTOMAS

lung
duodenum
pancreas
liver

SKELETAL

cortical thickening
bony islands

CUTANEOUS

adenoma sebaceum (angiofibromas) (80%)
shagreen patches (30%)
hypomelanotic patches

10.10 VON HIPPEL–LINDAU SYNDROME (vHL)

see Ch 08

SECTION 3

1. NORMAL

1.1 ABBREVIATIONS

CCA: common carotid artery
CN: cranial nerve or nerves
ECA: external carotid artery
HD: Hodgkin's disease
IAC/IAM: internal auditory canal / internal auditory meatus
ICA: internal carotid artery
IJV: internal jugular vein
NHL: non Hodgkin's lymphoma
SCC: squamous cell carcinoma

1.2 ANATOMICAL VARIANTS – PARANASAL SINUSES

Septal deviation, spur

Concha bullosa
pneumatized middle concha

Paradoxical middle concha
lower edge curves medially rather than laterally
usually bilateral and symmetrical

Haller cell
an ethmoidal cell extending under anteromedial orbital floor
rarely cause of orbital pathology if diseased

Agger nasii cell
anterior ethmoidal cell that lies anterior to frontonasal duct

Extended sphenoid pneumatization
into lateral sphenoid bone, pterygoid plates, middle cranial fossa floor or clinoid processes

Pneumatized petrous apex
if aerated, obvious on CT and a signal void on MR
if fluid filled, produces low T1W and high T2W signal on MR

1.3 DENTAL NOTATION

Orientation
mesial: closer to midline
distal: closer to condyle

buccal or labial: closer to cheek or lip
lingual or palatal: closer to tongue (mandible) or palate (maxilla)

Palmer's (UK) notation
written notation: angle for side and jaw (drawn as if facing patient), tooth numbered
QUADRANT: ⌐ right upper; ⌐ left upper; ⌐ right lower; ⌐ left lower
NUMBER: adult 1–8, child A–E

FDI notation
QUADRANT: 1–4 adult, 5–8 child
facing patient, starting upper right and progressing clockwise
NUMBER: tooth numbered

Examples
⌐2 = 3–2 = left lower 2nd incisor
⌐6 = 2–6 left upper 1st molar
E⌐ = 8–5 right lower 2nd deciduous molar
3⌐ = 1–3 = left upper canine

1.4 HARNSBERGER HEAD AND NECK SPACES

Suprahyoid neck
PARAPHARYNGEAL
fat, pharyngeal venous plexus, branches of CN V3

PHARYNGEAL MUCOSAL
tonsils, adenoids, constrictor muscles and pharyngobasilar fascia, distal auditory tube

MASTICATOR
masticator muscles: masseter and temporalis, lateral and medial pterygoids; inferior alveolar nerve and motor branch of CN V3; mandible

PAROTID
parotid gland and duct, facial nerve, retromandibular vein and external carotid/superficial temporal artery, lymph nodes

CAROTID
internal carotid artery, internal jugular vein, CN IX to XII, lymph nodes

RETROPHARYNGEAL
fat, retropharyngeal nodes

PERIVERTEBRAL
vertebrae, disks, spinal canal; prevertebral muscles and spinal muscles; scalenus anterior, brachial plexus, scaleni medius and posterior; vertebral artery

Oral cavity
TONGUE, SUBLINGUAL SPACE
interface to submandibular space: mylohyoid muscle; the two spaces communicate posteriorly around mylohyoid posterior border
hyoglossus muscle separates deep from superficial parts
deep to hyoglossus: tongue muscles (genioglossus, styloglossus, intrinsic muscles), CN IX, lingual artery
superficial to hyoglossus: lingual nerve, CN XII, submandibular duct, sublingual gland, mucosa

SUBMANDIBULAR SPACE
submandibular gland, anterior loop of CN XII, lymph nodes, digastric (anterior belly)

BUCCINATOR SPACE
buccinator muscle, buccopharyngeal raphe, parotid duct, lymph nodes, mucosa

ORAL MUCOSA

Infrahyoid neck
LARYNX, TRACHEA

PHARYNX, ESOPHAGUS

THYROID

CAROTID

RETROPHARYNGEAL SPACE
NOTE: communicates with mediastinum

POSTERIOR CERVICAL SPACE
(i.e. posterior triangle)
CN XI, lymph nodes
brachial plexus (in transit from perivertebral space to axilla)

PERIVERTEBRAL SPACE

1.5 LARYNX REGIONS

Supraglottis (supraglottic larynx)
epiglottis
aryepiglottic folds
false cords
upper arytenoid cartilages
paraglottic space
preglottic space

Glottis
true cords
anterior and posterior commissures (each <1 mm of soft tissue)
vocal process of arytenoid cartilage

Infraglottis (infraglottic larynx)

conus elasticus

cord undersurface

mucosa

Hypopharynx (see pharynx)

Lymphatic drainage patterns

watershed is at the cord epithelium, which is
relatively free of lymphatics (as a result,
true cord SCC metastasize late)

supraglottis – upper deep nodes

glottis, infraglottis – lower deep nodes

1.6 PHARYNX REGIONS

Nasopharynx

POSTEROSUPERIORLY: roof of nasopharynx
at the skull base, posterior to posterior
bony choanae

LATERALLY: lateral wall including fossa of
Rosenmuller and torus tubarii/tubal
orifice

INFERIORLY: superior surface of soft palate

Oropharynx

ANTERIORLY: base of tongue, valleculae

LATERALLY: tonsil and palatoglossal and
palatopharyngeal folds

POSTERIORLY: posterior pharyngeal wall

SUPERIORLY: inferior surface of soft palate
and uvula

Hypopharynx (= laryngopharynx)

ANTERIORLY: post cricoid area

ANTEROLATERALLY: pyriform fossa and
pyriform apex (inferiorly)

POSTEROLATERALLY AND POSTERIORLY:
posterior wall (extends from one thyroid
cartilage edge to the other) and
cricopharyngeus

1.7 ORBIT COMPARTMENTS

GLOBE

OPTIC NERVE COMPLEX

MUSCULAR CONE AND INTRACONAL
SPACE

EXTRACONAL SPACE AND LACRIMAL
GLAND

1.8 ORBIT MEASUREMENTS

Optic canal

diameter 4–6 mm; side–side difference
<1 mm

Optic nerve

normal diameter 2.5–4.5 mm

length: intraocular 1 mm, intraorbital 30 mm
over 25 mm, intracanalicular 10 mm,
intracranial 10 mm

1.9 LYMPH NODE GROUPS

Superficial horizontal chain

SUBOCCIPITAL NODES

POST AURICULAR AND PREAURICULAR
NODES

PAROTID NODES

SUBMANDIBULAR NODES

SUBMENTAL NODES

Superficial vertical chain

FACIAL NODES (i.e. buccinator nodes)

ANTERIOR JUGULAR NODES

PRELARYNGEAL AND PRETRACHEAL
NODES

PARATRACHEAL NODES

Deep vertical chain

INTERNAL JUGULAR NODES (FROM
JUGULODIGASTRIC TO
JUGULOOMOHYOID NODE)

POSTERIOR CERVICAL SPACE NODES (TO
SUPRACLAVICULAR FOSSA) (i.e. posterior
triangle or spinal accessory nodes)

Deep horizontal chain

RETROPHARYNGEAL (LATERAL OR
MEDIAL) NODES

lateral retropharyngeal nodes extend from
the level of the hard palate to the skull
base

medial retropharyngeal nodes extend from
the palate to the hyoid

Level of node in vertical chains

HIGH (or UPPER)–ABOVE HYOID

MID (or MIDDLE)–HYOID TO CRICOID

LOW (or LOWER)–BELOW CRICOID

Surgical level classification

LEVEL I

submental and submandibular nodes

IA: submental; IB: submandibular

LEVEL II

upper internal jugular nodes

IIB: posterior to IJV and not touching it; IIA:
all others

LEVEL III

middle internal jugular nodes

LEVEL IV

lower internal jugular nodes

LEVEL V

posterior triangle (posterior cervical space,
spinal accessory) nodes

VA: upper and middle nodes; VB: lower
nodes

LEVEL VI

anterior jugular nodes,
prelaryngeal/pretracheal and
paratracheal nodes

LEVEL VII

upper mediastinal nodes inferior to
suprasternal notch

1.10 SALIVARY GLANDS

Gland secretory type

PAROTID:	serous
SUBMANDIBULAR:	mixed seromucinous
SUBLINGUAL:	mixed mucoserous
MINOR:	mucous

Age related change

gradual fatty replacement

scattered oncocyte metaplasia

Imaging

CT

variable amount of intraglandular fat

usually heterogeneous low density (between
muscle and fat); fat content increases
with age or post irradiation

occasionally (children, young adults) density
same as muscle

enhances with contrast

MR

PAROTID GLAND

heterogeneous high T1W signal (not as high
as pure fat) that follows the same rules
as low density on CT

heterogeneous intermediate T1W and PD
signal (higher than muscle)

enhances with contrast

SUBMANDIBULAR GLAND

signal closer to muscle (compared with parotid gland)

enhances with contrast

PAROTID GLAND CROSS SECTIONAL ANATOMY

ANTERIOR TO POSTERIOR

ramus of mandible, gland and contents, styloid process (stylomastoid foramen laterally), carotid sheath

SUPERFICIAL TO DEEP

parotid duct, superficial part of gland, CN VII, retromandibular vein, superficial temporal artery, deep part of gland

FACIAL NERVE POSITION

facial nerve course is stylomastoid foramen, lateral to styloid process, lateral to retromandibular vein

1.11 THYROID DIMENSIONS

LOBE SIZE <2 X 3 X 4 CM

1.12 THYROID NUCLEAR MEDICINE SCANNING

Iodine

I-131

tracer dose: 5 to 50 microCuries

(do pregnancy test)

post thyroidectomy diagnostic dose: 2–3 mCi

I-123

diagnostic radioiodine of choice because of: half-life of 13 hours, photon energy of 159 keV, no beta emissions

tracer dose: 100–400 mCi (do pregnancy test)

NORMAL DISTRIBUTION

thyroid

salivary glands

oral cavity and swallowed saliva

lacrimal (minor) gastric mucosa, colon

faint liver (radioiodine T3/T4 de-iodination)

kidneys, bladder, urine contamination

24 HOUR NORMAL THYROID UPTAKE 10–30% OF TOTAL DOSE

Pertechnetate

20 MINUTE UPTAKE 1–4% OF TOTAL DOSE

THYROID TO SUBMANDIBULAR RATIO 2:1 to 5:1

THYROID TO BACKGROUND RATIO 6:1 to 11:1

1.13 THYROID I-131 THERAPY (overview)

In all patients

exclude pregnancy (beta hCG)

stop antithyroid medications for 2 weeks

Graves' disease

confirm Graves' disease (i.e. autoantibodies, thyrotoxicosis, increased thyroid uptake)

dose range 5–10 mCi

does not treat extrathyroid autoimmune manifestations

may give beta blockers to avoid thyroid storm

side effects: pain, swelling, thyroid storm (T4 release from damaged follicles) – treat with steroids

may undertreat if aiming for euthyroidism, requiring a repeat dose

eventual hypothyroidism highly likely (natural history of both treated and untreated disease) – monitor with TFTs, will require replacement therapy

Toxic nodule

dose range is 5–10 mCi

prognosis of cure is excellent; normal thyroid tissue is usually not affected if it is suppressed on the diagnostic scan (low risk of late hypothyroidism)

Toxic multinodular goiter

doses range between 5 and 15 mCi (depends on gland size and uptake and patient's history and cardiac status)

may give beta blockers to avoid thyroid storm

side effects: pain, swelling, thyroid storm (T4 release from damaged follicles) – treat with steroids

very rarely, acute thyroid inlet syndrome occurs secondary to swelling of retrosternal goiter

may require several treatments as suppressed follicles become dominant in turn

eventual hypothyroidism likely – monitor with TFTs, will require replacement therapy

Thyroid tissue ablation post thyroidectomy

routinely done after (near) total thyroidectomy to eliminate all thyroid tissue

wait till TSH >50 mU/L (or at least 6 weeks post surgery)

choice of empiric dose versus whole body dosimetry (with calculation of estimated radiation delivery to tumor) is controversial, as dosimetry is difficult, imprecise and theoretically may cause stunning

diagnostic study (I-123 or low dose I-131, beware of stunning with I-131)

avoid pregnancy and breastfeeding for at least 6 months post treatment

NO METASTASES OBVIOUS

empiric dose 70–100 mCi

TREATMENT OF IODINE AVID METASTASES

dose varies from 150 to 300 mCi

risk of leukemia starts increasing after a cumulative dose of 1000 mCi

treatment of multifocal lung metastases carries the theoretical risk of radiation induced pulmonary fibrosis

treatment of cerebral metastases carries the risk of acute cerebral edema (may cover with steroids)

FOLLOWUP SCANS (off thyroxine)

regular thyroglobulin levels (thyroglobulin is very sensitive for carcinoma recurrence after thyroid ablation)

scanning may not be necessary in low risk patients (thyroglobulin levels only)

first scan at 6 months, then yearly for ~5 years

after negative scan, restart thyroxine to suppress TSH to near absent levels

1.14 THYROID COLD IODINE BLOCKING

Application

used whenever I-131 is used as a tracer or therapeutic nuclide chelated to organic molecule (e.g. MIBG, antibodies)

Sample protocol

supersaturated potassium iodide solution (Lugol's iodine) with 5% I2 and 10% KI

10 drops tds, start 2–3 days in advance, continue for 7–10 days

2. GAMUTS

2.1 HEAD AND NECK SPACES GAMUTS

(all modalities)

these gamuts are organized by head and neck Harnsberger space

2.1.1 CAROTID SPACE

CCA/ICA
ANEURYSM

FALSE ANEURYSM

DISSECTION

INFRAHYOID MASS: 2ND BRANCHIAL CLEFT CYST

IJV
NORMAL ASYMMETRY

THROMBOSIS

MEDIASTINAL OBSTRUCTION, DILATION

Lymphoid (jugular chain nodes)
BENIGN

REACTIVE LYMPHADENOPATHY

INFECTIVE LYMPHADENOPATHY

LYMPH NODE ABSCESS

MALIGNANT

SCC METASTASES

NHL

INFRAHYOID MASS: HODGKIN'S DISEASE; THYROID METASTASES

Cranial nerves IX–XII
BENIGN

PARAGANGLIOMA

NERVE SHEATH TUMOR

MENINGIOMA

2.1.2 CYSTIC MASS
(any compartment)

Congenital
BRANCHIAL CLEFT CYST

1st BRANCHIAL CLEFT CYST

    INTRAPAROTID AND RARE

2nd BRANCHIAL CLEFT CYST

    95% OF ALL BRANCHIAL CLEFT CYSTS

    INTERCAROTID (anywhere along course of cleft)

3rd BRANCHIAL CLEFT CYST

    POSTERIOR CERVICAL SPACE

THORNWALT'S CYST

MIDLINE HIGH PHARYNGEAL MUCOSAL SPACE CYST

THYROGLOSSAL DUCT CYST

LYMPHANGIOMA/HEMANGIOMA

EPIDERMOID/DERMOID

Acquired
SALIVARY RETENTION CYST/SIALOCELE

RANULA (sublingual gland retention cyst/mucocele)

THYROID CYST

PARATHYROID CYST

LARYNGOCELE

look for SCC obstructing ventricle as cause

PHARYNGEAL DIVERTICULUM

Cystic necrosis
ABSCESS

NECROTIC SCC METASTASIS

(cystic degeneration in salivary tumor)

2.1.3 JAW GAMUTS

2.1.3.1 Lytic lesions in jaws
in dental/OPG radiology, 'CYST' = cavity (lined by epithelium or not) and containing amorphous or acellular material

indolent cyst pushes teeth, aggressive erodes teeth

INFECTION RELATED 'CYSTS'
APICAL GRANULOMA (smaller)

APICAL CYST (larger)

LATERAL CYST (rare)

RESIDUAL CYST (post extraction)

INFECTION RELATED NON CYSTS
CARIES

APICAL OSTEOMYELITIS

TRAUMA
(POST) TRAUMATIC BONE CYST

DEVELOPMENTAL CYSTS
DENTIGEROUS CYST = FOLLICULAR CYST

contains a tooth crown

ODONTOGENIC KERATOCYST = PRIMORDIAL CYST

keratinising cyst of dental lamina origin, with a regular basal cell layer and internal keratinisation; high recurrence rate

association: Gorlin syndrome (rare)

NASOPALATINE DUCT CYST

specific site at nasopalatine duct

PITFALL
Stafne bone cavity = impression by submandibular gland

2.1.3.2 Jaw specific tumors
ORAL SCC

AMELOBLASTOMA (adamantinoma)

benign, locally agressive tumor of odontogenic epithelium with a fibrous stroma

BURKITT'S LYMPHOMA

2.1.3.3 Lytic lesions at mandibular angle
ODONTOGENIC KERATOCYST

CT: dense nodules of keratin

MR: medium-high T1W signal, medium-low T2W signal

DENTIGEROUS CYST

contains a tooth crown

AMELOBLASTOMA

MR: low T1W signal, high T2W signal, thick wall; mural papillary nodules with dense contrast enhancement

GENERIC LYTIC LESION

2.1.4 MASTICATOR SPACE

Mandible, teeth
BENIGN

ABSCESS, OSTEOMYELITIS

BENIGN BONE TUMOR

MALIGNANT

OSTEOSARCOMA

MALIGNANT BONE TUMOR

Muscles of mastication
BENIGN

HYPERTROPHY OR ATROPHY

MALIGNANT

RHABDOMYOSARCOMA

Lymphoid/vascular
BENIGN

HEMANGIOMA, LYMPHANGIOMA

MALIGNANT

EXTRANODAL NHL

CN V3/Inferior alveolar nerve
BENIGN

NERVE SHEATH TUMOR

MALIGNANT

PERINEURAL SPREAD FROM ELSEWHERE

MALIGNANT NERVE SHEATH TUMOR

Mucosa in contact

MALIGNANT

SCC FROM ORAL MUCOSA

Parotid duct

BENIGN

ACCESSORY PAROTID GLAND

STONE, INFLAMMATION

2.1.5 ORAL CAVITY MUCOSAL SPACE

Mucosa

BENIGN

DENTAL INFECTION, CELLULITIS

LUDWIG ANGINA, ABSCESS

LINGUAL THYROID

MALIGNANT

SCC

Minor salivary glands

MALIGNANT

MUCOEPIDERMOID CARCINOMA

ADENOID CYSTIC CARCINOMA

2.1.6 PARAPHARYNGEAL SPACE

most masses in this space push in from outside

ASYMMETRIC PHARYNGEAL VENOUS PLEXUS

ACCESSORY SALIVARY GLAND TUMOR

ABSCESS

2.1.7 PAROTID SPACE

Parotid gland

BENIGN

ABSCESS, STONE

ACCESSORY GLAND

BENIGN SALIVARY TUMOR

BENIGN HYPERPLASIA (often related to alcohol abuse)

MALIGNANT

SALIVARY CARCINOMA

Lymphoid

BENIGN

REACTIVE LYMPHADENOPATHY

AIDS LYMPHADENOPATHY

HEMANGIOMA, LYMPHANGIOMA

1st BRANCHIAL CLEFT CYST

MALIGNANT

NHL

SCC METASTASES

Facial nerve

BENIGN

NERVE SHEATH TUMOR

MALIGNANT

PERINEURAL SPREAD

2.1.8 PERIVERTEBRAL SPACE

Brachial plexus (including phrenic nerve)

BENIGN

NERVE SHEATH TUMOR

MALIGNANT

PERINEURAL SPREAD FROM AXILLA

Vertebral vessels

BENIGN

FOCAL EXTRAOSSEOUS LOOP (normal variant)

ANEURYSM/DISSECTION

Vertebrae, disks

BENIGN

TRAUMA, DISK PROTRUSION

OSTEOMYELITIS/DISCITIS

BENIGN BONE TUMOR

MALIGNANT

MYELOMA, LYMPHOMA, METASTASIS

CHORDOMA, OTHER TUMOR

2.1.9 PHARYNGEAL MUCOSAL SPACE

Mucosa

BENIGN

ASYMMETRICAL MUCOSA

HEMATOMA

RETENTION CYST, BULLA

MALIGNANT

SCC

Lymphoid tissue

BENIGN

TONSILLAR HYPERTROPHY

TONSILLAR ABSCESS

RETENTION CYST

MALIGNANT

EXTRANODAL MUCOSAL NHL

Accessory salivary glands

BENIGN

PLEOMORPHIC ADENOMA

MALIGNANT

MALIGNANT SALIVARY TUMOR

2.1.10 POSTERIOR CERVICAL SPACE

CN XI

BENIGN

NERVE SHEATH TUMOR

Lymphoid

BENIGN

HEMANGIOMA, LYMPHANGIOMA

3rd BRANCHIAL CLEFT CYST

REACTIVE OR INFECTIVE LYMPHADENOPATHY

ABSCESS

MALIGNANT

SCC METASTASIS

NHL

HD

2.1.11 RETROPHARYNGEAL SPACE

Lymphoid

BENIGN

REACTIVE LYMPHADENOPATHY

CELLULITIS, ABSCESS

LYMPHATIC ENGORGEMENT

HEMANGIOMA, LYMPHANGIOMA

MALIGNANT

NHL

SCC OR OTHER METASTASES

2.1.12 SUBLINGUAL SPACE, TONGUE

BENIGN

MOTOR ATROPHY

HEMANGIOMA–LYMPHANGIOMA

MALIGNANT

SCC (invading from mucosa)

SUBMANDIBULAR TAIL AND DUCT

same as for submandibular gland

2.1.13 SUBMANDIBULAR SPACE

Muscles

BENIGN

MOTOR ATROPHY

2nd BRANCHIAL CLEFT CYST

THYROGLOSSAL DUCT CYST

Submandibular gland

BENIGN

STONE, OBSTRUCTION

INFECTION, ABSCESS

PLEOMORPHIC ADENOMA

DIVING RANULA

MALIGNANT

SALIVARY CARCINOMA

Lymphoid

BENIGN

REACTIVE, INFECTIVE ADENOPATHY

CELLULITIS, ABSCESS

DERMOID, EPIDERMOID

HEMANGIOMA, LYMPHANGIOMA

LIPOMA

MALIGNANT

SCC METASTASES

SCC DIRECT EXTENSION

NHL

Parotid tail

ANY PAROTID MASS

Cystic mass differential

ranula, diving ranula

abscess

lymphangioma

2.1.14 VISCERAL COMPARTMENT OF NECK

Thyroid

BENIGN

PYRAMIDAL LOBE

THYROGLOSSAL DUCT CYST

GOITRE, COLLOID CYST

THYROIDITIS

ABSCESS

ADENOMA

MALIGNANT

CARCINOMA

NHL

Parathyroid

ADENOMA

CARCINOMA

DIFFERENTIAL: fold of esophageal mucosa

Pharynx

PHARYNGEAL (ZENKER'S) DIVERTICULUM

SCC

NHL

Larynx, trachea

POST TRAUMATIC DEFORMITY

LARYNGOCELE (AIR OR FLUID)

PAPILLOMA

WEGENER'S GRANULOMA

SCC

Lymphoid

REACTIVE OR INFECTIVE ADENOPATHY

ABSCESS

METASTASIS (SCC, thyroid)

NHL

2.2 SINONASAL AND TEMPORAL BONE GAMUTS (all modalities)

2.2.1 CONDUCTIVE HEARING LOSS

TRAUMA

OSSICULAR CHAIN DISRUPTION

TYMPANIC MEMBRANE TEAR

HEMATOMA

OTITIS MEDIA

OTITIS MEDIA WITH EFFUSION

TYMPANIC MEMBRANE PERFORATION

FENESTRAL OTOSCLEROSIS

CHOLESTEATOMA

MIDDLE EAR TUMOR

MIDDLE AND EXTERNAL EAR
    MALFORMATIONS

EXTERNAL EAR

ATRESIAS

KERATOSIS OBTURANS

CHOLESTEATOMA

TUMOR

2.2.2 FACIAL NERVE PALSY

Intraaxial

MASS

INFARCT (including diabetic microinfarct)

DEMYELINATION

Cerebellopontine angle

MASS (usually schwannoma or meningioma)

POST RESECTION OF IAM TUMOR

ANY CAUSE OF MULTIPLE CRANIAL NERVE PALSY

Intratemporal

BELL'S PALSY (probable post viral)
shows mild facial nerve enhancement on MR

TEMPORAL BONE FRACTURE

MIDDLE EAR CHOLESTEATOMA WITH INVASION

AGGRESSIVE OTITIS MEDIA

Extratemporal

PAROTID CARCINOMA WITH PERINEURAL SPREAD

SCC WITH PERINEURAL SPREAD

POST PAROTID SURGERY

DIRECT TRAUMA

2.2.3 MIDDLE EAR MASS

PSEUDOMASS

HIGH AND/OR DEHISCENT JUGULAR BULB

ABERRANT INTERNAL CAROTID ARTERY

OTITIS MEDIA WITH EFFUSION
(OTOSPONGIOSIS)

CHOLESTEATOMA

TUMOR

GLOMUS TYMPANICUM/
JUGULOTYMPANICUM

SCC WITH DIRECT INVASION

PERINEURAL SPREAD (esp parotid
carcinoma)

CN VII NERVE SHEATH TUMOR OR
MENINGIOMA

2.2.4 PETROUS APEX LESIONS

Cholesterol granuloma

CT
possibly rim enhancement, no central
enhancement

MR
high T1W and high T2W signal (may be
heterogeneous or patchy), smooth
margins, possibly rim enhancement

Primary cholesteatoma

CT
no enhancement

MR
low T1W and high T2W signal, no
enhancement, scalloped borders

Mucocele

CT
iso or low density, possibly rim
enhancement, no central enhancement

MR
low T1W and high T2W signal, no
enhancement, smooth borders
can be high T1W signal and low T2W signal
if chronic and inspissated

Fatty bone marrow

CT
iso or low density (same as bone marrow)

MR
follows fatty marrow signal on all sequences

Pneumatized temporal apex

CT
unambiguous

MR
signal void

Fluid filled temporal apex

CT
fluid density inside a clearly cortically
marginated air cell

MR
low T1W, high T2W signal, well marginated,
no mass effect, no enhancement

Metastasis

Petrous apex primary chondrosarcoma

2.2.5 PULSATILE TINNITUS

ABERRANT ICA

DEHISCENT JUGULAR BULB

TEMPORAL BONE AVF

GLOMUS TUMOR

HIGH GRADE ICA STENOSIS

2.2.6 SENSORINEURAL HEARING LOSS

Cochlear

DEGENERATIVE/INDUSTRIAL

TRAUMA

LABYRINTHITIS/MENINGITIS

OSSIFICATION
COCHLEAR OTOSCLEROSIS
LABYRINTHITIS OSSIFICANS
TEMPORAL BONE PAGET'S DISEASE

ENDOLYMPHATIC HYDROPS

MÉNIÉRES SYNDROME

ENDOLYMPHATIC LEAK (erosion by
cholesteatoma/tumor)

LABYRINTHINE SCHWANNOMA

CONGENITAL
APLASIA (Michel syndrome)
HYPOPLASIA/MALFORMATION (Mondini
syndrome)

Retrocochlear

CEREBELLOPONTINE ANGLE MASS

INTRAAXIAL LESIONS
MICROVASCULAR INFARCT
TUMOR

ANY CAUSE OF MULTIPLE CRANIAL
NERVE PALSY

2.2.7 SINONASAL IMAGING PATTERNS

Indolent mass
expansile
pressure deossification, bony remodelling
may be water density

Aggressive mass
focally destructive
invasive

Infection (without cavity obstruction)
destructive but no tumor mass

Mucosal patterns
flat/concave mucosa = thickening
horizontal = air–fluid level
convex–long gamut of infiltrations, infections
and tumors

Enhancement patterns

MUCOSA, MUCOSAL POLYP
CT: may enhance mildly
MR: moderate uniform enhancement

MUCUS, MUCOCELE, OBSTRUCTED
SECRETIONS
no enhancement
(thin uniform rim enhancement allowed)

MUSCLE
no appreciable enhancement

TUMOR (in general)
mild enhancement with CT and with MR

VASCULAR TUMOR
CT: vivid enhancement
MR: vivid enhancement or flow voids

INFECTIVE MASS
CT: enhances

FUNGUS OR INSPISSATED
SECRETIONS IN SINUS
CT: may calcify
NO SIGNAL ON MR

2.2.8 SINONASAL MASS

MUCOCELE

INFLAMMATORY SINONASAL
POLYPOSIS

MALIGNANT TUMOR
SCC
ACCESSORY SALIVARY CARCINOMA
MELANOMA
NHL

PLASMACYTOMA

ESTHESIONEUROBLASTOMA

CHONDROSARCOMA

OSTEOSARCOMA

RHABDOMYOSARCOMA (children)

BENIGN TUMOR

PAPILLOMA OR INVERTING PAPILLOMA

JUVENILE ANGIOFIBROMA

OSTEOMA

NON TUMOR MASS

SPORADIC POLYP

ANTROCHOANAL POLYP

FIBROUS DYSPLASIA

NASAL GLIOMA

WEGENER'S GRANULOMATOSIS

MUCORMYCOSIS/ASPERGILLOSIS

2.2.9 SMALL OR ABSENT SINUSES

Absent frontal sinuses

NORMAL VARIANT

DOWN'S
90% of Down's syndrome have absent frontal sinuses

KARTAGENER'S SYNDROME

HYPOTHYROIDISM

Hypoplastic/absent maxillary sinus (overgrown wall)

POST CALDWELL–LUC PROCEDURE

FIBROUS DYSPLASIA

ANEMIAS WITH BONE MARROW EXPANSION

PAGET'S DISEASE

2.3 ORBIT AND SKULL BASE GAMUTS (all modalities)

2.3.1 'BARE ORBIT' ON PLAIN FILM

With mass

MENINGIOMA

METASTASIS

BONE PRIMARY

Without mass

SPHENOID WING DYSPLASIA

2.3.2 CONAL AND INTRACONAL ABNORMALITIES

Trauma

HEMATOMA

FOREIGN BODY

Infection

POST SEPTAL CELLULITIS

Vascular

CAROTICOCAVERNOUS FISTULA

VENOUS VARIX

SUPERIOR OPHTHALMIC VEIN THROMBOSIS

Tumor

CAVERNOUS HEMANGIOMA

LYMPHANGIOMA

ORBITAL LYMPHOMA

METASTASIS

Autoimmune

ORBITAL PSEUDOTUMOR

DYSTHYROID OPHTHALMOPATHY

WEGENER'S GRANULOMATOSIS

2.3.3 EXTRACONAL ABNORMALITIES

Lacrimal

INFLAMMATORY

POST VIRAL

SJÖGREN'S SYNDROME

SARCOIDOSIS

TUMOR

PLEOMORPHIC ADENOMA

ADENOID CYSTIC CARCINOMA

LYMPHOMA

Bone mass

FIBROUS DYSPLASIA

PAGET'S DISEASE

EOSINOPHILIC GRANULOMA

NF1, SPHENOID WING DYSPLASIA OR PLEXIFORM NEUROFIBROMA

Mass pushing into orbit from outside

MUCOCELE

SUBPERIOSTEAL ABSCESS

SPHENOID WING MENINGIOMA

SINONASAL SCC

BONY METASTASIS

SCALP SCC

DERMOID

EPIDERMOID

2.3.4 GLOBE ABNORMALITIES

Trauma

VITREOUS HEMORRHAGE

CHOROIDAL/SUPRACHOROIDAL HEMORRHAGE

CHOROIDAL DETACHMENT

RETINAL DETACHMENT

Infection

CHORIORETINITIS

ENDOPHTHALMITIS

IMPLANT INFECTION

Tumor

UVEAL METASTASIS

UVEAL MELANOMA

CHOROIDAL HEMANGIOMA

Autoimmune

PSEUDOTUMOR INVOLVING SCLERA

Degenerative

DISC DRUSEN

2.3.5 MULTIPLE CRANIAL NERVE PALSIES

Tumor

LEPTOMENINGEAL CARCINOMATOSIS

LEPTOMENINGEAL LYMPHOID INFILTRATION

LYMPHOMA

LYMPHOMATOID GRANULOMATOSIS

HISTIOCYTOSIS X

MENINGIOMATOSIS

PERINEURAL TUMOR SPREAD

Infection

BASAL CISTERN MENINGITIS OR SARCOIDOSIS

CAVERNOUS SINUS INFECTION OR THROMBOSIS (or tumor)
(CN III, IV, VI, possibly optic nerve and divisions of V1, V2)

Brainstem intraaxial lesion

constellation of cranial nerve palsies and long tract signs has to be concordant!

Other

SUPERFICIAL SIDEROSIS

Aneurysm

posterior communicating artery aneurysm: CN III

2.3.6 OPTIC CANAL GAMUTS

2.3.6.1 Enlarged optic canal

OPTIC NERVE GLIOMA

OPTIC NERVE MENINGIOMA

RETINOBLASTOMA IN OPTIC NERVE (child)

OPHTHALMIC ARTERY ANEURYSM

2.3.6.2 Defect in wall of canal

ADJACENT DURAL OR BONY TUMOR

SPHENOID MUCOCELE

NEUROFIBROMATOSIS

AVM, HEMANGIOMA

2.3.7 OPTIC NERVE

Malformation

OPTIC NERVE HYPOPLASIA

SEPTOOPTIC DYSPLASIA

ENLARGED SUBARACHNOID SPACE (hydrocephalus)

Tumor

OPTIC NERVE GLIOMA (80%)

OPTIC SHEATH MENINGIOMA (20%)

LYMPHOMA

METASTASIS

Optic neuritis/multiple sclerosis

2.3.8 ORBITAL HYPEROSTOSIS

Meningioma

Diffuse bone disease

FIBROUS DYSPLASIA

PAGET'S DISEASE

OSTEOPETROSIS

Sclerotic tumor

SCLEROTIC METASTASIS

TUMOR POST RADIATION THERAPY

2.3.9 SKULL BASE

Tumor

FROM BELOW

NASOPHARYNGEAL CARCINOMA

FROM ABOVE

MENINGIOMA

PITUITARY ADENOMA

FROM WITHIN NEURAL FORAMINA

GLOMUS TUMOR

NERVE SHEATH TUMOR

NERVE SHEATH MENINGIOMA

PERINEURAL TUMOR SPREAD

METASTATIC

BONE PRIMARY

FIBROUS DYSPLASIA

OSTEOSARCOMA

CHORDOMA

Pseudotumor

HIGH JUGULAR BULB

JUGULAR BULB FLOW ARTIFACT ON MR

ABERRANT ICA

PETROUS APEX AIR CELLS FILLED WITH FLUID

Retention 'tumor'

MIDDLE EAR CHOLESTEATOMA

FRONTAL MUCOCELE

SPHENOID MUCOCELE

PETROUS APEX CHOLESTEROL GRANULOMA

FISSURAL DERMOID/EPIDERMOID

Congenital 'tumor'

CEPHALOCELES

FRONTONASAL

FRONTOETHMOIDAL

COMPLEX SKULL BASE

Infection

OTITIS MEDIA

MASTOIDITIS

ETHMOID OR FRONTAL SINUSITIS

PETROUS APICITIS

Diffuse skull base bone abnormality

PAGET'S DISEASE

HEMOGLOBINOPATHIES, BONE MARROW INVOLVEMENT

OSTEOPETROSIS, ETC

Trauma

TEMPORAL BONE FRACTURES

SPHENOID BONE FRACTURES

ANTERIOR CRANIAL FOSSA FRACTURES

BASIOCCIPITAL FRACTURES

POST TRAUMATIC MENINGITIS, CSF LEAK

POST TRAUMATIC LEPTOMENINGEAL CYST

2.4 THYROID GAMUTS
(all modalities)

2.4.1 GOITER

SIMPLE GOITRE/DIETARY GOITRE

MULTINODULAR GOITRE (non toxic, toxic)

GRAVES' GOITRE (toxic)

GOITRE OF ACUTE THYROIDITIS

2.4.2 HYPOTHYROIDISM

Thyroid cause

AGENESIS

CONGENITAL BLOCK IN SYNTHESIS

SURGERY/RADIOIODINE
  ABLATION/NECK RADIOTHERAPY

AUTOIMMUNE THYROIDITIS

IODINE DEFICIENCY

ANTITHYROID DRUGS

Hypopituitarism

Hypothalamic hypothyroidism

Thyroxine (Triiodothyronine) peripheral resistance

2.4.3 THYROID NODULE

Gamut

COLLOID NODULE (cystic, solid, mixed)

ABSCESS

TRUE NEOPLASM

ADENOMA

CARCINOMA

LYMPHOMA

METASTASIS (rare)

INTRATHYROID PARATHYROID
  GLAND OR ADENOMA

Imaging findings

based on combination of US and Nuc Med

US

PURELY CYSTIC = COLLOID CYST

SOLID OR COMPLEX

  HIGH RISK
  >2 cm solid
  internal vascularity
  growth pattern fits neoplasm
  stippled internal microcalcification

  UNHELPFUL FINDINGS
  coarse calcification
  cystic change
  hemorrhage
  internal echoes

US GUIDED FINE NEEDLE ASPIRATION
high sensitivity, low specificity, can not
    distinguish follicular carcinoma from
    adenoma

NUC MED THYROID SCAN
  (pertechnetate)

HOT NODULE
dominant nodule in multinodular goitre
adenoma
1% or less risk of carcinoma

COLD NODULE
<20% risk of carcinoma
most common cause of solitary solid cold
    nodule is an adenoma

  DIFFERENTIAL
    COLLOID CYST
    COLD NODULE IN A MULTINODULAR GOITRE
    ADENOMA
    CARCINOMA
    ABSCESS/FOCAL THYROIDITIS
    LYMPHOMA, METASTASIS

PERTECHNETATE – IODINE DISCORDANCE
rarely, iodine organification block with
    normal iodine trapping will lead to an
    iodine cold nodule that is warm or hot on
    pertechnetate (and therefore can not be
    successfully ablated with radioiodine)

2.4.4 THYROTOXICOSIS

Definition
elevated levels of thyroxine/triiodothyronine
  of any cause

Gamut

HYPERTHYROIDISM

GRAVES' DISEASE

TOXIC ADENOMA

TOXIC MULTINODULAR GOITRE

THYROIDITIS WITH HYPERTHYROIDISM

ECTOPIC THYROID STIMULATING
  HORMONE

PITUITARY THYROTROPHIC ADENOMA (rare)

THYROXINE FROM ELSEWHERE

THYROID DAMAGE WITH THYROXINE LEAK
  (subacute thyroiditis)

EXOGENOUS THYROXINE OR STRUMA
  OVARII

Imaging

based on sequence of TFTs, thyroid US and
  thyroid Nuc Med scan

TSH HIGH
?pituitary thyrotrophic adenoma
?ectopic TSH

TSH LOW

US – DIFFUSELY ABNORMAL ECHOTEXTURE
  OR NORMAL
TcO4 uptake high – Graves' disease

TcO4 uptake low – thyroiditis with thyroxine
  leak or exogenous thyroxine

US – SOLITARY NODULE
TcO4 or I for ?toxic nodule
fine needle aspiration

US – UNEQUIVOCAL MULTINODULAR
  GOITER
TcO4 or I for suitability for radioiodine
  therapy

3. CONDITIONS OF THE ORAL CAVITY AND PHARYNX

3.1 IMPACTED THIRD MOLAR

IMAGING

OPG/PLAIN XR/CT

IMPACTION DEFINITE IF
crown of third molar directed into second
  molar
horizontal/near horizontal third molar
  position

IMPACTION IS LIKELY TO OCCUR IF
delayed eruption compared to contralateral
  side
root formation exceeds crown formation
root formation is complete and the apex is
  closed but tooth not erupted

IMPACTION TYPES

MESIOANGULAR IMPACTION (MOST
  COMMON)
long axis of third molar directed anteriorly
VERTICAL IMPACTION
long axis of third molar is craniocaudal
(DIFFERENTIAL: delayed eruption versus
  impaction)
DISTOANGULAR IMPACTION (RARE)
long axis of third molar directed posteriorly
HORIZONTAL IMPACTION

INFERIOR DENTAL CANAL PROBABLY
  INVOLVED IF (OPG)
canal lies close to or above third molar roots
canal distorted or constricted as it passes
  third molar roots

third molar roots grooved by canal
dental CT unequivocally shows canal and
root positions

3.2 ORAL SQUAMOUS CELL CARCINOMA (SCC)

CLINICAL

painless mass or ulcer
painful mass or ulcer (invasion, perineural
extension, superinfection)
dysphagia, otalgia (referred)
floor of mouth > anterior tongue > post
tongue > palate
60% have nodal metastases at presentation

Spread

wide submucosal in continuity
perineural along CN V3 (floor of mouth), V2
(palate), CN XII
lymphatic: ipsilateral nodes, contralateral
nodes approximately in order
late hematogenous: lungs, bones, liver

IMAGING (locoregional)

Plain XR

little to see unless mandible eroded

CT

mucosal only disease invisible even if
extensive
invasive or exophytic mass visible, but
mucosal extent very hard to define

PRIMARY MASS (mucosal space mass)

usually same or minimally higher density
than tongue or floor of mouth muscle
has no normal fat planes compared to
muscle
mucosal thickening only with mass effect or
mucosally based ulcerated mass or
extension into deeper muscle or
erosion of mandible or palate

enhances slightly with contrast, either
diffuse or peripheral enhancement
invasion of bone definite if erosion present
or marrow fat replaced by solid soft
tissue
no invasion of bone if fat plane exists
invasion vs adherence hard to judge if
contiguous to bone without erosion
extension across midline is clinically
relevant (contralateral nodal disease,
feasibility of hemiglossectomy)

SPREAD

enlarged lymph nodes, may have necrotic
low density core and ring enhancement
fuzzy nodal margin (extracapsular extension)
loss of fat or cortex of mandibular nerve
canal, rarely of greater palatine
foramen/canal

MR

same difficulty with mucosal only disease or
superficial spread as for CT

PRIMARY MASS

low T1W signal often comparable to muscle,
higher T2W signal than muscle
mucosal thickening only with altered signal
and mass effect or
mucosally based ulcerated mass or
extension into deeper tissues with mass
effect and altered signal

enhances with contrast, with better
demarcation of interface with muscle
(mucus or retained secretions do not
enhance)
cortical bone erosion hard to tell on MR
bone marrow edema suggestive of invasion,
but may also be reactive
extension across midline is clinically
relevant (see CT)

SPREAD

enlarged lymph nodes, usually high on T2W
high T2W core (necrotic core) and ring
enhancement
enhancing nodes without necrotic core
fuzzy nodal margin (extracapsular
extension)
loss of perineural fat planes in mandibular
canal, rarely greater palatine
foramen/canal, around CN V3 in
masticator space, in foramen ovale and
foramen rotundum
asymmetrical, thickened or beaded
enhancement in the same perineural
locations (differential for foramina:
asymmetrical emissary companion veins)
involvement of trigeminal cave in extreme
cases

US

involved lymph nodes are enlarged, usually
hypoechoic (may be hyperechoic to
muscle if intense fibrotic response) and
may have low density necrotic center
color or power Doppler vascularity may be
increased
used for lymph node biopsy guidance

PET (FDG)

vast majority of primaries have increased
FDG uptake

most sensitive modality for nodal staging
(increased FDG uptake)
monitoring: decreased FDG uptake with
treatment indicates good metabolic
response
most sensitive modality for identifying
potential sites of primary SCC in cases of
occult head and neck SCC (SCC
metastasis/metastases in head and neck
lymph nodes with no mucosal primary on
clinical examination)

3.3 PHARYNGEAL SQUAMOUS CELL CARCINOMA (SCC)

CLINICAL

dysphagia, painful swallowing
painful throat, slurred speech
lower CN involvement (esp V3)
referred otalgia
nodal mass, occult primary (commonly tonsil)

Spread

SUBSITES: see pharynx regions
in continuity
nodal (more than ½ at presentation)
perineural
distant metastases

IMAGING

See imaging of oral SCC

3.4 PHARYNGEAL (ZENKER'S) DIVERTICULUM

see Ch 06

3.5 SALIVARY STONES

CLINICAL

submandibular > parotid >> other salivary
glands
asymptomatic or recurrent painful
obstruction with eating or ductal
infection, chronic sialadenitis or acute
obstruction with distal acute
superinfected sialadenitis

IMAGING (stone)

Plain XR

shows the larger dense stones
intraoral occlusal view very helpful for distal
submandibular stone

Sialography

requires sufficiently large duct orifice for
cannulation
parotid easier than submandibular, even if
normal
complications of cannulation and contrast
injection include pain, perforation of duct
wall, contrast extravasation, rarely
sialadenitis
cardinal sign: filling defect or intraductal
mass with obstruction to contrast flow

US

submandibular duct accessible to
submandibular approach and intraoral
floor of mouth approach ('hockey stick'
probe)
parotid duct accessible to external US
approach
stone shows as intrasalivary or intraductal
reflector with shadowing

CT

stone dense on CT
located along the course of the parotid or
the submandibular duct
may have dilation, gland atrophy or gland
inflammation upstream (including
fulminating sialadenitis with cellulitis)
small stones in sialectasis may show as
multiple punctate intrasalivary
calcifications

MR

future role for MR sialography (non contrast
demonstration of ducts on T2W weighted
sequences)

NUC MED (TcO4)

salivary flow study quantitates the degree of
salivary obstruction

3.6 SALIVARY TUMORS

GROUP CHARACTERISTICS

~1/2 benign

~80%	PLEOMORPHIC ADENOMA
~20%	ADENOLYMPHOMA (WARTHIN TUMOR)
1%	ONCOCYTOMA

~1/2 malignant

~35%	MUCOEPIDERMOID CARCINOMA
~20%	ADENOID CYSTIC CARCINOMA
~20%	ADENOCARCINOMA NOS
~10%	MIXED
~1%	ACINIC CELL CARCINOMA

LYMPHOMA (SECONDARY, PRIMARY)
SECONDARIES TO LYMPH NODES

Gland involvement

parotid commonest (~3/4), most primary
tumors benign
submandibular intermediate
sublingual and minor: rare, most tumors
malignant

Imaging

hyperdense mass within fat containing gland
or mass with altered signal (with possible
central cystic or necrotic change)

BENIGN (general features)

sharp margins; displaces and stretches ducts

MALIGNANT (general features)

irregular margins; invades and cuts off ducts
central area of necrosis
DIRECT INVASION OF OTHER STRUCTURES
PERINEURAL SPREAD
DISTANT METASTASES

3.6.1 PLEOMORPHIC ADENOMA ('benign mixed tumor')

CLINICAL

40–60 years, female > male, parotid >>
other
slow growing painless mass; most are in
superficial part of the gland
25% recur from residual nests

MORPHOLOGY

solid multinodular gray-blue, mucinous and
chondroid like areas with a possibly
incomplete fibrous capsule
parenchyma: 2 cell layer epithelium in
strands and ducts; stroma: amorphous
hyalinized, myxoid, mucoid, chondroid,
fibrous (i.e. pleomorphic)

IMAGING

Parotid space mass

usually superficial to stylomandibular notch
usually superficial to plane of CN VII
rarely involves deep lobe of parotid gland:
either dumbbell shape passing through
the stylomandibular notch, or totally
deep to stylomandibular notch and
extending into parapharyngeal space
from posterolaterally
very rarely, primary parapharyngeal space
mass (with thin cuff of fat separating it
from deep lobe of parotid)

Submandibular space mass

arising from submandibular gland

CT

rounded or lobulated well marginated mass
denser than normal gland, but may have
cystic spaces
cystic central change occurs as tumor
enlarges
minimal enhancement
may contain clumpy calcification, which is
characteristic

MR

heterogeneous T1W and high T2W/PD signal
mass, with sharp demarcation from
normal gland
may have cystic spaces, cystic central
change occurs as tumor enlarges
minimal contrast enhancement

3.6.2 ADENOLYMPHOMA (Warthin's tumor)

CLINICAL

histologically bimodal oncocytic and
lymphoid benign salivary tumor
60–80 years, male > female
parotid >>> elsewhere; 10% bilateral
slow growing painless benign mass
cured by adequate excision

IMAGING

CT

well circumscribed superficial parotid lobe
soft tissue density mass, may have
central cystic degeneration

MR

well circumscribed, intermediate T1W and
high T2W signal mass, may have central
cystic change

NUC MED (TcO4)

accumulates and retains pertechnetate

3.6.3 ONCOCYTOMA (salivary)

CLINICAL

rare benign salivary tumor composed of columns of oncocytes without a lymphoid component

IMAGING

CT/MR

parotid well circumscribed mass

NUC MED (TcO4)

accumulates and retains pertechnetate

3.6.4 MUCOEPIDERMOID CARCINOMA

CLINICAL

slow growing salivary malignancy with moderate malignant potential
parotid and minor salivary glands
LOW GRADE (common) slow growing mass; 10% have both lymph nodal and hematogenous metastases
HIGH GRADE (uncommon) rapidly growing ulcerating mass with pain and CN VII palsy; 2/3 have lymph nodal metastases, 1/3 hematogenous metastases

MORPHOLOGY

pale gray-white mass with small cystic spaces and invasive margins
mucus secreting cells around cystic spaces (predominant in low grade) AND
sheets of squamous epidermoid cells with keratin pearls (predominant in high grade)

IMAGING

CT

lobulated or nodular parotid or submucosal mass
appearance varies with grade
low grade – well circumscribed, rarely with calcifications
high grade – invasive edge, homogenous

MR

low grade – similar to pleomorphic adenoma

high grade – intermediate T1W and T2W signal intensity
LOOK FOR perineural spread (CN VII for parotid tumors, V3/V2 for minor salivary tumors)

3.6.5 ADENOID CYSTIC CARCINOMA ('cylindroma')

CLINICAL

commonest malignant salivary tumor with long history of slow growth, local infiltration and late distant metastases
commoner in submandibular gland than mucoepidermoid carcinoma
presents with ulceration and pain
direct invasion characteristic: bone, nerve
late hematogenous and lymphatic metastases
tends to recur locally because of perineural spread outside of surgical and/or radiotherapy field
CRIBRIFORM TYPE; TUBULAR TYPE; SOLID TYPE

IMAGING

PERINEURAL SPREAD CHARACTERISTIC OF THIS TUMOR

CT/MR

relatively homogeneous mass of variable aggressivity
may have evidence of adjacent bone erosion (especially minor mucosal glands)
perineural spread is along CN VII for parotid masses, and CN V2/V3 for submucosal minor salivary glands

SIGNS OF PERINEURAL SPREAD
mass extension along the course of a nerve
'skip' mass further along the course of a nerve with no macroscopic continuity
loss of perineural fat in mandibular canal, greater palatine foramen/canal, foramen ovale and foramen rotundum
may extend as far as trigeminal cave
MR: nodular or asymmetrically prominent perineural contrast enhancement (beware of asymmetric normal emissary veins passing through skull base foramina)

3.6.6 ACINIC CELL CARCINOMA

CLINICAL

rare acini forming tumor of moderate malignant potential, almost always parotid
usually slow growing painless mass
high grade tumors have invasion, pain, ulceration
metastases in 10%

IMAGING

CT/MR

non specific mass, often of non aggressive appearance

3.7 SIALADENITIS (bacterial)

3.7.1 ACUTE SIALADENITIS

ascending oral infection, often secondary to reduced salivary flow

3.7.2 CHRONIC SIALADENITIS

chronic infection distal to stone or stricture

3.7.3 CHRONIC RECURRENT PAROTITIS

recurrent episodes of acute parotitis, no single clear cause isolated

IMAGING (all bacterial sialadenitis)

CT

swelling of one gland, surrounding edema and fat infiltration
increased gland density (swelling, inflammatory infiltrate)
may develop an abscess (focal complex cyst)
may show dilated duct
may show stone

Sialography
not done acutely
demonstrates strictures, sialectasis, stones

MR
future role for MR sialography

NUC MED (Gallium)
asymmetrically increased gallium uptake

3.8 SIALADENITIS
(non bacterial)

3.8.1 VIRAL

Mumps

Other viral parotitis

CMV (immunosuppressed parotitis)

IMAGING

swollen one or more glands, usually
    bilateral parotid glands
increased gland density

3.8.2 SARCOIDOSIS

CLINICAL (uveoparotid fever)

EPONYMOUS TERM: HEERFORDT
    SYNDROME

UVEAL TRACT INFLAMMATION

LACRIMAL GLAND INFLAMMATION

SALIVARY GLAND INFLAMMATION

CRANIAL NERVE SARCOIDOSIS

IMAGING

CT
multiple or all gland enlargement
multiple punctate foci of high density

NUC MED (Gallium)
markedly increased Ga avidity, usually in all
    four major glands ('panda sign')
quite specific if associated with increased
    hilar and paratracheal nodal Ga uptake
    ('lambda sign')

3.8.3 RADIATION SIALADENITIS

CLINICAL

acute sialadenitis (rare) – acute pain and
    swelling of gland with reduced salivary
    flow
chronic radiation atrophy – volume loss, fat
    replacement, reduction in salivary flow

IMAGING

Any modality
reduced gland volume with progressive
    atrophy and fat replacement

3.9 SIALECTASIS

DEFINITION

radiological definition: multiple dilated ducts
    and acini presenting as multiple
    cylindrical or cystic spaces at sialography

ETIOLOGY

ACUTE SIALADENITIS (but sialography
    contraindicated)
CHRONIC SIALADENITIS, STONES
CHRONIC RECURRENT PAROTITIS
    (CHILDHOOD SIALECTASIS)
SJÖGREN'S SYNDROME
ASYMPTOMATIC SIALECTASIS OF IMMUNE
    COMPLEX DISEASE (i.e. SILENT
    SJÖGREN'S SYNDROME)

IMAGING

Sialography
variable degree of main duct dilation, one
    dominant or multiple strictures
may show major duct stones
variable degree of saccular dilation and
    pruning of secretory ducts ('globular')
may have irregular cavities in
    communication with the ductal system
    ('cavitary')

CT
gland atrophy
ductal system seen only if grossly dilated
may show stones

3.10 SJÖGREN'S SYNDROME

DEFINITION

chronic autoimmune sialadenitis and
    lacrimal gland inflammation leading to
    xerostomia and keratoconjunctivitis
    sicca; commonly associated with other
    autoimmune disease

CLINICAL

female:male 10:1, usually >50 years
HLA DR3 or DR4 associated
50% primary; 50% secondary (rheumatoid
    arthritis 90%, SLE, other autoimmune
    states)
may evolve to salivary lymphoma
diffuse lymphocytic infiltration and gland
    enlargement

IMAGING

Sialography
sialectasis, starting with small ducts
    (punctate, globular)

CT
enlarged glands
may have multiple well defined areas of low
    attenuation (DIFFERENTIAL: AIDS
    lymphoproliferative lesions)

NUC MED (TcO4)
decreased pertechnetate uptake

DIFFERENTIAL
acute viral sialadenitis
atrophy from chronic obstruction
radiation atrophy

3.11 STAGING OF SCC
(TNM and summary)

T STAGING (except NPC)

Oropharynx/hypopharynx
see pharynx regions in normal

T STAGE – OROPHARYNX AND ORAL CAVITY/LIP
T1 size 2 cm or smaller
T2 2 cm <size <4 cm
T3 size >4 cm
T4 invades adjacent structures (mandible,
    hard palate, masticator or tongue
    muscle, larynx, maxillary sinus, nerve,
    skin of face)

T STAGE – HYPOPHARYNX
T1 one subsite, size <2 cm
T2 tumor in more than one subsite, or 2 cm
    <size <4 cm
T3 fixation of hemilarynx or size >4 cm
T4 invades adjacent structures (laryngeal
    cartilages, carotid sheath, esophagus,
    prevertebral space, neck soft tissues)

Larynx

see larynx regions in normal

T STAGING – SUPRAGLOTTIS

T1 one subsite, normal cord mobility

T2 more than one adjacent subsite of supraglottis or glottis, or extends outside the larynx without larynx fixation

T3 larynx tumor with cord fixation or invades post cricoid area, base of tongue, preepiglottic tissues

T4 extends through thyroid cartilage, or involves neck soft tissues, thyroid gland, esophagus

T STAGING – GLOTTIS

T1 limited to vocal cord (with/without commissure) with normal cord mobility

T2 impaired cord mobility or supraglottic or infraglottic extension

T3 vocal cord fixation, tumor limited to larynx

T4 invasion through thyroid cartilage, or extends beyond larynx

T STAGING – INFRAGLOTTIS

T1 limited to infraglottis

T2 extends to cord with normal or impaired mobility

T3 vocal cord fixation, tumor limited to larynx

T4 invasion through cricoid or thyroid cartilage or extends outside of larynx

Paranasal sinuses

T STAGE – MAXILLARY SINUS

T1 antral mucosa only

T2 bone destruction

T3 posterior maxillary wall, floor/medial wall of orbit, cheek

T4 orbit beyond T3, nasopharynx, base of skull, sphenoid or frontal sinus, cribriform plate

N STAGING AND STAGE GROUPING (except NPC)

Morphologic criteria

the usual size cutoff is >1.0 cm short axis

CT

nodes with SCC metastases enhance

low density core = necrotic core

fuzzy margin = extracapsular spread

MR

high T2W signal, contrast enhancing

ring enhancement = necrotic core

fuzzy margin = extracapsular spread

N stage

N1 single ipsilateral node <3 cm

N2a single ipsilateral node, 3 cm <size <6 cm

N2b multiple ipsilateral nodes, 3 cm <size < 6 cm

N2c bilateral/contralateral nodes <6 cm

N3 node or nodes >6 cm in size

Stage grouping

STAGE I	T1 N0 M0
STAGE II	T2 N0 M0
STAGE III	T3, up to N1, M0
	N1, up to T3, M0
STAGE IVA	T4, up to N1, M0
	any T, N2, M0
STAGE IVB	any T, N3, M0
STAGE IVC	any T, any N, M1

STAGING (nasopharyngeal carcinoma)

T STAGE

T1 nasopharynx only

T2 extends to soft tissue of nose or oropharynx

T2a without parapharyngeal invasion

T2b with parapharyngeal invasion

T3 involves bone or paranasal sinuses

T4 intracranial or orbital extension; CN involvement; infratemporal fossa or hypopharynx involvement

N STAGE

N1 unilateral node/nodes above supraclavicular fossa, size <6 cm

N2 bilateral node/nodes above supraclavicular fossa, size <6 cm

N3a nodes >6 cm in size

N3b supraclavicular nodes

STAGE GROUPING

STAGE I	T1 N0 M0
STAGE IIA	T2a N0 M0
STAGE IIB	T2b up to N1 or N1 up to T2b, M0
STAGE III	T3 up to N2, or N2 up to T3, M0
STAGE IVA	T4 up to N2, M0
STAGE IVB	N3 any T, M0
STAGE IVC	M1

GENERAL FEATURES – PRIMARY

Recurrence vs second primary

RECURRENCE IS DEFINED AS <2 YEARS POST TREATMENT

SECOND PRIMARY IS DEFINED AS >2 YEARS POST TREATMENT

Search for occult primary

USE FDG PET

CT features (general)

soft tissue density mass

may have necrotic core

minimal or mild contrast enhancement

bone invasion is definite if contiguous and erosion of bone or soft tissue in bone marrow

no bone invasion if fat plane separates

perineural invasion if filling and erosion of bony neural canals

MR features (general)

soft tissue mass, isointense on T1W, high on T2W sequences

mild contrast enhancement (with or without fat sat)

tumor to retained mucus margin: shows signal edge and mucus does not enhance

perineural spread: loss of perineural fat, nodular/beaded/thickened perineural enhancement (beware of emissary companion veins) or frank perineural mass

Clinical blind spots

NASOPHARYNX

TONSIL

PYRIFORM FOSSA

Perineural spread along

V3

V2 (BEWARE CAVERNOUS SINUS)

CN VII

4. CONDITIONS OF THE ORBIT

4.1 CHOROIDAL HEMANGIOMA

CLINICAL

usually present in Sturge–Weber syndrome

hemangioma located in choroidal layer, with variable mass effect and retinal elevation

IMAGING

CT

flat or biconvex mass based on globe wall
intense contrast enhancement

MR

flat or biconvex mass with base on sclera
low T1W, high T2W signal
intense contrast enhancement

4.2 DERMOID – EPIDERMOID SPECTRUM

DEFINITION

congenital ectodermal inclusion cyst
(extraconal, intraorbital) without
(epidermoid) or with (dermoid) dermal
appendages

CLINICAL

commonest location is upper lateral orbit
adjacent to sutures, but may be located
elsewhere in the orbit, usually extraconal
EPIDERMOID is lined by keratinizing
squamous epithelium and contains
keratin debris
DERMOID has dermal appendages (hair
follicles, sebaceous glands) and contains
sebum or complex fatty material
with/without hair or teeth

IMAGING

US (if can be reached by beam)

well encapsulated avascular rounded or
lobulated mass
homogenous or heterogeneous internal
debris, but also increased posterior
through transmission (i.e. complex cyst)

CT

well encapsulated extraconal mass,
commonly upper outer
epidermoid: low soft tissue density (usually
hypodense to muscle); no contrast
enhancement
dermoid: fat density mass, no contrast
enhancement (thin rim of marginal
enhancement possible)

MR

same location as above

epidermoid: low T1W, high T2W signal (but
usually can be differentiated from fluid
on T2W or PD); no contrast
enhancement; may have high T1W signal
if dense protein content
dermoid: high T1W signal that usually does
not saturate with fat sat; variable on
T2W (SE vs FSE); no contrast
enhancement

4.3 (DYS)THYROID OPHTHALMOPATHY

CLINICAL

usually follows clinical Graves' disease, but
may rarely precede it
may occur in euthyroid Graves' patients on
successful treatment
proptosis, restricted extraocular muscle
movement, diplopia, optic nerve
compression

MICRO

lymphocyte and plasma cell infiltrate of
involved muscle; later fat may be
involved

IMAGING

CT/MR

80% have bilateral, and often symmetrical
involvement
only 10% or so have single muscle
involvement
inferior recti most commonly involved, then
medial and superior recti, less commonly
lateral recti
swollen extraocular muscle/muscles
DOES NOT INVOLVE TENDON (in contrast to
pseudotumor or myositis)
swollen hypertrophic orbital fat, proptosis,
possibly optic nerve stretching

4.4 IMPLANTED OCULAR PROSTHESIS

CLINICAL

implanted after globe enucleation
deep implant ('coral') may be of various
materials, placed in Tenon's capsule, and
moves together with the other eye

later, a cosmetic superficial insert is placed
in conjunctival sac

IMAGING (?infected prosthesis)

no single reliable differentiator

MR

unequivocal if a collection or fistulous track
demonstrated
granulation tissue normally grows into
implant over many months, therefore
geographic or patchy enhancement of
implant is expected

NUC MED (WBC scan)

strongly suggestive of infection if focus of
white cell accumulation corresponds to
implant on delayed post surgical scans

4.5 RETINAL AND CHOROIDAL DETACHMENT/ HEMATOMA

CLINICAL

Traumatic (both)

choroid hemorrhage, suprachoroid space
hematoma, choroid detachment
penetrating trauma or ocular surgery, ocular
hypotonia, suprachoroid space effusion/
hematoma
subretinal hemorrhage, retinal detachment

Degenerative (retinal)

macular degeneration, retinal degeneration
retinal tear, subretinal transudate or
exudate

Traction (retinal)

vitreoretinopathy of diabetes in adults
vitreoretinopathy of prematurity, toxocara
enophthalmitis, Coats' disease (children)

Secondary to retinal tumor (retinal)

melanoma in adults
retinoblastoma in children

Inflammatory (choroid)

uveitis, scleritis produce a suprachoroid
effusion

IMAGING

CT/MR (retinal detachment)

subretinal fluid outlines extent of detachment and displacement

retina lies at the interface with vitreous and is itself invisible

retina remains attached at optic disc, and forms a semilunar or folded line elsewhere

density of subretinal fluid depends on its etiology:

blood (traumatic) is dense and has blood product signal

exudate (traction and tumor causes) is relatively dense and has high T1W signal

transudate (retinal degenerative tear, fluid ingress from vitreous) is of fluid density/signal

CT/MR (choroidal detachment)

may be impossible to differentiate from retinal detachment on imaging or

detached choroid often does not converge on the optic disc because of its wider anchoring by posterior ciliary nerves and arteries

suprachoroid hematoma is a biconvex-shaped mass of blood density/signal that is focal rather than involves entire suprachoroid space

suprachoroid effusion is crescentic, follows the same density/signal rules as subretinal effusion and may be difficult to differentiate from it (or may have inflamed thickened choroid at its margin)

4.6 RETINOBLASTOMA

see Ch 20

4.7 OPTIC DISC DRUSEN

CLINICAL

hyaline material accumulation on surface of optic disc

may be asymptomatic or may cause visual defects

75% bilateral

IMAGING

CT

discrete flat bilateral calcifications on optic disc

4.8 OPTIC NERVE GLIOMA

see Ch 11 astrocytomas

CLINICAL

80% of optic nerve tumors

75% are <10 years, and the glioma is usually a pilocytic astrocytoma

25% are adult, and the glioma is usually a glioblastoma multiforme

1/3 of patients with optic nerve glioma have NF1

15% of NF1 patients have optic nerve glioma

NF 1 features in the orbit

optic nerve glioma

optic nerve hemangioblastoma

optic sheath meningioma

optic sheath schwannoma

plexiform neurofibroma

sphenoid wing dysplasia (absence, abnormal shape, hypo or hyperplasia)

IMAGING

CT/MR

tubular or fusiform or nodular optic nerve enlargement

may be kinked or buckled as the nerve enlarges

no calcification

low on T1W, mixed high on T2W (areas of cystic change)

enhance with contrast (better shown with gadolinium), may have internal non enhancing areas

extend along optic pathway and may involve chiasm, or extend along optic tract into lateral geniculate body

often originate in chiasm, and then involve both optic nerves

bilateral optic nerve gliomas indicate NF 1

4.9 OPTIC NEURITIS

see Ch 11 multiple sclerosis

4.10 ORBITAL CELLULITIS

CLINICAL

spectrum of pyogenic infection of the orbit from cellulitis to abscess formation

commonest cause is adjacent ethmoidal sinusitis, with direct spread through medial orbital wall

Complications

visual deficit, diplopia, reduced eye movement, proptosis

ophthalmic and cavernous sinus thrombosis or septic thrombophlebitis

IMAGING

CT/MR

PRESEPTAL CELLULITIS

edema of eyelids and preseptal tissues, adjacent sinusitis

SUBPERIOSTEAL (SUBPERIORBITAL) PHLEGMON/ABSCESS

adjacent sinusitis

fluid or complex fluid density collection (low on T1W, high on T2W) elevating medial periorbita and compressing muscle cone from medially

irregular marginal enhancement, swollen adjacent muscle

ORBITAL CELLULITIS/ABSCESS

edema and masking of conal/extraconal fat

conal/extraconal collections with peripheral enhancement

air bubbles quite specific (unless post operative or trauma)

4.11 ORBITAL HEMANGIOMA/ LYMPHANGIOMA

4.11.1 HEMANGIOMA

CLINICAL

capillary hemangioma is common <1 year, and slowly involutes

cavernous hemangioma presents in children but also in young adults, and slowly enlarges

IMAGING

CT/MR

capillary hemangioma: usually extraconal, upper nasal quadrant mass of variable aggressivity

cavernous hemangioma: intraconal, well circumscribed mass

blood density on CT, may contain phleboliths
low T1W and high T2W signal on MR
uniform contrast enhancement

NUC MED (RBC)

if large enough, can be demonstrated on RBC study (SPECT)

4.11.2 LYMPHANGIOMA

CLINICAL

orbital mass of children and young adults
slowly growing
complete excision difficult, and recurrence common

IMAGING

CT/MR

multiloculated cystic mass
intraconal, conal, extraconal
infiltrative, occasionally better marginated
fluid density; low T1W and very high T2W signal (fluid signal)
mild rim enhancement with contrast
may contain internal hematomas

4.12 ORBITAL INFLAMMATORY PSEUDOTUMOR

DEFINITION

orbital polyclonal lymphocytic infiltrate of unknown etiology responding to steroids

CLINICAL

commonest cause of orbital mass
rapid unilateral painful ophthalmoplegia +/–proptosis in a previously well person
lasting response to steroids
75% involve orbital fat
50% involve muscles (INVOLVES TENDONS (in contrast to dysthyroid ophthalmopathy))
30% involve optic nerve or sclera

IMAGING

CT/MR

ANTERIOR ORBITAL PSEUDOTUMOR
uveitis, sclerotenonitis (involvement of Tenon's capsule and space)
thickening, diffuse edema of fat, enhances with contrast

DIFFUSE ORBITAL PSEUDOTUMOR (tumefactive)
intraconal/extraconal retrobulbar mass without invasion or destruction of structures
high density on CT, relatively low T2W signal
enhances with contrast
DIFFERENTIAL: true tumor, lymphoma (differentiation not always possible)
lymphoma does not enhance
true tumor tends to be high on T2W

MYOSITIC ORBITAL PSEUDOTUMOR
inflammatory infiltrate of one or more muscles
medial and superior rectus commonly involved
single muscle involvement suggestive
tendons involved, muscle margin indistinct
DIFFERENTIAL: dysthyroid ophthalmopathy
painless at onset
bilateral and symmetric
systemic signs of Graves' disease
tendons not involved
muscle margin sharply defined

4.13 ORBITAL LYMPHOMA

CLINICAL

usually non Hodgkin lymphoma in an adult
varies from discrete mass to diffuse infiltration, often bilateral
may involve lacrimal gland, cone, intraconal space, optic nerve complex

IMAGING

differential is (depending on appearance) either orbital mass or infiltrative process; orbital pseudotumor and dysthyroid ophthalmopathy in particular

CT/MR

relatively high density mass or masses, low–intermediate T1W and intermediate–high T2W signal
mild contrast enhancement
sharply defined edge, encases and envelops structures
usually not destructive

4.14 ORBITAL VENOUS VARIX

CLINICAL

usually congenital massive dilation of one or more orbital veins

IMAGING

MR/CT

greatly dilated superior ophthalmic vein
enlarges with Valsalva maneuver
+/–areas of thrombosis and phleboliths
no arterialized flow

4.15 OPTIC SHEATH MENINGIOMA

see Ch 11 meningioma

CLINICAL

20% of optic nerve tumors
middle aged adult, female > male
neurofibromatosis 2 is likely if in a child

IMAGING

CT

tubular, fusiform or nodular expansion of optic nerve complex
stippled calcification, marked contrast enhancement (may be 'tram track' in shape)
+/–optic canal expansion
+/–hyperostosis of optic canal and surrounding bone
minimal extension beyond canal

MR

morphology as for CT
optic nerve complex runs through mass and may be identifiable as such
mass intermediate–low on T1W and intermediate–low on T2W sequences
vividly enhances with contrast, and may have an optic sheath tail

4.16 SUPERIOR OPHTHALMIC VEIN THROMBOSIS

CLINICAL

usually occurs with cavernous sinus thrombosis (beware!), and so with multiple upper cranial nerve palsies

IMAGING

CT

vein contains thrombus, with a thin rim of peripheral enhancement

MR

thrombus within vein, with signal characteristics time dependent

4.17 UVEAL MELANOMA

CLINICAL

commonest globe primary in adults
initially uveal, eventually breaks through membrane between choroid and retina and grows into the subretinal space in a mushroom shape

IMAGING

CT/MR

soft tissue mass arising from globe wall and bulging inwards, sharply marginated and often mushroom shaped
may penetrate globe with retrobulbar soft tissue mass
CT: dense (hyperdense to vitreous), has contrast enhancement
MR: high T1W signal (melanin) and mixed or low T2W signal (hypointense to vitreous)
differential on MR: proteinaceous exudate or hematoma

Differential

choroidal metastasis
choroidal hemangioma
choroidal hematoma
proteinaceous suprachoroid fluid
neurofibroma/schwannoma

5. SINONASAL CONDITIONS

5.1 FACIAL BONE TRAUMA

5.1.1 BILATERAL FRACTURES

5.1.1.1 Isolated alveolar process

5.1.1.2 Le Fort I (floating teeth)
ALVEOLAR PROCESSES
LOWER PTERYGOID PROCESSES
+/–HARD PALATE
(hematoma in pharynx)

5.1.1.3 Le Fort II (floating maxillae)
associated with tripod fracture on side of impact
MAXILLARY ANTRA
INFERIOR ORBITAL MARGINS, ORBITAL FLOOR
HIGH MEDIAL ORBITAL WALLS
LOWER PTERYGOID PROCESSES
(hematoma)

5.1.1.4 Le Fort III (floating face)
HIGH LATERAL ORBITAL WALLS
BASES OF PTERYGOID PROCESSES
HIGH MEDIAL ORBITAL WALLS
ZYGOMATIC ARCHES
(severe pharyngeal hematoma, loss of airway)

5.1.1.5 Craniofacial bilateral
complex fractures
CSF fistulas and meningitis may occur

5.1.1.6 Mandibular
FRACTURES OCCUR IN TWO LOCATIONS
mandible and the TMJs form a rigid ring

ANATOMICAL LOCATION
NECK OR CONDYLAR FRACTURE
difficult to see on plain film
may need OPG or CT to exclude
RAMUS OR BODY OF MANDIBLE
oblique fracture, pull of masseter impacts fracture: favorable
oblique fracture, pull of masseter distracts fracture: unfavorable
teeth on either side allows dental wiring fixation

the fracture is an open fracture if a tooth socket is involved

ASSOCIATED INJURIES
TEMPOROMANDIBULAR JOINT DISLOCATION
EXTERNAL AUDITORY MEATUS FRACTURES
TEMPORAL BONE FRACTURES

5.1.2 MIDLINE FRACTURES

5.1.2.1 Nasal skeleton fractures

5.1.2.2 Nasoethmoidal fractures +/–cribriform plate fractures
complications: CSF rhinorrhea, meningitis

5.1.3 UNILATERAL

5.1.3.1 Isolated zygomatic arch

5.1.3.2 Isolated antrum

5.1.3.3 Tripod
FRACTURES THROUGH ORBITAL PROCESS OF MAXILLA, ZYGOMATIC ARCH, INFERIOR ANTRUM
IF SEVERE, INVOLVES POSTERIOR MAXILLARY ANTRUM + PTERYGOID PROCESS (+/– MAXILLARY ARTERY)

5.1.3.4 Isolated orbit
MEDIAL (?blowout)
beware of muscle entrapment and diplopia
LATERAL
INFERIOR (no blowout)
BLOWOUT FRACTURE
floor of orbit displaced down by orbital contents
floor fractures and a 'flap' of floor runs superomedial to inferolateral
soft tissue mass in fracture is orbital fat with or without inferior rectus (?diplopia)
'teardrop' in roof of maxillary antrum on plain film
CT direct coronal or coronal reformats shows position of defect and flap, and course of inferior rectus

5.1.3.5 Craniofacial isolated

5.2 FACIAL DYSMORPHIC SYNDROMES AND MALFORMATIONS

see Ch 20

5.3 INFLAMMATORY MASSES

5.3.1 RETENTION CYST

CLINICAL

mucus trapped behind blocked neck of a mucosal duct
raised epithelium over a dome like collection of retained secretions

IMAGING

CT/MR

non aggressive, semicircular, low density or fluid MR signal mass arising from one wall of a sinus (usually maxillary sinus) with no contrast enhancement

5.3.2 ANTROCHOANAL POLYP

CLINICAL

complex maxillary retention cyst pushing out into the middle meatus through the infundibulum

IMAGING

CT/MR

non aggressive, low density or fluid MR signal mass widening infundibulum, filling maxillary sinus and pushing through ostium along middle meatus into nasopharynx

5.3.3 RETAINED SECRETIONS BEHIND TUMOR

IMAGING

CT/MR

may be impossible to differentiate on CT
on MR, signal is usually different (secretions higher on PD and T2W sequences)
tumor has variable but solid contrast enhancement; secretions do not enhance or have a thin regular enhancing rim only

5.3.4 SINONASAL POLYPOSIS

DEFINITION

chronic allergic hyperplastic edematous proliferation of non malignant mucosa

CLINICAL

multiple bilateral edematous polyps arising from nasal mucosa and preferentially filling nasal vault

Local effects
obstruction, superinfection
bony pressure erosion
cavity expansion

IMAGING

CT/MR

inflammatory polyps tend to be of low density on CT, and of low T1W and high T2W signal
FINDINGS ARE BILATERALLY SYMMETRICAL (unless postoperative)
polypoid masses in nasal vault + sinuses
enlarged infundibula
bulging ethmoid + maxillary walls
bone shows pressure deossification
distal obstructive disease

5.4 INFLAMMATORY SINONASAL DISEASE

5.4.1 ACUTE SINUSITIS, PYOCELE

CLINICAL

usually bacterial superinfection of viral rhinitis in an obstructed sinus (maxillary sinusitis can come from a periapical abscess)
presents with fever, acutely painful and tender facial bones

COMPLICATIONS

ORBITAL ABSCESS
SUBDURAL EMPYEMA
INTRACRANIAL ABSCESS
CAVERNOUS SINUS THROMBOSIS

IMAGING

Plain XR
acute sinusitis: air–fluid level

CT
air–fluid level, mucoperiosteal thickening
osteomyelitis: bony wall destruction without mass
orbital abscess: medial crescentic soft tissue mass with possible rim enhancement

MR
orbital abscess: medial crescentic collection with rim enhancement
meningeal enhancement (frontal, ethmoidal, sphenoidal)
subdural empyema: see Ch 11; subdural collection with some mass effect and different signal from CSF with rim enhancement
focal cerebritis/brain abscess: see Ch 11
cavernous sinus thrombosis: modest mass effect, blood product signal, patchy enhancement

5.4.2 CHRONIC BACTERIAL SINUSITIS

CLINICAL

sinusitis with flora often mixed aerobic/anaerobic
often follows acute sinusitis in obstruction; complications same
osteomyelitis: patchy destruction of bony nasal walls with minimal mass

5.4.3 FUNGAL SINUSITIS

CLINICAL

Sinonasal aspergillosis

5.4.3.1 ASPERGILLOMA
fungus ball in a sinus

5.4.3.2 ALLERGIC SINONASAL ASPERGILLOSIS
extensive mucus superinfected with fungus, and containing eosinophils

5.4.3.3 CHRONIC GRANULOMATOUS ASPERGILLOSIS
slow fungal invasion of paranasal tissue
massive reaction (neutrophils, eosinophils, giant cells, granulomas, fibrosis)

5.4.3.4 ANGIOINVASIVE SINONASAL ASPERGILLOSIS
angioinvasion, thrombosis, infarction, necrosis
rapid, severe destruction of sinonasal structures with extension to orbit or thrombosis of cavernous sinus
diabetics, immunocompromised patients

5.4.3.5 Sinonasal mucormycosis

angioinvasive necrotizing mass forming infection
diabetic patients
rapid, severe destruction with extensive infarction
extension to orbit, anterior and middle cranial fossas, cavernous sinus thrombosis
similar to angioinvasive aspergillosis

IMAGING

CT
fungus ball may be high density
nodular mucoperiosteal thickening +/–calcification
may have aggressive bone destruction with mass

MR
low T1W, very low T2W signal
bone destruction if invasive

5.4.4 CHRONIC OBSTRUCTIVE DISEASE

CLINICAL

presentation is with symptoms of sinusitis
mucociliary drainage is inhibited where opposing mucosal surfaces touch and obstructed where mucosa is swollen or inflammatory mass develops
distal sinus becomes inflamed or filled with retained secretions

IMAGING

CT
thickened mucosa (concave and uniform)
(differential is retention cysts, which are convex)
fluid density filling sinus
air–fluid level (proof: shifts with changing position) indicates acute sinusitis, often purulent bacterial

MR
thickened mucosa is low on T1W, high on T2W sequences
fluid signal in sinus
fungal mass in a sinus may have no signal

Sporadic sinusitis
sporadic opacification or mucosal thickening of isolated sinuses that can not be grouped into a pattern

Sinusitis in an obstructive pattern

5.4.4.1 INFUNDIBULAR PATTERN
maxillary sinus only to level of infundibulum
narrowed/obstructed/diseased infundibulum

5.4.4.2 OSTIOMEATAL COMPLEX PATTERN
frontal, maxillary, anterior and middle ethmoid cells
obstruction/narrowing/mass at ostiomeatal recess with or without obstruction of middle nasal meatus

5.4.4.3 SPHENOETHMOIDAL RECESS PATTERN
sphenoid and posterior ethmoidal cells
obstruction or mass in sphenoethmoidal recess (axial scans)

5.4.4.4 FRONTONASAL DUCT PATTERN
frontal sinus with/without agger nasii or anterior ethmodial cells
especially common postoperatively
obstruction of distal frontonasal duct or very anterior ostiomeatal recess

Sinusitis behind postoperative synechiae

5.5 SINONASAL MUCOCELES

DEFINITION
mucus-containing sinus, expanded secondary to obstruction without infection

ETIOLOGY
INFLAMMATORY OBSTRUCTION
POST SURGICAL
SECONDARY TO TUMOR

LOCATION
FRONTAL (>> OTHERS)
MAXILLARY
SPHENOID
ETHMOID POLYPOID MUCOCELE
expanded opacified ethmoid complex

IMAGING

CT
dilated sinus containing mucus: watery low density, inspissated higher density
no contrast enhancement
thinned remodeled bone, may have areas of pressure atrophy and cortical push-through (sharp margin)

MR
watery mucus is fluid signal: high or isointense on T1W, high on T2W sequences
inspissated mucus: low on T1W, low on T2W sequences
no contrast enhancement
DIFFERENTIAL: polyp or tumor

5.6 POSTOPERATIVE CHANGE

5.6.1 CALDWELL–LUC PROCEDURE

CLINICAL

access to maxillary sinus from anterior
aspect with elevation of facial skin and
muscle just above maxillary alveolar
ridge and formation of antrostomy

IMAGING

bony window in anterolateral maxillary
sinus wall

5.6.2 INFERIOR MEATAL ANTROSTOMY

drainage pathway between maxillary sinus
and inferior nasal meatus (in lateral wall
of nose below inferior concha)

5.6.3 FESS (functional endoscopic sinus surgery)

goal is to resect structures obstructing
drainage pathways
UNCINECTOMY
BULLECTOMY
ETHMOIDECTOMY
SPHENOIDECTOMY

5.6.4 SYNECHIAE

usually invisible themselves, but cause
recurrent obstruction

5.7 TUMORS (benign)

5.7.1 SPORADIC POLYP

5.7.2 ANGIOMATOUS POLYP

5.7.3 JUVENILE ANGIOFIBROMA

CLINICAL

benign fibrovascular tumor arising in region
of sphenopalatine foramen

adolescent males presenting with epistaxis
mass pushing through sphenopalatine
    foramen into pterygopalatine fossa
extends back into nasopharynx and
    forwards into anterior nose
may push along foramen rotundum into
    middle cranial fossa

IMAGING

CT/MR

mass with extent and spread as above
strongly contrast enhancing, flow voids on
    MR

Angio
dense contrast blush

5.7.4 INVERTED PAPILLOMA

CLINICAL

lateral nose papillomatous mass
    invaginating under mucosa
may calcify

IMAGING

mass in lateral nasal wall, often centered on
    ostiomeatal unit

5.7.5 EVERTED PAPILLOMA

CLINICAL

squamous papilloma arising from nasal
    septum
non specific non aggressive mass

5.7.6 OSTEOMA

see Ch 05

5.7.7 FIBROUS DYSPLASIA

see Ch 05
isolated sphenoid wing or temporal bone, or
    multiple facial bones (cherubism)

5.8 TUMORS (malignant)

5.8.1 SINONASAL SCC

CLINICAL

90% of all sinonasal tumors
4/5 maxillary, 1/5 ethmoidal

IMAGING

CT/MR

destructive soft tissue mass, usually low on
    T1W, intermediate to high on T2W, with
    mild to moderate uniform contrast
    enhancement
retained secretions behind mass
spreads along cranial nerves (perineural
    mass, loss of perineural fat, nodular
    expansion of nerve, asymmetrical or
    nodular contrast enhancement)
centered on sinus of origin but invading
    other spaces and structures in continuity

5.8.2 NASOPHARYNGEAL CARCINOMA

DEFINITION

aggressive, undifferentiated SCC arising
    from nasopharynx

CLINICAL

male:female 2:1
Southern China > Africa > Europe
associated with Epstein–Barr virus (EBV)
nodal metastases in 90% at presentation
presents with: serous otitis media, nasal
    airway obstruction, epistaxis, CN palsies

IMAGING (locoregional)

CT

PRIMARY MASS (mucosal space mass)
mass isodense to nasopharyngeal
    mucosa/adenoids
mucosal thickening only with mass effect or
mucosally based mass or
extension into prevertebral muscle,
    parapharyngeal fat, or

erosion of skull base (basisphenoid)
opacified middle ear if Eustachian tube
obstructed

enhances slightly with contrast, either
diffuse or peripheral enhancement
invasion of bone definite if erosion present
or marrow fat replaced by solid soft tissue
no invasion of bone if fat plane exists
invasion vs adherence hard to judge if
contiguous to bone without erosion

SPREAD
enlarged lymph nodes, may have necrotic
low density core and ring enhancement
fuzzy nodal margin (extracapsular invasion)
loss of fat or cortex of foramen ovale,
possibly rotundum

MR

PRIMARY MASS (mucosal space mass)
low T1W signal often comparable to muscle,
higher T2W signal than muscle
mucosal thickening only with altered signal
and mass effect or
mucosally based mass or
extension into prevertebral muscle or
parapharyngeal fat with mass effect and
altered signal

enhances with contrast, with better
demarcation of interface with muscle
(mucus or retained secretions do not
enhance)
cortical bone erosion hard to tell on MR
bone marrow edema suggestive of invasion,
but may also be reactive

SPREAD
enlarged lymph nodes, usually high on T2W
high T2W core (necrotic core) and ring
enhancement
enhancing nodes without necrotic core
fuzzy nodal margin (extracapsular
extension)
loss of perineural fat planes around CN V3
in masticator space, in foramen ovale
and foramen rotundum
asymmetrical, thickened or beaded
enhancement in the same perineural
locations (differential for foramina:
asymmetrical emissary companion veins)
involvement of trigeminal cave

US
of little use for the primary
involved lymph nodes are enlarged, usually
hypoechoic (may be hyperechoic to
muscle if intense fibrotic response) and
may have low density necrotic center

color or power Doppler vascularity may be
increased
used for lymph node biopsy guidance

NUC MED (MDP)
MDP SPECT of skull base demonstrates
whether bony invasion is present

PET (FDG)
vast majority of primaries have increased
FDG uptake
most sensitive modality for nodal staging
(increased FDG uptake)
monitoring: decreased FDG uptake with
treatment indicates good metabolic
response
most sensitive modality for identifying
potential sites of primary carcinoma in
cases of occult head and neck SCC (SCC
metastasis/metastases in head and neck
lymph nodes with no mucosal primary on
clinical examination)

5.8.3 SINONASAL LYMPHOMA

5.8.4 ESTHESIO-NEUROBLASTOMA

CLINICAL

uncommon tumor of neuroendocrine origin
arising in superolateral nose
sheets of small round blue cells
highly aggressive with early distant
metastases

IMAGING

CT/MR
destructive mass in roof of nose with
moderate contrast enhancement
extension into anterior cranial fossa, orbits,
sphenoid and ethmoid sinuses

5.8.5 RHABDOMYOSARCOMA

see Ch 05

5.9 WEGENER'S GRANULOMATOSIS

see Ch 15

6. CONDITIONS OF THE LARYNX

6.1 LARYNGEAL MUCOSAL SCC

CLINICAL

stridor, cough, hoarseness, hemoptysis

Supraglottic
presents later, at higher stage, with greater
incidence of nodal metastases (~50%);
nodal metastases to upper neck

True cord
presents relatively early, low incidence of
metastases (~10%)

Infraglottic
lower incidence of metastases than
supraglottic SCC, metastases to lower
neck nodes

IMAGING (primary)

does not evaluate mucosal only involvement,
and does not exclude tumor if normal

Aims to assess deep extent
transglottic spread (feasibility of horizontal
hemilaryngectomy)
spread across midline (feasibility of vertical
hemilaryngectomy)
cartilage invasion

CT/MR
?do coronal reformats from thin section
helical multislice runs on CT
soft tissue density mass with variable
exophytic and variable invasive
component, mild contrast enhancement,
low (soft tissue) T1W signal,
moderate–high T2W signal

SUPRAGLOTTIC
mass arises from aryepiglottic folds, false
cords
mass extends down from epiglottis
may obstruct ventricle (leading to secondary
laryngocele)

REMAINS SUPRAGLOTTIC IF:
paralaryngeal fat is preserved in at least one
slice or delimits tumor from true cord on
coronal images

TRANSGLOTTIC IF:

extends to involve thyroarytenoid muscle (i.e. cord) or beneath cord

CARTILAGE INVASION:

unequivocal if tumor extends through cartilage

very likely if uniformly ossified cartilage is eroded by soft tissue mass in continuity with tumor

likely if persistent MR signal edge extends through unossified cartilage at the tumor/cartilage interface (tumor is higher on T2W than cartilage as TE increases, and an edge may show after contrast enhancement)

equivocal if cartilage is patchily ossified and tumor is contiguous

equivocal if cartilage is unossified and tumor is contiguous

not present if tumor separated from cartilage by paralaryngeal fat

cartilage sclerosis on CT is not a sign of invasion and may be reactive

GLOTTIC

mass arises directly from cord and may only be visible as cord thickening

REMAINS GLOTTIC IF:

limited to cord and does not cross anterior commissure

TRANSGLOTTIC:

extends to involve false cord

INFRAGLOTTIC:

extends through cord to endocricoid mucosa

CARTILAGE INVASION:

same guidelines as for supraglottic tumor

MIDLINE SPREAD:

more than 1 mm of soft tissue at anterior commissure or unequivocal bulky spread to other cord

bulky spread across posterior commissure with/without arytenoid cartilage involvement

INFRAGLOTTIC

mass arising from mucosa of lower vocal cone or cricoid cartilage

cartilage invasion: same guidelines as for supraglottic tumor

6.2 LARYNGEAL PAPILLOMA/ PAPILLOMATOSIS

CLINICAL

Papilloma

adults with hoarseness, hemoptysis

exophytic benign papilloma of the true cords, usually <1 cm

fibrovascular papillae covered with stratified epithelium

Papillomatosis

children with multiple laryngeal papillomas

associated with HPV (human papilloma virus) infection

frequently recur

IMAGING

usually does not progress beyond laryngoscopy

6.3 LARYNGEAL TRAUMA

6.3.1 INTUBATION TRAUMA

CLINICAL

difficult or blind intubation

presents with features of vocal cord palsy

IMAGING

anteriorly displaced arytenoid cartilage

immobile vocal cord

6.3.2 BLUNT TRAUMA

CLINICAL

external blunt impact

hyoid bone fracture

thyroid cartilage fracture (most commonly dislocation of one lamina under the other)

cricoid cartilage fracture (usually undisplaced fracture in at least two points)

tracheal ring fracture

Associated injuries

arytenoid dislocation

cricothyroid joint dislocation/cricothyroid cartilage separation

mucosal hematoma

airway compromise (displacement or hematoma)

surgical neck emphysema

6.4 LARYNGOCELE

DEFINITION

pathological enlargement of the laryngeal ventricle with/without outlet obstruction and with/without superinfection

CLASSIFICATION

Internal

enlarged ventricle confined to paraglottic space (in supraglottis)

External (mixed)

ventricle herniates through the thyrohyoid membrane

presents as a lateral neck mass of laryngeal origin

Simple (physiological)

air filled dilation of ventricle

no obstructing SCC

Secondary

laryngocele caused by ventricle outlet obstruction by supraglottic SCC

Superinfected (pyolaryngocele)

contains fluid, pus, secretions, air–fluid level

IMAGING

XR

simple external laryngocele: air filled lateral neck cavity level with the ventricle

superinfected laryngocele: air–fluid level

CT

simple internal laryngocele: air filled dilation of ventricle in paraglottic space

air filled external laryngocele herniates between hyoid bone and thyroid cartilage (lateral neck air filled sack, 'waist' in thyrohyoid membrane)

obstructed/superinfected laryngocele: internal debris, fluid, air fluid level, surrounding inflammatory change; thyrohyoid 'waist' if external

LOOK FOR SUPRAGLOTTIC SCC

MR

simple internal laryngocele: may not be visible (no signal), else air void

air filled external laryngocele: signal void

superinfected/obstructed: simulates soft
   tissue mass; rim contrast enhancement;
   thyrohyoid 'waist' if external

LOOK FOR SUPRAGLOTTIC SCC

6.5 VOCAL CORD PARALYSIS AND RECURRENT LARYNGEAL NERVE PALSY

ETIOLOGY

High vagal palsy

SURGERY

TUMOR

glomus jugulare, glomus vagale
skull base metastases
carotid sheath involvement

Recurrent laryngeal nerve palsy

TRAUMA

SURGERY
thyroidectomy/parathyroidectomy
neck dissection

PENETRATING TRAUMA

TUMOR

HEAD AND NECK
thyroid carcinoma
SCC

LUNG (RIGHT OR LEFT RECURRENT
   LARYNGEAL NERVE)
apical sulcus carcinoma with involvement of
   loop (right RLN) or ascending recurrent
   laryngeal nerve

METASTASES TO AORTOPULMONARY
   NODES (left recurrent laryngeal nerve)
lung primary, other primary
invasive metastases involving loop of left
   RLN

Differential diagnosis: arytenoid dislocation

IMAGING (larynx)

CT/MR

immobile cord is proven by scans in quiet
   breathing and in breathholding
   (demonstrating no change in position)
immobile anteromedial arytenoid cartilage

cord muscle atrophy (thinning, replacement
   by fat)
enlarged ipsilateral ventricle and pyriform
   sinus
paramedian cord position with or without
   lateral displacement by ventricle from
   below
other cord normal, and moves in
   breathing/breathholding;
   overcompensates (crosses midline)

7. CONDITIONS OF THE TEMPORAL BONE

7.1 CHOLESTEATOMA

DEFINITION

chronically enlarging collection of exfoliated
   keratin inside a squamous epithelial sac

CLINICAL

congenital (rare, ?2%): rests of squamous
   epithelium within middle ear, temporal
   bone, intracranial (analogous to
   epidermoid cysts)
acquired (vast majority): retraction pocket of
   tympanic membrane (usually of superior
   pars flaccida) which becomes sealed and
   separated from tympanic membrane,
   often after repeated episodes of otitis
   media
keratin desquamated into cyst, and cyst
   grows by expansion and pressure erosion
presents with hearing loss, ear discharge,
   labyrinthine fistula, facial palsy,
   meningitis

IMAGING

CT/MR

soft tissue density middle ear and mastoid
   mass
low T1W, high T2W signal
no enhancement with contrast (may have
   enhancement at margins only on MR)

DIFFERENTIAL

CHOLESTEROL GRANULOMA
high T1W and T2W signal, contrast
   enhancement at margins only

GRANULATION TISSUE
low T1W and high T2W signal, vivid
   contrast enhancement

classically originates in Prussak's space

scutum inferiorly
malleus head medially
attic lateral wall laterally

BEHAVIOR

erodes scutum, displaces and then erodes
   ossicles
as mass grows, fills and expands attic and
   middle ear cavity
accompanying bone erosion and expansion
differentiation from debris and effusion
   difficult if no bone erosion or expansion
   is present

INVOLVED STRUCTURES

ossicular chain
lateral semicircular canal (?labyrinthine
   fistula)
sinus tympani and facial nerve recess
   (?facial nerve)
tegmen tympani (?fistula, meningitis)

7.2 CHOLESTEROL GRANULOMA

CLINICAL

collection of hemorrhagic debris and
   granulation tissue within the temporal
   bone, often at petrous apex; NOT A
   CHOLESTEATOMA

IMAGING

CT

soft tissue or fluid density expansile mass

MR

expansile mass, high T1W and mixed T1W
   signal (blood products)
rim enhancement, no central enhancement

7.3 OTITIS + MASTOIDITIS

7.3.1 ACUTE OTITIS MEDIA

IMAGING

CT

fluid filled middle ear, with or without
   air–fluid levels
osteomyelitis: erosions of bony cortices

7.3.2 CHRONIC OTITIS MEDIA

CLINICAL

beware of obstructing tonsillitis or nasopharyngeal carcinoma as cause

Complications

hearing loss; tympanosclerosis; cholesteatoma; osteomyelitis; sigmoid sinus thrombosis; subdural empyema; brain abscess

IMAGING

see entries for acute otitis media (for imaging of the middle ear) and for cholesteatoma in this chapter and subdural empyema, sinus thrombosis and brain abscess in Ch 11

7.3.3 ACUTE MASTOIDITIS

CLINICAL

Complications

transverse or sigmoid sinus thrombosis; intradural abscess; petrous apicitis
Gradenigo syndrome (petrous apicitis with CN VI palsy)

IMAGING

CT

fluid-filled mastoid air cells, may have air–fluid levels
osteomyelitis: erosion of bony cortex

MR

fluid filled mastoid air cells
dural sinus thrombosis: see under CNS
extradural abscess, brain abscess: see under CNS
petrous apicitis: fluid signal in petrous apex, contrast enhancement

7.3.4 CHRONIC MASTOIDITIS

CLINICAL

abnormal development of mastoid air cells, often associated with chronic otitis media or chronic middle ear effusion

IMAGING

CT

sclerotic small mastoid air cells

7.4 OTOSCLEROSIS
(otospongiosis)

7.4.1 FENESTRAL OTOSCLEROSIS

CLINICAL

resorption of normal dense inner ear bone with replacement by vascular spongy bone
affects bone just anterior and lateral to oval window; may cause stapes fixation
presents with conductive hearing loss

IMAGING

CT

focal demineralization and expansion of bone at the anterolateral margin of oval window

7.4.2 COCHLEAR OTOSCLEROSIS

CLINICAL

resorption of normal dense inner ear bone with replacement by vascular spongy bone
affects cochlear bony walls
presents with sensorineural hearing loss

IMAGING

CT

demineralization of bone surrounding the cochlea (otic capsule demineralization)
DIFFERENTIAL: otic capsule Paget's disease

7.5 TEMPORAL BONE FRACTURES

7.5.1 (80%) LONGITUDINAL

risk of ossicular dislocation

~25% have CN VII palsy (usually due to edema and potentially reversible)

7.5.2 (20%) TRANSVERSE

~50% have CN VII palsy (usually due to transsection and not reversible)

7.5.3 MIXED (most fractures have mixed features)

STRUCTURES AT RISK

OSSICULAR CHAIN
dislocation, conductive hearing loss

COCHLEA
sensorineural hearing loss

VESTIBULAR LABYRINTH
CSF FISTULA
LABYRINTHITIS

FACIAL NERVE
EDEMA VS TRANSSECTION

CAROTID CANAL
LACERATION
DISSECTION

JUGULAR FOSSA

TEGMEN TYMPANI
CSF FISTULA
MENINGITIS

SPHENOID SINUS
CSF FISTULA
MENINGITIS

TEMPOROMANDIBULAR JOINT

7.6 TMJ DISC DERANGEMENT

CLINICAL

Normal

disc has posterior and anterior bands, and a thin central portion
condylar head lies between the two in the lower compartment
most rotation in lower joint space (condyle on disc)
most translation in upper joint space (disc on glenoid fossa)

IMAGING (anterior displacement)

Plain film

late degenerative change: osteophytes, sclerosis, deformity

Arthrography

posterior band displaced anteriorly, with disc 'bunched up'

reduction: condyle moves forward over posterior band in mouth opening

posterior attachment perforation: free contrast flow between compartments

MR

NORMAL

disc low on T1W and T2W sequences

posterior disc attachment higher T1W signal than disc

closed mouth: posterior band above condyle

open mouth: 'bow tie' configuration with thin portion between condyle and glenoid eminence

DISPLACEMENT WITH REDUCTION

posterior band of disc anterior to condyle in closed mouth position

disc may be rounded or deformed

rotational deformity if only medial or lateral part of disc displaced

in open mouth position disc returns to 'bow tie' configuration

DISPLACEMENT WITHOUT REDUCTION

ASSOCIATED ABNORMALITIES

disc deformity

'pseudodisc' (fibrosis of posterior disc attachment)

joint effusion with tear of posterior disc attachment

bone marrow edema

osteophytes

stuck disc

8. THYROID CONDITIONS

8.1 ABBREVIATIONS

T3:   triiodothyronine (active form of thyroid hormone)

T4:   thyroxine, tetraiodothyronine (converted to T3)

TSH: thyroid stimulating hormone

TcO4:   Tc-99m pertechnetate

TFT's: thyroid function tests (free thyroxine, T3, TSH levels)

Tg: thyroglobulin

8.2 CRETINISM

see Ch 20

8.3 GRAVES' DISEASE

also see dysthyroid ophthalmopathy

DEFINITION

syndrome of autoimmune hyperthyroidism, diffuse goitre and thyroiditis, ophthalmopathy and other manifestations

EPIDEMIOLOGY

30–50 years old, female > male

HLA DR3 associated

part of thyrogastric cluster (Graves' disease, Hashimoto's thyroiditis; Addison's disease, vitiligo; autoimmune gastritis, pernicious anemia)

PATHOGENESIS

antiTSH receptor antibody, hyperthyroidism

diffuse epithelial hyperplasia; reduced colloid with marginal scalloping

+/–features of Hashimoto's thyroiditis

CLINICAL

high T3, T4, low TSH, antiTSH receptor antibodies

thyroid disease eventually 'burns out' with destruction of functioning thyroid tissue, producing eventual hypothyroidism

THYROID MANIFESTATIONS (90%)

painful modest size goitre

HYPERTHYROIDISM

(DYS)THYROID OPHTHALMOPATHY

OTHER

pretibial myxedema

thyroid acropachy: manifestations are the same as in hypertrophic osteoarthropathy (see Ch 01 gamut 2.1.6); may occur after treatment of hyperthyroidism and does not depend on endocrine status

IMAGING

US

diffusely enlarged gland, hypervascular on color Doppler

may be heterogeneous or have multifocal nodularity (in general, less so than multinodular goitre)

NUC MED (TcO4 or I)

hypervascular gland (on perfusion phase)

massively uniformly increased uptake, markedly increased relative to background and salivary uptake

prominently elevated 20 minute TcO4 and 24 hour I uptake

NUC MED (I-131 therapy)

see I-131 therapy entry

8.4 MULTINODULAR GOITER (MNG)

DEFINITION

diffusely nodular thyroid enlargement by variably hyperplastic (non neoplastic) thyroid follicles

CLINICAL

very common; female:male 8:1

incidence of malignancy same as in general population

FOLLICULAR HETEROGENEITY

cuboidal non neoplastic lining with papillary infolding or ingrowths

PRESENTS WITH MASS (euthyroid)

PRESENTS WITH ENDOCRINOPATHY

hypothyroid

hyperthyroid (~50%) = Plummer's syndrome

IMAGING

XR

usually normal

soft tissue mass, tracheal deviation or compression (on CXR or neck XR for soft tissues)

superior mediastinal mass with no upper border (i.e. continuous with thoracic inlet)

thyroid calcification (coarse; eggshell in a follicle)

US

enlarged nodular gland

thickened isthmus, bilateral enlargement (may be asymmetrical)

coarse echotexture with multiple heterogeneous nodules

partly cystic, partly solid nodules

thyroid cysts (may contain debris)

coarse calcification

beware of a size dominant nodule: ?carcinoma

CT

DO NOT ADMINISTER IV CONTRAST IF PLANNING NUCLEAR MEDICINE INVESTIGATION OR THERAPY (or delay nuclear medicine studies by 4–6 weeks post contrast CT)

heterogeneously enlarged gland with focal hypoechoic nodules

gland density higher than muscle (intrinsic iodine content)

INTRATHORACIC/RETROSTERNAL EXTENSION

in-continuity soft tissue mass extending from one or both lobes of thyroid through the thoracic inlet, frequently extends into tracheoesophageal groove

may deviate, distort, surround or compress trachea, great vessels and esophagus

inferior border may be at sternal notch, retrosternal, or at aortic arch

MR

morphology same as for CT, but coronal plane allows direct demonstration of retrosternal extension continuity

hemorrhagic follicles have high T1W signal

NUC MED (TcO4 or I)

MULTINODULAR GOITRE

TcO4 or I, use pinhole collimator

enlarged gland, often asymmetric

patchy uptake with focal warmer and cooler areas

20 minute TcO4 and 24 hour I uptake within normal range overall

MNG WITH TOXIC NODULE (Plummer's syndrome)

signs of MNG and

one nodule has focally increased uptake, with the rest of the gland variably suppressed

degree of suppression of remaining gland not as profound as in functioning adenoma

NUC MED (I-131 therapy)

see I-131 therapy entry

PET (FDG)

no elevated uptake above soft tissue levels (unless a toxic nodule is also present)

8.5 SIMPLE GOITER

DEFINITION

diffuse hyperplastic thyroid enlargement secondary to inadequate T3/T4 levels

CLINICAL

diffuse hyperplasia; uniform fleshy lobules with cuboidal cells and little colloid

ENDEMIC

iodine deficiency

commonest cause of goitre worldwide

SPORADIC

female:male 8:1

PRESENTS WITH MASS (euthyroid)

PRESENTS WITH ENDOCRINOPATHY

subclinical hypothyroid

clinical hypothyroid

IMAGING

US/CT/MR

diffuse uniform enlargement of thyroid gland

may have coarse echotexture

NUC MED (TcO4 or I)

enlarged gland, uniform uptake

20 minute TcO4 or 24 hour I uptake normal (impaired synthesis) or high (dietary deficiency)

8.6 THYROID ADENOMA

DEFINITION

benign and often hormonally functional neoplasm

CLINICAL

common cause of cold nodule (and a more common cause than carcinoma), and of nearly all solitary toxic nodules

PRESENTS WITH: incidental US finding, thyroid mass, hyperthyroidism

MORPHOLOGY

solid gelatinous or fleshy mass 3–10 cm

+/–hemorrhage or cystic change

delimited by fibrous capsule

NO INVASION

histological differential is follicular carcinoma

IMAGING

US

solitary nodule (but may arise on a background of multinodular goitre since it is so common)

may have cystic areas or a prominent vascular color ring

used for fine needle biopsy guidance

NUC MED (TcO4 or I)

cold nodule (differential is carcinoma, if solid)

OR

warm nodule OR

hyperfunctioning nodule, with suppression of remainder of gland (almost certainly benign)

NUC MED (I-131 therapy)

see I-131 therapy entry

8.7 THYROID CARCINOMA

8.7.1 (70%) PAPILLARY CARCINOMA OF THYROID

CLINICAL

well differentiated thyroid carcinoma with tendency to lymphatic spread and a good prognosis

female:male 3:1; association with radiation

mass, cold nodule
extremely rarely a hot nodule
lymph nodal metastases in neck ('aberrant lateral thyroid' of old surgical textbooks)
hematogenous metastases (lung, bone, brain) late and uncommon
excellent prognosis even untreated

MACRO

irregular hard white mass with ill defined invasive edge
20% multifocal (spread via intrathyroid lymphatics)

MICRO

neoplastic cystic follicles with papillary ingrowths (fibrovascular core)
calcified psammoma bodies (diagnostic)
ORPHAN ANNIE EYES: malignant cells with ground glass nuclei that have grooves or intranuclear inclusions

8.7.2 (20%) FOLLICULAR CARCINOMA OF THYROID

CLINICAL

moderately well differentiated thyroid carcinoma with tendency to hematogenous spread
40–70 years old (older than papillary), female:male 3:1
mass or cold nodule
HEMATOGENOUS spread: LUNGS, BONES

MORPHOLOGY

gelatinous or fleshy mass with cystic change, hemorrhage; may show frank invasion
small neoplastic follicles
invasion into blood vessels (poor prognosis) or neighboring structures diagnostic

8.7.3 (5%) MEDULLARY CARCINOMA OF THYROID

DEFINITION

carcinoma of parafollicular (APUD) cells associated with multiple endocrine neoplasia

EPIDEMIOLOGY

75% sporadic
solitary often large mass in a 50–70 year old

25% familial
younger adults
MEN II [mnemonic PMP] (parathyroid adenoma, medullary carcinoma of thyroid, pheochromocytoma)
MEN III [mnemonic MPM] (medullary carcinoma of thyroid, pheochromocytoma, mucosal neuromas)
von Hippel Lindau syndrome
neurofibromatosis 1

CLINICAL

solitary mass or multiple smaller masses
hemorrhage, calcification, cystic change

Endocrinopathy
calcitonin, ACTH, serotonin
AE type AMYLOIDOSIS

8.7.4 ANAPLASTIC CARCINOMA OF THYROID

DEFINITION

rare aggressive carcinoma of older females

CLINICAL

hard thyroid mass with rapid thyroid enlargement
rapidly progressive course despite treatment
death from local invasion, compression, metastases
small cell, spindle cell, giant cell variants

IMAGING (group)

XR
CXR may show thoracic inlet mass
thyroid metastases to bone classically expansile lytic

US
thyroid mass, may be very large
may have complex internal vascularity
may have punctate internal calcification

NUC MED (TcO4 or I)

usually a cold mass or nodule, but carcinoma is <20% of solitary cold nodules
very rarely a warm or a hyperfunctioning nodule (well differentiated carcinoma)
medullary carcinoma always cold (by definition)

NUC MED (In-111 octreotide)

medullary carcinoma is octreotide avid

NUC MED (whole body I scanning)

well differentiated and moderately well differentiated papillary and follicular carcinoma take up iodine; as they take up iodine less efficiently than normal thyroid tissue, the carcinoma usually presents as a cold nodule on a background of functional thyroid tissue
after ablation of all functioning thyroid tissue, metastases manifest as iodine avid foci or masses
in time, carcinoma metastases dedifferentiate and are no longer iodine avid
ablative or treatment doses of I-131 may demonstrate small volume or poorly avid metastases not visible with a diagnostic dose of I-131 or I-123

THYROID STUNNING
'thyroid stunning' is controversial: postulated reduced avidity of normal thyroid tissue or well differentiated carcinomatous tissue for radioiodine after a diagnostic dose of I-131
evidence for stunning incomplete
theoretically eliminated if no diagnostic scan done before ablative dose given
theoretically minimized if I-123 is used for diagnosis, or if I-131 diagnostic dose is kept to a minimum (at risk of missing small metastases) and if therapy dose is given as soon as possible after the diagnostic I-131 dose

NORMAL I-131 UPTAKE
salivary glands, and in secreted saliva
saliva outlines oral cavity and may outline esophagus (scan after a drink of water)
renal and urinary
stomach and colon
faint liver (de-iodination of radiothyroxine)
diffuse very low grade whole body

NUC MED (I-131 therapy)

see I-131 therapy entry

PET (FDG)

very FDG avid, but focal increased thyroid FDG uptake is not specific for carcinoma

8.8 THYROID LYMPHOMA

CLINICAL

usually non Hodgkin's B lymphoma
primary thyroid lymphoma develops on a background of autoimmune thyroiditis

IMAGING

US

focal mass or diffuse enlargement

NUC MED (TcO4 or I)

lymphoma does not take up TcO4 or I, but may not be visible if there is no normal thyroid uptake in the background

PET (FDG)

FDG avid

8.9 THYROIDITIS

DEFINITION

THYROIDITIS: autoimmune or infectious inflammation of thyroid

CLASSIFICATION OF THYROIDITIS

Acute infective non viral

BACTERIAL (+/–ABSCESS)

TB, FUNGAL

Viral/subacute post viral

SUBACUTE GRANULOMATOUS (De Quervain's thyroiditis)

RARE IMMUNOLOGICAL: RIEDEL'S THYROIDITIS

Autoimmune

HASHIMOTO'S THYROIDITIS AND RELATED CONDITIONS

HASHIMOTO'S THYROIDITIS

ATROPHIC THYROIDITIS

FOCAL LYMPHOCYTIC THYROIDITIS

coexistent GRAVES' DISEASE

Radiation thyroiditis

8.9.1 HASHIMOTO'S THYROIDITIS AND RELATED CONDITIONS

CLINICAL

incidence peaks in 30–60 year olds, female:male 5:1
part of thyrogastric autoimmune cluster
associated with Graves' disease ('Hashitoxicosis' if both are simultaneously present)
painful normal size thyroid or painful small goitre
hyperthyroid early (leak of T4 from damaged follicles)
eventually hypothyroid–subclinical or clinical; increased lymphoma risk

MICRO

Hashimoto's thyroiditis (chronic lymphocytic thyroiditis)

lymphocyte and plasma cell infiltrate, lymphoid follicles
patchy destruction of thyroid follicle walls

Atrophic thyroiditis (late manifestation of autoimmune thyroiditis)

Focal lymphocytic thyroiditis

asymptomatic subacute variant, clinically latent

IMAGING

FOCAL LYMPHOCYTIC THYROIDITIS usually has no imaging findings

US

early: diffusely swollen gland, may have altered echotexture (coarsened, hypoechoic, hyperechoic)
late: variably shrunken gland, may be hyperechoic
may be totally normal

NUC MED (TcO4 or I)

diffusely reduced uptake
reduced 20 minute TcO4 or 24 hour I uptake

8.9.2 SUBACUTE GRANULOMATOUS (DE QUERVAIN'S) THYROIDITIS

CLINICAL

acute or subacute self limiting post viral thyroiditis, with histology characterized by neutrophils, giant cells and granulomas
prodromal upper respiratory infection 2–3 weeks prior
sudden onset of painful thyroid gland (but up to 1/3 may be pain-free)
hyperthyroidism in 50% (damaged gland) followed by hypothyroidism in 5% (dysfunction)

IMAGING

US

may be normal
slightly swollen, diffusely hypoechoic gland
beware of asymmetric ('focal') thyroiditis simulating malignancy (rare!!)
eventually normal as thyroiditis resolves

NUC MED (TcO4 or I)

diffusely decreased uptake, may see 'shadow' of gland only
beware of focal thyroiditis simulating a cold nodule (rare!)
restored to normal once thyroiditis resolves

9. PARATHYROID CONDITIONS

9.1 HYPER-PARATHYROIDISM

see Ch 02

9.2 HYPO-PARATHYROIDISM, PSEUDO, PSEUDOPSEUDO

see Ch 02

9.3 PARATHYROID MASSES

9.3.1 PARATHYROID ADENOMA

CLINICAL

female > male

presents with endocrinopathy or osteoporosis, only rarely presents with neck mass

solitary tan/red mass with or without a well defined capsule

atrophy of own gland and other glands

commoner in inferior glands, may be ectopic

9.3.2 PARATHYROID CARCINOMA

irregular mass with or without a fibrous capsule

only criterion of malignancy is local invasion or metastases

part of multiple endocrine neoplasia spectrum

9.3.3 PARATHYROID HYPERPLASIA

CLINICAL

usually a renal dialysis patient or renal transplant recipient with secondary or tertiary hyperparathyroidism

asymmetrical enlargement of several or all parathyroid glands

IMAGING (group)

XR

see entries on hyperparathyroidism and osteoporosis in Ch 2

US

more successful if targeted by nuclear medicine study

parathyroid gland expected locations: upper parathyroid: behind upper part of thyroid lobe; lower parathyroid: posterior or inferior to thyroid lobe

hypoechoic rounded mass, solid or mixed solid/cystic

usually lies behind thyroid, but may be physically separate and may be intrathyroidal

echotexture may be indistinguishable from thyroid tissue

very vascular, and a color Doppler 'ring' may show it separately from thyroid tissue

US will not see mediastinal parathyroid adenomas

lateral fold of esophagus is a cause of false positives

CT

enhancing nodule in the same location as for US

helpful in showing anterior mediastinum

MR

Gd enhancing soft tissue mass (use fat saturation)

particularly useful in mediastinal adenoma

NUC MED (MIBI)

variable protocols exist, which depend on two phenomena:

parathyroid adenomas take up and retain MIBI relative to thyroid tissue which washes out;

parathyroid adenomas do not take up TcO4

TcO4/MIBI subtraction protocols rely on showing MIBI avid tissue not shown with TcO4

MIBI early/MIBI late protocols rely on preferential MIBI retention by the adenoma (done with SPECT)

Nuc Med studies useful in demonstrating ectopic adenomas, but are usually negative in parathyroid hyperplasia

overall sensitivity (adenomas) is 70–80%, specificity is ~90%

MIBI may be used for radioguided neck dissection

9.4 PARAGANGLIOMAS

DEFINITION

tumors of neural crest origin sharing a common histology that occur in a wide but predictable distribution

CLASSIFICATION

Paraganglia

clusters of cells of neural crest origin innervated by the autonomic nervous system

homologues of autonomic GANGLIA but the cells are not post ganglionic neurons

tend to form GLOMERA (conglomerations of cells and small blood vessels)

may function as hormone secreting endocrine glands (e.g. adrenal gland, organ of Zuckerkandl) or as chemoreceptors (carotid and aortic bodies)

Naming is by location

functioning paraganglioma is termed a pheochromocytoma (extra or intraadrenal)

unnamed, non functioning paraganglioma is termed a paraganglioma

ADRENAL MEDULLA
PHEOCHROMOCYTOMA

CHEMORECEPTOR BODIES
CAROTID BODY TUMOR (CHEMODECTOMA)

MEDIASTINAL PARAGANGLIOMA (aortic body)

ABDOMEN
PARAGANGLIOMA or PHEOCHROMOCYTOMA

PARASYMPATHETIC CRANIAL OUTFLOW
GLOMUS TYMPANICUM
associated with recurrent tympanic branch of CN IX

GLOMUS JUGULARE
associated with mastoid branch of CN X

GLOMUS VAGALE
associated with CN X

ORBITAL GLOMUS

PARASYMPATHETIC VISCERAL OUTFLOW
VISCERAL PARAGANGLIOMAS

EPIDEMIOLOGY

may be familial

CLINICAL

wide range of ages, peak 20–40 years, female > male; may be familial

multicentric in up to 20%

tan or red vascular mass that may have a bruit

neuroendocrine type cells with large nuclei

unpredictable behavior

IMAGING FINDINGS – ANY MODALITY (head and neck tumors only)

Carotid body tumor (carotid space)

rounded vascular mass in carotid bifurcation or adjacent to it

usually splays the carotid arteries, may wrap around either carotid artery

may displace or compress internal jugular vein

Glomus tympanicum (middle ear)

middle ear cavity vascular mass arising from cochlear promontory, extending to tympanic membrane, often produces a red or a blue mass behind the eardrum on visual inspection

glomus jugulotympanicum: mass is in continuity between middle ear and jugular bulb

BEWARE of dehiscent high jugular bulb (normal variant) or aberrant ICA (normal variant) mimicking a glomus tympanicum

Glomus jugulare (jugular bulb)

vascular mass within/pushing through the jugular canal and fossa (and extending caudally)

may compress internal jugular vein or appear to arise from jugular bulb

punctate calcifications and surrounding permeative-type loss of bone cortex (CT bone windows)

Glomus vagale (carotid space)

vascular mass along the course of the high ICA (by definition, just below skull base but above carotid bifurcation)

COMMON IMAGING CHARACTERISTICS IN ALL HEAD AND NECK LOCATIONS

Plain XR

usually non contributory

US

useful for carotid body tumor
very vascular well circumscribed mass

CT

rounded, well circumscribed very vascular mass with arterial phase vivid contrast enhancement (demonstrated to advantage on CT angiography especially in the neck)

punctate calcification and permeative jugular bone erosion in glomus jugulare

MR

low T1W and intermediate T2W signal with characteristic 'salt and pepper' flow voids (larger tumors)

well shown on MR angiography

vividly contrast enhancing, but flow voids remain

Angio

classic appearance is of highly vascular mass fed by multiple abnormal vessels, with a tumor blush

if feeding vessels can be identified, used for preoperative embolization (ascending pharyngeal artery for glomus tympanicum in particular, or other branches of external carotid or maxillary artery)

NUC MED (octreoscan)

In-111 octreotide
most have vivid uptake

NUC MED (CERETEC or ECD)

vivid uptake because of vascularity

10. SKIN MALIGNANCIES

10.1 MELANOMA

DEFINITION

malignant melanocytic tumor with incidence related to sunlight exposure and with a highly unpredictable behavior

CLINICAL

geographically variable, increasing overall, incidence related to sunlight exposure (UV)

particularly common in Australia

association: dysplastic nevus syndrome (mean age at diagnosis is 35 years)

Presentation

DE NOVO

IN PREEXISTING NEVUS (ALTERATION OR GROWTH)

METASTATIC MELANOMA, PRIMARY NOT FOUND

RARE LOCATIONS: IRIS; ORAL, VAGINAL AND ANAL MUCOSA; INTERNAL: ESOPHAGUS, MENINGES

Spread

into dermis, then unpredictable

LYMPHATIC: locoregional and distal

hematogenous: liver, lung, brain, etc

locations unusual for carcinoma: muscle and skeletal soft tissues; spleen; subcutaneous nodules

Staging

for Clark levels, and Breslow thickness see section on prognosis

T STAGE

pTis	melanoma in situ (Clark level I)
pT1	<0.75 mm thick and invades papillary dermis (Clark level II)
pT2	<1.5 mm thick and/or invades papillary/reticular dermis junction (Clark level III)
pT3	<4.0 mm thick and/or invades reticular dermis (Clark level IV)
pT4	>4.0 mm thick and/or invades subcutaneous tissue (Clark level V) and/or satellites within 2 cm

N STAGE

| N1 | regional lymph node <3 cm |
| N2 | regional node >3 cm or in transit metastasis or both |

MORPHOLOGY

SUPERFICIAL SPREADING MELANOMA (>70%)

flat spreading pigmented lesion

NODULAR MELANOMA (~20%)

focal bulky tumor with downward growth

LENTIGO MALIGNA

slow growing pigmented patch in an elderly patient

ACRAL LENTIGINOUS

subungual, palms and soles

IMAGING (melanoma specific)

CT

regional lymphadenopathy

soft tissue density masses in unusual locations: muscle, subcutaneous soft tissues, spleen

soft tissue density masses in locations prone to metastases (liver, brain, lungs, bone)

may have ring or solid enhancement

MR

morphology as for CT

melanin is intermediate to high T1W signal, if expressed, and melanoma deposits may be relatively high on T1W (esp brain)

(differential is hemorrhage into melanoma metastases)

for orbital melanoma, see orbit section

NUC MED (Gallium)

melanoma is Ga avid and Ga can be used for staging

(lack of Ga uptake does not rule out melanoma metastases)

NUC MED (lymphoscintigraphy)

CHOICE OF COLLOID

antimony colloid has ideal dimensions (approx 30 nm) but not FDA approved

sulfur colloid is large (200 nm) unless microfiltered

TECHNIQUE AND RATIONALE

intradermal injection around melanoma excision scar

demonstration of draining lymph channels and draining nodes

by definition, first node or echelon of nodes are sentinel node(s)

selective radioguided (and/or blue dye guided) excision of sentinel nodes and histology very accurately predict status of entire lymph node basin

lymphoscintigraphy also shows patterns of drainage for ambiguous regions (e.g. trunk) and how many lymph node basins are involved

PET (FDG)

accurate staging and monitoring of therapy

melanoma is FDG avid

10.2 SQUAMOUS CELL CARCINOMA (SCC)

DEFINITION

common well differentiated skin malignancy with strong causal relationship to sunlight

ETIOLOGY

DNA damage by UV radiation or otherwise; smoking and alcohol in head and neck SCC

HPV acts as promoter (involved in the spectrum papilloma–carcinoma) with or without UV

progression to SCC accelerated with suppressed cell mediated immunity

RARE associations: xeroderma pigmentosum, topical cyclic hydrocarbons

CLINICAL

orderly progression: solar keratosis, Bowen disease, atypical warts to SCC in situ to invasive SCC

presents early unless neglected

raised, warty or ulcerated mass or thickening

lymphatic spread occurs only following dermal invasion

hematogenous spread late

MICRO

mass of dysplastic epithelium with loss of stratification; preserved keratinization and keratin pearls

clearly invasive (differential is carcinoma in situ, and keratoacanthoma)

IMAGING

usually none required for simple skin tumors

Thorax

1. NORMAL

1.1 LUNG ON HRCT

Density of lung tissue

DEPENDENT GRADIENT: dependent lung denser because of crowding and vascular filling

EXPIRATORY–INSPIRATORY GRADIENT: expiratory lung denser because of crowding

HRCT lobule = secondary lobule

3–15 acini

1–2 cm in diameter

limited by interstitial septa (interlobular septa) with pulmonary veins and lymphatics

supplied by small bronchiole and its artery (centrilobular structures)

Peripheral extent of central structures (HRCT)

bronchi to within 2–3 cm of pleura

centrilobular structures to within 5–10 mm of pleura

Peripheral vessel size

the diameter of an artery accompanying a normal bronchus is usually between 1x and 1.5x the diameter of the bronchus

1.2 DEFINITION OF AIRSPACE/ AIRSPACE PATTERN

Airspace

air containing compartment of lung (including all interstitial structures too thin to resolve)

Airspace opacity

fluffy or solid, patchy or confluent opacity

no mass effect by definition

partly obscures vessels (groundglass opacity) or fully obscures vessels (consolidation)

outlines air in bronchi (air bronchograms)

patchy/multifocal airspace pattern merges into NODULAR pattern

1.3 DEFINITION OF NODULE/ NODULAR PATTERN

Nodule

circumscribed soft tissue density, sharply or fuzzily marginated

nodules have mass effect by definition

may be airspace nodule (centered on airspace) or interstitial nodule (centered on interstitial structures)

Nodular pattern

nodular pattern may be INTERSTITIAL or AIRSPACE (depending on isocenter of nodules), MILIARY (random, implying arterial embolic spread) or nodules may be too big to tell

1.4 DEFINITION OF INTERSTITIUM/INTER- STITIAL PATTERN

Interstitium

connective tissue compartment of the lung, carrying bronchi, arteries, veins, lymphatics

Central interstitium = peribronchovascular and centrilobular interstitium

follows bronchi and arteries (and centrilobular/peribronchovascular lymphatics) from major bronchi and arteries to the centrilobular structures

Peripheral interstitium = septal and subpleural interstitium

follows pleura and subpleural septa on periphery of lobules, and follows veins and perivenular lymphatics

Interstitial pattern

CLASSIFICATION BY DISTRIBUTION

PERIBRONCHOVASCULAR/CENTRILOBULAR

PERIPHERAL

PERILYMPHATIC (combination of the above two)

CLASSIFICATION BY CONTOUR

SMOOTH

accentuation and thickening of interstitial markings

RETICULOLINEAR on CXR

interstitial fluid (e.g. edema) does not produce nodules on CXR!

NODULAR

nodules centered on interstitium

NODULAR on CXR

nodular interstitial pattern merges into lung nodules

MIXED

RETICULONODULAR on CXR

HRCT CAVEAT

superimposed airspace pattern carries the differential diagnosis of acute airspace component (implies active disease) vs fibrosis that is too fine to resolve!

2. GAMUTS

2.1 GENERIC (all modalities)

2.1.1 AIRSPACE OPACITY

Transudate ('acute pulmonary edema')

CARDIOGENIC

NEUROGENIC

CIRRHOTIC

NEPHROTIC

PANCREATIC

Exudate ('adult respiratory distress syndrome')

DIFFUSE ALVEOLAR DAMAGE

ALVEOLAR PROTEINOSIS

Blood

CONTUSION

INFARCTION

e.g. WEGENER'S GRANULOMATOSIS

HEMORRHAGE

e.g. GOODPASTURE'S SYNDROME, EXCESSIVE WARFARINIZATION

Pus

CONVENTIONAL INFECTIVE CONSOLIDATION

EOSINOPHILIC PNEUMONIA

ACUTE INTERSTITIAL PNEUMONIA (esp viral)

PNEUMOCYSTIS PNEUMONIA (groundglass)

LIPOID PNEUMONIA (low density by definition)

Cancer

BRONCHIOLOALVEOLAR CARCINOMA

LEUKEMIA, LYMPHOMA

Interstitial gone airspace (= 'IGA')

initially interstitial process that secondarily involves the airspace, or produces that impression on imaging

DIP-RBILD; NSIP; AIP

ORGANIZING PNEUMONIA

VASCULITIS, WEGENERS, SLE

SARCOIDOSIS

2.1.2 ASYMMETRICAL/ UNILATERAL PULMONARY EDEMA

Increased congestion on one side only ('edema, this lung abnormal')

PULMONARY EDEMA AND GRAVITY (e.g. prolonged decubitus position)

UNILATERAL MECHANICAL VENOUS OBSTRUCTION

AFTER EXPANSION OF ONE LUNG

classic cause: rapid unilateral pleural effusion drainage

Pulmonary edema, decreased congestion on one side ('edema, other lung abnormal')

ARTERIAL HYPOPERFUSION

UNILATERAL PULMONARY EMBOLISM

PULMONARY ARTERY COMPRESSION

usually tumor

UNILATERAL PULMONARY ATRESIA/HYPOPLASIA

e.g. McLeod/Swyer–James syndrome

Asymmetric lung, but not edema at all

UNILATERAL LYMPHANGITIS

implies central tumor at hilum of abnormal lung

UNILATERAL ARDS

unilateral aspiration, radiation pneumonitis

CONTRALATERAL HYPERLUCENT HEMITHORAX

see its own gamut

UNILATERAL LUNG TRANSPLANT

CYSTIC FIBROSIS OF NATIVE LUNG

SEVERE EMPHYSEMA OF NATIVE LUNG

2.1.3 BRONCHIAL OBSTRUCTION

Causes

LUMEN

FOREIGN BODY

MUCUS

CLOT

TUMOR

WALL

FRACTURE

STRICTURE

INFECTION

SARCOIDOSIS

TUMOR

WEGENER'S GRANULOMATOSIS

AMYLOID

EXTRINSIC COMPRESSION

CANCER

NON CANCER

LYMPH NODES

VESSELS

Sequelae of proximal obstruction

NO SEQUELAE

DISTAL COLLAPSE

DISTAL AIR TRAPPING

DISTAL DROWNING

BRONCHOCELE (bronchus only)

BRONCHUS AND LUNG (endogenous lipoid pneumonia)

2.1.4 COLLAPSE

Non obstructive (iso T1W, low T2W signal)

PASSIVE COMPRESSIVE

DISTAL ATELECTASIS

SCARRING

ROUND ATELECTASIS

Obstructive (iso T1W, high T2W signal)

LOBAR SIGNS

FISSURE SHIFT AND HILAR ROTATION

VESSEL CROWDING

(increased opacity depends on fluid content of collapsed lobe)

VOLUME LOSS

MEDIASTINAL AND DIAPHRAGM SHIFT

RIB CROWDING

COMPENSATORY HYPERINFLATION

Funny collapses

LUL

WITH ANTERIOR R LUNG HERNIATION

WITH LUFTSICHEL (superior LLL herniation)

WITH PERIPHERAL ADHESIONS

WITH ACCESSORY HORIZONTAL FISSURE

RUL AND RML

(looks like LUL)

RML AND RLL

loss of oblique and horizontal fissures

PA: loss of diaphragm and R heart border

Lat: loss of entire R diaphragm

2.1.5 CYST

a cyst is a focal air collection with a truly thin wall ('THIN AIR, THIN WALL')

BULLA

POST LACERATION CYST

POST INFECTIVE PNEUMATOCELE

BRONCHIECTATIC 'PSEUDOCYST'

RUPTURED HYDATID

2.1.6 INTRACAVITARY MASS

Cavity developed first

MYCETOMA

CLOT

Mass developed first

see nodule or mass (CASH TRAP)

CLASSIC CAVITATING MASSES:

ABSCESS

TB

INVASIVE ASPERGILLOSIS/OTHER FUNGI

HAS AIR CRESCENT SIGN

SEPTIC EMBOLISM (really an abscess)

HYDATID

RUPTURES, DOES NOT TRULY CAVITATE

BRONCHOGENIC CARCINOMA, ESPECIALLY SQUAMOUS

METASTASIS (LESS COMMON)

HEMATOMA, BLAND INFARCT, WEGENER'S INFARCT

MASSIVE CONTUSIONS/LACERATIONS (need evidence of trauma)

2.1.7 LUNG MASS IN A CHILD

see Ch 21

2.1.8 LYMPHADENOPATHY

see Ch 14

2.1.9 MASSIVELY INCREASED LUNG DENSITY

METASTATIC CALCIFICATION

HYPERPARATHYROIDISM, RENAL DISEASE, HYPERCALCEMIA

AMIODARONE LUNG

LOOK FOR HYPERDENSE LIVER AND SPLEEN

ALVEOLAR MICROLITHIASIS

2.1.10 NODULE OR MASS: SOLITARY/OLIGOFOCAL, INTRAPARENCHYMAL

Mnemonic: CASH TRAP

C-ANCER (1ry, 2ry) AND C-ARCINOID

A-BSCESS

S-EQUESTRATION (LL) AND S–ARCOIDOSIS (UL)

H-YDATID AND H-AMARTOMA

T-B (and fungus)

R-HEUMATOID AND WEGENER'S

A-VM AND ROUND COLLAPSE (vessel tail)

P-MF AND P-EDIATRIC ROUND P–NEUMONIA

Unifocal vs oligofocal

MOST COMMONLY UNIFOCAL

healed infective focus (granuloma)

reactivated TB/fungus

round atelectasis

round pneumonia

bronchogenic carcinoma

carcinoid

hamartoma

sequestration

MOST COMMONLY OLIGOFOCAL

metastases

lung abscesses (assuming vascular spread)

sarcoidosis

progressive massive fibrosis

Wegener's and other causes of infarction (e.g. SLE)

rheumatoid lung nodules

EITHER UNIFOCAL OR OLIGOFOCAL

AVM

hydatids

2.1.11 NODULE: MULTIFOCAL/DIFFUSE

see under CXR gamuts if on CXR
see under HRCT if on CT

2.1.12 NODULE: MULTIFOCAL/DIFFUSE CALCIFIED

OLD INFECTION

varicella pneumonia

histoplasmosis

other viral or fungal disease

MITRAL STENOSIS WITH HEMOSIDEROSIS

METASTASES

OSTEOSARCOMA METASTASES (ossified not calcified)

METASTATIC CALCIFICATION

CHRONIC RENAL FAILURE

HYPERPARATHYROIDISM

SILICOSIS

CALCIFICATION IN MINORITY OF CASES

ALVEOLAR MICROLITHIASIS

very fine calcified nodules <1 mm different in appearance from the rest of this group

may produce 'white out'

2.1.13 PLEURALLY BASED MASS

Truly pleural

LOCULATED FLUID

EFFUSION/HEMATOMA/PYOTHORAX

PLEURAL PLAQUE

PLEURAL TUMOR (fibroma or mesothelioma)

PLEURAL SEEDING

METASTASES

LYMPHOMA

SPLENOSIS OR ENDOMETRIOSIS

Parenchymal, looks pleural

INFARCT (i.e. Hampton's hump)

ROUND ATELECTASIS

SUBPLEURAL MASS OF PARENCHYMAL ORIGIN

Chest wall, looks pleural

METASTASIS TO RIB

PLASMACYTOMA, LYMPHOMA

NEUROFIBROMA

CHEST WALL PRIMARY BONE OR SOFT TISSUE TUMOR

EXTRAMEDULLARY HEMOPOIESIS

2.1.14 REVERSE PULMONARY EDEMA PATTERN (reverse batswing)

EOSINOPHILIC PNEUMONIA (chronic), LOEFFLER'S SYNDROME (acute)

DRUG REACTION AND RELATIONS

SARCOIDOSIS (atypical in the absence of other findings)

ATYPICAL TB/FUNGAL INFECTION (unilateral!)

BRONCHIOLOALVEOLAR CARCINOMA (unilateral!)

ORGANIZING PNEUMONIA

2.2 CXR

2.2.1 ABNORMAL TRAUMATIC AIR

Pneumothorax, hemopneumothorax

HORIZONTAL BEAM FILM

ERECT CXR (inspiratory/expiratory)

DECUBITUS

CROSS TABLE LATERAL

VERTICAL BEAM FILM

PNEUMOTHORAX OBVIOUS

DEEP SULCUS SIGN ONLY

NO CXR FINDINGS

CT

always demonstrates

Tension (hemo) pneumothorax

MEDIASTINAL SHIFT

EXPIRATION

EXPIRATION AND INSPIRATION

!pneumothorax may not show if hemothorax is also present

!beware tracheal or bronchial injury

Pneumomediastinum

SIGNS

gas at mediastinal contours

continuous diaphragm sign, V sign

gas in root of neck

mediastinal gas on lateral film

CAUSES

tracheobronchial injury

esophageal injury

medial pneumothorax

2.2.2 DIFFUSE OR MULTIFOCAL INTERSTITIAL PATTERN

gamut includes scarring in same pattern
also see Lung Machine

Upper lobe predominance

MNEMONIC: THIS APEX

T-B

H-ISTOPLASMOSIS, HISTIOCYTOSIS X

I-BD AND ANKYLOSING SPONDYLITIS

S-ARCOIDOSIS

A-LLERGIC BRONCHOPULMONARY ASPERGILLOSIS

P-NEUMOCONIOSES (NOT ASBESTOSIS)

E-XTRINSIC ALLERGIC ALVEOLITIS

X- RADIATION

Lower lobe predominance

MNEMONIC: BACIL

B-RONCHIECTASIS

A-SBESTOSIS

C-RYPTOGENIC FIBROSIS

I-MMUNE COMPLEX DISEASE (rheumatoid arthritis, CREST)

L-YMPHANGITIS CARCINOMATOSA

2.2.3 ELEVATED DIAPHRAGM

Elevated diaphragm

VOLUME LOSS ABOVE – COLLAPSE

PHRENIC NERVE PALSY

EVENTRATION (focal or entire)

COLLECTION, DISTENSION OR TUMOR BELOW

Conditions simulating elevated diaphragm

SUBPULMONIC EFFUSION

PLEURALLY BASED TUMOR

SCOLIOSIS

2.2.4 FUNNY RIBS (ON CXR) [MPS NOT ACHONDROPLASIA]

exclude previous surgery or trauma first
confirm this is not notching

Mnemonic: MPS not achondroplasia

MUCOPOLYSACCHARIDOSES (MPS)

N-EUROFIBROMATOSIS

O-STEOGENESIS IMPERFECTA

T-HALASSEMIA

ACHONDROPLASIA

2.2.5 HYPERRADIANT HEMITHORAX

!the abnormal side cycles least in expiratory–inspiratory views

Technical

ROTATION

BUCKY OR GRID CUTOFF

INTERPOSED DENSITY (e.g. plaster)

CHEST WALL

MASTECTOMY

in children, asymmetrical breast development

POLAND SYNDROME OR CHEST WALL SURGERY

e.g. pectoralis major rotation flap to neck

CONTRALATERAL BREAST PROSTHESIS

CONTRALATERAL MASS

Pleural space

PNEUMOTHORAX

CONTRALATERAL EFFUSION

Vessels

PULMONARY EMBOLISM (normal size lung)

McLEOD/SWYER-JAMES SYNDROME (small lung)

CONGENITAL PULMONARY ARTERY HYPOPLASIA (small lung)

Bronchi

LUNG SIZE SYMMETRICAL

CONGENITAL LOBAR EMPHYSEMA

BULLA

COMPENSATORY HYPERINFLATION (entire lung smaller)

LOBAR COLLAPSE ON SAME SIDE

LOBECTOMY ON SAME SIDE

AIR TRAPPING (entire lung larger)

FOREIGN BODY

MUCUS PLUG (collapse much more likely)

EXTRINSIC COMPRESSION (collapse much more likely)

2.2.6 MULTIFOCAL OR MILIARY SMALL NODULES

CXR definition of miliary

SMOOTH WELL DEFINED (SMALL) NODULES

RANDOM AND UNIFORM

SOME RELATE TO VESSELS

Gamut

MILIARY INFECTION

SOFT TISSUE DENSITY

  TB, FUNGAL, VIRAL

CALCIFIED

  OLD VIRAL (varicella)

  OLD FUNGAL (histoplasmosis)

MILIARY METASTASES

PNEUMOCONIOSES/ HEMOSIDEROSIS

SILICOSIS, ANTHRACOSIS
silicotic nodules may calcify

HEMOSIDEROSIS (2ry, 1ry)
dense nodules by definition (iron)
expect cardiac signs of mitral disease to be the dominant CXR finding in 2ry hemosiderosis (see cardiac chapter)

SARCOIDOSIS

2.2.7 RIB NOTCHING

Arterial

NORMAL HEART ON CXR

AORTIC COARCTATION

ENLARGED BRONCHIAL ARTERIES (non cardiac cause)

  cystic fibrosis

  other chronic parenchymal disease

ABNORMAL HEART ON CXR

BLALOCK–TAUSSIG SHUNT (see Ch 21)

PULMONARY ARTERY HYPOPLASIA, DILATED BRONCHIAL ARTERIES (see Ch 21)

UNILATERAL NOTCHING ONLY

RIGHT ONLY

  aortic coarctation which is BEFORE the origin of the left subclavian artery

  UNILATERAL Blalock–taussig shunt

LEFT ONLY

  aortic coarctation with anomalous right subclavian artery origin AND coarctation

before the anomalous origin (i.e. a rocking horse dung condition)

UNILATERAL Blalock–Taussig shunt

Venous

CHRONIC SVC OBSTRUCTION

Neural

NEUROFIBROMA

2.3 CT

2.3.1 TRAUMA CHEST CT CHECKLIST

Mediastinal windows

MEDIASTINAL HEMATOMA

VASCULAR FLAPS OR TEARS (use contrast)

Lung windows

PNEUMOTHORAX

BRONCHIAL WALL CONTINUITY

Bone windows

RIB AND SPINAL FRACTURES

SHOULDER GIRDLE FRACTURES

Diaphragm

2.4 HRCT

2.4.1 AIRSPACE OPACITIES

HRCT/CT signs

compare with air in bronchi

GROUND GLASS OPACITY

= no obscuration of underlying architecture
geographic or regional increase in airspace density
may progress to consolidation

beware partial volume effects if fibrosis is present (fine fibrosis simulating an airspace process)
if true airspace opacity is present in fibrosis this indicates disease activity
DIFFERENTIAL: MOSAIC PERFUSION, AIR TRAPPING

CONSOLIDATION

= obscuration of underlying architecture, airbronchograms
geographic or regional increase in airspace density

Differential: same as airspace opacity differential in generic gamuts

2.4.2 INTERSTITIAL OPACITIES

Centrilobular/peribroncho-vascular interstitial

SIGNS (changes may be smooth or nodular)
peribronchovascular thickening
traction bronchiectasis
centrilobular thickening
centrilobular traction bronchiolectasis
cardinal sign: interface sign (irregular surface of interstitial structures)

DIFFERENTIAL

CELLS

  LYMPHANGITIS, LYMPHOMA
no distortion of architecture
smooth or nodular; 'beaded septa'

FLUID (always smooth)

  PULMONARY INTERSTITIAL EDEMA

  ACUTE PULMONARY EDEMA

FIBROSIS

  MNEMONIC: PISA

  P-NEUMOCONIOSES
SILICOSIS: peribronchovascular changes dominant
ASBESTOSIS: peripheral changes dominant; central changes late
conglomeration in silicosis and mixed pneumoconioses, NOT in asbestosis

  I-DIOPATHIC FIBROSIS AND IMMUNE COMPLEX DISEASE
peripheral changes dominant

  S-ARCOIDOSIS (DIFFERENTIAL: TB)
peribronchovascular > centrilobular
nodular, conglomeration

  A-LLERGIC ALVEOLITIS (CHRONIC)

DIFFERENTIAL OF FIBROSIS: SMALL AIRWAYS DISEASE

  BRONCHOPNEUMONIA/TB

  BRONCHIECTASIS/CYSTIC FIBROSIS

  BOOP, PANBRONCHIOLITIS

Peripheral interstitial

SIGNS (changes may be smooth or nodular)

interlobular septal thickening

pleural and fissural thickening

subpleural bands or lines

parenchymal bands (scars, atelectasis, gross fibrosis)

intralobular thickening (fibrosis may be too small to resolve – then produces peripheral apparently airspace opacities)

honeycombing (late)

DIFFERENTIAL

CELLS

LYMPHANGITIS, LYMPHOMA

studded > smooth; 'beaded septa' typical

AMYLOID

FLUID (always smooth)

INTERSTITIAL PULMONARY EDEMA

ACUTE PULMONARY EDEMA

FIBROSIS

MNEMONIC: PISA

P-NEUMOCONIOSES

ASBESTOSIS (intralobular thickening, subpleural bands)

ALL ELSE (nodular changes)

I-DIOPATHIC FIBROSIS AND IMMUNE COMPLEX DISEASE

intralobular thickening early, honeycombing late

S-ARCOIDOSIS

subpleural, nodular

A-LLERGIC ALVEOLITIS

intralobular thickening early, honeycombing late

2.4.3 MULTIPLE LUNG CYSTS

Bullous disease NOS

histiocytosis

lymphangioleiomyomatosis, tuberous sclerosis

PCP pneumatoceles

2.4.4 MOSAIC PERFUSION VS GROUNDGLASS

Mosaic oligemia with air trapping

small vessel reflex vasoconstriction in underventilated lung

air trapping usually present

underlying BOOP or BRONCHIECTASIS SPECTRUM

IDENTIFIED BY INCREASE IN DIFFERENCE TO NORMAL LUNG ON EXPIRATORY SCAN

normal areas have normal expiratory crowding

abnormal areas air trap, remain lucent, and become more obvious

Mosaic oligemia without air trapping

PULMONARY EMBOLISM

decrease in difference on expiratory scan (no air trapping) SIMILAR TO GROUNDGLASS OPACITY

Groundglass opacity

IDENTIFICATION BY DECREASE IN DIFFERENCE TO NORMAL LUNG ON EXPIRATORY SCAN

normal areas have normal expiratory crowding

abnormal areas have groundglass opacity and become less obvious

2.4.5 NODULAR OPACITIES

nodules may be interstitial or airspace

Random nodules (miliary nodules)

MILIARY METASTASES

MILIARY TB OR FUNGAL OR VIRAL INFECTION

MILIARY ABSCESSES

Perilymphatic distribution = peribronchovascular and centrilobular nodules

fluid does not produce peribronchovascular nodular opacities

CELLS

LYMPHANGITIS

LYMPHOMA, LYMPHOCYTIC INTERSTITIAL PNEUMONITIS (AIDS)

–merges with interstitial thickening

FIBROSIS

PNEUMOCONIOSES (not asbestosis)

centrilobular and subpleural

nodules can conglomerate (UL > LL)

SARCOIDOSIS

peribronchovascular and subpleural

merges with interstitial disease

nodules can conglomerate (UL > LL)

Centrilobular only

CELLS

SMALL AIRWAYS INFECTION

BRONCHOPNEUMONIA NOS

TB BRONCHOPNEUMONIA

BRONCHIECTASIS, CYSTIC FIBROSIS

MERGES WITH BRONCHIOLITIS

BRONCHIOLOALVEOLAR CARCINOMA

FLUID

early stages, later merges into airspace opacities

AIRSPACE PULMONARY EDEMA

ALLERGIC ALVEOLITIS (acute)

HEMORRHAGE, VASCULITIS

FIBROSIS

BOOP

Conglomeration

LARGE MASSES OF SAME ETIOLOGY AS SMALLER NODULES

SARCOID

PROGRESSIVE MASSIVE FIBROSIS

TUBERCULOSIS

(Wegener's granulomatosis)

DIFFERENTIAL: ROUND ATELECTASIS (peripheral, evidence of asbestosis)

2.5 NUC MED

2.5.1 DEMONSTRATION OF OTHER ORGANS ON V/Q PERFUSION

Brain

R to L shunt; usually intracardiac, may be intrapulmonary (e.g. AVM)

Thyroid

free pertechnetate

Liver/spleen (no brain)

colloid size too small – usually failure of MAA particle formation and formation of reduced hydrolyzed Tc instead

Kidneys

DTPA aerosol absorption

Hot clumping in lungs

MAA aggregates (settling or blood admixture for too long)

2.5.2 DIFFUSE LUNG GALLIUM UPTAKE

Immunosuppressed

PNEUMOCYSTIS PNEUMONIA TILL PROVEN OTHERWISE

Non immunosuppressed

Ga uptake is evidence of active pneumonitis

ACTIVE AUTOIMMUNE PNEUMONITIS

DIFFUSE INFECTION (usually viral)

CHEMOTHERAPY OR DRUG INDUCED PNEUMONITIS

SARCOIDOSIS, DIFFUSE LUNG INVOLVEMENT

ACTIVE DIFFUSE PNEUMOCONIOSIS

DIFFUSE NEOPLASTIC INVOLVEMENT

LYMPHOMA, less likely lymphangitis carcinomatosa

2.5.3 FOCAL/OLIGOFOCAL GALLIUM UPTAKE

SARCOIDOSIS

classically 'panda' and 'lambda' signs

symmetrical and confined to lymph nodal areas

LYMPHOMA (always do SPECT)

Hodgkin's disease (>90% are Ga avid)

Non hodgkin lymphoma (low grade may not be Ga avid)

BRONCHOGENIC CARCINOMA

MELANOMA METASTASES

RADIOTHERAPY CHANGE (conforms to radiation portal)

2.5.4 LOSS OF NORMAL POSITIONAL GRADIENT OR GRADIENT MISMATCH

Normal

ventilation done supine

MAA injection done supine

anterior (less intense) to posterior (more intense) perfusion gradient, ventilation gradient concordant but not as apparent

Loss of perfusion gradient (no focal abnormalities)

injection done upright

left ventricular failure, vascular congestion

Loss of perfusion and ventilation gradients

usually multifocal defects that obscure any underlying residual normal gradient

2.5.5 V/Q MISMATCH INVOLVING WHOLE LUNG

Ensure that there is lung present!

No perfusion/reduced perfusion

TUMOR COMPRESSION

MASSIVE UNILATERAL ONLY PE

PULMONARY ARTERY HYPOPLASIA (see above)

SURGICAL SYSTEMIC TO PULMONARY SHUNT

need to know anatomy and degree of circulation mixing to determine flow of tracer

No ventilation/reduced ventilation

MUCUS PLUG, OTHER CAUSE OF BRONCHIAL OBSTRUCTION (see obstruction in gamuts)

ENDOTRACHEAL TUBE IN THE OPPOSITE BRONCHUS

2.5.6 V/Q MISMATCH, PERFUSION ABNORMALITY > VENTILATION ABNORMALITY

these apply to INTRAPULMONARY defects only (i.e. EXTRAPULMONARY defects such as pleural effusions, hilar masses, pacemakers, aortic aneurysms not considered)

1. Pulmonary embolism

ACUTE

CHRONIC

(beware of septic embolism before airspace abnormality becomes visible)

2. Mimickers

TUMOR COMPRESSION

MULTIFOCAL VASCULITIS/PULMONARY INFARCTION

Wegener's

microscopic variant of PAN

Takayasu's arteritis

SLE

NON THROMBOTIC EMBOLISM

fat embolism

IV drug use

foreign bodies

3. Congenitally reduced pulmonary perfusion

PULMONARY ARTERY APLASIA/ HYPOPLASIA

McLEOD/SWYER-JAMES SYNDROME

4. Radiation therapy

perfusion defect conforms to radiation portal

may have CXR/CT evidence of radiation pneumonitis

2.5.7 V/Q MISMATCH, VENTILATION ABNORMALITY > PERFUSION ABNORMALITY (reverse mismatch or shunt)

COAD/COPD

air trapping, bullae, diffuse emphysematous change

MUCUS PLUG

POSTOPERATIVE

ASTHMA

CYSTIC FIBROSIS

COLLAPSE WITH RESIDUAL PERFUSION

EARLY AIRSPACE CONSOLIDATION OF ANY CAUSE

2.5.8 V/Q MISMATCH, VENTILATION = PERFUSION

COAD/COPD

CONSOLIDATION OF ANY CAUSE

COLLAPSE OF ANY CAUSE

PULMONARY MASSES OF ANY CAUSE

2.5.9 PIOPED AND BIELLO CRITERIA

PIOPED data (JAMA 1990; 263:2753–2759)

DEFINITIONS OF UNMATCHED PERFUSION DEFECTS

large is > 75% of a segment

moderate is 25% < of a segment < 75%

small is < 25% of a segment

unmatched is: perfusion abnormality substantially larger than ventilation or CXR abnormality

PROBABILITY CATEGORIES (abridged)

high probability is two or more large segmental defects or arithmetic equivalent in moderate defects

low probability is:

non segmental

any defect with ventilation > perfusion

four or fewer matched defects per lung

single moderate unmatched perfusion defect

very low probability is three or fewer small segmental defects

normal is normal

intermediate probability is anything that does not fit into one of the above or is too difficult to categorize

INCIDENCE OF PE IN EACH PROBABILITY GROUP

prevalence in study	PE on angio
high 13%	85%
mid 40%	33%
low 33%	15%
norm 14%	< 3%

PIOPED criteria modified by Gottschalk (J Nucl Med 1993; 34:1119–1126)

high probability is two or more large unmatched perfusion defects or arithmetic equivalent in moderate defects

intermediate probability is:

one moderate to two large mismatched defects with clear CXR (or arithmetic equivalent)

single matched defect with clear CXR

anything too difficult to categorize

low probability is:

non segmental defects

any defect with CXR abnormality >> perfusion

matched defects with normal CXR

any number of small perfusion defects with normal CXR

normal is normal

Biello criteria (abridged, AJR 1979; 133:1033–1037)

high probability is:

One or more large or two or more moderate unmatched perfusion defects with clear CXR

perfusion defects >> CXR abnormalities

intermediate probability is:

severe COAD/COPD

single moderate unmatched perfusion defect, CXR clear

perfusion defects matched to CXR abnormalities

low probability is:

small unmatched defects with any CXR

matched perfusion and ventilation defects, CXR clear

perfusion defects << CXR abnormalities

normal is normal

2.5.10 XENON IN LIVER

FATTY LIVER (any cause)

HEPATITIS

2.5.11 XENON TRAPPING

Classically area that traps xenon is cold on washin phase

COAD/COPD (ANY CAUSE)

ASTHMA

CYSTIC FIBROSIS, ABPA

FOREIGN BODY, BALL VALVE OBSTRUCTION

2.6 PET

see Ch 25

2.7 SOLITARY PULMONARY NODULE WORKUP

1. LOOK AT PREVIOUS CXR

no change in 2 years or very rapid change = benign (this rule is not infallible; the longer the time period the better)

2. ASSESS RISK FACTORS

FOR CANCER (age, smoking, known primary)

OTHER RISK FACTORS (infection, trauma, known PE)

this gives a Bayesian estimate of malignancy risk

3. CHARACTERIZE BY CT AND PET

PATHOGNOMONIC CT FINDINGS

If there are no parenchymal changes

MULTIPLE MASSES (disclosed on CT) = metastases; other causes of multifocal lung nodules (see gamut)

FAT = HAMARTOMA

POPCORN CALCIFICATION = HAMARTOMA

VESSELS, VASCULAR ENHANCEMENT = ARTERIOVENOUS MALFORMATION

VESSELS, COMET TAIL = ROUND COLLAPSE

If parenchymal changes are present

the features of the nodule have to be concordant with the features of parenchymal lung disease before Occam's razor can be used

carcinoma and TB are common in many parenchymal lung diseases despite Occam's razor!

IF NO PATHOGNOMONIC CT FINDINGS, DO

Histology

SPUTUM CYTOLOGY

CT GUIDED BIOPSY (if nodule peripheral)

BRONCHOSCOPY (if nodule central)

FDG PET for metabolic activity

sensitivity and specificity both high

increased FDG uptake compared with mediastinal bloodpool is positive

SUV(max) >2.5 is the most commonly used cutoff for malignancy (this is as imperfect as visual interpretation)

no activity in an SPN of 1.5 cm or above on PET may obviate the need for tissue diagnosis (needs to be validated for a particular patient population)

FALSE POSITIVES

active TB, active fungal infection

abscess

sarcoidosis

FALSE NEGATIVES

small nodule (in general, <1.5 cm) because of partial volume artifact

malignancy with a low metabolic rate (particularly bronchioloalveolar carcinoma and carcinoid)

Dynamic CT for vascularity

see further discussion in bronchogenic carcinoma entry

classic criterion is enhancement >10 HU which implies activity

specificity poor

practical differential becomes neoplasm vs active infection (TB or fungal)

2.8 LUNG MACHINE

COMMENT

the lung machine is a conceptual approach to classifying diffuse lung disease to reach a diagnosis or differential diagnosis

the lung machine is CXR based and does not differentiate different types of interstitial pattern that can be further characterized on HRCT

see DEFINITIONS in the normal section for terms used in the lung machine

DECISION MAKING TREE

1. IS THE CXR CHANGE CHRONIC OR ACUTE?

get previous CXR

2. IS THE PATIENT IMMUNOSUPPRESSED?

see AIDS lungs overview

3. IS THE DIFFUSE PATTERN PREDOMINANTLY AIRSPACE OR PREDOMINANTLY INTERSTITIAL?

4. IS THERE LYMPHADENOPATHY?

FURTHER ANALYSIS OF AIRSPACE PATTERN

MNEMONIC: material that can cause airspace opacity: transudate, exudate, blood, pus, cancer, 'IGA'

AIRSPACE PATTERN, ACUTE CHANGE, NO LYMPHADENOPATHY

Transudate (APO)

airspace pulmonary edema of some cause:

CARDIOGENIC

NEUROGENIC

CIRRHOTIC

NEPHROTIC

PANCREATIC

Exudate (ARDS)

airspace exudate secondary to:

DIFFUSE ALVEOLAR DAMAGE

Blood

CONTUSION

INFARCTION

DIFFUSE HEMORRHAGE (GOODPASTURE'S SYNDROME, EXCESS WARFARIN)

VASCULITIS

Pus

INFECTIVE CONSOLIDATION

BACTERIAL, VIRAL, FUNGAL CAUSES

EOSINOPHILIC PNEUMONIA

Interstitial gone airspace ('IGA')

initially interstitial process that either secondarily involves airspace or appears to do so on imaging

VIRAL PNEUMONIA

ACUTE INTERSTITIAL PNEUMONIA

DIP OF UIP

SARCOIDOSIS

AIRSPACE PATTERN, ACUTE CHANGE WITH LYMPHADENOPATHY

Lymphadenopathy came first, consolidation is secondary to compression or direct extension

versus

Consolidation came first, lymphadenopathy developed second

CLASSICAL TB, FUNGAL INFECTIONS

(less commonly EBV, mycoplasma, anthrax)

AIRSPACE PATTERN, CHRONIC CHANGE, NO LYMPHADENOPATHY

IS THERE A CENTRAL UNDERLYING MASS?

Transudate

IN GENERAL, TRANSUDATE DOES NOT CAUSE CHRONIC AIRSPACE OPACITIES; EITHER THE OPACITY RESOLVES OR THE CONDITION EVOLVES

Exudate

ALVEOLAR PROTEINOSIS

DELAYED RESOLUTION OF ARDS, ORGANIZING PNEUMONITIS

Blood

VASCULITIS

WEGENER'S GRANULOMATOSIS

Pus

LIPOID PNEUMONIA

CHRONIC EOSINOPHILIC PNEUMONIA

TB OR FUNGAL BRONCHOPNEUMONIA

Cancer

BRONCHIOLOALVEOLAR CARCINOMA

LEUKEMIA, LYMPHOMA

Interstitial gone airspace ('IGA')

CHRONIC VIRAL PNEUMONIA

LYMPHOCYTIC INTERSTITIAL
PNEUMONITIS

VASCULITIS

BOOP

SARCOIDOSIS

DIP PHASE OF UIP

AIRSPACE PATTERN, CHRONIC CHANGE WITH LYMPHADENOPATHY

(is there a central underlying mass?)

Preexisting consolidation, lymphadenopathy developed second

TB, FUNGAL INFECTION

BRONCHIOLOALVEOLAR CARCINOMA

Lymphadenopathy came first, consolidation developed later

SARCOIDOSIS, LYMPHOMA

FURTHER ANALYSIS OF INTERSTITIAL PATTERN

MNEMONIC: causes of interstitial opacity (cells, fluid, fibrosis)

INTERSTITIAL PATTERN, ACUTE CHANGE

Cells

INFECTIVE: VIRAL, MYCOPLASMAL, CHLAMYDIAL

Fluid

TRANSUDATE (APO)

interstitial pulmonary edema of some cause:

CARDIOGENIC

NEUROGENIC

CIRRHOTIC

NEPHROTIC

PANCREATIC

EXUDATE (ARDS)

interstitial exudate secondary to:

DIFFUSE ALVEOLAR DAMAGE (interstitial phase)

Fibrosis

EARLY FIBROSIS/DIP

DRUG REACTION, OTHER

ACCELERATED FIBROSIS

HAMMAN–RICH SYNDROME

INTERSTITIAL PATTERN, CHRONIC CHANGE

Cells

LYMPHANGITIS CARCINOMATOSA, LANGERHANS CELL HISTIOCYTOSIS, LYMPHOMA

(INFECTIVE CAUSES OF CHRONIC INTERSTITIAL PATTERN LESS COMMON: VIRAL INFECTION, MYCOPLASMA, CHLAMYDIA)

Fluid

in general, fluid does not cause chronic interstitial pattern; either the condition evolves or the fluid is resorbed

Fibrosis

MNEMONIC: PISA DIT A FAAART

DIFFUSE FIBROSIS, INHALED CAUSE

(PISA)

P-NEUMOCONIOSES

    SILICOSIS

    ANTHRACOSIS

    ASBESTOSIS

    BERYLLIUM/ZIRCONIUM

    MIXED

I-NFECTION

    ADENOVIRUS

    OTHER VIRAL

    CHLAMYDIA, MYCOPLASMA

S-ARCOIDOSIS

A-LLERGENS

    HYPERSENSITIVITY PNEUMONITIS (EAA)

DIFFUSE FIBROSIS, CIRCULATED CAUSE

(DIT)

D-RUGS

    PARTICULARLY CYTOTOXICS AND AMIODARONE

    SEE DRUGS AND LUNGS ENTRY IN LUNG CONDITIONS

I-MMUNE COMPLEXES

    I-DIOPATHIC

    SCLERODERMA/CREST

    ANKYLOSING SPONDYLITIS

    SLE

    RHEUMATOID ARTHRITIS

T-OXINS

    e.g. PARAQUAT

FAILURE OF A-RDS TO RESOLVE

(A)

FOCAL OR MULTIFOCAL FIBROSIS

(FART)

F-UNGUS

    ASPERGILLOSIS

    HISTOPLASMOSIS

    BLASTOMYCOSIS/CRYPTOCOCCOSIS/COCCIDIOMYCOSIS

A-BNORMAL AIRWAY, BRONCHIECTASIS

    CYSTIC FIBROSIS

    BRONCHIECTASIS NOS

    STRICTURE

A-SPIRATION

A-LLERGIC BRONCHOPULMONARY ASPERGILLOSIS (ABPA)

R-ADIOTHERAPY

T-B

Mimickers of fibrosis

MNEMONIC: LATS

L-YMPHANGIOLEIOMYOMATOSIS

A-MYLOIDOSIS

T-UBEROUS S-CLEROSIS

CONDITIONS ASSOCIATED WITH LYMPHADENOPATHY

MNEMONIC: TALISMAN

T-B, fungi, viruses (especially EBV), mycoplasma, chlamydia

A-IDS: CONSIDER TB, MAC (non TB mycobacteria), Kaposi's sarcoma, lymphoma

L-ymphoma

I-nhalational disease (pneumoconioses)

S-arcoidosis

M-etastases

A-myloidosis

CASTLEMA-N'S DISEASE
(angiofollicular hyperplasia)

3. PULMONARY CONDITIONS

3.1 AIDS LUNGS OVERVIEW

* indicates statistically major

CMI (cell mediated immunity) dependent infections

PROTOZOAL INFECTION

*PNEUMOCYSTIS CARINII PNEUMONIA (PCP)

INTERSTITIAL OR AIRSPACE PATTERN, NO LYMPHADENOPATHY, CYSTS, PNEUMOTHORACES

VERY HOT ON GALLIUM

TOXOPLASMOSIS

variable airspace or nodular pattern

MYCOBACTERIAL/FUNGAL

*TB/MAC (+/− lymphadenopathy)

FIBROCASEOUS TB

TB BRONCHOPNEUMONIA

MILIARY TB

MAC BRONCHOPNEUMONIA

FUNGAL INFECTION (+/− lymphadenopathy)

*HISTOPLASMOSIS

COCCIDIOMYCOSIS

*CRYPTOCOCCOSIS

*ASPERGILLUS (classical angioinvasive)

ANGIOINVASIVE (!Aspergillus) – PARTICULARLY IN NEUTROPENIC ONCOLOGY PATIENTS

SEMIINVASIVE (!Aspergillus nodular)

FUNGAL BRONCHOPNEUMONIA

CONSOLIDATIVE (unreactive granulomatous)

VIRAL

CYTOMEGALOVIRUS (CMV) PNEUMONITIS

INTERSTITIAL OR GROUNDGLASS PATTERN, OBSCURED BY CHANGES OF PCP

Humoral immunity dependent infections

BACTERIAL PNEUMONIA (classical presentation)

Autoimmune (?) processes

LYMPHOCYTIC INTERSTITIAL PNEUMONITIS

UIP/IDIOPATHIC PULMONARY FIBROSIS

DRUG REACTION

all these produce an interstitial pattern on CXR

Neoplasms

*KAPOSI'S SARCOMA

LYMPHADENOPATHY, LUNG BRONCHOCENTRIC MASSES, FLAME SHAPED HEMORRHAGES; COLD ON GALLIUM

B cell NHL

EXTENSIVE LYMPHADENOPATHY COMMON – DIFFERENTIAL IS TB

Bronchogenic carcinoma (usually aggressive)

3.2 ALVEOLAR MICROLITHIASIS

CLINICAL

rare condition with small foci of calcification within alveoli

familial in 50%

asymptomatic for a long time; may progress to pulmonary fibrosis and right heart failure

IMAGING

XR/CT

widespread sand-like calcified uniform particles <1 mm in size

may produce massively increased lung density ('white out')

3.3 ALVEOLAR PROTEINOSIS

DEFINITION

rare failure of surfactant clearance from alveoli leading to progressive respiratory deterioration

CLINICAL

usually middle aged adult with insidious dyspnea and cough

postulated macrophage clonal failure with secondary failure of alveolar clearance

alveoli filled with homogenous eosinophilic proteinaceous fluid (surfactant)

secondary fungal infection (nocardia is the most common) is the principal cause of death

IMAGING

CXR

diffuse perihilar ground glass

diffuse or patchy multifocal airspace consolidation

all changes chronic by definition

perihilar densities may simulate pulmonary edema

chronicity, lack of fever and relatively mild symptoms suggestive

HRCT

INTERSTITIAL PATTERN (peripheral)
smooth septal thickening

AIRSPACE PATTERN (geographic)
bilateral groundglass
GEOGRAPHIC DISTRIBUTION

CRAZY PAVING (combination of above two)
mosaic of ground glass filled lobules interspersed with normal lobules, and separated by smoothly thickened interlobular septa

3.4 AMYLOIDOSIS (pulmonary manifestations)

type AL amyloid ('primary' amyloid) involves lung in 30–70%

type AA amyloid ('reactive' amyloid) rarely involves lung

IMAGING

CXR/CT

diffuse tracheobronchial wall thickening or distortion

nodular form with single ('amyloidoma') or multiple masses

diffuse interstitial deposition

may mimic sarcoidosis

3.5 ANKYLOSING SPONDYLITIS (pulmonary manifestations)

IMAGING

CXR

bilateral upper lobe predominant fibrosis with a reticulonodular interstitial pattern

may coalesce into larger linear and nodular opacities
! evidence of ankylosis in thoracic spine !

3.6 ARDS (adult respiratory distress syndrome)

see diffuse alveolar damage entry

3.7 ASBESTOSIS

CLINICAL

lung fibrosis caused by inhalation of asbestos fibers
asbestosis present in ~1/2 of those with evidence of asbestos exposure
pattern distinct from other pneumoconioses

Associated conditions of asbestos exposure

see specific entries for each

PLEURAL DISEASE
FOCAL PLAQUES
DIFFUSE FIBROTHORAX
BENIGN SMALL EFFUSIONS
ROUND ATELECTASIS

BRONCHOGENIC CARCINOMA (risk synergistic with smoking: x55)

MESOTHELIOMA

PATHOLOGY

peripheral interstitial pulmonary fibrosis
centered on respiratory bronchioles, extends peripherally
asbestos bodies (ferruginous bodies) – parenchyma, sputum

IMAGING

CXR
peripheral fine fibrosis, LL > UL
other signs of asbestos exposure (calcified pleural plaques)

HRCT
INTERSTITIAL PATTERN (peripheral > centrilobular)
LOWER LOBES
peripheral smooth interstitial pattern
subpleural lines (run parallel to pleura in lower lobes)

subpleural dots
intralobular thickening (may appear as airspace)
parenchymal bands
visible intralobular bronchioles

FIBROSIS
honeycombing
visible bronchioles distally
traction bronchiectasis

OTHER FINDINGS OF ASBESTOS DISEASE
round atelectasis
parietal pleural plaques
effusions

3.8 ASPERGILLOSIS (all forms)

GROUP ETIOLOGY

inhaled Aspergillus flavus/fumigatus/niger
mycelial growth as saprophyte (45 degree slender hyphae) or invades
see Ch 12 for sinonasal aspergillosis

3.8.1 ASPERGILLOMA (fungus ball)

superinfection of preexisting cavity (usually TB) with saprophytic fungal growth as a mass

IMAGING

XR/CT
soft tissue density mass within a cavity, freely mobile
mobility best shown with decubitus CXR or supine/prone CT
air crescent around mass
cavity requires diagnosis on its own merits (TB versus malignant)

Angio
role in bronchial artery embolization

3.8.2 ALLERGIC BRONCHOPULMONARY ASPERGILLOSIS (ABPA)

strong association with asthma; may present as asthma +/– fever; also colonizes asthmatic lungs

PATHOGENESIS

Acute form (type I hypersensitivity)
fungus colonizes asthmatic airways and mucus
type I hypersensitivity to fungal protein
bronchospasm, mucus hypersecretion, eosinophilic mucus
mucus plugging of airways (finger in glove)
distal patchy collapse or hyperinflation (air trapping)

Chronic form (type III hypersensitivity)
serum antibodies to fungal protein ('precipitins')
local immune complex deposition
chronic inflammatory and lymphocytic infiltrate with weakening of bronchial wall, reactive fibrosis
central bronchiectasis, surrounding and distal fibrosis (upper lobes > lower lobes)

Bronchocentric granulomatosis (type IV hypersensitivity)
bronchial wall centered granulomatous inflammation, low grade aspergillus invasion of bronchial wall, necrotizing granulomas centered on bronchioles

IMAGING

XR/CT

ACUTE
fleeting patchy consolidation
patchy hyperinflation and collapse
finger in glove bronchoceles
segmental/lobar collapses (mucus plugging)

CHRONIC
reticulolinear interstitial pattern (UL > LL)
volume loss in fibrosis
chronic hyperinflation otherwise
superimposed acute component (if any)

HRCT
as above and:
central bronchiectasis with mucus plugging and distal collapses
mosaic perfusion (decreased perfusion of non ventilated lobules) in acute ABPA
mosaic perfusion is accentuated by expiration

3.8.3 INVASIVE ASPERGILLOSIS

neutropenic patients (especially chemotherapy); AIDS
angioinvasive: very unwell rapidly deteriorating patient, septic, hypoxic, dyspneic

PATHOGENESIS AND HISTOLOGY

Semiinvasive

usually starts as aspergilloma or seeding of cavity
slow direct fungal invasion of cavity wall
no angioinvasion by definition

Invasive (angioinvasive)

multifocal or diffuse direct invasion of lung parenchyma
infective vasculitis with neutrophilic response
thrombosis and hemorrhage of involved blood vessels
extensive local destruction and infarction

IMAGING (invasive)

XR/CT

patchy multifocal rapidly progressive consolidation with cavitation
wedge shaped infarcts possible

HRCT

pulmonary nodules/masses with air bronchograms
miliary (i.e. vascular) distribution of nodules
'halo' sign (groundglass opacity around focus of consolidation, presumed hemorrhage) +/– central necrosis
crescentic cavitation (?central necrotic mass retraction)
wedge shaped suggests infarcts
fuzzy edge suggests invasion and hemorrhage
may be as less well defined consolidation

3.9 ASTHMA

DEFINITION

abnormal bronchial hyperreactivity leading to paroxysmal dyspnea and wheezing and to chronic airflow limitation

EPIDEMIOLOGY

Extrinsic atopic (type I hypersensitivity)

childhood onset, male > female, paroxysmal, family history
atopy, eczema, hayfever

Intrinsic

later onset, female > male
allergens/precipitants often not isolated
chronic airflow limitation

Extrinsic non atopic (type III hypersensitivity)

usually occupational asthma
symptoms delayed (behaves like extrinsic allergic alveolitis)

PATHOGENESIS

Common pathway

bronchial hyperreactivity
mucosal hyperemia, edema, swelling
increased mucus secretion and retention
distal collapse or air trapping
decreased airflow and increased work of breathing

CLINICAL FEATURES

Precipitants:

plant and animal proteins, dust, gaseous irritants, cold air, viral infections, exercise, emotional stress

Presentation

ACUTE: mild wheeze through to status asthmaticus; pneumothorax
CHRONIC: cough, shortness of breath, reduced exercise capacity

COMPLICATIONS

COAD (COPD)
ABPA (allergic bronchopulmonary aspergillosis)
superinfection
growth failure
complications of treatment

IMAGING

XR/fluoro

most commonly normal
hyperinflation (see under COAD)
simple collapses (subsegmental, segmental, lobar)
pneumothorax

IF COMPLICATED (e.g. ABPA)

bronchial wall thickening
bronchoceles
superinfection (consolidation, etc)
see COAD

AIR TRAPPING ON EXPIRATION

in pneumothorax (implies tension)
distal to flap valve obstruction (e.g. mucus plug)

NUC MED

most commonly normal
severe asthma classically has a patchy ventilation scan
perfusion may be matched patchy
very severe bronchospasm and bronchial mucus plugging show segmental ventilation defects

3.10 BENIGN PLEURAL DISEASE

3.10.1 PLEURAL PLAQUES

DEFINITION

benign pleural reaction following (occupational) dust exposure (especially asbestos); not premalignant

MORPHOLOGY/IMAGING

firm white raised smooth or nodular plaques, often calcified
normally <5 mm thick
acellular parallel bundles of collagen
basal > apical
symmetrical
posterior sulcus, diaphragmatic surfaces, mid and lower zones
'holly leaf' pattern on CXR
indicator of asbestos exposure not asbestosis
may have microscopic/imaging/macro signs of asbestosis as well

3.10.2 BENIGN PLEURAL FIBROMA

DEFINITION

rare benign solitary fibrous pleural tumor, usually of occupational etiology (asbestos related)

MORPHOLOGY/IMAGING

pedunculated or sessile white fibrous mass
with whorled cut surface
fibroblast (not mesothelial) origin, spindle
cells, collagen, few mitoses

3.10.3 FIBROTHORAX

asbestos related, post TB, post empyema
usually <1 cm thick
may be difficult to differentiate from
mesothelioma
may calcify

3.10.4 ROUND ATELECTASIS

DEFINITION

failure of pleural adhesions to separate with
residual area of collapsed lung following
re-expansion

CLINICAL

asymptomatic
associations: asbestosis, pleural effusions,
hemothoraces
significance is that it is a differential
diagnosis of carcinoma

IMAGING

CXR/CT

peripheral subpleural rounded mass, usually
LL
may have strands of peripheral linear
collapse
cardinal sign: 'comet tail' of vessels +/-
bronchus leading to mass, may be curved
or deformed
evidence of etiology (e.g. asbestos plaques)
enhances on dynamic CT – as expected of
collapsed lung
stable on serial imaging

3.11 BRONCHIECTASIS

DEFINITION

abnormal permanent dilation of bronchi

ETIOLOGY

Focal bronchiectasis

foreign body
bronchial obstruction (internal, external –
see gamuts)
aspiration (LL > UL)

Diffuse/multifocal bronchiectasis

ABNORMAL HOST

cystic fibrosis (UL > LL)
ABPA (see ABPA) – (UL>LL)
immotile cilia (LL > UL)
immunosuppressed (immunodeficiency
syndromes)

NORMAL HOST, VIRULENT INFECTIONS

Staphylococcus bronchitis/pneumonia
adenovirus
pertussis
TB (cicatrisation and traction
bronchiectasis)

MACRO

Cylindrical

cylindrical dilation, transverse ridging
abnormal, collapsed, consolidated or
fibrosed distal lung

Saccular (+ varicose)

varicose: beaded bronchi
cystic dilation, wall thick or thin
obliteration of distal airways and airspace

NATURAL HISTORY

Complications

LOCAL

distal bronchopneumonia
lung abscess
erosion of (enlarged) bronchial arteries,
hemoptysis
squamous cell carcinoma

SYSTEMIC

septic embolism
pulmonary hypertension, cor pulmonale
clubbing
type AA amyloidosis

IMAGING

XR/Fluoro

dilated bronchi

'tram tracks' (thickened bronchial walls in
parallel)
'rings' (thickened bronchial walls end-on)
bronchiectatic cysts (often in bunches)
air–fluid levels
bronchoceles
distal volume loss, collapse, patchy or
segmental consolidation, fibrosis
signs of pulmonary hypertension (see under
cardiac)

FOCAL

look for underlying central cause

MULTIFOCAL/DIFFUSE

look for underlying lung abnormality, e.g.
cystic fibrosis

CT/HRCT

normal bronchus size is < accompanying
artery size
dilation of bronchi, 'signet ring' of dilated
bronchus next to its artery
bronchial wall thick (usual) or thin
grape like cystic clusters of cylindrical
bronchiectasis (differentiation from
parenchymal cysts by location)
air–fluid levels
bronchoceles
demonstration of bronchi too distally in lung
parenchyma (usually no bronchi visible
within 2 cm of pleura)
distal collapse, fibrosis, patchy oligemia,
patchy air trapping
peribronchial consolidation, distal
consolidation
DIFFERENTIAL: TRACTION
BRONCHIECTASIS (this diagnosis
requires fibrosis to be present)

Angio

role in bronchial artery embolization

NUC MED

with COAD, cause of indeterminate V/Q scans
reverse mismatch (perfused, non aerated
lung)
matching defects, may be segmental
central airway aerosol clumping

3.12 BRONCHIOLITIS OBLITERANS AND ORGANIZING PNEUMONIA

DEFINITIONS

chronic inflammatory process of lower
respiratory tract with granulation tissue

obstructing bronchiolar lumen (OBLITERATIVE BRONCHIOLITIS) or predominantly filling acini and airspaces (ORGANIZING PNEUMONIA or CRYPTOGENIC ORGANIZING PNEUMONIA – COP) without obstructing bronchioles

acronym BOOP (BRONCHIOLITIS OBLITERANS ORGANIZING PNEUMONIA) has become synonymous with ORGANIZING PNEUMONIA (same as CRYPTOGENIC ORGANIZING PNEUMONIA – COP)

some classifications define a continuum: obliterative bronchiolitis – organizing pneumonia

ETIOLOGY

3.12.1 OBLITERATIVE BRONCHIOLITIS

adenovirus infection

graft versus host disease; lung transplant rejection

others: inhalation (SO_2, NO_2, NH_3), chronic infection, allergic bronchiolitis/alveolitis, autoimmune disease

3.12.2 ORGANIZING PNEUMONIA

usually cryptogenic ('COP')

immune complex disease

organizing infections or aspiration pneumonia

extrinsic allergic alveolitis

drug reactions

should really be termed 'ORGANIZING PNEUMONITIS'

responds to steroids, but may relapse with steroid cessation

PATHOGENESIS

epithelial necrosis and desquamation

healing of bronchiolar necrotic areas by excessive polypoid granulation tissue with luminal obstruction (obliterative bronchiolitis)

failure of distal airspace clearance, healing by organization into granulation and then connective tissue (organizing 'pneumonia')

organizing pneumonia may have a good response to steroids

IMAGING

CXR

OBLITERATIVE BRONCHIOLITIS

classically normal

ORGANIZING PNEUMONIA

normal; or subpleural patchy groundglass opacity; or subpleural patchy consolidation (bilateral)

HRCT

OBLITERATIVE BRONCHIOLITIS

patchy areas of reduced perfusion (reduced density) +/– attenuated vessels

mosaic perfusion and air trapping accentuated by expiratory HRCT

ORGANIZING PNEUMONIA

AIRSPACE pattern: patchy bilateral subpleural consolidation or groundglass opacity, LL>UL; air bronchograms

centrilobular/peribronchovascular nodules

larger subpleural nodular like areas of consolidation

bronchial wall thickening +/– bronchiolectasis

3.13 BRONCHOGENIC CARCINOMA

DEFINITION AND CLASSIFICATION

malignant bronchogenic neoplasm largely caused by smoking, with a number of different morphological presentations

Classified by histological type

non small cell lung carcinoma (NSCLC)

small cell lung carcinoma (SCLC)

EPIDEMIOLOGY

Australian AntiCancer Council data 1997: 6% of all deaths

leading cause of cancer deaths (28%)

Lifetime risk of lung carcinoma:

smoker 1/6 to 1/14

non smoker 1/360

passive smoke exposure 1/280

ETIOLOGY

smoking (98%)

all others (asbestos, radioactive ores, polycyclic hydrocarbons, pulmonary fibrosis, familial cytochrome P450 mutation)

PATHOGENESIS

probably an ordered premalignant to malignant progression; difficulty of access to bronchial epithelium limits studies

bronchial epithelium origin: squamous cell carcinoma (SCC), small cell carcinoma

bronchiolar epithelium origin: adenocarcinoma, bronchioloalveolar carcinoma

CLINICAL FEATURES

Presentation (presents late)

MASS EFFECT

collapse, recurrent infection, dyspnea

cough, wheeze, stridor

dysphagia, SVC syndrome

DIRECT INVASION

bronchi (hemoptysis)

neural (recurrent laryngeal, phrenic, Horner's palsies)

pleural (pleural effusion, rarely bronchopleural fistula)

chest wall (pain)

PARANEOPLASTIC SYNDROMES

MNEMONIC: SCLC Hypercalcemia

syndromes usually caused by small cell lung carcinoma (SCLC)

S-IADH

syndrome of inappropriate anti diuretic hormone secretion

C-ushing's

adrenocorticotrophic hormone or pro-ACTH

L-ow calcium (Calcitonin)

C-arcinoid (Serotonin)

HYPERCALCEMIA

caused by squamous carcinoma (parathyroid hormone related protein)

CONSTITUTIONAL

loss of weight, anemia, myopathy

clubbing, hypertrophic osteoarthropathy

METASTASES PRESENTING FIRST

Tissue diagnosis

DIFFICULT AND SUBJECT TO SAMPLING ERROR

Spread

SCLC (15%) usually widely disseminated at diagnosis

NSCLC (85%)

direct invasion
locoregional nodes
hematogenous: adrenals, brain, liver, bones, other lung

STAGING (TNM)

STAGING T

Tx: occult, Tis: in situ, T0: no evidence of primary
T1: <3 cm isolated
T2: >3 cm isolated, or to visceral pleura, or to main bronchus @ >2 cm to carina, or distal collapse to hilum
T3: chest wall, or superior sulcus, or diaphragm, or mediastinal pleura, or main bronchus @ <2 cm to carina, or collapse of whole lung
T4: invades vital structures (including carina), or vertebral bodies, or malignant effusion, or separate tumor masses in the same lobe

STAGING N

N0: nil
N1: ipsilateral hilar (10–14)
N2: ipsilateral mediastinal/subcarinal (1–9)
N3: supraclavicular/scalene or contralateral (1–9)

STAGING M

M0: nil
M1: distant metastases including tumor in any other lobe of lung

STAGE GROUPING

S0:   Tis N0 M0
SIa: T1 N0 M0
SIb: T2 N0 M0
SIIa: T1 N1 M0
SIIb: T2 N1 M0 or T3 N0 M0
SIIIa: T1 N2 M0 or T2 N2 M0 or T3 N1–2 M0
SIIIb: any T N3 M0 or T4 any N M0
SIV: any T any N M1
SUMMARY OF STAGE GROUPING
SI: T1 or T2 N0 M0
SII: T1 or T2 N1 M0 or T3 N0 M0
SIIIa: up to T3, up to N2
SIIIb: any N T4, any T N3
SIV: M1
in general, SIIIa is the watershed for surgical/radiotherapy treatments

AJCC-UICC LYMPH NODE STATIONS 1996

1 R/L highest mediastinal (above L brachiocepahlic V)
2 R/L upper paratracheal (above aortic arch upper margin)
3A prevascular (above aortic arch upper margin)
3P retrotracheal (above aortic arch upper margin)
4 R/L lower paratracheal (aortic arch upper margin to right upper lobe bronchus or left main bronchus)
5 aortopulmonary
6 anterior mediastinal (below aortic arch upper margin)
7 subcarinal
8 R/L paraesophageal (below carina)
9 R/L pulmonary ligament
10 R/L hilar (distal to mediastinal pleural reflection)
11 R/L interlobar (between lobar bronchi)
12 R/L lobar (with distal lobar bronchi)
13 R/L segmental nodes (with segmental bronchi)
14 R/L subsegmental nodes

MACRO

upper lobes more than lower lobes
white/yellow firm mass with lobulated or spiculated edge
cheesy (keratinizing SCC) or with central keratin
may cavitate (more commonly SCC)
may be diffuse mucinous consolidation (bronchioloalveolar)

MICRO

type by best differentiated, grade by least differentiated
Australian data 1990

Squamous cell (SCC) (40%)

central, cavitates, male predominance
well differentiated (keratin pearls, tight junctions)
mod differentiated (tonofilaments)

Adenocarcinoma (30%)

incidence rising
peripheral with fibrosis, female predominance, brain metastases
recapitulates glands, PAS+

Bronchioloalveolar

special subset of adenocarcinoma
sheet of adeno cells (?type II ?Clara) along septa

peripheral, presents in two forms:

classic nodular mass
diffuse type with mucus, resembling consolidation

Large cell (10%)

poorly differentiated end of entire spectrum

Mixed (5%)

Small cell (SCLC) (15%)

central, aggressive, early hematogenous metastases
extensive paraneoplastic endocrinopathy
small round blue cells, neurosecretory granules

IMAGING

XR/fluoro

UTILITY

initial detection
2 year stability rule (i.e. stable >2 years = no carcinoma) is very good but not infallible!

SIGNS

PERIPHERAL/PARENCHYMAL MASS
soft tissue density mass
may cavitate
lobulated or spiculated contour
may retract pleura
may have distal collapse
may have calcium!
if pleural/subpleural (e.g. Pancoast) may simulate pleural thickening
CENTRAL/HILAR MASS
abnormal hilar contour
increased hilar density
abnormal air bronchogram
collapse distal to hilum with obscuration of hilum
drowned lung/bronchocele distal to hilum
Golden's S sign: hilar mass with distal lobar collapse (each responsible for one half of the S)
failure of distal pneumonia to resolve
recurrent pneumonia, same segment
GROWING MASS
LYMPHADENOPATHY
BRONCHIOLOALVEOLAR CARCINOMA
ill defined airspace consolidation – may be rounded, may be multifocal
DIFFERENTIAL: any other causes of airspace opacity
pattern evolution over time more specific

CT

UTILITY

first line cross sectional modality
resolution of nodes and especially parenchyma superior to MR

accurate T staging (problems with chest wall)
nodal staging on size criteria only
    (inaccurate)
invasion undercalled unless gross

SIGNS

PULMONARY NODULE (often defined as
    <3 cm)
  BENIGN
heavily calcified (i.e. old scar)
fat density (i.e. hamartoma)
vascular enhancement, draining vessel
    (i.e. pulmonary AVM)
totally stable over many years
  MORE LIKELY BENIGN
smooth rounded margin
coarse calcification
enhancement <10 HU on dynamic CT
no mass component (i.e. lung parenchymal
    scar without mass)
  MORE LIKELY MALIGNANT
spiculated margin, 'tails'
satellite nodules
strong enhancement on dynamic CT
    (differential: active TB, infection,
    sarcoidosis, fungus)
PULMONARY MASS (often defined as >3 cm)
high likelihood of malignancy if true mass
    (i.e. mass effect and not airspace
    consolidation)
see differential diagnosis for pulmonary
    nodule/mass in gamuts
  UNEQUIVOCAL SIGNS OF MALIGNANCY
invasion of structures with destruction or
    change of contour
distant metastases
  SIGNS OF PROBABLE MALIGNANCY
bronchial compression/invasion
distal changes: collapse, consolidation,
    'drowning' (i.e. fluid buildup)
bronchus encased in mass
possible invasion if in contiguity (i.e. loss of
    intervening air or fat) – not definite
cavitation
other signs as for nodule
NODAL STAGING
relies on size criteria
commonest is transverse diameter >10 mm
see lymphadenopathy in gamuts

MR

UTILITY

better at vascular hilum anatomy/invasion
better than CT for chest wall, mediastinal,
    and suprapleural membrane/root of neck
    invasion (i.e. superior sulcus)
nodal staging on size criteria only
    (inaccurate)

SIGNS

similar to CT
high T2W signal may reflect edema without
    microscopic invasion or may indicate
    microscopic invasion
coronal plane useful for carina, thoracic
    inlet, diaphragm

NUC MED

UTILITY

gallium: some carcinomas avid Ga but not
    sufficiently specific to exclude carcinoma
thallium: carcinomas often avid; poor
    resolution and penetration makes most
    studies uninterpretable

PET (FDG)

UTILITY

lung carcinoma staging is a cardinal
    indication for PET
? lung carcinoma recurrence is a cardinal
    indication for PET
characterization of indeterminate lung
    nodule or mass (solitary or multiple) is a
    cardinal indication for PET
proven best modality for N staging
PET stage better predictor of overall survival
    than imaging stage without PET
negative PET of a solitary pulmonary nodule
    allows biopsy to be avoided (this has to
    be validated for each specific patient
    population)

SIGNS

increased FDG uptake compared with
    mediastinal blood pool
not reliable with masses < approx 1.5 cm
    (depends on machine) – valid if positive
SUV(max) >2.5 is most commonly used
    cutoff for malignancy (this is as imperfect
    as visual interpretation)
may have central necrosis
DIFFERENTIAL: sarcoidosis, tuberculosis,
    fungal infections (and post surgical
    change – usually linear and low grade)
DIFFERENTIAL: other malignancies
post radiotherapy change: diffuse low grade
    activity in area of radiation portal and
    active pleural uptake
recurrence: uptake in excess of radiation
    change or increasing over time

3.14 CAPLAN'S SYNDROME

*see rheumatoid lung disease and anthracosis
(under pneumoconioses)*

3.15 CHEST TRAUMA

3.15.1 CHEST WALL TRAUMA

Sternal fractures
beware cardiac injury, bronchial laceration

Rib fractures

COMPRESSION
pneumothorax unlikely (fragments point out)

DIRECT TRAUMA
pneumothorax likely (inward crush)

3.15.2 PULMONARY CONTUSIONS

Contusion
greatest at 24 hours
starts clearing at 48–72 hours

Hematoma

Laceration

Post traumatic pneumatocele

3.15.3 TRAUMATIC PNEUMOTHORAX

3.15.4 BRONCHIAL INJURY

Fractured bronchus or trachea

'FALLEN LUNG'
displaced lung as pedicle disrupted

PERSISTENT TENSION
    PNEUMOTHORAX ON DRAINAGE

PNEUMOMEDIASTINUM

Foreign body or flap
DO INSPIRATORY AND EXPIRATORY VIEWS
    (LOOKING FOR AIR TRAPPING)

3.15.5 AORTIC INJURY

see aortic injury in Ch 15

3.15.6 CARDIAC INJURY

see Ch 14

3.16 CHOLESTEROL PNEUMONITIS

another term for endogenous lipoid (lipid) pneumonia
see under pneumonia entry

3.17 COAD (or COPD: chronic obstructive airways (pulmonary) disease)

3.17.1 CHRONIC BRONCHITIS

DEFINITION

>2 years with >3 months per year of daily sputum

ETIOLOGY

smoking (>90%)
occupational
asthma
abnormal airways (cystic fibrosis, immotile cilia syndromes)
recurrent infections (immune deficiency syndromes)
recurrent aspiration (neurological deficit)

IMAGING

CXR

commonest: normal
hyperinflation
bronchial wall thickening
patchy distal collapses
patchy bronchopneumonia
evidence of pulmonary hypertension

3.17.2 EMPHYSEMA

DEFINITION AND CLASSIFICATION

destruction and permanent enlargement of all or part of an acinus

Classification

centrilobular (UL > LL, smoking/dusts)
panacinar (LL > UL, smoking/alpha 1 antitrypsin deficiency)

paraseptal (subpleural, paraseptal, associated with pneumothorax)
irregular/pericicatricial (surrounding scarring)

ETIOLOGY

smoking
alpha 1 antitrypsin (a1AT) deficiency

IMAGING

CXR

changes manifest late in disease
spirometry detects disease much earlier!

OVERINFLATION

increased number of cleared ribs
enlarged prevascular clear space on lateral
decreased cardiothoracic ratio
blunting of costophrenic angles, no effusions
FOCAL
look for other underlying cause
MULTIFOCAL/DIFFUSE
UPPER > LOWER
ABPA (allergic bronchopulmonary aspergillosis)
cystic fibrosis
LOWER > UPPER
classically alpha 1 antitrypsin deficiency
EQUAL
any cause

DIAPHRAGMATIC FLATTENING AND REDUCED MOVEMENT

abnormally flat diaphragm (see normal)
fluoro diaphragm motion <3 cm

INCREASED TRANSLUCENCY (subjective)

SIGNS OF PULMONARY HYPERTENSION (see under cardiac)

LOSS OF NORMAL DISTAL VASCULAR MARKINGS

BULLAE AND CYSTS

large avascular air filled spaces
may air trap or have mass effect
UL: usual COAD
LL: sign of alpha 1 AT deficiency
may be superinfected (air–fluid levels)
may rupture

Coexistent disease manifestations

silicosis/other pneumoconioses
TB (old, less likely active)

HRCT

lung hyperexpansion
decreased parenchymal density
centrilobular emphysema: centrilobular lucencies, reduction in number of visible centrilobular structures
panacinar emphysema: extensive destruction of septal and interstitial structures, irregular residual spaces
paraseptal emphysema: subpleural/ subfissural bullae
bulla formation

NUC MED

V/Q DEMONSTRATES EXTENT OF MISMATCH AND EXTENT OF PULMONARY HYPOPERFUSION

matched defects (segmental or non segmental)
poor ventilation phase (poor distal tracer penetration)
central aerosol clumping (turbulent central flow)
reverse mismatch (perfused not ventilated, i.e. a right to left shunt and a cause of hypoxia)

Q PHASE ALONE PROVIDES QUANTITATIVE ASSESSMENT OF LOCATION AND SYMMETRY OF PULMONARY PERFUSION

commonest: symmetrical right–left unless dominant bullae, and better perfusion to lower lobes
allows planning of lung volume reduction surgery (i.e. resection of non perfused emphysematous air trapping lung)

3.17.3 AIRWAY HYPERREACTIVITY

ASTHMA

see asthma entry

REVERSIBLE COMPONENT OF COAD

often present in smoking related COAD
bronchial hyperreactivity behaves similarly to asthma
empirically treated with bronchodilators and steroids, etc

3.18 COLLAPSE

see under gamuts – generic

3.19 CONNECTIVE TISSUE DISEASE

3.19.1 RHEUMATOID ARTHRITIS

see rheumatoid lung disease entry

3.19.2 SCLERODERMA, MIXED CONNECTIVE TISSUE DISEASE, POLYMYOSITIS, DERMATOMYOSITIS

see pulmonary fibrosis entry
essentially similar to idiopathic pulmonary fibrosis

3.19.3 SYSTEMIC LUPUS ERYTHEMATOSUS

see SLE entry in Ch 15

3.20 CRYPTOCOCCOSIS

DEFINITION

granulomatous fungal infection –
 Cryptococcus neoformans
PRIMARY PULMONARY COMPLEX
CRYPTOCOCCOMA
DISSEMINATED CRYPTOCOCCOSIS
CRYPTOCOCCAL MENINGITIS

EPIDEMIOLOGY

Normal host, endemic
particularly prevalent in North America

Immunocompromised host
AIDS, Hodgkin's disease
invasive lung cryptococcosis (massive
 edema, consolidation, hemorrhage)
generalized miliary dissemination

CLINICAL

Primary pulmonary complex
chronic immune type non caseating
 granuloma
lymphocytes, macrophages, giant cells, yeasts
chronic inflammatory and granulomatous
 response
yeasts carried to lymph nodes – regional
 lymphadenopathy
usually heals with fibrotic scar, may calcify

Cryptococcoma
inflammatory granulomatous mass

Cryptococcal meningitis
CSF: yeasts black with Grocott's stain or
 stand out in Indian ink
see Ch 11 CNS 7.4 and 7.5

IMAGING

XR/Fluoro/CT

PRIMARY PULMONARY COMPLEX
non specific pulmonary nodule or mass, may
 calcify
lymphadenopathy possible but unusual

INVASIVE CRYPTOCOCCOSIS
consolidation, fluffy hemorrhage

MILIARY
like TB

MR
see Ch 11 CNS

3.21 CYSTIC FIBROSIS (CF)

DEFINITION

autosomal recessive syndrome of exocrine
 gland and respiratory failure caused by
 defective chloride (Cl) transmembrane
 transport protein

EPIDEMIOLOGY

1/2000 live Caucasian births, infrequent in
 Asians/Africans
variable severity, median survival 25 years,
 death of respiratory failure or cor
 pulmonale

ETIOLOGY

CF gene on 7q (multiple variations of
 variable severity) – coding abnormal
 membrane Cl transport protein
 (autosomal recessive)
70% is deltaF508 deletion
homo deltaF508 – commonest combination,
 classical severe disease
deltaF508, other mutation – milder disease

PATHOGENESIS

failure of Cl transport with resulting viscid
 abnormal exocrine secretions (including
 bronchial mucus) leading to obstruction,
 distal atrophy, superinfection

MACRO/MICRO

Lungs (100%) – most morbidity and mortality
inspissated dry mucus with failure of
 clearance
distal air trapping, collapse
bronchiectasis, fibrosis, pulmonary
 hypertension, cor pulmonale
Pseudomonas (mucoid colonies),
 Staphylococcus (abscesses)
secondary ABPA, autoimmune
 hypersensitivity disease

Vas deferens (100%)
obstruction, atresia, sterility

Pancreas (90%)
obstruction of small ducts with distal fibrotic
 atrophy, eventual exocrine pancreatic
 failure

Paranasal sinuses
chronic sinusitis, failure of clearance

Salivary glands
gradual fibrotic atrophy

Liver (5%)
obstruction of small bile ducts, jaundice,
 secondary biliary cirrhosis

Gut (neonate)
meconium ileus, ileal atresias, meconium
 peritonitis

Gut (adult)
(rare) meconium ileus equivalent

Sweat glands
asymptomatic failure of Cl resorption with
 salty sweat
basis for SWEAT TEST

IMAGING (lungs)

*see Ch 06 for gut manifestations, Ch 07 for
pancreatic manifestations*

SECTION 4

CXR/CT

early: no findings
childhood: recurrent chest infections,
    bronchial wall thickening, lung volume
    increase, patchy overinflation/collapse

ESTABLISHED FINDINGS IN CHILDHOOD/ADOLESCENCE/ADULTHOOD

multifocal bronchiectasis (UL > LL)
mucus plugs, distal collapses
patchy infection, lung abscesses
overinflation

HRCT

BRONCHIECTASIS

cylindrical and cystic
UL > LL
thickened bronchial wall
mucus plugs, distal collapses, distal
    overexpansion

MOSAIC PERFUSION WITH AIR TRAPPING

NUC MED

V/Q: bilateral patchy grossly abnormal
    perfusion and ventilation, classically
    matched but may have reverse mismatch
    (i.e. perfusion no ventilation)
ventilation scintigram usually more severe
    than CXR

3.22 DESQUAMATIVE INTERSTITIAL PNEUMONIA (DIP)

see pulmonary fibrosis/interstitial pneumonitis entry

3.23 DIFFUSE ALVEOLAR DAMAGE (DAD)

clinical manifestations are the adult
    respiratory distress syndrome (ARDS)
overlaps with non cardiogenic pulmonary
    edema

DEFINITION

non immune or immune and usually acute
    loss of (or damage to) type I pneumocytes
    and capillary endothelial cells with
    resulting intraalveolar edema

ETIOLOGY

Inhalation

gas (e.g. SO2, nitrogen oxides and smoke
    inhalation)
gastric content aspiration (Mendelson's
    syndrome) – very high mortality
near drowning
viral pneumonia
allergen/massive hypersensitivity (extrinsic
    allergic alveolitis, other e.g. eosinophilic
    pneumonia)

Circulation

pulmonary toxins (e.g. paraquat, salicylates,
    snake venom)
uremia/cirrhosis (but see Pulmonary Edema)
disseminated intravascular
    coagulation/septicemia/septic shock
transfusion reaction
fat embolism (pancreatitis or trauma)
autoantibodies (Goodpasture's syndrome)
NB chronic immune complex disease
    (rheumatoid arthritis, systemic lupus
    erythematosus, systemic sclerosis all very
    unlikely to produce acute DAD)

Radiation

Unclear

neurogenic pulmonary edema
amniotic fluid embolism
altitude sickness

PATHOGENESIS, MICRO

INJURY PHASE (hours to days)
diffuse damage or loss of both pulmonary
    capillary endothelium and alveolar
    epithelium in variable proportion (direct
    cell injury or immune system mediated)
HYALINE MEMBRANES

EDEMA PHASE (days)
proteinaceous or hemorrhagic exudate
    flooding airspace ('non cardiogenic
    pulmonary edema')
HYALINE MEMBRANES: eosinophilic bland
    layer of cell debris and exudate adherent
    to alveolar/alveolar sac walls
mixed cellular infiltrate (at approximately
    3 days) expanding interstitium and
    spilling into airspace
clinical features manifest in this phase as
    gas exchange fails

RECOVERY WITH CLEARANCE OR
    ORGANIZATION AND FIBROSIS

clearance of exudate by macrophages
regeneration of alveolar epithelium by type
    II pneumocytes (starting at
    approximately 7 days)
usually a fibroblastic response with fibrosis
    (see outcomes)

CLINICAL FEATURES

= adult respiratory distress syndrome
acute severe dyspnea, reduced lung
    compliance
central cyanosis and hypoxia, not responsive
    to oxygen
overall mortality >60%, many from
    superimposed pneumonia

OUTCOMES

RESOLUTION

exudate/edema cleared, reticulin framework
    intact
successful alveolar re-expansion

ORGANIZING PNEUMONIA

poor clearance and re-expansion
macrophage activation//fibroblast activation
exudate organization and membrane
    incorporation

BRONCHIOLITIS OBLITERANS

patchy bronchiolar damage
granulation overgrowth

LATE FIBROSIS

see 3.50

IMAGING

CXR sequence

cardinal sign: airspace diffuse or multifocal
    bilateral patchy opacity with a
    characteristic delay after injury
may have same appearance as cardiogenic
    pulmonary edema, or be more patchy

0 to 12 hours	no findings
12 to 24 hours	patchy airspace opacity
24 hours to 3 days	maximal opacification
3 to 7 days	patchy clearance

HRCT

AIRSPACE PATTERN

diffuse or patchy ground glass, then
    consolidation
eventual progression to fibrosis if patient
    survives

3.24 DRUGS AND LUNGS

'standard' list

drugs: cytotoxics, amiodarone, gold
produce: diffuse alveolar damage/BOOP
/fibrosis

'special' list

opioids (APO)
methysergide (pleural fibrosis)
paraquat (DAD)
sulfasalazine/nitrofurantoin/pyrimethamine
(eosinophilia)
amphotericin/anticoagulants/cytotoxics
(hemorrhage)
nitrofurantoin (interstitial fibrosis)

3.25 EXTRINSIC ALLERGIC ALVEOLITIS (EAA)

DEFINITION

alveolar centered allergic reaction to foreign
protein leading to acute dyspnea or
chronic fibrosis (other term:
'hypersensitivity pneumonitis')

ETIOLOGY

many allergens and occupational diseases
described
fungus on mouldy hay (farmer's lung)
mushrooms (mushroom worker's lung)
bird droppings/feathers (pigeon fancier's
lung)
etc

PATHOGENESIS

type III (immune complex) and type IV
(delayed type hypersensitivity) reaction to
foreign protein reaching distal airspace
neutrophil and lymphocyte acute response,
inflammation, edema
loss of alveolar epithelium and bronchiolitis
eventual distal fibrosis with repeated
episodes

CLINICAL

dyspnea, fever, dry cough 6–12 hours post
exposure; ARDS if massive
ultimate evolution to pulmonary fibrosis

IMAGING

XR/fluoro

ACUTE
no findings
diffuse ground glass pattern
non cardiogenic pulmonary edema

CHRONIC
no visible findings until fibrosis becomes
apparent
fine reticulonodular interstitial pattern,
UL > LL
eventual volume loss, traction
bronchiectasis, pattern of
undifferentiated pulmonary fibrosis

HRCT

CHRONIC PHASE
may have acute changes superimposed
INTERSTITIAL PATTERN (centrilobular and
peripheral)
smooth fibrosis
patchy distribution
mid and upper zones involved

ACUTE PHASE
AIRSPACE PATTERN
patchy groundglass opacity
NODULAR PATTERN
centrilobular nodules

3.26 GAUCHER'S (and NIEMANN-PICK) DISEASES (manifestations)

*produce a diffuse interstitial pattern with
reticulolinear, reticulonodular or coarse
reticulonodular pattern*

3.27 GRANULOMAS

a pathological entity, defined as a focal
collection of monocyte/macrophage cells
(see Ch 26 general pathology:
granulomatous inflammation for
classification)
radiological 'granuloma' is shorthand for
'pulmonary nodule'

3.28 HAMMAN–RICH SYNDROME

see pulmonary fibrosis entry

3.29 HISTIOCYTOSIS X (LANGERHANS CELL HISTIOCYTOSIS) (pulmonary manifestations)

*see histiocytosis X and eosinophilic
granuloma in Ch 05
Ch 11 for neurohistiocytosis*

IMAGING (lung)

CXR

UL > LL
reticulonodular pattern
nodules small, 1–3 mm
irregular air cysts
increased lung volume
pattern may mimic fibrosis
sometimes recurrent spontaneous
pneumothoraces

HRCT

LUNG CYSTS
cysts have walls and mass effect: not
emphysema!
thin wall cysts +/– confluence
UPPER ZONES

NODULAR PATTERN
centrilobular nodules

INTERSTITIAL PATTERN
(peribronchovascular)
peribronchial nodularity

3.30 HISTOPLASMOSIS

DEFINITION

granulomatous fungal infection by
Histoplasma capsulatum; frequent cause
of solitary pulmonary nodule

CLINICAL

most prevalent in North America, usually
self limiting

Primary pulmonary complex

pulmonary subapical mass, regional
lymphadenopathy (analogous to TB)
immune type granulomas, usually non
caseating
reactive fibrosis, may calcify, may cavitate

Chronic form

cavitation, extensive fibrosis, diffuse apical infiltrate

mass difficult to differentiate from carcinoma

Miliary disease

immunocompromised host, analogous to miliary TB

IMAGING

XR/fluoro/CT

PRIMARY PULMONARY COMPLEX

solitary or oligofocal pulmonary nodule/mass

concentric calcification very suggestive if present

rounded well defined indolent appearance usual

may be more atypical with aggressive edge

may cavitate or grow

lymphadenopathy possible, calcifies

CHRONIC FORM

fibrocaseous histoplasmosis

appearance as for TB

MULTIFOCAL FORM

massive exposure required

multiple pulmonary nodules

heal with calcification (similar to healed varicella)

INVASIVE FORM

immunocompromised host

non specific consolidation of any pattern

PET (FDG)

active histoplasmosis is FDG avid and can be impossible to differentiate from malignancy

3.31 HYDATID DISEASE

also see hydatid disease in Ch 07

DEFINITION

accidental infestation by cysts of Echinococcus granulosus (canine tapeworm), rarely other Echinococcus spp

PATHOGENESIS

cysts in dog feces; intermediate host: sheep, cattle, horses

ova swallowed, larvae hatch, penetrate gut wall, carried by portal blood, lodge in liver or lungs or other organs

cysts grow slowly by secretion of hydatid fluid

cysts may die – collapse, mild host inflammatory response

seeding of spaces/cavities if live cyst ruptures

anaphylaxis if presensitized and cyst fluid enters blood

MACRO

liver > lung>kidney > other visceral > skeletal

LAYERS

host capsule: pericyst

echinococcal outer capsule: ectocyst

echinococcal inner layer: endocyst (has germinal epithelium)

scolices in endocyst (bud from germinal epithelium)

loose hooks and scolices form 'hydatid sand'

daughter cysts in endocyst

IMAGING

XR/CT

INTACT CYST

rounded water or soft tissue density pulmonary parenchymal mass

often lobulated/deformed by adjacent structures

may erode into ribs or vertebrae

inner daughter cysts along wall

lung cysts virtually never calcify

liver cysts have a calcific wall

RUPTURED PERICYST

round smooth edge mass inside cystic wall, air crescent

RUPTURED INNER MEMBRANES

water lily (air–fluid level, floating crumpled membranes, floating daughter cysts)

serpent (crumpled membranes only)

empty cyst (all contents expectorated)

superinfected cyst (like any other superinfected cavity)

US/CT

liver hydatids: see in Ch 07

3.32 KAPOSI'S SARCOMA
(pulmonary manifestations)

IMAGING

CXR/CT/HRCT

peribronchovascular masses (1–2 cm)

classic 'flame shaped' appearance

endobronchial masses, may grow along bronchus

parenchymal nodular metastases

parenchymal lymphangitis

hilar lymphadenopathy (approx 1/2)

effusions (approximately 1/2)

pulmonary hemorrhage

NUC MED

classically gallium negative and thallium or PET positive

Differential diagnosis

bacillary angiomatosis – eminently curable with antibiotics

produced by Bartonella Henselli – cause of cat scratch disease !

3.33 KARTAGENER'S SYNDROME

CLINICAL

autosomal recessive syndrome of absent dynein arms in cilia, with defective cilial motion

resutant bronchiectasis, sinusitis, infertility

IMAGING

classically: dextrocardia with bronchiectasis and recurrent bronchopneumonias AND absent frontal sinuses, sinusitis

3.34 LUNG ABSCESS

ETIOLOGY

Aspiration

see ASPIRATION PNEUMONIA 3.46.8

Septic embolism/septic infarct

IV drug use

infected cannulas

commonly Staphylococcus aureus – aggressive abscess

Superinfection of cavity

cavitating carcinoma (esp squamous), TB, ruptured hydatid

Obstructive pneumonia, superinfection

foreign body, endogenous tumor, extrinsic compression

Virulent primary pneumonia

Staphylococcus aureus, Klebsiella pneumoniae, Pseudomonas spp, Escherichia coli

Abnormal lung

e.g. cystic fibrosis, bronchiectasis

Abnormal host

(immunosuppressed)

(see invasive aspergillosis and TB)

Transdiaphragmatic

amebic abscess

NATURAL HISTORY

Complications

chronicity
septic embolism (brain, kidneys)
pyopneumothorax, empyema, bronchopleural fistula

IMAGING

XR/fluoro/CT

cavity, air–fluid level
wall of variable thickness, usually thinner than in cancer
rapid progression
may be multiple
starts as consolidation unless preexisting cavity

PET (FDG)

often FDG avid – lung abscess can simulate cancer

3.35 LUNG PRIMARIES

(not bronchogenic carcinoma)

3.35.1 BENIGN

CENTRAL

3.35.1.1 SQUAMOUS PAPILLOMA

3.35.1.2 PLEOMORPHIC ADENOMA

3.35.1.3 HEMANGIOMA

PERIPHERAL

3.35.1.4 HAMARTOMA

CLINICAL
presentation: usually adults around 50 years old
solitary mass 90% peripheral, usually <4 cm, average 2.5 cm
10% endobronchial
cartilage (with chondroid calcification), fat (50%), clefts lined by bronchial epithelium
CARNEY'S TRIAD
pulmonary hamartomas, gastric leiomyosarcomas, extra adrenal functional paragangliomas
IMAGING
round smoothly lobulated mass
cardinal sign is fat in mass or chondroid (popcorn) calcification (avoids biopsy, but minority)

3.35.2 MALIGNANT

3.35.2.1 BRONCHIAL CARCINOID

CLINICAL
younger adults, not related to smoking
neuroendocrine (APUD) cell origin
obstruction, endocrinopathies (Cushing's, carcinoid), distant metastases
90% central dumbbell tumor through bronchial wall, may calcify; endocrine rosettes
IMAGING
central bronchial mass with obstruction and distal changes
if peripheral – non specific mass
often calcifies
may be cold on FDG PET
usually has some degree of In-111 octreotide uptake (see carcinoid entry in Ch 06)

3.35.2.2 SALIVARY CARCINOMA (rare)

3.35.2.3 LYMPHOMA (rare)

3.35.2.4 PRIMARY BRONCHIAL MELANOMA (rare)

3.35.2.5 KAPOSI'S SARCOMA (AIDS)

3.36 LYMPHANGIOLEIO-MYOMATOSIS

DEFINITION

rare congenital idiopathic proliferation of perilymphatic smooth muscle cells leading to distal airspace air trapping and development of lung cysts; virtually exclusively in females

IMAGING

rarely, tuberous sclerosis may have identical CXR/HRCT changes

CXR

may be normal
lung volume increased
UL > LL cystic change
differential diagnosis fibrosis, histiocytosis
secondary pneumothoraces

HRCT

thin wall lung cysts +/– confluence
lung cysts have walls and mass effect: not emphysema!
interspersed normal parenchyma
diffuse HRCT distribution
pleural effusions (chylous; probably secondary to lymphatic obstruction)

3.37 LYMPHANGITIS CARCINOMATOSA

DEFINITION

not a separate entity but manifestation of many malignancies
diffuse lymphatic infiltration of lung parenchyma by malignant cells, usually of carcinoma

ETIOLOGY

Focal/lobar

bronchogenic carcinoma (in continuity)
mesothelioma
Hodgkin's disease (in continuity with lymph node disease)

Diffuse

breast carcinoma
prostate carcinoma
adenocarcinoma of other origin (colon, stomach, lung, cervix, pancreas, thyroid)
lymphoma/leukemia (rare)

IMAGING

CXR

reticulonodular interstitial pattern
classically bilateral lower zone
chronic with slow evolution
may have lymphadenopathy or evidence of primary tumor

HRCT

INTERSTITIAL PATTERN (perilymphatic)

smooth or nodular peribronchovascular
cuffing
peripheral reticulonodular interstitial
thickening
centrilobular nodules
normal lung architecture (i.e. no evidence of
fibrosis)
pleural effusions

NODULAR PATTERN (miliary)

miliary pattern often coexists

3.38 LYMPHOCYTIC INTERSTITIAL PNEUMONITIS ('pseudolymphoma')

CLINICAL

common in HIV (especially in children)
extensive infiltration of lung interstitium by
mature polyclonal lymphocytes and
plasma cells originating from resident
MALT (mucosa associated lymphoid
tissue), NOT a pneumonitis

IMAGING

causes an interstitial pattern on CXR/CT

3.39 LYMPHOMATOID GRANULOMATOSIS

*see in pulmonary vasculitides and non
vasculitides entry*

3.40 MCLEOD/SWYER–JAMES SYNDROME

DEFINITION

postnatal secondary unilateral pulmonary
hypoplasia

ETIOPATHOGENESIS

severe childhood bronchiolitis (often
adenovirus) with arrest of distal acinar
growth and with bronchiolitis obliterans

IMAGING

CXR

unilateral small hypovascular hyperlucent
lung with/without air trapping (cycles
least in inspiration/expiration)
usually first manifests in childhood
ipsilateral pulmonary artery hypoplasia

3.41 MESOTHELIOMA

DEFINITION

malignant pleural tumor (rarely arises in
mesothelium elsewhere) with strong
association with asbestos, bipotent
morphology and very aggressive local
behavior

ETIOLOGY

non asbestos ?1/1 000 000 per year
asbestos: heavy exposure lifetime risk 10%,
long lag time; 80% give industrial history,
20% have asbestosis
tumor induction proportional to durability
and length:width of fibers (long straight
crocidolite worst, soft curled chrysotile
best)

CLINICAL

Presentation

dull chest pain, dyspnea, effusion, cough,
weight loss
effusion which is often bloody and commonly
recurs
most commonly irresectable at presentation
rare locations: peritoneum (abdominal pain,
bloody ascites); pericardium (recurring
bloody effusion, may tamponade);
scrotum

Spread

locally invasive (chest wall, diaphragm)
lymphatic spread to nodes and lymphangitis,
hematogenous metastases (liver,
adrenals, lung) late

MICRO

electron microscopy: long microvilli
EPITHELIOID (50%): cuboidal cells
(cytokeratin) with microvilli, less
aggressive

SARCOMATOID (25%): spindle cells
(vimentin), hyalinized stroma with
necrosis, more aggressive
BIPHASIC (25%)

IMAGING

CXR/CT

pleurally based soft tissue mass/rind,
commonly >1 cm, nodular or smooth
may enter fissures
collapse of underlying lung
associated effusion
evidence of diaphragm or chest wall
invasion

MR

best modality for showing local invasion
(particularly diaphragm)

PET (FDG)

FDG avid – allows monitoring of therapy and
differentiation from benign fibrothorax

3.42 NEUROFIBRO-MATOSIS (lung manifestations)

see neurofibromatosis in Ch 11

IMAGING

CXR

approximately 10% of NF patients >30 years
old
interstitial bibasal reticulolinear pattern
large upper lobe bullae

3.43 PLEURAL EFFUSION

Transudate (<3 g protein/l)
cardiac
cirrhotic
nephrotic
pancreatic

Exudate – infective
(purulent/serofibrinous)
secondary to lung infection
secondary to subphrenic abscess
primary bloodborne

Exudate – autoimmune
(serofibrinous)
immune complex disease (including SLE)
vasculitis

lung infarct
sympathetic (includes paraneoplastic)

Exudate – neoplastic

(hemorrhagic)
direct extension
pleural metastases
mesothelioma

Chylous

3.44 PLEURAL TUMORS

see the following:
benign pleural disease entry
mesothelioma entry

3.45 PNEUMOCONIOSES

GROUP DEFINITION

inorganic dust deposition diseases with
variable amount of inflammatory
reaction, immunologic reaction, reactive
fibrosis and superinfection

CLASSIFICATION

SIMPLE PNEUMOCONIOSES (ANTHRACOSIS,
SILICOSIS, MIXED)
PROGRESSIVE MASSIVE FIBROSIS
SILICOTUBERCULOSIS
IMMUNE GRANULOMATOUS
PNEUMOCONIOSES (BERYLLIOSIS,
ZIRCONIUM DISEASE)
ASBESTOS DISEASE

3.45.1 SILICOSIS

DEFINITION

high free silica dust content; forms hard
fibrotic nodules sometimes going on to
progressive massive fibrosis (PMF)

ETIOLOGY

SiO2 – quartz mining, sandblasting,
quarrying, etc; average time to clinical
disease is 20 years
acute silicoproteinosis may develop with
high silica dust exposures (timecourse
5 years)

PATHOGENESIS

SiO2 particles toxic (via silicic acid which
causes cell membrane injury) but not
immunogenic
macrophages ingesting silica stimulated to
secrete interleukins and fibroblastic
growth factors leading to a non specific
inflammatory response
development of fibrotic, non immune
granulomas

MACRO

Simple

small hard whorled fibrotic nodules, UL > LL
lymphadenopathy, lymph node fibrosis and
eggshell calcification
dilated bronchioles and focal emphysema
surround parenchymal fibrosis

PMF = complicated

large confluent fibrotic masses UL >>> LL
(by definition, >1cm)

ACUTE SILICOPROTEINOSIS

alveolar accumulation of lipoproteinaceous
material (morphologically same as
alveolar proteinosis)

NATURAL HISTORY

progression usually slow
increased incidence of emphysema,
especially in smokers
increased incidence of TB (silicotuberculosis)
PMF progresses to respiratory failure, cor
pulmonale

IMAGING

CXR

imaging findings do not correlate well with
clinical severity

SIMPLE
no early findings
interstitial nodular pattern UL > LL
size of nodules variable, by definition <1 cm
lymphadenopathy (bilateral), eggshell
calcification

STAGES
I   early disease, nodules faintly visible
II 2–3 mm nodules
III nodules >3 mm with coalescence

PMF
slowly growing and slowly retracting, often
symmetrical upper lobe masses

(classically move towards hila or retract
hila into themselves)
classically 'discoid' in shape, flattened in
plane of fissures and thin in the sagittal
plane with an elongated outer margin
paralleling the rib cage
may have eggshell calcification/engulf
calcified nodes
may cavitate (thick walled cavity), may have
TB

surrounding fibrosis, spiculation, retraction,
subpleural scarring, emphysema
volume loss of fibrotic areas, usually
emphysema of rest of lung results in
overall expansion
by definition of conglomeration (see
definitions) there are surrounding
nodules

differentiation from carcinoma may be very
hard morphologically (try FDG PET)

ACUTE SILICOPROTEINOSIS
similar to alveolar proteinosis
upper lobe predominance

CT/HRCT

INTERSTITIAL PATTERN (nodular)
see nodular pattern 1.3, 1.4
linear markings not prominent
eventual fibrosis
UL > LL

NODULAR PATTERN (perilymphatic)
small perilymphatic nodules, centrilobular >
peribronchovascular, also subpleural
UL > LL

CONGLOMERATION (PMF)
coalescence of similar masses into a bigger
mass
see CXR appearance
often cavitates

EMPHYSEMA
focal centrilobular emphysema
cicatricial emphysema

LYMPHADENOPATHY
usually discrete multiple non confluent nodes
may calcify; eggshell calcification

3.45.2 ANTHRACOSIS
(<5% free SiO2)

DEFINITION

coal dust; interstitial nodule formation and
occasional development of progressive
massive fibrosis

ETIOLOGY

pure or near pure coal dusts (coal mining)

PATHOGENESIS

dust ingestion by alveolar macrophages, deposition in interstitium and lymph nodes

low fibrotic potential, carbon dust does not incite an inflammatory response; non immune granulomas with relatively little collagen

MACRO

Simple

soft black stellate macules, UL > LL

peripheral cuff of dilated bronchioles /emphysema

black carbon filled hilar nodes, may enlarge

PMF

by definition >1 cm

soft black confluent masses, little fibrosis or cellularity, UL > LL

may cross fissures, may cavitate

Rheumatoid pneumoconiosis
(Caplan's syndrome)

combination of coal pneumoconiosis and rheumatoid arthritis

CAPLAN'S NODULES

rheumatoid nodule (central fibrinoid necrosis, concentric dust laminations with inflammatory cells, peripheral lymphocytes and plasma cells)

tend to accompany subcutaneous rheumatoid nodules

NATURAL HISTORY

usually asymptomatic or slow

PMF progresses to respiratory failure

may have coexistent emphysema

increased susceptibility to TB and incidence of TB

IMAGING

CXR

SIMPLE

interstitial nodules, UL > LL

by definition, <1 cm

may have lymphadenopathy

PMF

see PMF imaging in silicosis entry above

CAPLAN'S NODULES

multifocal pulmonary masses, larger than usual nodules, smaller than PMF, 0.5 to 5 cm

may cavitate, may regress, UL or LL, subpleural or more central

CT

centrilobular and peripheral interstitial nodules

PMF: conglomeration, cavitation, spiculated masses, calcification (see CXR)

HRCT

see silicosis (pattern similar)

3.45.3 MIXED SILICOANTHRACOSIS

commonest form; see Coal Worker's Pneumoconiosis

3.45.4 COAL WORKER'S PNEUMOCONIOSIS

TERMINOLOGY

term has been used to denote either pure anthracosis only OR a pneumoconiosis that occurs in a specific occupational group irrespective of degree of dust admixture

CLINICAL

found mainly in hard coal (anthracite) workers

degree of pathology relates to degree of silica exposure

progressive massive fibrosis in approximately 1/3

3.45.5 ASBESTOSIS

see its own entry

3.45.6 BERYLLIOSIS

beryllium particles act as haptens – immune granulomas, fibrosis, lymphadenopathy

3.46 PNEUMONIA

GROUP IMAGING

AIRSPACE PNEUMONIA
(broncho or lobar)

LOBAR/SEGMENTAL

more or less uniform consolidation of entire segment or lobe, usually bounded by septa or pleural surfaces (pathologic mechanism – distal airspace spread through pores of Kohn)

bulging implies massive exudate formation, but is also suspicious for bronchioloalveolar carcinoma

BRONCHOPNEUMONIA

patchy peribronchial consolidation without filling of segmental airspace and with less regard for septal boundaries

INTERSTITIAL PNEUMONIA

HRCT (not cause specific)

AIRSPACE PATTERN

(acutely) groundglass, possibly consolidation

3.46.1 PNEUMOCOCCAL PNEUMONIA

DEFINITION

acute primary bacterial pyogenic lobar pneumonia, non necrotizing, non fibrosing

ETIOLOGY

Streptococcus pneumoniae: Gram+ coccus (capsule has multiple serotypes)

CLASSIC HISTOLOGIC STAGES (pre antibiotic era)

Inflammatory edema

congestion, bacteria, neutrophil exudate

Red hepatisation (24 hours on)

congestion and pyogenic hemorrhagic fibrinous exudate

Gray hepatisation

as above but reduced congestion

Resolution (1 week on)

successful bacterial kill as capsule specific
antibodies appear
slow resolution of exudate/fibrin/debris

IMAGING

CXR

preradiographic stage
classic airspace pneumonia, segmental or
lobar, airbronchograms
radiographic resolution lags behind
symptoms

3.46.2 STAPHYLOCOCCAL PNEUMONIA

DEFINITION

acute (usually) secondary bacterial pyogenic
bronchopneumonia, necrotizing and
abscess forming

ETIOLOGY

Staphylococcus aureus: Gram+ coccus with
capsule, coagulase
often post viral (esp influenza), cystic
fibrosis, alcoholism, neonate and child
direct destruction; necrotic, thick walled
abscesses; secondary septic embolism

IMAGING

bronchopneumonia
abscess formation
EMPYEMAS, PYOPNEUMOTHORAX
PNEUMATOCELES (air containing thin
walled cysts; develop in recovery phase
possibly by ball–valve air trapping)

3.46.3 PRIMARY 'ATYPICAL' PNEUMONIA

DEFINITION

acute primary chlamydial or mycoplasmal
pneumonia with bronchopneumonic and
interstitial components, no necrosis and
with a lymphocyte predominant response

CLINICAL/MORPHOLOGY

endemic/epidemic (especially young adults)
patchy bronchopneumonic changes
interstitial lymphocytic, monocytic, plasma
cell infiltrate
often radiographically occult

3.46.4 ROUND PNEUMONIA

see Ch 21 pediatric thorax, 4.5.2

3.46.5 VIRAL PNEUMONIA

DEFINITION

acute viral interstitial pneumonia with
variable degrees of hemorrhage and
necrosis

ETIOLOGY – NORMAL HOST

influenza: necrotizing bronchiolitis, diffuse
alveolar damage; parainfluenza
adenovirus (can be severe; 25% go to
bronchiectasis, bronchiolitis obliterans)
Coxsackie viruses, echoviridae

ETIOLOGY – IMMUNE SUPPRESSED

CMV: AIDS
HSV: burns, other immune suppression
VZV: immunosuppression, malignancy

MICRO

patchy epithelial viral infection and loss,
interstitial edema and infiltrate
(lymphocytic/monocytic), +/– alveolar
exudate or hemorrhage

IMAGING

variable: from nothing to maximal (any or
none of below)
patchy bronchopneumonia
soft miliary nodules (esp VZV) that later may
calcify
confluent airspace opacities
diffuse alveolar damage pattern

3.46.6 PNEUMOCYSTIS CARINII PNEUMONIA (PCP)

DEFINITION

diffuse secondary sporozoite
bronchopneumonia particularly seen in
AIDS; airspace exudate with minor
interstitial infiltrate

ETIOLOGY

Pneumocystis carinii: sickle shaped non
invasive sporozoite (fungus)
CD4 usually <200

MICRO

frothy pink exudate in alveoli (periodic acid
Schiff positive)
non staining sickle shaped PC cysts in
exudate (stain with silver stains)
diffuse mononuclear type interstitial
infiltrate, of variable extent

IMAGING

CXR

variable: may have no findings
CLASSIC: fine reticular ill defined interstitial
perihilar symmetrical pattern
OTHER:
miliary interstitial pattern
patchy bronchopneumonic pattern
non specific segmental consolidation
upper zones if on aerosol prophylaxis

lymphadenopathy and effusions very
uncommon
pneumatoceles (40%)
pneumothoraces common, difficult to treat

HRCT

AIRSPACE (groundglass)
diffuse or mosaic groundglass opacity;
progresses on to consolidation

CYSTIC DISEASE
thin wall cysts, pneumatoceles
thick wall cysts
smooth interstitial thickening
pneumothoraces

Gallium

classic diffuse massively intense bilateral
early (24 hours, 48 hours) uptake

3.46.7 LIPID PNEUMONIA
(exogenous, endogenous)

Endogenous

CLINICAL

other terms: cholesterol pneumonitis, endogenous lipid pneumonia

sequel of airway obstruction (foreign body, mucus plug, tumor)

lipid laden macrophages in damaged collapsed alveoli

IMAGING

unifocal, segment subtended by obstructed bronchus

volume loss but no complete collapse by definition

consolidation +/–

water density: 'drowned lung'

lipid density: 'lipid pneumonia'

Exogenous

CLINICAL

sequel of inhalation of lipid material (usually laxatives)

chronic chemical pneumonitis with consolidation of parenchyma, lipid containing macrophages and progressive reactive fibrosis

3.46.8 ASPIRATION PNEUMONIA (adult)

DEFINITION

acute severe mixed bacterial focal pneumonia, usually with focal destruction, necrosis, hemorrhage, +/– abscess formation

ETIOPATHOGENESIS

unconsciousness, general anesthesia, alcoholism

reflux; achalasia (low volume chronic aspiration with basal fibrosis)

esophageal stricture

dysfunctional swallowing (usually pseudobulbar palsy)

dysfunctional airway protection (often recurrent laryngeal nerve palsy)

Chemical only pneumonitis

sterile stomach acid: Mendelson's syndrome

Mixed flora

aerobic: Escherichia coli, Streptococcus viridans or fecalis

anaerobic (responsible for abscess formation and smell): Bacteroides spp, coliforms

Food solid bodies

obstruction, chronic foreign body granulomas, abscess formation

MACRO AND IMAGING

typically apical or posterior basal segment RLL > LLL, posterior segment RUL

focal edematous pneumonia with abscess formation and putrefaction

3.46.9 CHRONIC BACTERIAL (SUPPURATIVE) PNEUMONIA

Actinomycosis

Actinomyces spp (gram+ rod, not a fungus)

MACRO

lower lobe predominance

dense fibrotic mass with network of abscess cavities containing 'sulfur granules'

IMAGING

consolidation or focal mass with possible architectural distortion and fibrosis

empyema common

Nocardiosis

Nocardia spp

usually opportunistic infection in immunocompromised host

MACRO

multiple focal abscesses, progresses to consolidation

IMAGING

as for actinomycosis

3.46.10 FUNGAL PNEUMONIA

see cryptococcosis, histoplasmosis, aspergillosis

3.46.11 EOSINOPHILIC PNEUMONIA

DEFINITION

symptomatic or asymptomatic inflammatory disease with eosinophil dominant lung infiltrates and often no identifiable etiology

ETIOLOGY

tropical – related to nematode larvae

allergic; drug reaction

no cause identified (usual)

CLINICAL

Acute

usually asymptomatic with diffuse peripheral airspace consolidation and eosinophilia (Loffler's syndrome)

Chronic

by definition, >4 weeks

course variable, may remit, may progress to fibrosis

IMAGING

CXR

classic appearance of 'reverse bats wing' consolidation involving peripheral airspace, usually symmetrical, often UL

or non specific consolidation

3.46.12 MELIOIDOSIS PNEUMONIA

tropical bacterial infection by Pseudomonas pseudomallei classically with aggressive multifocal cavitating bronchopneumonia, muscle abscesses, and septic emboli

3.46.13 ANTHRAX PNEUMONIA

CLINICAL

exotoxin producing Gram positive rod; inhaled spores germinate in regional lymph nodes, incubation period ~1 week

viral-like symptoms, malaise, cough, fever, myalgia

dyspnea, hypoxia, headache, meningitis

IMAGING

CXR/CT

mediastinal and hilar lymphadenopathy, possibly hyperdense (hemorrhage)

interstitial perilymphatic pattern, peribronchovascular thickening (exudate, hemorrhage, lymphatic obstruction)

large progressive pleural effusions, compressive atelectasis

3.46.14 ORGANIZING PNEUMONIA

see bronchiolitis obliterans

3.47 PULMONARY AV MALFORMATIONS

see Ch 15 vascular, hereditary hemorrhagic telangiectasia

3.48 PULMONARY EDEMA

also see Lung Machine

DEFINITION AND CLASSIFICATION

abnormal accumulation of fluid in interstitial or airspace compartments
INTERSTITIAL vs AIRSPACE
HYDROSTATIC vs PERMEABILITY
WITHOUT DIFFUSE ALVEOLAR DAMAGE vs WITH

ETIOLOGY

TRANSUDATE

CARDIOGENIC
LVF
valve disease
venoocclusive disease or pulmonary venous hypertension

NEUROGENIC
really an exudate
includes narcotic overdose

CIRRHOTIC
(oncotic)

NEPHROTIC
(oncotic)
acute renal failure, fluid overload without dialysis, etc

PANCREATIC
acute pancreatitis – probably an exudate

EXUDATE

for simplicity, the entire diffuse alveolar damage/ARDS group is placed here irrespective of mechanism
see diffuse alveolar damage – etiology

PATHOGENESIS

Hydrostatic edema
CARDIOGENIC OR
ONCOTIC (cirrhotic/nephrotic)
imbalance of hydrostatic and oncotic pressures
interstitial accumulation of transudate (septal lines)
lymphatic clearance capacity overwhelmed
airspace fills at mean pulmonary capillary pressure of 25 mmHg
central hypoxia, alveolar collapse

Permeability edema
overlaps with ARDS/diffuse alveolar damage
without endothelial damage – exudate, but behavior similar to hydrostatic edema with potentially fast reversibility (e.g. neurogenic, narcotic overdose, altitude)
WITH DIFFUSE ALVEOLAR DAMAGE: see 3.23

IMAGING

CXR
see Lung Machine

INTERSTITIAL PULMONARY EDEMA
pulmonary congestion (dilated veins, equalization of upper and lower lobe vessel caliber, engorged vascular markings reaching abnormally far peripherally)
peribronchovascular cuffing
reticulolinear pattern, lower > upper (but no interstitial nodules by definition)
Kerley lines:
A: long lines running to hila (central lymphatics)
B: interlobular septa (LL > UL, peripheral, at right angles to pleura)
C: (not seen on CXR) subpleural lymphatic plexus

AIRSPACE PULMONARY EDEMA
(DAD does not have to proceed through interstitial stage)
soft fluffy airspace nodules or ground glass opacity early
frank airspace consolidation later (usually perihilar 'bats wing')
pulmonary effusions

CT
reticulolinear pattern, LL > UL
engorged interlobular septa and subpleural lymphatics
groundglass opacity, LL > UL
frank consolidation, perihilar distribution
pleural effusions

HRCT
usually a problem when it is unrecognized at time of HRCT and mimics other pathology

INTERSTITIAL PATTERN (central and peripheral)
smooth peribronchovascular thickening
smooth septal thickening
(fluid does not cause nodules)
preserved lung architecture (i.e. no fibrosis)
dependent lung more affected

AIRSPACE PATTERN
ground glass or consolidation
same rules as for CXR

NUC MED
if hydrostatic: reversal of normal gravity perfusion gradient on V/Q
if right heart pressures elevated, delayed right heart transit or jugular reflux

3.49 PULMONARY EMBOLISM and INFARCTION

DEFINITION

PULMONARY EMBOLISM (PE): lodgment of solid material in pulmonary circulation sufficient to produce adverse effects
PULMONARY INFARCTION: hemorrhagic infarct resulting from pulmonary artery obstruction

ETIOLOGY

Thromboembolism
(deep venous thrombosis)
total embolus load relevant to risk/severity/outcome

LEG DVT
immobilization, trauma, surgery, plane travel
venous stasis or compression (e.g. tumor)
hypercoagulable state, anticoagulation cascade factor deficiencies, malignancy, estrogens (OCP), polycythemia
isolated below knee DVT of questionable risk
superficial DVT virtually never embolizes

ARM DVT
indwelling catheters, infuser ports
pacemakers
may produce lifethreatening PE

Fat or tissue embolism
trauma, surgery, pancreatitis?

Foreign body embolism

clinically relevant if diffuse or repeated
(e.g. talc in IV drug use)
diffuse granulomatous arteritis
eventual pulmonary hypertension

Septic embolism

IV drug use
systemic sepsis
cardiac source (bacterial endocarditis)

Amniotic fluid embolism

not true embolism (not a solid)
induces pulmonary vasospasm and
disseminated intravascular coagulation

In situ thrombosis

Wegener's granulomatosis
Churg–Strauss syndrome
microscopic variant of polyarteritis nodosa
(PAN)
all uncommon to rare

PATHOGENESIS

Bland emboli

pulmonary artery obstruction
MASSIVE: acute right heart failure and
death
LARGE: acute right heart failure, central
hypoxia, collapse
SEGMENTAL: segmental hemorrhagic
infarct, pleurisy; NOT hypoxia
SMALL: silent

MECHANISM OF HYPOXIA IN PE

total cardiac output is diverted into residual
patent pulmonary vascular bed, with
increased recruitment and speed of flow
RBC capillary dwell time (next to gas
exchange membranes) drops below that
required for adequate oxygen exchange
only at very high velocities
therefore, non massive PE usually does not
produce hypoxia

Septic emboli

multiple parenchymal abscesses
pale (neutrophil infiltrated, consolidated)
infarcts
often cavitate

Infarct

HEMORRHAGIC INFARCTION (often wedge
shaped)
patchy alveolar damage
collateral supply via bronchial arteries
maintained

congestion and airspace hemorrhage from
collateral circulation
TRUE PALE INFARCT only if lung already
compromised or if septic embolism
fibrinous pleurisy leads to pleuritic chest
pain

NATURAL HISTORY

Evolution of thromboembolism

clot breakup, incorporation into vessel wall,
web formation

Evolution of bland infarct

resolution with restoration of normal
architecture (if necrosis minimal and
reticulin skeleton preserved)
cavitation, healing by scarring (if necrosis
extensive)

Long term outcomes

no adverse long term effect
silent pulmonary hypertension (thrombotic
arteriopathy) – recurrent silent PE

IMAGING

CXR

cardinal sign of PE is normality
other signs:
dilated pulmonary artery leading up to an
oligemic segment (Westermark sign) or
lung (Fleischner sign)
(segmental) hemorrhage
non specific linear or subsegmental
collapses
pleurally based consolidation with smooth
rounded inner margin (Hampton's hump)
– sign of established organizing infarct
pleural effusion possible

US

used for DVT diagnosis
DVT is not a proxy for PE (clot may have all
embolized)
3/4 of all PE have no evidence of DVT

CTPA

have to see pulmonary artery before it can
be 'cleared'
need to differentiate arteries from
pulmonary veins
poor subsegmental PE pickup, good central
PE pickup
acute embolism: intraluminal filling defect
(often sausage shaped) or abrupt vessel
cutoff

chronic embolism: webs, mural masses,
bands
distal airspace may show collapses or
airspace consolidation (usually
hemorrhage)
negative CTPA is in error 2%, similar to
normal V/Q (assuming technically
satisfactory study)
combination of V/Q that is positive and CTPA
that is negative usually indicates previous
recurrent PE with residual perfusion
abnormalities at segmental/subsegmental
level

CT

INFARCT
pleurally based segmental/subsegmental
area of consolidation +/– air
bronchogram
may cavitate (uncommon in bland)
resolves by resorption from outside in

CHRONIC PE
mosaic oligemia
multiple infarcts of variable age

SEPTIC EMBOLISM
multifocal nodules in miliary distribution,
often directly related to vessels
distal triangle shaped opacities (hemorrhage
and infarction) extending to margin of
lung segment
nodules frequently cavitate

HRCT

mosaic oligemia (mosaic perfusion)
not changed or even accentuated by
expiratory scans (cf. groundglass opacity)

MRPA

not widespread; may be with/without Gd
signs analogous to CTPA

Angio

gold standard
mortality/morbidity low despite common
misconceptions
filling defect (preferably in >1 projection) or
abrupt vessel cutoff
failure of segmental/subsegmental capillary
phase perfusion
before an artery can be cleared, it has to be
identified
relatively poor interobserver agreement on
subsegmental PE
chronic PE: webs, irregularities of vessel
caliber, mural masses; absence of
capillary phase perfusion, delays in
capillary phase perfusion,
segmental/subsegmental vessel cutoff

NUC MED

first line modality ventilation/perfusion (with macroaggregated albumin) scanning

ventilation done with Xe or DTPA aerosol in USA; most commonly with Technegas (fine carbon particle suspension in air) in Europe/Australia

advantages of aerosol/Technegas: can do multiple static views

disadvantage of aerosol: severe central clumping in COAD (more than with Technegas)

SPECT can demonstrate segments not visible otherwise (especially medial and anterior basal segments of LL)

INTERPRETATION

cardinal sign is segmental absent perfusion with normal or relatively preserved segmental ventilation ('unmatched' or 'mismatched' perfusion defect)

RIM SIGN

peripheral presence of perfusion around a defect – makes acute PE very unlikely (chronic PE possible)

REVERSE MISMATCH

relatively preserved segmental/non segmental perfusion with poor or absent ventilation (and often collapse on CXR)

produces shunt (unoxygenated blood from perfused non ventilated lung)

!! commonest cause of hypoxia and tachypnea in hospitalized patients

NON SEGMENTAL DEFECTS

multitude of causes, including pleural effusions, ectatic aorta, fissural fluid, lung masses, pacemaker artifact, poorly ventilated areas in COAD with secondary vasoconstriction and reduced perfusion

INTERPRETATION CRITERIA

interpretation is unfortunately couched in probabilistic terms – hangover from PIOPED

multitude of diagnostic criteria and plethora of PIOPED criteria modifications confuse the issue: see 2.5.9 (and all these apply to planar imaging)

ACUTE vs CHRONIC PE

can not tell acute from chronic PE without previous scans

more likely chronic if rim sign present; defects subsegmental, with fuzzy margins, partial density of MAA

positive V/Q and negative CTPA are probably the result of chronic recurrent PE with segmental/subsegmental residual perfusion abnormality

---

3.50 PULMONARY FIBROSIS and INTERSTITIAL PNEUMONITIS

also see Lung Machine, and a useful reference is Am J Respir Crit Care Med (2002); 165:277-304

DEFINITION AND CLASSIFICATION

distal pulmonary interstitial inflammation with loss of type I pneumocytes (whether direct injury or immunologically driven) leading to fibrosis, loss of gas exchange surface, loss of diffusing capacity and eventual honeycomb lung

TERMINOLOGY

equivalent terms: IDIOPATHIC PULMONARY FIBROSIS (IPF), CRYPTOGENIC FIBROSING ALVEOLITIS (CFA), USUAL INTERSTITIAL PNEUMONITIS (UIP)

other term for interstitial pneumonitis: interstitial pneumonia

CLASSIFICATION – PULMONARY FIBROSIS

PRIMARY: IDIOPATHIC PULMONARY FIBROSIS (IPF) OR UIP

always diffuse

either 'lone' or associated with immune complex disease

SECONDARY

diffuse or focal depending on cause

multiple systemic or local causes exist: see etiology

CLASSIFICATION – IDIOPATHIC INTERSTITIAL PNEUMONITIS OTHER THAN IPF/UIP

always diffuse

NON SPECIFIC INTERSTITIAL PNEUMONITIS (NSIP)

DESQUAMATIVE INTERSTITIAL PNEUMONITIS (DIP)

same as respiratory bronchiolitis associated interstitial lung disease (RB-ILD)

ACUTE INTERSTITIAL PNEUMONITIS (AIP)

same as Hamman-Rich syndrome

MIMICKERS

LYMPHOCYTIC INTERSTITIAL PNEUMONITIS (LIP)

lymphocytic infiltrate, not a pneumonitis – see its own entry 3.38

GIANT CELL INTERSTITIAL PNEUMONITIS (GIP)

manifestation of hard metal pneumoconiosis

ETIOLOGY

pulmonary fibrosis is a common condition overall, with secondary more common than primary

idiopathic interstitial pneumonitis is relatively uncommon, with UIP most common and NSIP second most common

secondary pulmonary fibrosis has many well documented causes, each numerically minor

MNEMONIC: PISA DIT A FAAART

DIFFUSE FIBROSIS [PISA DIT A]

CAUSATIVE AGENT INHALED

P-neumoconioses

silicosis, anthracosis, asbestosis: non immune

berylliosis, zirconium disease: immune granulomatous (Be, Zr act as haptens)

I-nfection (eg adenovirus)

direct injury

S-arcoidosis

postulated infectious agent with immune mediated damage

A-llergens (EAA – hypersensitivity pneumonitis)

immune mediated

CAUSATIVE AGENT CIRCULATED

D-rugs

chemotherapy, toxins: direct injury

amiodarone, idiopathic reactions: immune mediated

I-mmune complex / I-diopathic

systemic sclerosis, mixed connective tissue disease, polymyositis/dermatomyositis, rheumatoid lung, ankylosing spondylitis and other immune complex disease and (presumably) IDIOPATHIC PULMONARY FIBROSIS are all immune mediated

T-oxins (eg Paraquat)

direct injury

FAILURE OF A-RDS/DAD TO RESOLVE

see 3.23 diffuse alveolar damage

FOCAL OR MULTIFOCAL FIBROSIS [FAAART]

F-ungal bronchopneumonia

A-BPA

A-spiration

A-bnormal Airway
e.g. cystic fibrosis and bronchiectasis

R-adiotherapy

T-B bronchopneumonia/fibrosis

PATHOGENESIS

Fundamental requirements for pulmonary fibrosis

Loss of type I pneumocyte epithelium (direct injury or immune driven)

Loss of reticulin framework (by collapse or destruction)

Lymphocyte/ macrophage infiltrate (reactive or autoimmune)

Fibroblasts/fibroblast activating factor/collagen deposition

Chronicity: persistence of stimulus or failure to clear

Endstage changes

Terminal bronchiole dilation – honeycombing

Loss of exchange surface

Thickened diffusion distance

Loss of diffusion capacity

Fibrotic pulmonary vasculopathy

Restrictive lung disease

CLINICAL AND MICRO

SECONDARY PULMONARY FIBROSIS

see entries for the underlying conditions (3.5, 3.7, 3.8, 3.9, 3.11, 3.17, 3.20, 3.21, 3.23, 3.24, 3.25, 3.45, 3.53, 3.56, 3.60)

IDIOPATHIC INTERSTITIAL PNEUMONITIS

variable mixtures of inflammatory infiltrate and fibrosis

within each entity, better prognosis if inflammatory infiltrate is dominant and worse prognosis if fibrosis is dominant

3.50.1 USUAL INTERSTITIAL PNEUMONITIS (UIP)

60 year olds, male > female

insidious onset of dyspnea, malaise, lung crackles, clubbing

slowly progressive, poor response to steroids, high mortality (median survival 3 years)

interstitial foci of actively proliferating fibroblasts

collagen deposits with thickened alveolar septa

honeycombing (enlarged air spaces separated by thick fibrotic walls)

inflammatory component mild – few interstitial lymphocytes

pathognomonic criterion is SPATIAL and TEMPORAL HETEROGENEITY: coexistence of normal lung, fibroblast foci and collagen scarring at the same time

3.50.2 NON-SPECIFIC INTERSTITIAL PNEUMONITIS (NSIP)

50 year olds, female : male 1:1

subacute onset of dyspnea and cough, lung crackles; may have fever and weight loss

good response to steroids, low mortality (10%)

temporally uniform chronic lymphocytic and plasmacyte interstitial infiltrate

mild interstitial fibrosis, fibroblast foci not dominant

3.50.3 DESQUAMATIVE INTERSTITIAL PNEUMONITIS AND RESPIRATORY BRONCHIOLITIS ASSOCIATED INTERSTITIAL LUNG DISEASE (DIP AND RB-ILD)

rare disease of heavy smokers, male>female

insidious dyspnea and cough

good response to steroids, good survival

misnomer: no desquamation; cells in airspace are macrophages

DIP: macrophage accumulation in alveoli

RB-ILD: macrophage accumulation around respiratory bronchioles

septal infiltrate and collagen deposition relatively minor

3.50.4 ACUTE INTERSTITIAL PNEUMONITIS (AIP)

rare rapidly progressive pulmonary fibrosis (months)

acute onset, fulminating dyspnea, death

poor response to steroids

active diffuse interstitial fibrosis similar to UIP, but temporally uniform

rapid development of honeycombing, similar to organizing stage of diffuse alveolar damage

IMAGING

SECONDARY PULMONARY FIBROSIS

see entries for the underlying conditions (3.5, 3.7, 3.8, 3.9, 3.11, 3.17, 3.20, 3.21, 3.23, 3.24, 3.25, 3.45, 3.53, 3.56, 3.60)

CXR (BOTH IDIOPATHIC AND SECONDARY FIBROSIS)

no findings (till quite late) – about 30% of patients with biopsy proven pulmonary fibrosis have a normal CXR

RARELY, ill defined groundglass opacity (represents airspace acute component)

CARDINAL SIGN: FOCAL, MULTIFOCAL OR DIFFUSE INTERSTITIAL PATTERN

focal/multifocal: look for local abnormality

reduced lung volume (unless coexistent emphysema in pneumoconioses or hyperinflation in ABPA and cystic fibrosis)

earlier: fine reticulolinear pattern, often peripheral/subpleural

idiopathic/immune complex disease and drug reactions in particular produce a regular symmetrical diffuse pattern

airspace component suggests acute episode ('interstitial gone airspace')

later: ring shadows, coarser fibrosis (honeycombing)

usually no pleural effusions

CLASSIFICATION BY LOCATION: see CXR gamuts

USUAL INTERSTITIAL PNEUMONITIS:

interstitial reticulolinear pattern, usually basal

decreased lung volume

MIMICKERS ON CXR

LYMPHANGITIS

lower>upper on CXR

reticulonodular and nodular pattern

subpleural and perilymphatic

pleural effusions possible

HISTIOCYTOSIS

irregular air cysts

increased lung volume

see histiocytosis

LYMPHANGIOLEIOMYOMATOSIS / TUBEROUS SCLEROSIS / NEUROFIBROMATOSIS

perfectly rounded air cysts

interspersed normal parenchyma

AMYLOIDOSIS

LYMPHOCYTIC INTERSTITIAL PNEUMONITIS

HRCT (IDIOPATHIC PULMONARY FIBROSIS, INTERSTITIAL PNEUMONITIS)

UIP

INTERSTITIAL PATTERN (peripheral)

peripheral bilateral smooth reticulolinear pattern with honeycombing

LL > UL, starts subpleurally

intralobular thickening (may mimic groundglass)

smooth peripheral septal thickening, dilated air spaces

honeycombing with overall volume loss

visible intralobular bronchioles

traction bronchiectasis

AIRSPACE PATTERN ('interstitial gone airspace')

superimposed groundglass (when active)

POINTERS TO SPECIFIC CAUSES in UIP

dilated esophagus – ?scleroderma / MCTD

UL > LL, with cystic change ?ankylosing spondylitis

pleural effusions, destroyed shoulders ?rheumatoid

SHORT DIFFERENTIAL DIAGNOSIS

asbestosis, chronic extrinsic allergic alveolitis, sarcoidosis – can usually all be differentiated

NSIP

AIRSPACE PATTERN ('interstitial gone airspace')

patchy peripheral bilateral groundglass opacity, LL>UL

dominant HRCT finding; soliltary finding in 1/3

INTERSTITIAL PATTERN (peripheral)

mild peripheral septal thickening

honeycombing absent or minimal

DIP/RB-ILD

AIRSPACE PATTERN ('interstitial gone airspace')

patchy bilateral groundglass opacities

LL>UL, tend to be peripheral

centrilobular nodules or centrilobular groundglass opacities

AIP

similar progression to diffuse alveolar damage (see 3.23)

3.51 PULMONARY HYPERTENSION and ARTERIOPATHY

DEFINITION

pulmonary hypertension (HT) is persistently elevated pulmonary arterial pressure above 30/15 mmHg; pulmonary venous HT is >12 mmHg

pulmonary arteriopathy is the vascular changes associated with pulmonary HT

ETIOLOGY/PATHOLOGY

Hypoxic

commonest cause of pulmonary HT

COAD, emphysema, asthma, obstructive sleep apnea

chronic hypoxic arteriolar vasoconstriction, distal arteriolar muscularization

Thromboembolic

silent or clinically overt recurrent thromboembolism

embolus incorporation into arterial walls and recanalization produces septa, webs, bands

Volume overload: left to right heart shunts

CLASSIC PLEXOGENIC ARTERIOPATHY

proximal to distal muscularization of arterioles, onion skin intimal hypertrophy

DILATION LESIONS (wide thin walled ballooned vessels)

PLEXIFORM LESIONS (plexi of wide capillary like channels inside dilated arteries, ?recanalization)

rarely, pulmonary schistosomiasis or portal hypertension and cirrhosis produce identical histology

Congestive/pulmonary venooclusive

MITRAL VALVE DISEASE, CHRONIC LVF

PRIMARY PULMONARY VENOOCCLUSIVE DISEASE

VENOUS arterialization, arterial fibrosis

Fibrotic

occurs in response to pulmonary fibrosis of any cause (not just idiopathic pulmonary fibrosis)

fibrosis has to be extensive before clinically significant pulmonary HT follows

Unexplained pulmonary HT

USUALLY: silent thromboembolism, pulmonary venooclusive disease, or undiagnosed cardiac left to right shunt

primary pulmonary HT/primary plexogenic arteriopathy is a diagnosis of exclusion

IMAGING

also see pulmonary embolism (PE)

CXR/CT

early: normal

dilation of central pulmonary arteries (up to segmental/subsegmental divisions), tortuosity

calcification of pulmonary arteries is pathognomonic

reduction in diameter and prominence of small pulmonary arteries ('peripheral pruning') with oligemia of peripheral 1/2–1/3 of lung parenchyma

may see evidence of acute or chronic PE on CT

may see evidence of mitral valve disease (see cardiac)

may see evidence of cardiac shunts (see cardiac)

in volume overload, progression from plethora to peripheral pruning (Eisenmenger's reaction) implies underlying pulmonary hypertension with constrictive/obliterative arterial disease

NUC MED

V/Q

classically, appearance of chronic PE

segmental and subsegmental unmatched perfusion defects with fuzzy and shrinking edges and corners and rim sign

serial progression from sharp well marginated segmental perfusion defects (acute PE) to chronic PE appearance

!without previous V/Q for comparison, it is impossible to age the appearance despite suggestive findings

combination of V/Q that has segmental and subsegmental perfusion defects and negative CTPA is suggestive of recurrent chronic pulmonary embolism

3.52 PULMONARY VASCULITIDES and NON VASCULITIDES

3.52.1 WEGENER'S GRANULOMATOSIS

see Ch 15 vascular, Wegener's granulomatosis

3.52.2 ALLERGIC ANGIITIS and GRANULOMATOSIS

(Churg–Strauss syndrome)

rare syndrome of pulmonary eosinophilic vasculitis, interstitial granulomatosis, peripheral blood eosinophilia and asthma

3.52.3 MICROSCOPIC VARIANT OF POLYARTERITIS NODOSA

has lung involvement
see Ch 15 vascular, microscopic variant of PAN

3.52.4 RHEUMATOID VASCULITIS

very rare
see rheumatoid lung disease

3.52.5 GRANULOMATOUS NON VASCULITIDES

3.52.5.1 Bronchocentric granulomatosis

see ABPA

3.52.5.2 LYMPHOMATOID GRANULOMATOSIS

not a vasculitis, and not a granulomatosis!
T cell lymphoproliferative disorder
necrotizing angiocentric infiltrate with multiple bilateral lung masses (mid, lower) + skin involvement
CNS involvement as leptomeningitis/cranial nerve infiltration

3.52.6 GOODPASTURE'S SYNDROME

CLINICAL

not a vasculitis
type II hypersensitivity (antiglomerular basement membrane antibodies) causing acute glomerulonephritis and diffuse alveolar damage with pulmonary hemorrhages
produces diffuse or multifocal pulmonary airspace opacities (see imaging of diffuse alveolar damage and Lung Machine)

3.53 RADIATION PNEUMONITIS

also see diffuse alveolar damage and lung machine

DEFINITION

lung parenchymal changes (acute: radiation pneumonitis; chronic: radiation fibrosis) from radiotherapy

CLINICAL

manifests where relatively large lung volumes are covered
not a linear dose response curve; there is usually no change for 20 Gy, with most patients developing change after 45 Gy

PATHOLOGY

Acute radiation pneumonitis

(days–weeks)

mechanism and progression is that of diffuse alveolar damage, but extent is limited by radiation portals

Chronic radiation fibrosis

(starting 1–6 months)

progressive interstitial fibrosis with incorporation of hyaline membranes
thickening of interstitial space, loss of alveolar architecture
gas exchange mismatch and increased diffusion distance
traction bronchiectasis

IMAGING

cardinal sign: all changes are confined to radiation portals and have straight margins

CXR/CT/HRCT

ACUTE RADIATION PNEUMONITIS

groundglass opacity (variable severity)
usually not visible on CXR

CHRONIC FIBROSIS

progressive linear scarring and strands extending from irradiated hilum or mediastinum into lung parenchyma
progressive volume loss with hilar rotation and possibly diaphragm elevation
traction bronchiectasis
changes of coarse reticulolinear pattern within radiation portal

NUC MED

V/Q

straight edged non segmental area of reduced perfusion and ventilation
both perfusion and ventilation affected to a variable extent, but often perfusion more abnormal
NOT pulmonary embolism (for reasons of morphology)

PET (FDG)

classic appearance is of uniform area of moderately FDG avid uptake corresponding to radiotherapy portal (with straight edges)
diffuse moderate intensity pleurally based uptake in irradiated field which can persist for months
if radiotherapy successful, hot central primary uptake disappears and does not recur (i.e. no focally elevated FDG uptake)

3.54 RELAPSING POLYCHONDRITIS

uncommon and probably autoimmune recurrent inflammation of structural cartilage (airway cartilage, ear cartilage, nasal cartilage), particularly trachea
multifocal/diffuse narrowing and abnormal MR signal in trachea and major bronchi
differential includes intubation induced, postoperative or post traumatic stenosis, Wegener's granulomatosis

3.55 RHEUMATOID LUNG DISEASE

also see rheumatoid arthritis in Ch 03

DEFINITION

lung or pleural involvement in rheumatoid arthritis, multiple pathological forms

EPIDEMIOLOGY

male > female
high rheumatoid factor titers
usually follows rather than precedes joint disease

MANIFESTATIONS

Pleural effusions/pleurisy (in 50%)

unilateral > bilateral, large, fluctuating

Interstitial pneumonitis/ fibrosis (in 1%)

same clinical presentation and histology as idiopathic fibrosis
follows joint disease by ~5 years, poor prognosis

Necrobiotic nodules (uncommon)

subpleural, multiple, discrete, size varies, may cavitate
central fibrinoid necrosis, peripheral palisading fibroblasts/histiocytes

RHEUMATOID PNEUMOCONIOSIS

see 3.45.2 anthracosis

3.56 SARCOIDOSIS

also see entry in Ch 11 CNS conditions and Ch 12 head and neck

DEFINITION

multisystem disease of uncertain etiology (but perhaps infective?) with multiple immune non caseating granulomas

EPIDEMIOLOGY

younger patients (more often <40 at first onset)
female slightly > male
black > white

THORACIC SARCOIDOSIS

CLINICAL

speed of onset variable; may be asymptomatic
acute (dyspnea, erythema nodosum, arthritis, uveitis) – better prognosis
insidious (dyspnea, pulmonary fibrosis) – worse prognosis
ACE raised, hypercalcemia
often proceeds to spontaneous resolution (few years)
may progress to pulmonary fibrosis

GRADING

I   hilar lymph nodes only
II hilar lymph nodes + reticular lung pattern
III reticular lung pattern only
IV pulmonary fibrosis (UL > LL)
0   extrathoracic
better prognosis in grades I and II

MACRO

small (2–3 mm) fleshy yellow–white nodules in lung parenchyma, may coalesce
hilar lymphadenopathy

MICRO

non caseating IMMUNE granulomas with reticulin and collagen – conglomerate
Schaumann bodies (CaFe mucoprotein)
asteroid bodies (lipoprotein)
interstitial pneumonitis

IMAGING (pulmonary manifestations)

CXR

BILATERAL (80%) OR UNILATERAL (5%) THORACIC NODES

LUNG CHANGES IN 50% (UL > LL, USUALLY BILATERAL)

ill defined nodules (90%)
patchy airspace (10%)
endobronchial nodules (5%)
large nodules (1%)
eventually 1/3 proceed to fibrosis (UL > LL)

CT/HRCT

INTERSTITIAL PATTERN (peribronchovascular and peripheral)

peribronchovascular > peripheral
UL > LL
nodular peribronchovascular thickening
interstitial peripheral nodules
fibrosis (eventually, and not inevitably)

NODULAR PATTERN

UL > LL
small nodules in perilymphatic distribution (merges into above)
larger nodules/masses

CONGLOMERATION

association of smaller masses into larger masses of the same character (DIFFERENTIAL: PMF, TB, sarcoidosis)

AIRSPACE PATTERN

groundglass

MEDIASTINUM AND HILA

bilateral hilar, paratracheal and mediastinal lymphadenopathy
non confluent, non cavitating, may calcify

NUC MED

GALLIUM

typically intense symmetrical uniform uptake in:
salivary glands and lacrimal glands ('Panda sign')
hilar, paratracheal ('lambda sign') +/– subcarinal nodes
Hodgkin's disease is a differential on Ga

PET (FDG)

may be FDG avid
pattern of low grade bilateral mediastinal and hilar nodal uptake suggestive of sarcoidosis
parenchymal masses may be mistaken for carcinoma when hot

EXTRATHORACIC SARCOID (20% to 30%)

Skin + parotids

see Ch 12
(uveoparotid fever – Heerfordt's syndrome)

Lymph nodes, spleen, liver

Eye + CNS
see Ch 11

BONES + JOINTS
lacework of granulomas
see Ch 02

3.57 SCLERODERMA (lung manifestations)

interstitial pulmonary fibrosis analogous to idiopathic pulmonary fibrosis
dilated esophagus with disordered motility; reflux, aspiration, basal lung fibrosis

3.58 SPONTANEOUS PNEUMOTHORAX

3.58.1 PRIMARY

DEFINITION

spontaneous pneumothorax occurring in healthy young adults (usually male > female) related to rupture of apical blebs

CLINICAL

20–40 year olds, male > female
tall, thin (exaggerated pressure gradient in lung)
1/3 recur within 3 years

IMAGING

pneumothorax of any size
by definition, no underlying hilar mass
may show an apical 'bleb'
CT may show paraseptal emphysema

Non tensioning vs tensioning

tensioning: mediastinal deviation to other side or evidence of air trapping (i.e. movement away from pneumothorax on expiration) – usually progressive unless relieved and may be catastrophic

3.58.2 SECONDARY

cavitating infection, bronchopleural fistula

PCP, rupture of blebs
asthma, emphysema, COAD
lymphangioleiomyomatosis, histiocytosis
pulmonary fibrosis
Marfan's syndrome
cavitating tumor, bronchopleural fistula
sarcoma metastases (classically osteosarcoma)

3.59 SYSTEMIC LUPUS ERYTHEMATOSUS (lung manifestations)

see Ch 15
half of patients have pulmonary or pleural involvement at some time during disease
commonest are pleurisy and pleural effusions, usually bilateral
pericardial effusion may occur
pulmonary fibrosis (see pulmonary fibrosis entry) uncommon
in children pulmonary hemorrhage is common and has high mortality

3.60 TUBERCULOSIS

DEFINITION AND CLASSIFICATION

commonest manifestation of tuberculous infection characterized by caseating granulomas and a wide spectrum of immune response

EPIDEMIOLOGY AND RISK FACTORS

major disease of the third world: crowding/poor sanitation/malnutrition
alcoholism
increasing incidence with increasing AIDS prevalence

ETIOLOGY

Mycobacterium tuberculosis (fastidious aerobe)
acid fast rods (or auramine–rhodamine stain) that grow on Lowenstein–Jensen medium
no exotoxins/endotoxins, induces little acute inflammation
slow (18 hours) doubling time

BUT
waxy envelope resists lysosomal killing and induces both cell mediated immunity and delayed type (IV) hypersensitivity; organism survives inside cells and induces granulomas

PATHOGENESIS – PRIMARY TB

1. Inoculation (naive host)
usually apical segment of LL or lower part UL (Ghon focus)

2. Non specific response
non specific acute inflammation
non specific chronic inflammation
non immune granulomas (no cell kill)
macrophages with viable ingested organisms travel to regional lymph nodes
humoral immune response unhelpful

3a. If cell mediated immunity (CMI) adequate
CMI activated specific immune granulomatous response against TB
Ghon complex: immune granulomatous response at Ghon focus and draining lymph nodes, minor caseation, healing by fibrosis

OUTCOMES
full eradication (rare)
containment (common)
incomplete response, progression to secondary type TB ab initio (uncommon) – see secondary TB 2a

3b. If cell mediated immunity (CMI) inadequate
tuberculous bronchopneumonia or disseminated miliary TB
overwhelming infection with minimal containment
common because of AIDS

4. Development of delayed type hypersensitivity (DTH)
probably dissociated from CMI
histology of DTH is also immune granulomatous disease
BCG (bacille Calmette–Guérrin) vaccination confers both CMI and DTH

DTH RESPONSIBLE FOR
cutaneous response (Mantoux reaction)
erythema nodosum
?pleural effusions
?bystander cell destruction

PATHOGENESIS – SECONDARY TB

1. Immune host with deteriorating CMI or reinfection

usually subapical lung (high pO2)

2a. If CMI adequate for containment, immune type response

typical secondary cavitating fibrocaseous TB
fibrosis, caseation, immune type granulomas
DTH usually concurrently present

2b. If CMI inadequate, non immune type response

common in AIDS, other immune suppression
loss of capacity to produce immune granulomas
loss of DTH also occcurs, but may be dissociated
TB bronchopneumonia, miliary TB, overwhelming infection

MACRO/MICRO

Fibrocaseous TB (CMI adequate for containment)

caseation: cheesy white necrosis
thick ragged fibrotic wall of cavity
often communicates with bronchus
+/– pleural effusion
+/– regional lymphadenopathy (may caseate)

CASEATING IMMUNE GRANULOMA

epithelioid macrophages, Langhans giant cells (fused macrophages), lymphocytes, plasma cells
extensive destruction, central necrotic debris; microorganisms hard to find
peripheral dense fibrosis (fibroblast factor driven)

TB bronchopneumonia (partially inadequate CMI)

seeding via endbronchial spread or hematogenous
multifocal/diffuse caseous consolidation
lymphadenopathy
variable degrees of granuloma formation, fibrosis, caseation, containment (usually poor)

Disseminated miliary TB (inadequate CMI)

hematogenous spread by definition, extensive microorganisms
+/– lymphadenopathy

NON IMMUNE GRANULOMA

non activated macrophages filled with live organisms
extensive monocytic exudate

NATURAL HISTORY

depends on CMI response

Complications

LOCAL

massive hemoptysis
TB empyema (calcifies)
bronchopleural fistula
mediastinal fistulas
aspergilloma

METASTATIC TB FOCI

kidneys and adrenals
brain
testes
ovaries and Fallopian tubes
bones

IMAGING

XR/fluoro/CT

GHON FOCUS (HEALED)

round soft tissue density or calcified
location as in MACRO
no enhancement on dynamic CT

PRIMARY TB (non specific response)

peripheral nodule or consolidation
unilateral hilar lymphadenopathy
may have mediastinal lymphadenopathy
lymphadenopathy classically ring enhances
primary lung focus may be invisible
location as in MACRO
sympathetic effusion

FIBROCASEOUS TB

pulmonary nodule/mass or
irregular cavity with ragged wall
air–fluid level possible
usually apical
reactive pleural thickening, fibrotic architectural distortion
satellite nodules possible
bronchial communication likely
bronchopleural fistula/TB empyema occurs
TB empyema calcifies if longstanding
differentiation from cavitating cancer may be hard
usually no lymphadenopathy (if containment OK)

FUNGUS BALL (mycetoma)

see aspergillosis

SILICOTUBERCULOSIS

accelerated TB in silicotic lungs
features of silicosis, superimposed cavitation, conglomeration, collapse, fibrosis
differentiation from progressive massive fibrosis alone difficult

TB BRONCHOPNEUMONIA

no characteristic CXR features
see HRCT

MILIARY TB

miliary small nodules (e.g. <3 mm) on CXR
not a pattern specific to TB, but TB till proven otherwise!

TB IN AIDS

extensive mediastinal and hilar lymphadenopathy
often enhances (ring enhancement)
low density lymphadenopathy
effusions
bronchiectasis suggests MAC

HRCT

TB BRONCHOPNEUMONIA

NODULAR PATTERN (centrilobular)
classical tree-in-bud centrilobular nodules arising from small bronchi filled with content (endobronchial spread)

AIRSPACE PATTERN
patchy peribronchial consolidation
cavitation with thick walled cavities

progression to consolidation

MILIARY TB

miliary interstitial nodule pattern

Angio

may be relevant if hemoptysis requires bronchial artery embolization

PET (FDG)

variable intensity lung focus
may be avid enough to simulate lung cancer
may have hilar/subcarinal node pattern suggestive of granulomatous disease

3.61 UIP (usual interstitial pneumonitis)

see pulmonary fibrosis/interstitial pneumonitis overview

3.62 WEGENER'S GRANULOMATOSIS

see Ch 15 vascular

1. NORMAL

2. CARDIOMEDIASTINAL AND VASCULAR GAMUTS

CARDIAC AND MEDIASTINAL CONDITIONS

3. ACQUIRED AND ADULT

1. NORMAL

1.1 ABBREVIATIONS

AA: arteries
AoV: aortic valve
ASD: atrial septal defect
AVSD: atrioventricular septal defect,
    endocardial cushion defect
DORV: double outlet right ventricle
D-TGV: dextro-TGV ('uncorrected'
    transposition of great vessels)
EDV: end diastolic volume
ESV: end systolic volume
LA: left atrium
L-TGV: levo-TGV ('corrected' transposition of
    great vessels)
LV: left ventricle
LVF: left ventricular failure
LVOT: left ventricle outflow tract
MV: mitral valve
PA: pulmonary artery
PDA: patent ductus arteriosus
PFC: persistent fetal circulation
PFO: patent foramen ovale
PV: pulmonary (pulmonic) valve
RA: right atrium
RV: right ventricle
RVOT: right ventricle outflow tract
TGV: transposition of great vessels
TV: tricuspid valve
VSD: ventricular septal defect
VV: veins

1.2 AORTIC DIAMETERS

(approximate)
ASCENDING 3.5 cm
ARCH 3 cm
DESCENDING 2.5 cm

1.3 CARDIAC CHAMBERS AND VALVES

all values approximate adult values only!

Right atrium
broadbased trabeculated triangular auricle
pressure 5 mmHg
end diastolic volume 50–60 ml

Tricuspid valve

Right ventricle
infundibulum (crista supraventricularis)
    separating inflow and outflow; triangular

pressure 25/0 mmHg
end diastolic volume 150–160 ml
stroke volume 70 ml
ejection fraction >45%

Pulmonary valve

Pulmonary artery
pressure 25/10 mmHg

Left atrium
narrow based finger like auricle
pressure 2–8 mmHg
end diastolic volume 50 ml

Mitral valve
4–6 cm2

Left ventricle
inflow and outflow adjacent
elongated cavity, two papillary muscles
pressure 120–140/0 mm Hg
end diastolic volume 120–150 ml
stroke volume 70 ml
ejection fraction >55%

Aortic valve
3 cm2

Aorta
pressure 120–140/80 mmHg

1.4 CARDIAC SIZE ON CXR

Adult
PA projection, 2m film-focus distance, grid
90th centile is 15.5 cm male, 12.5 cm female
cardiothoracic ratio <50%
systolic–diastolic difference 1.5 cm

Child
cardiothoracic ratio <50%

Neonate
cardiothoracic ratio <60%

1.5 LYMPH NODE STATIONS

see in Ch13, bronchogenic carcinoma
    staging

1.6 PERICARDIUM

<3 mm thick; follows fibrous tissue on MR

(low on both T1W and T2W sequences);
    separates epicardial and pericardial fat

1.7 RESTING EJECTION FRACTION

Left ventricular ejection fraction (LVEF)
normal is >55% and (usually) <70%
a drop of 10% or a drop below normal is
    significant
earliest sign of chemotherapy cardiotoxicity
    is an apical lag and/or unexplained LV
    dilation

Right ventricular ejection fraction (RVEF)
normal is >45%

1.8 THYMUS

CT/MR
bilobed structure
lobes ovoid or triangular
maximal lobe thickness 13 mm
>40 years of age maximum lobe thickness
    7 mm
progressive fatty involution after puberty
    with decreasing density and usually full
    involution >40 years of age

2. CARDIO-MEDIASTINAL AND VASCULAR GAMUTS

2.1 GENERIC (all modalities)

2.1.1 AMBIGUOUS SITUS

see situs machine in Ch 21 pediatric thorax

2.1.2 MEDIASTINAL CYSTS

HYDATID

DUPLICATION
BRONCHIAL
ESOPHAGEAL
NEURENTERIC
PERICARDIAL
THYMIC

INCLUSION DERMOID/EPIDERMOID

MATURE TERATOMA

2.1.3 MEDIASTINAL LYMPHADENOPATHY

MNEMONIC: TALISMAN

T-B AND SIMILAR INFECTIONS

TB

FUNGAL

VIRAL (esp Epstein–Barr virus)

MYCOPLASMA or CHLAMYDIA

ANTHRAX

A-IDS LYMPHADENOPATHY

MYCOBACTERIUM AVIUM COMPLEX (MAC)

TB

FUNGAL

KAPOSI'S SARCOMA

L-YMPHOMA (and uncommonly LEUKEMIA)

I-NHALATIONAL DISEASE (pneumoconioses)

S-ARCOIDOSIS

M-ETASTASES

A-MYLOID (rare)

Castlema-N DISEASE
see its own entry

Low density lymphadenopathy

TB
classically show ring contrast enhancement

MYCOBACTERIUM AVIUM COMPLEX

FUNGAL

LYMPHOMA

TESTICULAR METASTASES

Calcifying lymphadenopathy

TB, FUNGAL

TREATED HODGKIN'S LYMPHOMA (possibly eggshell)

PNEUMOCONIOSES (possibly eggshell)

SARCOIDOSIS (possibly eggshell)

Vividly contrast enhancing lymphadenopathy

VASCULAR METASTASES

CASTLEMAN DISEASE

Eggshell nodes
circumferential calcification in normal size or enlarged nodes

SILICOSIS

SARCOIDOSIS

FUNGUS

AMYLOID

TREATED LYMPHOMA

2.1.4 PERICARDIAL MASS

Congenital

LIPOMA

PERICARDIAL DIVERTICULUM

LYMPHANGIOMA

PERICARDIAL CYST

INTRAPERICARDIAL BRONCHOGENIC CYST

Non tumor

CALCIFIED PLAQUE (TB, asbestos, postoperative)

HYDATID

Tumor

METASTASIS, LYMPHOMA

MESOTHELIOMA

BENIGN CYSTIC TERATOMA

Cardiac mass simulating pericardial mass

LV ANEURYSM

OTHER

2.1.5 PULMONARY VENOUS HYPERTENSION

see Ch 21

2.2 X-RAY/CT

2.2.1 AIR–FLUID LEVEL IN MEDIASTINUM

Truly mediastinal

HIATUS HERNIA

ACHALASIA

GASTRIC PULL-UP OR COLONIC INTERPOSITION

ESOPHAGEAL DIVERTICULUM

COMMUNICATING DUPLICATION CYST

Pulmonary

ABSCESS

INFECTED BULLA

EMPYEMA

HYDROPNEUMOTHORAX

INTRALOBAR SEQUESTRATION

2.2.2 AORTIC ARCH DILATED

Atherosclerosis, 'unfolding'

Ascending aorta/arch aneurysm

ATHEROSCLEROTIC

OLD AORTIC DISSECTION

MARFAN'S SYNDROME

INFECTIVE (SYPHILIS) OR AUTOIMMUNE AORTITIS

Aortic valve incompetence

Post stenotic dilation, aortic stenosis

2.2.3 AORTIC ARCH TOO SMALL

LEFT TO RIGHT SHUNT

AORTIC COARCTATION (long segment)

Ebstein's anomaly
variable, and other signs of Ebstein's anomaly have to be present

2.2.4 AORTIC VALVE CALCIFICATION

AGE RELATED DEGENERATIVE

BICUSPID AORTIC VALVE

RHEUMATIC HEART DISEASE

RENAL FAILURE, HYPERCALCEMIA

2.2.5 CARDIAC CALCIFICATION

Pericardium

INFECTIVE (esp TB)

ASBESTOS

AUTOIMMUNE

(beware constrictive pericarditis)

Coronary artery calcification

see coronary CT in 3.10

Atrial

CLOT

MYXOMA (RARE)

Atrioventricular valves

DEGENERATIVE

STENOSIS

RHEUMATIC FEVER

Ventricles

INFARCT

THROMBUS

ANEURYSM

ENDOMYOCARDIAL FIBROSIS

Ventriculoarterial valves

DEGENERATIVE

STENOSIS

Great arteries

HYPERTENSION

ATHEROMA

THROMBUS

2.2.6 CARDIAC CHAMBER ENLARGEMENT (acquired)

Classification by etiology

VOLUME OVERLOAD

ventricle dilates earlier than in pressure overload

SHUNT

CONGESTIVE CARDIAC FAILURE ('backwards' failure)

INFLOW VALVE INCOMPETENCE

OUTFLOW VALVE INCOMPETENCE

PRESSURE OVERLOAD

compared to volume overload, ventricle hypertrophies first and dilates later

---

HYPERTENSIVE HEART DISEASE

SYSTEMIC HYPERTENSION

PULMONARY ARTERIAL HYPERTENSION

SUBVALVULAR STENOSIS

e.g. subaortic membrane

OUTFLOW VALVE STENOSIS

OUTFLOW GREAT ARTERY STENOSIS

DYNAMIC OUTFLOW OBSTRUCTION

HYPERTROPHIC OBSTRUCTIVE CARDIOMYOPATHY

MYOCARDIAL FAILURE

MYOCARDIAL ISCHEMIA

CARDIOMYOPATHY

OTHER

CXR signs

GLOBAL

cardiothoracic ratio > 50%

BEWARE: depressed sternum or straight back; expiratory view

interval enlargement >1.5 cm

lesser change can be produced by variation in cardiac cycle

LEFT ATRIUM

left main bronchus elevation, displacement, carinal splaying

left atrial diameter (right margin of the left atrium to left main bronchus) >7 cm

double right heart border

LATERAL VIEW: esophageal and left main bronchus displaced posteriorly

prominent left auricle

BEWARE: resected left auricle from prior closed mitral valve surgery

LEFT VENTRICLE

elongated left heart border and heart axis

rounded and downpointing apex

left ventricle beyond esophagus and IVC in lateral view >2 cm

BEWARE: parallax errors from imperfectly lateral film

RIGHT ATRIUM

overprominent curved or square right heart border

right heart border too far to the right

enlarged right auricle over right ventricle outflow tract

RIGHT VENTRICLE

rounded and uppointing apex

upwards extension of cardiac soft tissue to beyond 1/3 or 1/2 of lower sternum

---

DIFFERENTIAL: depressed sternum, straight back syndrome

look for pulmonary artery dilation

Echo signs

Increased ESV and EDV of each chamber (see normal echo)

2.2.7 MEDIASTINAL WIDENING (in trauma)

Hematoma - lifethreatening

HEMATOMA ASSOCIATED WITH AORTIC INJURY

see aortic injury entry in Ch 15 vascular conditions

Hematoma–other

STERNAL FRACTURES

VERTEBRAL AND RIB FRACTURES

Spurious

POSITIONAL

LIPOMATOSIS

TUMOR

2.2.8 MITRAL VALVE CALCIFICATION

Age related degenerative

especially mitral valve ring

Rheumatic heart disease

2.2.9 VASCULAR CALCIFICATION

Arterial dystrophic

ATHEROMA

THROMBUS

MONCKEBERG'S SCLEROSIS

Arterial metastatic

RENAL OSTEODYSTROPHY

DIABETES MELLITUS

HYPERPARATHYROIDISM

Venous

PHLEBOLITHS

HEMANGIOMAS

AV MALFORMATION

2.2.10 WATERBOTTLE HEART

Pericardial effusion

Ebstein's anomaly

Severe congestive heart failure

Multivalve disease

2.3 NUCLEAR MEDICINE

2.3.1 DECREASED RESTING LV EJECTION FRACTION

Technical

poor angle, processing errors, selection of background, etc

problems with gating (e.g. wrong lead placement, atrial fibrillation, etc)

Ischemic heart disease

Cardiomyopathy

Chemotherapy toxicity

(oncology patients)

earliest sign: apical lag

Decompensating hypertensive heart disease

Decompensating valvular heart disease

Transplant rejection (transplant patients)

2.3.2 INCREASED RESTING LV EJECTION FRACTION

Resting LVEF >70%

Hyperdynamic circulation

febrile neutropenia, sepsis, other

Mitral incompetence

Athlete

Hypertrophic cardiomyopathy

Technical (see 2.3.1)

2.3.3 MYOCARDIAL PERFUSION STUDY FALSE NEGATIVE FOR ISCHEMIA

Technical

INADEQUATE EXERCISE OR DOBUTAMINE STRESS

UNABLE TO REACH ADEQUATE HEART RATE AND BP

BETA BLOCKADE

INADEQUATE PERSANTIN OR ADENOSINE STRESS

PRIOR METHYLXANTHINES (caffeine, theophylline, etc)

Physiological

BALANCED TRIPLE VESSEL DISEASE

INTERMITTENT CORONARY ARTERY VASOSPASM

2.3.4 MYOCARDIAL PERFUSION STUDY FALSE POSITIVE FOR ISCHEMIA

Technical

BREAST ATTENUATION ARTIFACT, VARIABLE STRESS TO REST

rotating projections and attenuation correction helpful

INFERIOR ATTENUATION ARTIFACT, VARIABLE STRESS TO REST

CARDIAC MOTION ARTIFACT

GROSS PATIENT MOTION

RESPIRATORY 'CREEP'

NORMALIZING TO NON CARDIAC MAXIMAL ACTIVITY

NON ALIGNED SLICES

RESPIRATORY ARTIFACT

symmetrical reduced activity in anterior and inferior wall, worse with greater respiratory amplitude

Physiological

LEFT BUNDLE BRANCH BLOCK, SEPTAL 'STRESS DEFECT' WITH EXERCISE OR DOBUTAMINE

use dipyridamole (Persantin) or adenosine in preference

VERY HIGH EXERCISE LEVELS, HETEROGENEOUS PERFUSION

CARDIOMYOPATHY, HETEROGENEOUS PERFUSION

2.3.5 MYOCARDIAL PERFUSION STUDY FALSE POSITIVE FOR INFARCTION

Technical

BREAST ATTENUATION ARTIFACT

rotating projections and attenuation correction helpful

INFERIOR ATTENUATION ARTIFACT

attenuation correction and prone imaging helpful

gated SPECT helpful

Physiological

'APICAL THINNING'

SELF ATTENUATION OF BASAL INFERIOR WALL

vertically positioned heart, particularly in athletes

'HOT SPOTS' RAISING POSSIBILITY OF ISCHEMIA ELSEWHERE

SEPTUM

SEVERE EMPHYSEMA

LATERAL WALL AND SEPTUM

RESPIRATORY ARTIFACT (LARGE RESPIRATORY EXCURSION): SYMMETRICALLY REDUCED ACTIVITY IN ANTERIOR AND INFERIOR WALLS, RELATIVELY INCREASED ACTIVITY IN LATERAL WALL AND SEPTUM

BASAL INFERIOR WALL

COMBINATION OF RELATIVELY VERTICAL HEART ORIENTATION AND ATTENUATION CORRECTION

Missed viable myocardium

SEVERE ISCHEMIA INTERPRETED AS INFARCTION

OPTIONS: 24 HOUR TL IMAGES OR FDG STUDY

2.3.6 MYOCARDIAL PERFUSION STUDY PATTERNS

	TL REDISTRIBUTION (OR REST PERFUSION STUDY)			
Stress perfusion	**normal***	**reduced†****		**absent**
normal*	normal or false negative for ischemia	reverse redistribution pattern		look for technical cause
reduced†**, gated wall motion normal	inducible ischemia or false positive for ischemia	fixed non transmural infarction or false positive for infarction		look for technical cause
reduced†, gated wall motion reduced	inducible ischemia, induced stunning	24 hour Tl or FDG concordant with rest study indicates fixed infarct (or false positive for infarction)	24 hour Tl or FDG shows greater extent of uptake than at rest indicates underestimated viable ischemic myocardium	reverse redistribution pattern
absent	severe inducible ischemia	infarct with residual inducible ischemia	24 hour Tl or FDG concordant with rest study (i.e. absent) indicates fixed infarct (scar)	24 hour Tl or FDG shows uptake not present at rest indicates underestimated viable hibernating myocardium

*: matching stress-rest; **: matching stress-rest; †: qualitative estimate

2.3.7 MYOCARDIAL PERFUSION STUDY SIGNS OF DIFFERENT MYOCARDIAL STATES

Normal
normal stress perfusion
normal rest perfusion
normal redistribution
normal regional wall motion (at rest)
normal FDG uptake at rest

Inducible ischemia
ischemia can be deliberately induced by stress (exercise, pharmacological), or occur spontaneously (i.e. 'hot' perfusion study done during presentation with acute chest pain)

reduced/absent stress perfusion
normal rest perfusion
normal redistribution
normal regional wall motion (at rest)
normal FDG uptake at rest
also see myocardial perfusion reserve

Stunned myocardium
acutely injured non contractile myocardium which usually occurs in the context of acute coronary occlusion with or without acute reperfusion; may infarct or improve depending on circumstances

reduced stress perfusion (or normal, if treated)
normal rest perfusion
normal redistribution
abnormal regional wall motion (at rest)
normal FDG uptake at rest

Hibernating myocardium
defined as chronically ischemic non contractile but live myocardium (absolute proof is restoration of contractility with revascularization)

absent stress perfusion
absent rest perfusion
absent redistribution (but definition varies and may include 4 and/or 24 hour thallium uptake in the absence of rest perfusion)
abnormal regional wall motion
FDG uptake present

Non transmural infarction/scar
degree of reduction in perfusion variable and depends on volume of remaining myocardium
sensitivity of perfusion studies for detection of non transmural infarction is therefore lower than of transmural infarction

reduced/absent stress perfusion
reduced/absent rest perfusion
reduced/absent redistribution (all match)
abnormal regional wall motion
reduced/absent FDG uptake

Transmural infarction/scar
sensitivity of perfusion imaging greatest for detection of transmural infarction

absent stress perfusion
absent rest perfusion
absent redistribution (all match)
abnormal or no regional wall motion (depends on extent of scar)
absent FDG uptake

Reperfusion, combination of viable and necrotic myocardium
classically, reverse redistribution pattern

Myocardial perfusion reserve and myocardial steal
exercise and dobutamine increase myocardial workload and myocardial oxygen demand; any perfusion defects with such stress are true ischemia (insufficient perfusion to meet tissue needs)
dipyridamole (Persantin) and adenosine cause coronary vasodilation in the absence of physiological tissue need

the increased perfusion caused by
dipyridamole and adenosine
demonstrates MYOCARDIAL PERFUSION
RESERVE

relative reduction in perfusion in an area of
myocardium during dipyridamole or
adenosine stress is therefore an area of
REDUCED CORONARY PERFUSION
RESERVE unless true CORONARY STEAL
occurs

if a stenosis is so critical that dilation of
other coronary vessels drops its perfusion
pressure enough to cause ischemia,
CORONARY STEAL is present (and may
manifest symptomatically or on ECG)

Signs of LV failure

INCREASED LUNG THALLIUM
UPTAKE

ACUTE STRESS LV DILATION

2.3.8 PARADOXICAL SEPTAL MOTION

Ischemia/infarction

Left bundle branch block

Post valve plane surgery

Paced rhythm

2.3.9 REVERSE REDISTRIBUTION (TI)

After myocardial injury

mixture of viable and damaged myocardial
cells, with washout of thallium from
damaged cells and retention in viable
cells

NON TRANSMURAL INFARCTION

ACUTE THROMBOLYSIS,
ANGIOPLASTY OR 'HOT' BYPASSES

Postulated differential washout rates

true ischemic myocardium
diverse other conditions

Artifactual

Unexplained

2.4 MEDIASTINAL MASS MACHINE

DOES THE MASS PASS THROUGH THE THORACIC INLET OR OUTLET?

Passes through inlet

GOITROUS THYROID

LYMPHANGIOMA (child)

Passes through outlet

DIAPHRAGMATIC HERNIA

EVENTRATION

RUPTURE

DIAPHRAGMATIC MASS

CAN THE MASS BE NOT OF MEDIASTINAL ORIGIN?

Pulmonary mass protruding into mediastinum

Cardiac mass occupying mediastinum

WHAT IS THE SHAPE AND DENSITY OF THE MASS?

Spheroid: may be a cyst (see mediastinal cyst gamut)

Complex shape: cyst unlikely

Any distinguishing characteristics?

MOST MEDIASTINAL MASSES ARE
SOFT TISSUE DENSITY

OTHER: ?AIR, ?FAT, ?CALCIUM,
?FLUID LEVEL

VASCULAR OR LYMPHANGIOMATOUS MASS MAY BE FOUND IN ANTERIOR, MIDDLE OR POSTERIOR MEDIASTINUM

Arterial

ABERRANT VESSEL

ECTASIA, ANEURYSM, DISSECTION

Venous

ABERRANT VESSEL

Hemangioma, lymphangioma (child)

LYMPH NODAL MASS TENDS TO ANTERIOR OR MIDDLE MEDIASTINUM

see mediastinal lymphadenopathy gamut

ANTERIOR MEDIASTINAL MASS

listed by structure of origin

Sternum

OSTEOMYELITIS

METASTASIS

PLASMACYTOMA/MYELOMA

EOSINOPHILIC GRANULOMA

PRIMARY TUMOR

Thymus

HYPERPLASIA

CYST

THYMOMA

THYMOLIPOMA

CARCINOMA

LYMPHOMA

Pericardium

CYST

LIPOMA

Germ cell tumor

Thyroid mass

should pass through the thoracic inlet

Lymph nodal mass (see above)

Vascular or lymphatic mass (see above)

MIDDLE MEDIASTINAL MASS

Mnemonic: BEDPAN

B-ronchogenic tumor

E-sophageal mass

DILATED ESOPHAGUS AND NOT A TRUE MASS

should have an air–fluid level

ESOPHAGEAL DIVERTICULUM

may have an air–fluid level

ESOPHAGEAL TUMOR

D-uplication cyst

see mediastinal cysts gamut

P-ericardial cyst or lipoma

A-ngioma

HEMANGIOMA

LYMPHANGIOMA

particularly common in infants

N-eural tumor

PARAGANGLIOMA

NERVE SHEATH TUMOR

OTHER

Lymph nodal mass (see above)

Vascular or lymphatic mass (see above)

POSTERIOR MEDIASTINAL MASS

listed by organ of origin

Esophagus

HIATUS HERNIA

usually has an air–fluid level, but not always

DILATED ESOPHAGUS AND NOT A TRUE MASS

should have an air–fluid level

ESOPHAGEAL DIVERTICULUM

may have an air–fluid level

ESOPHAGEAL TUMOR

ESOPHAGEAL DUPLICATION CYST

Germ cell tumor

Neural tumor

GANGLIAL

GANGLIONEUROMA

GANGLIONEUROBLASTOMA

NEUROBLASTOMA

PARAGANGLIAL

PARAGANGLIOMA

NERVE SHEATH TUMOR

DURAL ECTASIA

SCHWANNOMA

NEUROFIBROMA

Vertebral mass

OSTEOMYELITIS WITH PHLEGMON

METASTASIS, MYELOMA, EOSINOPHILIC GRANULOMA

VERTEBRAL PRIMARY

EXTRAMEDULLARY HEMOPOIESIS

Disk derived mass

DISCITIS WITH ABSCESS

Lymph nodal mass (see above)

Vascular or lymphatic mass (see above)

CARDIAC AND MEDIASTINAL CONDITIONS

3. ACQUIRED AND ADULT

3.1 ANGIOFOLLICULAR LYMPH NODE HYPERPLASIA (Castleman's disease) (AFH)

see entry in Ch 16 hematology

3.2 AORTIC VALVE DISEASE (acquired)

3.2.1 AORTIC STENOSIS

ETIOLOGY

NB 'Lambl's excrescences' is age related change only and are not pathological

Bicuspid valve degeneration

Tricuspid valve degeneration

Rheumatic fever

IMAGING

CXR

LV hypertrophy, AoV calcification, post stenotic dilation

Echo

cross sectional area <0.8 cm2 in clinically significant stenosis
(normal is 2–3 cm2)
estimated pressure gradient >50 mmHg

MR

stenotic jet visible on cine MR
valve area can be measured

3.2.2 AORTIC INCOMPETENCE

ETIOLOGY

Infective endocarditis

Rheumatic fever

Annuloaortic ectasia

MARFAN'S/EHLERS–DANLOS SYNDROMES

IMMUNE

SYPHILIS

HLA B27 RELATED

ANKYLOSING SPONDYLITIS

REITER'S SYNDROME

RHEUMATOID ARTHRITIS

(ATHEROMATOUS)

IDIOPATHIC

Prior aortic dissection

IMAGING

CXR
massive LV enlargement
(if acute aortic incompetence, CXR shows
acute pulmonary edema)

Echo
regurgitant jet (quantifiable)

MR
regurgitant jet on cine MR

3.3 CARDIAC TRAUMA

ETIOLOGY

Blunt
CAR ACCIDENTS

CRUSHING INJURIES

EXTERNAL CARDIAC COMPRESSION

Sharp
PENETRATING INJURY

SPECTRUM OF MANIFESTATIONS

HEMOPERICARDIUM, TAMPONADE

CORONARY ARTERY LACERATION,
DISSECTION, OCCLUSION

MYOCARDIAL HEMORRHAGE OR
NECROSIS

TRAUMATIC PSEUDOANEURYSM

TRAUMATIC VSD

ACUTE VALVULAR DISRUPTION (MR,
AR, TR)

IMAGING (myocardial contusion)

MR
areas of high T2W signal immediately post
trauma

3.4 CARDIAC TUMORS

3.4.1 METASTATIC (more common than primary)

Endomyocardial (hematogenous)
LYMPHOMA, LEUKEMIA

MELANOMA

OTHERS

Pericardial with effusion
(retrograde lymphatic spread)

BREAST

BRONCHUS

ESOPHAGUS

OTHERS

Intracavitary
IVC

RENAL CARCINOMA

HEPATOCELLULAR CARCINOMA

ADRENAL CARCINOMA (about 5%)

SVC

THYROID CARCINOMA

3.4.2 PRIMARY – BENIGN

3.4.2.1 Myxoma
30–60 years old, female > male
75% left atrium, 20% right atrium (can recur
or be locally invasive)
present with obstructive, embolic or
constitutional symptoms
systemic embolism common

IMAGING

ECHO
intraatrial relatively fixed solid mass with
fronds

CT
contrast outlined intraatrial mass

MR
inhomogeneous lobulated mass
may have areas of high T2W signal or
hemorrhage
enhances with Gd (unlike thrombus)

3.4.2.2 Intracavitary lipoma
extensions or projections of lipomatous
hypertrophy of the atrial septum

IMAGING

MR
high on T1W, low on T2W; saturates with fat
sat sequences

3.4.2.3 Fibroma
commoner in children
solitary, arise from septum or LV
myocardium

IMAGING

MR
low T1W and T2W signal

3.4.2.4 Hemangioma
rare

IMAGING

MR
characteristic low T1W and high T2W signal
with areas of necrosis and hemorrhage
high on T2W

3.4.2.5 Rhabdomyoma

CLINICAL
commonest childhood cardiac tumor
hamartomas rather than true neoplasms
associated with tuberous sclerosis
(approximately 50%)
arise from myocardium of interventricular
septum and ventricular walls
atria involved in 1/3
multiple in 90%

IMAGING

MR
mass with isocenter in myocardium
may be entirely intramuscular and difficult
to identify
frequently multiple
intermediate T1W signal, may have
increased T2W signal

3.4.3 PRIMARY – MALIGNANT

usually presents after 40 years of age with
murmur, cardiac failure, anemia, weight
loss
most patients die within 1 year of diagnosis

3.4.3.1 Angiosarcoma
irregular mass centered on myocardium
with central high T2W signal and
intermediate signal periphery
enhance with Gd

3.4.3.2 Pericardial mesothelioma

see mesothelioma in Ch 13 lung
irregularity and nodular thickening of pericardium and epicardium
hemorrhagic pericardial effusion

3.4.3.3 Fibrosarcoma/malignant fibrous histiocytoma

multiple, sessile masses usually involving left atrium

3.5 CARDIOMYOPATHY – DILATED

DEFINITION

abnormally reduced myocardial contractility with dilation of left ventricle
primary cardiomyopathy is idiopathic by definition; there are multiple causes of secondary cardiomyopathies; a number of conditions are specifically excluded by definition (see below)

ETIOLOGY

commonest are viral, alcohol related and chemotherapy related cardiomyopathies

Myocarditis related

INFECTIVE

VIRAL: Coxsackie, Echo, polio, influenza, AIDS

BACTERIAL: Chlamydia, Rickettsia, Meningococcus, Staphylococcus, diphtherial toxin

FUNGAL: Candida, Aspergillus

PROTOZOAL: Chagas (trypanosomiasis), Toxoplasma

METAZOAL: Trichinosis, hydatids

AUTOIMMUNE

RHEUMATIC FEVER

SARCOIDOSIS

IMMUNE COMPLEX DISEASE

   SLE

   RHEUMATOID ARTHRITIS

   CREST

VASCULITIS (polyarteritis nodosa)

Toxic

ETHANOL

CHEMOTHERAPY

Metabolic

HYPERTHYROIDISM, HYPOTHYROIDISM

BERI-BERI

HEMOCHROMATOSIS

Primary dilated cardiomyopathy

20–60 years
OCCASIONALLY POSTPARTUM
NO ISCHEMIC HEART DISEASE
NEGATIVE FOR ANY OF ABOVE
progressive congestive cardiac failure, 25% 5 year survival

Specifically excluded disease

ISCHEMIC HEART DISEASE

HYPERTENSIVE HEART DISEASE

VALVULAR HEART DISEASE

CLINICAL

presents with progressive heart failure, reduced exercise tolerance, dyspnea
dilation of all cardiac chambers
myocardial thickness may be increased or decreased
mural thrombi and endocardial scars common

IMAGING

CXR

cardiomegaly, often in left ventricular pattern
pulmonary venous congestion

Echo

uniform LV dilation with global hypokinesis
RV may be dilated
LV may contain mural thrombus
fractional shortening reduced
functional valvular regurgitation (secondary to valve ring dilation

NUC MED (gated blood pool scan)

dilated left ventricle
global hypokinesis without focal segmental abnormality in excess of other segments
reduced left ventricular ejection fraction
right ventricular ejection fraction may be normal or reduced

NUC MED (perfusion study)

normal perfusion or heterogeneous patchy pattern

no perfusion defects
may have obviously dilated LV
if gross LV failure, may have Tl lung uptake or stress LV dilation

CT/MR

dilated cardiac chambers (particularly LV)
normal myocardial thickness
may show mural thrombus
no specific myocardial signal characteristics on MR

3.6 CARDIOMYOPATHY – HYPERTROPHIC

DEFINITION

myocardial dysfunction with abnormal LV myocardial thickening
primary is idiopathic; a number of causes exist, with several conditions specifically excluded from definition

ETIOLOGY

Primary hypertrophic obstructive cardiomyopathy (HOCM)

Depositional disease

GLYCOGEN STORAGE DISEASE

MUCOPOLYSACCHARIDOSES

Dystrophies

DYSTROPHIA MYOTONICA

DUCHENNE MUSCULAR DYSTROPHY

FRIEDREICH'S ATAXIA

Specifically excluded disease

HYPERTENSIVE HEART DISEASE

second commonest cause of LV failure and contributing factor to ischemic heart disease

VALVULAR HEART DISEASE

CLINICAL (HOCM)

usually young adult, familial in 50%
no amyloid or hypertensive heart disease by definition
may present with angina, syncopal attacks, dyspnea; sudden death 2–5% per year

massive myocardial hypertrophy
LV outflow may be obstructed when the
hypertrophied myocardium contracts
myofiber disarray (disorganization of
myocytes and also of sarcomeres within
myocytes), massive myocyte hypertrophy
and glycogen buildup

IMAGING

CXR

may be normal
variable LV enlargement

Echo

small LV cavity
normal or increased fractional shortening
asymmetric septal hypertrophy (90%)
symmetric hypertrophy may be present
reflective myocardial echotexture
RV affected less
systolic anterior motion (SAM) of mitral
valve (excessive anterior motion
compared to lateral wall, associated with
pressure drop across LVOT)
septal thickness >30 mm is associated with
significant risk of sudden death from an
arrhythmia

NUC MED (RBC study)

small LV cavity, may be banana shaped
ejection fraction may be normal

CT/MR

shows extent and location of myocardial
hypertrophy
cine MR shows LVOT morphology
no specific myocardial signal characteristics
on MR

3.7 CARDIOMYOPATHY – RESTRICTIVE

DEFINITION

poor cardiac function secondary to impaired
diastolic relaxation of the left ventricle
primary is idiopathic; secondary is due to
several rare conditions; some conditions
are specifically excluded by definition

ETIOLOGY

Primary restrictive cardiomyopathy

Secondary restrictive cardiomyopathy

ENDOMYOCARDIAL FIBROSIS
LOEFFLER'S ENDOCARDITIS
INFANTILE ENDOCARDIAL
FIBROELASTOSIS
probably congenital or developmental
endocardial fibrous and elastic
thickening particularly involving LV and
valves (esp mitral)

Amyloid

CARDIAC ONLY AMYLOID
SYSTEMIC AMYLOID

Specifically excluded disease

HYPERTENSIVE HEART DISEASE
CONSTRICTIVE PERICARDITIS

IMAGING

Echo

restrictive filling pattern
LV cavity size normal
dilated atria

ENDOMYOCARDIAL FIBROELASTOSIS
cavity obliteration
retraction of papillary muscles and/or valves
increased endocardial reflectivity

NUC MED (gated study)

'diastolic failure' pattern: slow or irregular
filling on ventricular volume vs time
curve (analogous to echo findings)

MR

normal size LV and RV, often dilated atria
and systemic great veins
myocardium thickness may or may not be
increased
infiltration (e.g. amyloid) will increase
myocardial thickness
major utility is differentiation from
constrictive pericarditis (no signs of
pericardial thickening)

3.8 CONSTRICTIVE PERICARDITIS

DEFINITION

progressive fibrotic constriction of
pericardium leading to failure of diastolic
filling

ETIOLOGY

TB
post tuberculous fibrosis (inactive TB)
post bacterial pericarditis
postoperative
radiation
sarcoidosis
asbestos

CLINICAL

right heart failure
increased systemic venous pressure
diastolic heart failure

IMAGING

Full heart study

right atrial pressure = left atrial pressure
(demonstrated as equalization of
pressure between the RA and pulmonary
capillary wedge pressure)

CXR

small heart +/– pericardial calcification
distended systemic and pulmonary veins

MR/CT

pericardium thickened >4 mm
usually no excessive contrast enhancement
calcification suggests prior TB
no myocardial thickening
normal size ventricles and often dilated atria
CT DIFFERENTIAL: effusion
MR DIFFERENTIAL: restrictive
cardiomyopathy

3.9 INFECTIVE ENDOCARDITIS

DEFINITION

growth of viable microorganisms on
endocardium and valves with local
(destructive) and systemic (embolic,
immune complex) complications

ETIOLOGY

Microorganism

VIRULENT (no underlying structural
change)
Staphylococcus aureus (source: IV drug
abuse, lung abscess, deep abscess)
any overwhelming bacteremia

LOW GRADE BACTERIAL

Staphylococcus albus (sources: skin; associations: surgery, prosthetic valves)
Streptococcus viridans (association: dental work, prosthetic or abnormal valves)
Enterococci (sources: gut, urinary procedures)
Pseudomonas (immunosuppressed)

LOW GRADE OTHER

Candida (immune suppressed, IV drug abuse, prosthetic valves)
Coxiella (follows Q fever)

Host

normal host, virulent organism
ABNORMAL VALVE: rheumatic fever, degenerate calcified aortic valve, floppy mitral valve
PROSTHETIC VALVE
IMMUNOSUPPRESSED
IV drug abuse (R heart endocarditis in particular)

PATHOGENESIS

two absolute preconditions:
PRESENCE OF THROMBUS (focal agranulocytosis)
BACTEREMIA (seeding of thrombus with survival)
HALLMARK: VEGETATION (mass of thrombus and bacteria) – variable depending on organism; Staphylococcus particularly destructive

CLINICAL

FEVER + NEW HEART MURMUR
ACUTE CARDIAC DECOMPENSATION
SIGNS OF EMBOLISM: stroke, Osler nodes (skin), Roth spots (retina), visceral infarcts
SIGNS OF IMMUNE COMPLEX DISEASE: purpura (Janeway lesions), glomerulonephritis, splinter hemorrhages, vasculitis
LAB: blood culture is mandatory and may grow organism
MORTALITY 30% EVEN WITH THERAPY, 100% WITHOUT

IMAGING

Echo

independently mobile vegetations are pathognomonic
hypoechoic areas adjacent to the involved valve indicate development of paravalvular abscesses

transesophageal echo: independently mobile vegetations are pathognomonic (moving on the valve leaflet as well as with the valve leaflet)

MR

vegetations have high T2W signal and often enhance
calcification has signal voids

3.10 ISCHEMIC HEART DISEASE (IHD)

DEFINITION

spectrum of ischemic cardiac disease secondary to coronary atherosclerosis

EPIDEMIOLOGY

leading manifestation of atherosclerosis
leading cause of sudden (<6 hours) death

Risk factors

CONTROLLABLE

smoking
hypertension
dyslipidemia
diabetes

NOT CONTROLLABLE

male gender
age
adverse family history

OTHER

evidence of vascular disease elsewhere

ETIOLOGY

VAST MAJORITY – CORONARY ATHEROSCLEROSIS

EXACERBATED BY HYPERTENSION OR AORTIC STENOSIS

RARE CAUSES

CORONARY ARTERITIS
SYSTEMIC EMBOLISM TO CORONARY ARTERIES
UNRECOGNIZED LIGATION AT SURGERY
TRAUMA
AORTIC DISSECTION (with involved coronary arteries)
COCAINE INDUCED SPASM

PATHOGENESIS

Fibrofatty plaque vs complicated plaque

see atherosclerosis entry in Ch 15
complicated plaque more prone to sudden intraplaque hemorrhage, occlusion, fissuring, thrombosis

Concentric vs eccentric

media under plaque slowly atrophies
uninvolved media remains contractile in eccentric plaque

CLINICAL PRESENTATION SPECTRUM

Stable angina

stable plaques with exertional flow limitation
presents with long history of typical angina with predictable precipitating factors
angina not prolonged, and controlled by rest or nitrates

Unstable angina

indicates evolving plaque; usually fissuring with transient superimposed thrombosis
high risk of myocardial infarct (MI) from acute occlusion by propagating thrombus
increasing frequency of angina
prolonged angina (longer than few minutes)
angina not relieved by usual measures
angina at rest

Variant angina (Prinzmetal angina)

coronary vasospasm in eccentric plaque; same significance as unstable angina

Slow ischemic atrophy

chronic inadequate supply with slow fibrosis; ischemic cardiomyopathy

Myocardial infarction (MI)

usually thrombotic occlusion superimposed on complicated (fissured, hemorrhagic) plaque
less commonly stable plaque with hypotension
there is a spectrum of myocardial injury (depends on area subtended by occluded vessel, collateral supply)
majority reperfuse (either spontaneously or with thrombolysis)

Ischemic arrhythmia

usual cause of sudden death (mainly ventricular tachycardia)
usually develops in the setting of MI

IMAGING (acute presentation)

CXR

normal unless pulmonary edema supervenes

may show evidence of prior heart disease (cardiomegaly, prosthetic valves, coronary bypass clips and wires)

excludes alternative causes of pain

NUC MED ('hot MIBI' perfusion study)

MIBI injected during chest pain; no redistribution occurs

imaging can be performed within 4–6 hours of injection after stabilization

totally normal study excludes ischemia with a high degree of confidence, and confers a good (cardiac) prognosis

perfusion defects usually require a matching resting study

PERFUSION DEFECT DIFFERENTIAL

acute ischemia

acute MI

prior MI with (stable) scar

NUC MED (stress perfusion study)

usually performed to clarify significance of presenting pain if there is no evidence of infarction (ECG or biochemical)

graded exercise is the safest option

if there is evidence of infarction, stress (exercise or pharmacological) contraindicated, but a rest-redistribution study may be performed

NUC MED (rest-redistribution study)

either Tl (rest, then re-image with 4 or 24 hour delay) or MIBI/FDG pair

shows any resting ischemia and amount of perfused myocardium at rest

Echo

may be used in looking for wall motion abnormalities in the acute presentation with no ECG changes

Coronary catheter angiography

'HOT ANGIO; HOT ANGIOPLASTY'

see entries under imaging of stable IHD and imaging of myocardial infarction

IMAGING (stable IHD)

CXR

see acute presentation

CT (coronary calcium scoring)

most published studies have been performed with electron beam CT (EBCT); data on ECG-gated helical subsecond CT is accumulating

requires ECG gating to 'freeze' cardiac motion and software analysis of coronary calcium

principal use is screening of asymptomatic population (with or without risk factors)

resulting coronary artery calcium score is a surrogate measure of coronary plaque burden

negative EBCT makes presence of plaque very unlikely, and is associated with low short to medium term coronary event risk

positive EBCT confirms presence of atherosclerotic plaque

can not discriminate between hemodynamically significant plaque and calcification with no hemodynamic effects

underestimates total plaque burden (does not detect non calcified plaque)

USED FOR SCREENING

current EBCT data for asymptomatic patients (screening mode) have same or slightly greater positive and negative predictive values compared to predictive values derived from traditional multifactorial risk factor model

USED FOR DIAGNOSIS

sensitivity is comparable to perfusion scintigraphy and stress echocardiography (~90%)

specificity low (~50%) and significantly lower than for perfusion scintigraphy (~80–85%)

USED FOR MONITORING

there is evidence for considerable variation in calcium scores between measurements in the same patient – monitoring likely not to be accurate

CT coronary angiography/MR coronary angiography

both still not in routine clinical use

requires multislice CT with ECG gating or ultrafast MR with respiratory motion correction

Coronary catheter angiography

significant stenosis on angio taken to be >70% diameter reduction in one plane (but >50% for left main coronary artery)

OCCLUSIONS, CUTOFFS

COLLATERALS

TIMI FLOW CLASSIFICATION

see myocardial infarction

Dobutamine stress echo

inducible wall motion abnormality indicates functionally significant ischemia

NUC MED (perfusion study)

NUCLIDES (outline)

Thallium

behaves analogously to potassium ion

taken up by Na/K ATPase into viable cells

for a wide range of coronary flow rates myocardial uptake is proportional to flow, but reaches eventual saturation plateau

initial distribution reflects relative regional perfusion

Thallium redistributes (equilibrates) within the myocardium over a few hours

delayed (4 or even 24 hour) images reflect regional distribution of live myocardium

injected at peak exercise and imaged soon after

resting images obtained in 4 hours (often with reinjection to increase Tl pool available for uptake)

MIBI/tetrofosmin

complex organic chelates of technetium

irreversibly taken up by myocardial cells

myocardial uptake proportional to flow but saturation comes faster than with thallium

injected at peak exercise

small proportion washes out of myocardium early, and the rest is fixed – this allows delays in imaging

second injection necessary for rest study

stomach and liver uptake a potential confounder – delayed images performed to allow biliary and bowel clearance

Fluorodeoxyglucose

taken up by live cells via glucose active transport, and then trapped

shows viable myocardium

MEANS OF ACHIEVING CARDIAC STRESS (outline only)

graded exercise (treadmill or bicycle) (refer to specific guidelines/texts on performance)

can not be used if beta blocked

dipyridamole (Persantin)

coronary vasodilator (increases adenosine levels)

demonstrates limitations in relative regional
  perfusion reserve
if true steal occurs this produces true
  ischemia
contraindicated in asthma or heart block
antagonized by prior xanthines (caffeine,
  theophylline, etc)

adenosine
coronary vasodilator with short half-life
same comments as for dipyridamole

dobutamine
beta and alpha agonist
increases myocardial workload, contractility
  and heart rate
increases rate of arrhythmias
contraindicated in hypertension
can not be used if beta blocked

FINDINGS
see gamuts: myocardial perfusion study patterns
cardinal sign is regional reduced tracer
  activity at stress compared to rest,
  implying reduced perfusion at stress but
  not at rest
pitfall: balanced triple vessel disease (no
  regional normal to allow standardization)

3.11 MITRAL VALVE ACQUIRED DISEASE

3.11.1 STENOSIS

ETIOLOGY

Rheumatic fever
usually produces mixed mitral valve disease

IMAGING

CXR
LA enlargement (see under gamuts)
LA thrombus (may be visible if calcifies)
MV calcification (leaflets and/or annulus)
pulmonary venous congestion
pulmonary edema
pulmonary hemosiderosis and osseous
  nodules

Echo
valve area of 2 cm2 or less is clinically
  significant
(normal is 4–6 cm2)
estimated pressure gradient 6 mmHg

MR
cine MR shows stenotic jet
valve area can be measured

3.11.2 INCOMPETENCE

ETIOLOGY

INFECTIVE ENDOCARDITIS

RHEUMATIC FEVER

AUTOIMMUNE
SLE
LOEFFLER'S SYNDROME (endomyocardial
  fibrosis)

LEAFLET PROLAPSE
FLOPPY OR MYXOMATOUS MV
  MARFAN'S, EHLERS DANLOS SYNDROMES
  IDIOPATHIC
PAPILLARY ISCHEMIA, RUPTURE
CHORDAL RUPTURE

Mitral ring dilation
LEFT VENTRICULAR FAILURE OF ANY
  CAUSE
DILATED CARDIOMYOPATHY

IMAGING

CXR
LV enlargement
LA enlargement
LA thrombus (may be visible if calcifies)
MV calcification (leaflets and/or annulus)
pulmonary venous congestion
pulmonary edema
pulmonary hemosiderosis and osseous
  nodules

Echo
regurgitant jet (quantifiable)

MR
regurgitant jet on cine MR

3.12 MYOCARDIAL INFARCTION

DEFINITION

myocardial necrosis secondary to acute
  ischemia, overwhelmingly as part of
  ischemic heart disease (IHD)

EPIDEMIOLOGY, ETIOLOGY

See ischemic heart disease

PATHOGENESIS

Regional infarction
acute coronary occlusion (plaque fissuring,
  deroofing, hemorrhage with
  superimposed thrombus)
less commonly fixed stenosis and
  hypotension
many reperfuse spontaneously

TRANSMURAL VS SUBENDOCARDIAL
TRANSMURAL
infarction of entire myocardial thickness
increased risk of rupture
subsequent hypokinetic, akinetic or
  dyskinetic scar

SUBENDOCARDIAL (non transmural)
infarction of inner myocardial layers only
  where reduced perfusion pressure has
  been insufficient for myocardial needs
thickness variable, but does not involve full
  wall thickness by definition
may have no ECG changes
harder to detect with NUC MED perfusion
  studies
better prognosis

Diffuse infarction
usually fixed stenoses and hypotension
usually SUBENDOCARDIAL

CLINICAL

Classic presentation
crushing relentless severe central chest pain
  with possible neck or left arm radiation;
  sweating, tachycardia, arrhythmias,
  hypotension; cardiovascular collapse

Atypical presentation
atypical pain or no pain (especially if
  diabetic)

ECG
previous ECG very useful
diagnoses secondary rhythm disturbances
  (e.g. VT)
serial ECG over 6–12 hours

ACUTE
normal does not exclude myocardial
  ischemia or infarction
ST elevation ('ST elevation myocardial
  injury' = 'STEMI') indicates significant
  volume of damaged myocardium

ST depression classically is an indication of ischemia without major infarction

non-STEMI ('non ST elevation myocardial infarction') is diagnosed when there is biochemical evidence of infarction but no ECG ST elevation

'unstable angina' is diagnosed when there is no biochemical evidence of myocardial infarction

SUBACUTE/EVOLVING

ST depression classically resolves

ST elevation usually evolves through T wave inversion and subsequent development of Q waves

STABLE

Q waves in relevant leads (or equivalent in V1 and precordial leads); may eventually resolve over years

Serial enzymes

TROPONIN (serial measurement over 6–12 hours)

more sensitive and specific than CK-MB, but remains elevated for longer

false positives occur in renal failure and pulmonary embolism

no elevation of troponin over 12 hours suggests no infarction

what is a significant troponin level depends on the particular laboratory and varies from institution to institution (guideline: normal is <2 microgram/l)

correlation between amount of myocardial damage and troponin peak level is as yet not proven

CREATINE KINASE (CK), CK-MB (serial measurement over 6–12 hours)

small amounts of CK-MB occur in non cardiac muscle

false positives occur particularly with unfractionated CK

no elevation over 12 hours suggests no infarction

area under curve rather than peak of curve reflects amount of myocardial damage

guideline: normal total CK is <200 U/L; CK-MB index <4.5

MORPHOLOGY BY TIME

different areas are at different stages at any one time

speed of injury depends on relative preservation of blood supply, adequacy of collaterals and any reperfusion (spontaneous or therapeutic)

speed of repair depends on viability of connective tissue and blood vessels which form granulation tissue and then scar

Reversible injury (0 to 30 min)

cessation of contraction and aerobic glycolysis

anaerobic glycolysis, ATP and glycogen depletion (ATP reserves exhausted at 60 min); lactic acidosis

mitochondrial swelling

myocardial cells damaged first, endothelium and fibroblasts relatively resistant

Irreversible injury (30 min to 3 hours)

damaged cell membrane, K outflow, Na, Ca influx; mitochondrial rupture; sarcomere damage and locking; chromatin clumping

by light microscopy, dead fibers appear wavy (stretched by viable muscle)

infarcted myocardium fails to take up tetrazolinium at 3 hours

REPERFUSION INJURY (O2 and products of anaerobic metabolism, oxygen radicals, lipid oxidation of cell membrane and damage, Ca flooding and second messenger arrest)

Coagulative necrosis (3 to 24 hours)

progressive cell eosinophilia and swelling, nuclear pyknosis and lysis (reliably seen by light microscopy at 12 hours)

early edema and neutrophil infiltrate

Acute inflammation (24 hours to 4 days)

shrunken disintegrating necrotic cells, heavy neutrophil infiltrate; pale central area; hyperemic hemorrhagic patchy necrosis in areas of reperfusion

Macrophage response (4 to 10 days)

marked macrophage infiltrate with digestion of dead cells; fibrovascular response at margins; yellow-brown soft focus with hyperemic margins

Progressive granulation (10 days to a few weeks)

progressive replacement by granulation tissue; central infarct yellow and soft till replaced; eventual scarring

NATURAL HISTORY

Acute complications

ISCHEMIC ARRHYTHMIA, SUDDEN DEATH

ACUTE RUPTURE (most likely at 4–10 days)

EXTERNAL

INTERVENTRICULAR

PAPILLARY

ACUTE LV FAILURE, ACUTE PULMONARY EDEMA

from initial infarct

from papillary muscle rupture and acute MV incompetence

Subacute complications

HEART BLOCK (especially with RCA territory infarcts)

DRESSLER'S PERICARDITIS

ATRIAL FIBRILLATION, THROMBOSIS

Chronic

CHRONIC LVF

LV ANEURYSM WITH THROMBUS

PAPILLARY ISCHEMIA AND MV INCOMPETENCE

IMAGING

CXR

no findings other than secondary changes (e.g. acute pulmonary edema)

NUC MED (perfusion study)

also see NUC MED – ischemic heart disease
also see gamuts: 2.3.6 and 2.3.7

REST PERFUSION – VIABILITY STUDY

NUCLIDES

resting Tl – redistribution Tl (no reinjection) at 4 and 24 hours

MIBI/tetrofosmin and FDG pair

PERFUSION STUDY PATTERNS

see 2.3.6 and 2.3.7 in nuclear medicine gamuts

TRANSMURAL COMPLETED INFARCTION

TRANSMURAL INFARCTION WITH PERIINFARCT RESTING ISCHEMIA

NON TRANSMURAL INFARCTION

REPERFUSION, COMBINATION OF VIABLE AND NECROTIC MYOCARDIUM

STRESS PERFUSION – REST PERFUSION STUDY

safety of study depends on time since infarction, location and extent of infarct, and occurrence of arrhythmias (risk: arrhythmias and rupture of soft scar)

in general, the longer time interval, the safer (MI within 2 days is an absolute contraindication); if possible, wait 4–6 weeks before exercise

in general, if performed prior to discharge from hospital, submaximal exercise is safest

NUCLIDES
Tl stress/rest (with/without reinjection)
MIBI/tetrofosmin stress/rest
PERFUSION STUDY PATTERNS
TRANSMURAL COMPLETED INFARCTION
NON TRANSMURAL COMPLETED INFARCTION
PERIINFARCT ISCHEMIA
also: INCIDENTAL ISCHEMIA IN ANOTHER VASCULAR TERRITORY

NUC MED (gated study)

either gated perfusion study or gated blood pool study
reduced or absent contraction in area of infarction
degree of reduction depends on location and infarct size
dyskinesis: paradoxical motion
LV aneurysm

Echo

segmental wall motion abnormality in distribution of infarct
chronic infarct (as opposed to ischemia or acute infarct) is scarred and therefore has reduced wall thickness as well as segmental dyskinesia (normal LV wall thickness is ~2 cm)
echo also diagnoses complications

Coronary angio

'HOT ANGIO; HOT ANGIOPLASTY'
coronary occlusions, vessel cutoffs
TIMI flow grades 0, 1, 2
Abnormal segmental wall motion in distribution of ischemia or infarct on LV gram
LVEDP (left ventricular end diastolic pressure) is a measure of LV dysfunction

TIMI FLOW GRADES

'thrombolysis in myocardial infarction' trial classification
TIMI 0 NO FLOW
TIMI 1 SLUGGISH FLOW WITH INCOMPLETE FILLING OF VESSEL

TIMI 2 FILLS ENTIRE VESSEL TO TIP BUT SLOWER THAN NORMAL VESSELS
TIMI 3 NORMAL PERFUSION ON ANGIO

CORONARY STENOSES

significant stenosis on angio taken to be >70% diameter reduction (but >50% reduction for left main coronary artery)
stenosis in itself does not prove infarct distal to it

MR

area of increased T2W signal compared to normal myocardium
perfusion MR shows hypoperfusion acutely; in late stages shows hyperperfusion and extravasation of Gd into interstitial space
gated study findings comparable to NUC MED findings

3.13 PERICARDITIS, PERICARDIAL EFFUSION

ETIOLOGY (pericarditis/pericardial effusion)

INFECTIVE

VIRAL

BACTERIAL

TB
serous, then fibrinous, tubercle formation, calcification

FUNGAL (immune suppression)

AUTOIMMUNE

RHEUMATIC FEVER

SARCOIDOSIS

IMMUNE COMPLEX DISEASE

POST MYOCARDIAL INFARCT/POST SURGICAL (Dressler's syndrome)

TOXIC

UREMIC

RADIATION

ETIOLOGY (pericardial effusion, no pericarditis)

CONGESTIVE CARDIAC FAILURE

MALIGNANT

METASTASES, LYMPHOMA

MESOTHELIOMA

CLINICAL

asymptomatic if small or slow
symptoms of pericarditis, pericardial rub (e.g. viral)
reduced heart sounds (effusion)
raised JVP and reduced cardiac output if large or collects quickly (tamponade)
classic ECG changes of pericarditis: global ST segment elevation concave upwards

IMAGING

CXR

may have no findings
cardiomegaly with no specific features
'waterbottle' heart; recent change in heart size
may see epicardial and pericardial fat separated by >3 mm

Echo

shows location and amount of fluid, and whether the effusion is loculated or not
variable echogenicity and debris depending on type of effusion
RV collapse/LA collapse/LV collapse are evidence of progressively severe tamponade
variation of mitral and tricuspid inflow velocities of >50% with respiration indicates presence of tamponade

CT

non enhancing ring of variable density surrounding myocardium
may be loculated (e.g. TB effusion)
splits epicardial and pericardial fat
does not extend above pericardial attachments
density of effusion reflects presence of blood
contrast enhances myocardium, but not effusion
may have vivid pericardial and epicardial contrast enhancement (infective and inflammatory effusions)

NUC MED (RBC scan)

uniform area of photopenia around the LV and RV cavities in excess of expected myocardial thickness
present on all views (may vary in thickness)
DIFFERENTIAL: breast attenuation artifact

MR

normal pericardium is a thin line of low T1W and T2W signal separating pericardial fat from epicardial fat

signal of simple pericardial effusion follows free fluid

infected, proteinaceous, inflammatory effusions have intermediate T1W and T2W signal (differs from free fluid)

hemorrhagic effusion has variable signal of blood products

pericarditis may have thickened visceral and parietal pericardium with intermediate T2W signal (not low)

inflamed pericardium may have thickened contrast enhancement

3.14 PULMONARY VALVE ACQUIRED DISEASE

3.14.1 STENOSIS

ETIOLOGY

very rare
carcinoid syndrome (paraneoplastic fibrosis)

3.14.2 INCOMPETENCE

ETIOLOGY

IV DRUG ABUSE ENDOCARDITIS

3.15 RHEUMATIC FEVER

DEFINITION

acute systemic autoimmune illness secondary to immune cross-reactivity with group A Streptococcus (GpA Strep)

EPIDEMIOLOGY

rare; greatest incidence 5–8 year olds
very high risk of subsequent attacks with further GpA strep pharyngitis
ENDEMIC: Australian Aborigines, third world

CLINICAL

2–3 weeks post GpA Strep pharyngitis/tonsillits 3% develop:

Minor manifestations

elevated ESR, fever, myalgia, prolonged PR interval on ECG

Major manifestations

arthritis, erythema marginatum
cardiac disease
pericarditis
chorea (rare)

MORPHOLOGY

valve inflammation, fibroblast invasion, scarring; MV > AoV >> TV
myocarditis – usually resolves without sequelae
HALLMARK: Aschoff body (granuloma in any heart layer with fibrinoid necrosis, giant (Aschoff) cells and activated histiocytes (Anitchkow cells)
ENDOCARDIUM – McCallum's plaques

IMAGING

depends on which valves are affected and on severity of valvular disease
see individual valve and cardiac chamber enlargement entries

3.16 SUDDEN CARDIAC DEATH

ETIOLOGY

Ischemic heart disease

ACUTE CORONARY OCCLUSION

Other

AORTIC STENOSIS

CARDIOMYOPATHY

MYOCARDITIS

CONDUCTION DEFECT

CONGENITAL HEART DISEASE

PATHOGENESIS

the commonest mechanism is development of a lethal arrhythmia

IMAGING

only relevance is knowledge of conditions predisposing to sudden cardiac death
also see imaging of hypertrophic cardiomyopathy

3.17 SUPERIOR VENA CAVA SYNDROME

ETIOLOGY

Malignant compression

LUNG

NODAL OR MEDIASTINAL

Mediastinal fibrosis

TB

FUNGUS

SARCOIDOSIS

PROGRESSIVE MASSIVE FIBROSIS

Thrombosis

LINES AND CATHETERS

HYPERCOAGULABLE STATE

IMAGING

clinical and angiographic signs of SVC compression:
facial congestion, difficulty lying flat, severe headache, swelling of face, neck, arms
engorged neck, chest and arm veins, may thrombose
chest wall collaterals
high pressure in SVC tributaries
abnormally slow forwards flow

3.18 THYMIC HYPERPLASIA (pathological)

also see thymic rebound entry

DEFINITION

diffuse pathological thymic lymphoid follicular hyperplasia

ASSOCIATIONS

myasthenia gravis
Graves' disease
Addison's disease
systemic lupus erythematosus, CREST, rheumatoid arthritis

IMAGING

differential diagnosis of anterior mediastinal mass, thymic mass, thymoma, lymphoma

3.19 THYMIC REBOUND

CLINICAL

regrowth of involuted thymus following illness or chemotherapy

most common in childhood but may occur in adolescents

diagnostic problem if the differential is lymphoma recurrence

ultimate proof is by biopsy or long term followup

IMAGING

CT (and MR)
bilobed or bow tie soft tissue density in anterior mediastinum

rebound overgrowth documented in literature to 50% above prechemotherapy size

NUC MED (Ga)
takes up gallium in a triangular or cross-shaped pattern in anterior mediastinum (may occur at 2–12 months following chemotherapy)

diagnostic dilemma if differential is recurrence of gallium avid lymphoma

therefore, tends to be a diagnosis of exclusion or made on followup of stable uptake

may use CT to help differentiate (on size, density and morphology characteristics)

NUC MED (Tl)
thallium negative (but need prior proof lymphoma was thallium positive if lymphoma recurrence is the differential)

PET (FDG)
no FDG uptake very helpful (lymphoma unlikely)

thymic rebound usually has low grade or no FDG uptake

lymphoma has avid FDG uptake to the same extent as lymphoma elsewhere

pitfall: treated lymphoma with temporarily reduced FDG avidity

3.20 THYMOMA

DEFINITION

thymic neoplasm of variable malignant potential originating from thymic epithelial cells (not lymphocytes)

EPIDEMIOLOGY

commonest primary thymic tumor (and much less common than lymphoma and metastases)

>40 years old, male = female

40% of thymomas have myasthenia gravis

10% of myasthenia have thymomas

MORPHOLOGY

lobulated firm gray-white mass

cystic change, calcification, necrosis

75% encapsulated

25% macroscopically invasive

MEDULLARY TYPE (thin spindle cells, indolent)

CORTICAL TYPE THYMOMA (plumper cells, aggressive)

THYMIC CARCINOMA

IMAGING

CXR
anterior mediastinal mass

may show calcification

CT
anterior mediastinal mass

thymolipoma: low density

may have cystic and low density areas

often has calcifications

enhances with contrast

ill defined edge suggests invasion

MR
anterior mediastinal mass

low on T1W, high on T2W sequences

may have cystic areas

DIFFERENTIAL

MASS OF LYMPHATIC ORIGIN

THYMIC HYPERPLASIA

OTHER CAUSES OF ANTERIOR MEDIASTINAL MASS

3.21 TRICUSPID VALVE ACQUIRED DISEASE

3.21.1 STENOSIS

ETIOLOGY

RHEUMATIC FEVER

IMAGING

CXR
RA enlargement

Echo
enlarged RA

stenotic jet (quantifiable)

3.21.2 INCOMPETENCE

ETIOLOGY

IV DRUG ABUSE ENDOCARDITIS

RHEUMATIC FEVER

LEAFLET PROLAPSE

FLOPPY OR MYXOMATOUS TV

PAPILLARY MUSCLE ISCHEMIA

IMAGING

Echo
regurgitant non trivial jet

3. CONTRAST MEDIA

3.1 INTRAVASCULAR CONTRAST REACTIONS

EXPECTED EFFECT, NOT AN ADVERSE REACTION

vein distension, possibly stinging
hot flush, possible metallic taste

MINOR ADVERSE REACTION, NOT HYPERSENSITIVITY

nausea and vomiting

MINOR ATOPIC ADVERSE REACTION

skin rash or urticaria
usually develops within minutes of injection,
   but may develop within 24 hours
no evidence of any other adverse reaction
TREATMENT: observation only or
   promethazine (Phenergan) 25–50 mg
   orally or IV, or other antihistamine

MODERATE ATOPIC ADVERSE REACTION

bronchospasm, asthma attack
usually develops within minutes of injection
no evidence of more severe anaphylactoid
   change
in particular, airway NOT compromised;
   blood pressure normal
TREATMENT: salbutamol nebuliser or other
   bronchodilator nebuliser in oxygen; IV
   access; observe very closely for
   progression (?need for adrenaline
   (epinephrine)); consider steroids and
   antihistamines

SEVERE ANAPHYLACTOID ADVERSE REACTION

usually develops immediately or within
   minutes; very unlikely after 1 hour

Prodrome
itching, unexpected coughing and tickling in
   the throat, non definable feeling of
   'doom', urticaria

Reaction
bronchospasm, acute pulmonary edema
facial and laryngeal edema
hypotension, peripheral vasodilation,
   anaphylactic shock
loss of consciousness, fitting
cardiac arrhythmias or arrest

Treatment: this is a dire emergency; treat accordingly

check AIRWAY, BREATHING, CIRCULATION
IV ACCESS
ADRENALINE IM, OR SC, OR EVEN IV
   (monitor ECG) (do not delay if no IV
   access, give IM or SC)
ADRENALINE AMPOULES: 1 mg in 1 ml =
   1:1000 (for SC or IM, or dilute to 10 ml
   for IV); 1 mg in 10 ml = 1:10 000 (for IV)
ADRENALINE ALIQUOTS: 100 micrograms =
   1 ml of 1:10 000 (for IV); 0.1 ml of
   1:1000 (for SC or IM)
ADRENALINE DOSES: give 300–700
   micrograms of adrenaline if IM or SC
   (0.3–0.7 ml of 1:1000 depending on
   patient size); 100 micrograms at a time,
   slowly if IV (1ml of 1:10 000) - monitor
   ECG!
REPEAT ADRENALINE AS NECESSARY,
   usual adult total dose 500–1000
   micrograms, usual child total dose 10
   micrograms per kilogram; larger doses
   or infusion may be needed
OXYGEN with or without salbutamol
   nebuliser
MAINTENANCE OF AIRWAY: intubate if
   desperate; can try nebulized adrenaline
   (5 ml of 1:1000)
IV FLUID for hypotension
DIAZEPAM for fitting
ECG MONITORING, AND CARDIAC
   RESUSCITATION IF ARRHYTHMIA
CARDIOPULMONARY RESUSCITATION/
   DEFIBRILLATION IF NO CARDIAC
   OUTPUT OR ASYSTOLE
STEROIDS (e.g. hydrocortisone 100 mg IV)
   AND ANTIHISTAMINES (e.g.
   promethazine (Phenergan) 25–50 mg IV
   and ranitidine 50 mg IV)

3.2 COMPLICATIONS OF ANGIOGRAPHY

Contrast related complications

TOXICITY

CEREBRAL, CARDIAC, RENAL

OSMOTIC SHIFTS

PREDICTABLE REACTIONS

pain, burning, flushing, vasovagal attacks

IDIOSYNCRATIC REACTIONS

allergic, anaphylactoid and anaphylactic
   reactions

Catheter problems

FAILURE TO CATHETERIZE

DISSECTION

SPASM, TRANSIENT OCCLUSION

THROMBOSIS, PERMANENT
   OCCLUSION

EMBOLISM

air, foreign liquids or solids, thrombus

SEPSIS

Puncture problems

FAILURE TO GAIN ACCESS

DISSECTION

LOCAL DAMAGE TO OTHER
   STRUCTURES

EXTRAVASCULAR INJECTION

THROMBOSIS

ACUTE HEMORRHAGE

FALSE ANEURYSM, AV FISTULA

LOCAL SEPSIS

Complications of intervention

3.3 CONTRAST EXTRAVASATION

Frequency

CT 0.03–0.2%

FREQUENCY OF COMPLICATIONS IS
   1% OF EXTRAVASATIONS (estimates
   of 1/10 to 1/200)

Mechanism

SITE
old IV line (phlebitis, backflow)
butterfly needle ('cut-out')
multiple insertions (puncture holes,
   possibility of malposition)

PATIENT
venous, arterial, lymphatic insufficiency
unable to feel pain or communicate

MECHANISM
malinsertion
phlebitis, backflow, rupture
multiple holes, leakage
pressure overload, rupture

THERE IS NO RELIABLE PREDICTOR
OF WHETHER COMPLICATIONS
WILL OCCUR FOLLOWING
CONTRAST EXTRAVASATION

Pathogenesis

hyperosmolality producing acute
inflammation at 24–48 hours +/– slow
chronic inflammation after that
NECROSIS (direct injury, inflammation)
COMPARTMENT SYNDROME (volume of
injection, inflammatory swelling)
non ionic contrast better than ionic (lower
osmolality)

Injury spectrum

NO PERMANENT INJURY

SKIN ULCERATION/NECROSIS
1/2 heal with no sequelae
1/2 further neural or dermal problems,
problematic contractures

COMPARTMENT SYNDROME

Management

AIMS
clear protocol of management
minimization of secondary effects
adequate documentation
close followup

TREATMENT
aspirate back if possible

ELEVATE, COLD FOR 15–60 MIN THREE
TIMES/ DAY
no convincing evidence for local chemical or
pharmacological treatment

CALL PARENT UNIT/REFERRING DOCTOR

CLOSE OBSERVATION

FOLLOWUP: daily to resolution

CALL PLASTIC SURGEONS IF
>100 ml injected
blistering, increasing pain
neuropathy
decreased perfusion
?compartment syndrome

4. VASCULAR CONDITIONS

4.1 ANEURYSMS (outline)

DEFINITION

true aneurysm: abnormal dilation of all
layers of vessel wall

false aneurysm: partial or complete
penetration of wall by blood with blood
filled cavity in communication with lumen

ETIOLOGY

Aortic

THORACIC ASCENDING
atherosclerosis
trauma
Marfan's syndrome, Ehlers–Danlos syndrome
aortic dissection
ankylosing spondylitis
syphilitic aortitis

THORACOABDOMINAL
atherosclerosis
aortic dissection

ABDOMINAL
atherosclerosis (simple or inflammatory)

AORTOILIAC
atherosclerosis

Cerebral (Ch 11)

CIRCLE OF WILLIS
berry aneurysms

DEEP PERFORATING ARTERIES
Charcot–Bouchard aneurysms

OTHER
traumatic (e.g. anterior communicating
artery under falx)

Other locations

MYCOTIC

ARTERITIC

KAWASAKI'S DISEASE

POLYARTERITIS NODOSA

FALSE ANEURYSMS (trauma, iatrogenic)

IMAGING (generic)

All modalities

abnormal dilation of aorta or artery:
fusiform or saccular
may be outlined by dystrophic calcification
(especially on AXR)
contrast opacifying lumen may
underestimate aneurysm extent filled
with thrombus
cross sectional modalities show contents
(flowing blood, thrombus) and
surrounding tissues (normal fat; soft
tissue ?fibrosis, ?inflammation
?extravasated blood) as well as any
contrast extravasation

CT angio, angio, MR angio
(abdominal aortic aneurysm)

distance of neck to renal artery origins
critical
extension into iliac arteries important
caliber and tortuosity of iliac arteries
determine possibility of endovascular
access
origins of celiac axis, SMA, IMA (may be
thrombosed) need to be identified

4.2 ANTIPHOSPHOLIPID ANTIBODIES

ETIOLOGY

8% of normals, 75% of SLE, other
autoimmune disease, female:male 5:1;
HIV, syphilis

ASSOCIATIONS

peripheral DVT, silent PE, pulmonary
hypertension
cerebral venous thrombosis, intracranial
hypertension
bony avascular necrosis

4.3 AORTIC INJURY

CLINICAL

85% full thickness tear–exsanguination,
death
15% partial thickness (intima + media) tear
interscapular pain, dyspnea, dysphagia,
pulse differentials
if untreated, 50% die within 24 hours, 90%
die within 1 month; remainder: aortic
pseudoaneurysm

Location
85% isthmus (junction of arch and
descending aorta)
10% aortic root/ascending aorta

IMAGING

CXR
frequently normal

MEDIASTINAL HEMATOMA IS NOT
FROM BLOOD LEAKING THROUGH
THE TEAR

CXR SIGNS–BLOOD

HARRIS'S CRITERIA
loss of aortic arch, aortopulmonary window
widened or tall left paravertebral stripe
    (above aortic arch)
left apical pleural cap
abnormal right paratracheal stripe
20% of these patients have aortic injury
    (Harris, Radiology of Emergency
    Medicine)

OTHER
right apical pleural cap
left hemothorax

CXR SIGNS–MASS
mediastinal width >8 cm
left main bronchus depressed
trachea/esophagus deviated
paraaortic mass
aortic intimal calcification displaced

CXR SIGNS–SEVERE TRAUMA
thoracic inlet fractures
multiple l rib fractures

CT
mediastinal hematoma, effusions
completely negative: 100% negative
    predictive value
dynamic contrast CT may show focal dilation
    or subintimal contrast tracking

Angio
still the gold standard
need multiple views
intimal tear, subintimal contrast tracking
focal dilation (classically junction of arch
    and descending aorta)
traumatic pseudoaneurysm

BEWARE
resistance to catheter/wire advance (in an
    otherwise normal aorta) indicates entry
    into tear/dissection or false aneurysm
if in doubt, gentle hand injection and look

ANGIO DIFFERENTIAL: ductus diverticulum
10% of population
level with ligamentum arteriosum
regular contour, smooth intima

4.4 ATHEROSCLEROSIS

DEFINITION

diffuse proliferative process involving intima
    of major arteries with well understood
    late stages leading to predictable end
    organ disease

EPIDEMIOLOGY AND RISK FACTORS

commonest cause of death; silent in itself
    and therefore assessed on incidence and
    prevalence of clinical endpoints;
    decreasing (male), increasing (female)

Hard risk factors

CORRECTABLE
SMOKING
HYPERTENSION
DYSLIPIDEMIA
DIABETES MELLITUS

FIXED
MALE GENDER
AGE
ADVERSE FAMILY HISTORY

Soft risk factors
OBESITY
TYPE A PERSONALITY
HORMONAL DISORDERS
etc

CLINICAL

ischemic heart disease
cerebral infarcts
renal ischemia, renovascular hypertension
mesenteric ischemia
claudication, leg resting ischemia, impotence
aneurysms

MORPHOLOGY

Fatty streak
subintimal flat yellow collections of foam
    cells
occur at ostia, bifurcation points and points
    of turbulence
all children >10 years manifest some fatty
    streaks

Fibrofatty plaque (hallmark)
FIBROUS CAP: collagen, smooth muscle
    cells, ground substance (proteoglycans)
FATTY LAYER: foam cells (macrophages and
    smooth muscle cells), free lipid
    (cholesterol and triglycerides),
    incorporated thrombus, ground
    substance, activated macrophages and T
    lymphocytes, neovascularization (from
    periphery inwards)
underlying media slowly atrophies and thins
    out, eventually leading to aneurysmal
    disease
occur at points of hemodynamic turbulence,
    usually eccentric

number, size and extent proportional to
    severity and duration

Complicated plaque

CALCIFIED
patchy or extensive dystrophic calcification

ULCERATED
brittle plaque can fissure from
    hemodynamic changes, movement or
    intraplaque hemorrhage
break in the fibrous cap exposes soft
    amorphous necrotic core to arterial
    lumen
atheroembolism (carotid, renal, lower limb)
thrombogenesis with adherent mural
    thrombus (luminal occlusion)

HEMORRHAGIC
intraplaque neovascularity leading to
    intraplaque hemorrhage (sudden
    ulceration or lumen occlusion)

Distribution

AORTA
abdominal > thoracic
ostia of major branches (arch branches,
    renal and mesenteric arteries, iliac
    arteries) and smaller branches (e.g.
    segmental arteries)
aneurysmal disease of aorta itself
occlusive disease of branches
occlusion of distal aorta (Leriche syndrome:
    claudication and impotence)

ILIACS
external > internal
aneurysmal or occlusive disease

FEMORAL, POPLITEAL, RUNOFF
largely occlusive disease, also popliteal
    aneurysms
isolated or multiple, short or long segment
    stenoses
total occlusions
extensive collateral formation, distal
    reconstitution

RENAL
ostial stenoses
proximal occlusive atheroma

CAROTID AND INTRACEREBRAL ARTERIES
carotid bifurcation, ICA origin and bulb
    (occlusive)
aortic origin of CCA
intracerebral carotid (and vertebral) diffuse
    or focal atheroma (often calcifies)

CORONARY ARTERIES
isolated or multiple, focal or diffuse
    stenoses; origins and bifurcations

IMAGING (general comments)

X-ray

does not differentiate plaque from
dystrophic medial calcification
does not show degree of stenosis

US

PLAQUE CHARACTERIZATION

SMOOTH vs ROUGH

CALCIFIED (shadowing) vs SOFT

SOFT PLAQUE

INTIMAL THICKENING

HOMOGENEOUS

HETEROGENEOUS/COMPLEX

(FOCAL ANECHOIC AREAS INDICATE
HEMORRHAGE)

CROSS SECTIONAL LUMEN MEASUREMENT

COLOR OR POWER DOPPLER

visual detection of accelerated flow

THROMBOSIS

artery filled with echogenic material with no
color or Doppler signal

Doppler ultrasound

*also see: Ch 10 carotid Doppler, Ch 08 renal
artery Doppler*

TECHNICAL PITFALLS

aliasing
sample volume in wrong place or wrong size
too much wall filter
wrong color/2D write priority
breathing or movement artifact
insonation angle too close to 90 degrees
(above 60 degrees unreliable)
wrong angle correction (for absolute velocity
measurements)

PEAK SYSTOLIC VELOCITY (PSV) RATIOS (general comments)

assumption of laminar flow
PSV taken at or just through the stenosis
and above the stenosis
ratios <2:1 not hemodynamically significant
(i.e. <50%)
PSV ratio 2:1 implies ~50% stenosis
PSV ratio 3:1 implies >75% stenosis
PSV ratio 4:1 implies >90% stenosis
ratios not reliable downstream of a tight
stenosis where normal velocity profile
and waveform do not reconstitute
OCCLUSION: 'thump at the stump' (reflected
waveform); does not reliably differentiate
from critical stenosis with residual trickle
flow

WAVEFORM ANALYSIS (general comments)

NORMAL RESISTIVE
triphasic or biphasic with rapid upstroke
and falloff, little spectral broadening
high resistive index ((systolic velocity–
diastolic velocity)/systolic velocity)
fasting mesenteric, peripheral limb,
infrarenal aorta, external carotid

NORMAL CAPACITIVE
rapid upstroke, gentle downstroke with
persistent diastolic flow
largely silent 'acoustic window' under
waveform
low resistive index
internal carotid, renal, post prandial
mesenteric

MORPHOLOGY CHANGES AT STENOSIS
spectral broadening
elevation of PSV
elevation in diastolic velocity

MORPHOLOGY CHANGES POST STENOSIS
'tardus parvus' : slow upstroke, low volume
plateau
spectral broadening
loss of normal waveform
low velocity, poorly phasic flow

Electron beam CT (coronary calcium)

see Ch 14, ischemic heart disease

CT angiography (general comments)

large contrast load, multislice helical
volumetric acquisition
2D and 3D reformatting with post processing
subject to metal, breathing and motion
artifact
difficulty differentiating contrast from bone
(e.g. Circle of Willis)
allows demonstration of vessel wall and
atheromatous plaque as well as flowing
lumen

MR angiography

protocols evolving and depend on machine
specifics
'white blood' time of flight MRA (no
contrast) – may overestimate stenoses
3D contrast enhanced MRA currently best
technique
subject to metal, breathing and motion
artifact
interpretation (once artifacts excluded)
subject to same morphology criteria as
catheter angiography

Angio

SIMPLE PLAQUE

focal narrowing with smooth edge and
smooth even shoulders, may have
calcification

COMPLICATED PLAQUE

sharp shoulders, overhanging plaque
erosions and ulcers into plaque, central
craters
irregular uneven edge

HEMODYNAMICALLY SIGNIFICANT PLAQUE

'angiographically significant' coronary
stenosis is >70% diameter reduction (but
50% for main left coronary artery)
'angiographically significant' stenosis
elsewhere varies from 70% to 85%
diameter reduction
collaterals always indicate hemodynamic
significance
slow contrast flow through stenosis

COMPLETE OCCLUSION

no flow through a segment
possibly late reconstitution distally by
collaterals

4.5 AV MALFORMATIONS

see hereditary hemorrhagic telangiectasia

4.6 BLOOD VESSEL TUMORS (overview)

BENIGN

4.6.1 Hemangioma

4.6.1.1 CAPILLARY HEMANGIOMA

CUTANEOUS (strawberry nevus)

CNS CAPILLARY TELANGIECTASIA (Ch 11)

4.6.1.2 CAVERNOUS HEMANGIOMA

CNS HEMANGIOMA (Ch 11)

LIVER HEMANGIOMA (Ch 07)

SKELETAL HEMANGIOMA (Ch 05)

DEEP SOFT TISSUE HEMANGIOMA (Ch 05)

CUTANEOUS HEMANGIOMA

MUCOSAL HEMANGIOMA

4.6.2 Lymphangioma

INTERMEDIATE AGGRESSIVITY

4.6.3 Liver hemangioendothelioma (Ch 18)

4.6.4 Skeletal hemangioendothelioma (Ch 05)

4.6.5 Epithelioid hemangioendothelioma

4.6.6 Hemangioblastoma (Ch 11)

MALIGNANT

4.6.7 Angiosarcoma (Ch 05)

4.6.8 Hemangiopericytoma

CNS HEMANGIOPERICYTOMA

DEEP SKELETAL HEMANGIOPERICYTOMA

4.6.9 Kaposi's sarcoma (Ch 05)

4.7 DEEP VENOUS THROMBOSIS (DVT)

also see Ch 13 pulmonary embolism

ETIOLOGY

Immobilization
IMMOBILIZATION
PROLONGED TRAVEL
POSTOPERATIVE

Proximal obstruction
PELVIC MASS
PREGNANCY
OBESITY
RIGHT HEART FAILURE

Hyperviscosity
PREGNANCY
PARANEOPLASTIC
CONGENITAL (PROTEIN S DEFICIENCY)

Upper limb DVT
ASSOCIATED WITH PACEMAKERS AND CATHETERS

IMAGING

Fluoro (venography)
gold standard for iliac veins and IVC; gold standard for leg veins (but not first line)
bilateral arm venogram required for adequate brachiocephalic vein and SVC demonstration (may try to backfill internal jugular veins by using Valsalva maneuver)

ACUTE DVT
filling defect in two or more views
DVT forms acute angles with vein wall
abrupt vein cutoff
non opacification of vein lumen (DIFFERENTIAL: absent vein, other causes of non filling)

CHRONIC DVT
irregular lumen with murally based masses
webs, recanalization with multiple channels

US
first line investigation for DVT
graded compression US usually with color/power Doppler
accuracy above knee good; below knee depends on patient factors and is poorer in larger legs with edema
US has 'blind spots' in external iliac veins and IVC (overlying gas), behind the jaw (for IJV) and behind the medial clavicle

ACUTE DVT
hypoechoic solid material within vein lumen
non compressible (but soft acute thrombus may be deformable particularly in the jugular veins)
vein may be expanded
no Doppler or color flow; may have thin cuff of residual flowing blood around thrombus

CHRONIC DVT
irregular murally based masses with gradual restoration of flow
may develop deep venous incompetence
distinction between acute and chronic DVT difficult

CT
central thrombus, often with a thin ring of surrounding contrast enhanced blood

extensive collaterals in chronic SVC or IVC thrombosis

MR
persistently altered venous signal (classically high on T1W)
filing defects with contrast venography
phase contrast venography most accurate
see entry on cerebral sinus thrombosis Ch 11

Angio
intravenous filling defects, may be mobile, may be rounded and regular or irregular and thread-like
contrast flows around thrombus
prelude to thrombolysis or IVC or SVC filter insertion

PET (FDG)
differentiates bland from tumoral thrombus (tumoral thrombus FDG avid)

4.8 FIBROMUSCULAR HYPERPLASIA (FMH)

DEFINITION

fibrous cellular proliferation of uncertain etiology occurring in any layer of (large) arterial wall producing stenoses and predisposing to dissection

CLINICAL

younger adults (25–50 years), female > male, family history
carotid FMH associated with intracerebral aneurysms
RENAL ARTERIES (commonest) – renovascular hypertension
HEAD AND NECK (CAROTID AND VERTEBRAL) – associated with dissection
MESENTERIC ARTERIES

IMAGING

Angio
'string of beads': multifocal short stenoses alternating with focal areas of dilation
may show a dissection flap or occlusion related to dissection
renal artery: mid artery
carotid: distal internal carotid at base of skull

4.9 HEREDITARY HEMORRHAGIC TELANGIECTASIA (HHT, Osler–Weber–Rendu syndrome)

DEFINITION

autosomal dominant syndrome of angiodysplasia and multiple AV malformations

EPIDEMIOLOGY

autosomal dominant; strong (but incomplete) penetrance and variable expressivity
incidence 2/100 000
at least 80% of patients with pulmonary AV malformations (AVMs) and all patients with multiple pulmonary AVMs have HHT

CLINICAL

principal morbidity is from cerebroembolic complications of pulmonary AV malformations (bland or septic) and from repeated gastrointestinal or urinary blood loss

Skin and mucosal surfaces

oral and nasal mucosal telangiectasias
frequent epistaxes

GIT

gastrointestinal mucosal telangiectasias, telangiectatic polyps, AV malformations
upper and lower GIT hemorrhages

CNS

intracranial AV malformations (~30%)
intracranial hemorrhages
cerebral abscesses, cerebral infarcts

Lungs

pulmonary AV malformations
paradoxical embolism (bland or septic), hemoptysis
10% present in childhood: right to left shunt with cyanosis or heart failure
90% present as adults

Liver

AV malformations (~30%); possibly portal hypertension

Urinary

mucosal telangiectasias and AVMs
hematuria

IMAGING

CXR

solitary or multiple soft tissue masses often with vascular 'tails'

CT

chest AVMs, liver AVMs (hepatic artery origin)
pancreatic AVMs fed by dilated arteries

NUC MED

MAA deposition in systemic vascular beds (especially brain)
first pass autologous RBC study is done for quantitation of the shunt

Angio

CLASSICAL ARTERIOVENOUS MALFORMATION (AVM)
nidus with arterial phase vascular enhancement
arterial channels, early venous drainage (often dilated), feeder aneurysms, intranidal aneurysms, draining vein stenoses
CAPILLARY/SMALL VESSEL ANGIOMA
contrast blush in capillary phase
HEREDITARY HEMORRHAGIC TELANGIECTASIA, COLONIC ANGIODYSPLASIA

4.10 HYPERTENSION (HT)

DEFINITION

WHO DEFINITION

	NORMAL	BORDERLINE	DEFINITE HT
SBP	< 140	SBP 140–160	SPB > 160
DBP	< 90	DBP 90–95	DBP > 95

EPIDEMIOLOGY (primary HT)

Gaussian distribution with arbitrary cutoff
RISK FACTORS: family history, dietary (sodium intake, other)
prevalence female > male; black > white; complications male > female

ETIOLOGY (secondary HT)

Renal

RENOVASCULAR
GLOMERULONEPHRITIS
REFLUX NEPHROPATHY
ANALGESIC NEPHROPATHY
DIABETIC NEPHROPATHY
POLYCYSTIC KIDNEY DISEASE
PRIMARY RENINOMA

Endocrine

CUSHING'S SYNDROME
CONN'S SYNDROME
PHEOCHROMOCYTOMA
ADRENOGENITAL SYNDROMES

Preeclampsia, eclampsia

CLINICAL

Benign HT

hypertensive cardiac changes (LV concentric hypertrophy)
cerebral berry aneurysms, hypertensive hemorrhages
(eventually) granular small kidneys
atherosclerosis

Malignant (accelerated phase) HT

develops on background of benign HT, but may be first overt presentation
BP usually >220/140
headaches, visual disturbances
papilloedema, retinal hemorrhages
proteinuria, hematuria, renal failure
hypertensive encephalopathy, obtundation, fits

4.11 LYMPHEDEMA

DEFINITION

abnormal accumulation of tissue fluid secondary to lymphatic insufficiency

CLINICAL

Cancer related

TUMOR INFILTRATION

BLOCK LYMPH NODE DISSECTION

RADIOTHERAPY

Not cancer related

ACUTE POST OPERATIVE

MILROY'S DISEASE (congenital)

PRIMARY LYMPHEDEMA

SECONDARY LYMPHEDEMA

VENOUS INSUFFICIENCY

FILARIASIS

CHRONIC INFLAMMATION

IMAGING

US

increased subcutaneous tissue thickness

may have lymphoceles at sites of nodal
dissection

MR

heavily T2 weighted sequences show
increased T2W signal and swelling of
subcutaneous tissues and may show
abnormally dilated fluid filled lymphatic
channels ('MR lymphangiography') where
these are present (e.g. Milroy's disease)

NUC MED (colloid scan)

subdermal injection (classically toe web
spaces)

non demonstration of lymphatic channels
and nodes

delayed demonstration of lymphatic
channels and nodes

increased soft tissue colloid activity

(moderate liver activity is normal and colloid
may enter the circulation either via direct
venous absorption or via lymphatic
return to great veins)

4.12 MARFAN'S SYNDROME

autosomal dominant abnormality of collagen
and elastin

tall with arachnodactyly and high arched
palate

ocular lens subluxation

ligamentous laxity, joint subluxations

aortic dissection, aortoannular ectasia,
aortic valve insufficiency and
regurgitation

4.13 MONCKEBERG'S ARTERIOSCLEROSIS

age related progressive calcification of large
artery media unrelated to atherosclerosis

limbs, head and neck

medial hyalinization, calcification,
ossification

major differential is atheromatous
calcification

DOES NOT ENCROACH ON LUMEN

4.14 PULMONARY HYPERTENSION AND ARTERIOPATHY

see Ch 13

4.15 RETROPERITONEAL AND MEDIASTINAL FIBROSIS

CLINICAL

chronic inflammation centered on the aorta
(most likely caused by transudation of
antigenically abnormal lipids) with
eventual occlusion of adjacent structures

ATHEROSCLEROTIC (older, male > female)

OTHER: methysergide, drugs

inflammatory component may respond to
steroids

SUBTYPES

RETROPERITONEAL FIBROSIS (firm mass
symmetrically centered on aorta): medial
deviation of ureters, occlusion of adjacent
structures; fibrosis at base of mesentery

FIBROSING MEDIASTINITIS: centered on
descending aorta (rare)

INFLAMMATORY ANEURYSM

IMAGING

IVP

deviation of both ureters medially at lumbar
levels

variable degree of smooth extrinsic
compression

CT

soft tissue density mass centered on normal
diameter or aneurysmal lumbar aorta,
usually at lower lumbar levels

deviation of ureters into mass and loss of
intervening fat planes

compression or narrowing of IVC

soft tissue may enhance with contrast (slow
non vascular enhancement) when active
or be non enhancing when mature

DIFFERENTIAL DIAGNOSIS: scirrhous
retroperitoneal tumor

MR

mass low signal on T1W and T2W
sequences

variable enhancement with contrast (see
CT); generally enhances if in acute
inflammation phase

DIFFERENTIALS

hematoma from aortic hemorrhage is bright
on T2W

lymphomatous tissue may be bright on T2W

4.16 SPONTANEOUS AORTIC DISSECTION

ETIOLOGY

HYPERTENSION (up to 90%)

ABNORMAL COLLAGEN

Marfan's syndrome

Ehlers–Danlos syndrome

ABNORMAL AORTIC VALVE

stenosis

bicuspid valve

PREVIOUS AORTIC VALVE/AORTIC SURGERY

AORTIC COARCTATION

CLINICAL

chest or interscapular pain +/– unequal or
absent pulses

aortic regurgitant murmur

neurological deficit, acute renal failure

tamponade

exsanguination, sudden death

CLASSIFICATION

(2/3) Stanford A:
dissection involves ascending aorta or arch
entry commonly just above aortic valve
anterior and to the right

(1/3) Stanford B:
dissection involves descending aorta only
entry commonly distal to L subclavian artery
posteriorly and to the left

IMAGING

CXR
change in aortic diameter (>1 cm)
aortic calcification displaced away from
outer aortic contour by more than
expected wall thickness (DIFFERENTIAL:
mural thrombus)
left pleural effusion, acute pericardial
effusion

SIGNS OF MEDIASTINAL HEMATOMA
change in mediastinal contour
widened mediastinum (40–80%)
displaced trachea, left main bronchus, etc

Angio
depending on distal extent of dissection,
catheter entry is usually into true lumen
but occasionally may be into false lumen

ANGIO TECHNIQUE
gentle hand injection to differentiate true
from false lumen if in doubt
soft tip wire
can puncture other side if first puncture is
into false lumen

ANGIO SIGNS
cardinal signs: dissection flap, narrowed
true lumen, patent false lumen, double
lumen
distorted or compressed true lumen, major
branch cutoffs
false lumen spirals, opacifies slowly, washes
out late
'double lumen': false lumen has a re-entry
tear distally and may have same rate of
flow as true lumen (dissection flap
separates the two)
aortic valve regurgitation

BEWARE THROMBOSED DISSECTION
false lumen does not opacify with contrast
true lumen shape distortion and branch
cutoffs still present

CT angio
shows dissection flap well in cross section
patent false lumen: opacifies with flowing
blood (same or delayed compared to true
lumen)
thrombosed false lumen: clot (usually denser
than atheroma)
pericardial fluid or blood
contrast leaks
non opacification of major branch vessels (or
even dissection extending into them)
dilation of aorta
BEWARE MISSED AORTIC REGURGITATION
(not obvious on CT because of uniform
contrast enhancement)

Echo (transesophageal)
direct visualization of flap and lumens +/–
aortic regurgitation
shows flow in false lumen
access to descending aorta limited and does
not show origins of major abdominal
branches

MR
morphology as for CT
sagittal and coronal planes may show
dissection flap as well
cine MR shows aortic regurgitation

FALSE LUMEN CONTENTS
cobwebs (strands of medial elastin)
thrombus (with blood product signal)
flowing blood producing flow void

BEWARE CHEMICAL SHIFT ARTIFACT
apparent thickening of one aortic wall
mimicking compressed false lumen

4.17 SYSTEMIC LUPUS ERYTHEMATOSUS (SLE)

DEFINITION
immune complex disease with nephritis,
vasculitis and skin involvement
secondary to multiple autoantibodies

EPIDEMIOLOGY
variable incidence ~1/3000
female:male 9:1, black > white, young adult
peak
HLA DR4 associated
family history of SLE, monozygotic
concordance ~25%

CLINICAL
presentation highly variable

Classical
young female with malar skin rash,
inflammatory polyarthropathy,
polyserositis and glomerulonephritis;
relapsing and remitting course

Drug induced
caused by hydralazine, procainamide,
isoniazid, other
no nephritis
remits with cessation of drug

MORPHOLOGY
see indicated chapters for imaging

Mnemonic: MASH LUCK

M-yositis
small vessel arteritis, fibrinoid deposits in
arterial wall

A-rthritis with A-VN (Ch 02)
non erosive symmetric inflammatory
arthropathy, engorged infiltrated
synovium, effusions

AVN IN 30% (SLE or SLE and steroids)
femoral head, humeral head, knee, talus
(specific to SLE), hands and feet (specific
to SLE)

S-kin lesions (UV sensitive)
characteristic malar rash (50%)
variable edema and infiltration of dermis
fibrinoid small vessel vasculitis

and S-erositis
pericarditis
painful pleurisy

H-eart disease
Libman–Sacks endocarditis
pericarditis

and H-ematology
multiple autoantibodies (type III and type II
reactions)
antinuclear antibodies (these are not specific
to SLE)
anti double strand DNA antibodies (highly
specific)
antiphospholipid antibodies

lupus cells (neutrophils that have ingested a
    fragment of nucleus)
hemolytic anemia
leukopenia
lymphopenia
thrombocytopenia

LU-ng (Ch 13)

painful pleurisy with effusions
interstitial pneumonitis, eventual fibrosis

C-oagulopathy

anticoagulant effect in vitro
procoagulant effect in vivo
arterial thromboses, strokes
venous thromboses, DVT, PE, cerebral
    infarcts
midtrimester abortions

and C-NS (major morbidity) (Ch 11)

1. as a result of coagulopathy
2. postulated small vessel vasculitis
3. unknown mechanism neuropsychiatric
    syndromes

K-idney (major morbidity, mortality)

GLOMERULONEPHRITIS
hematuria, hypertension, nephritic
    syndrome, nephrotic syndrome
eventual renal failure

4.18 VASCULITIDES OVERVIEW

PULMONARY VASCULITIDES: see Ch 13

ETIOLOGY

Non infective vasculitis

PRIMARY VASCULITIS
numerically most common
'vasculitis' without any further qualification
    implies primary vasculitis

PART OF GENERALIZED IMMUNE
    COMPLEX DISEASE
SYSTEMIC LUPUS ERYTHEMATOSUS
SCLERODERMA VASCULITIS, CREST
ANKYLOSING SPONDYLITIS
RHEUMATOID VASCULITIS
BEHÇET'S SYNDROME

Infective vasculitis

MYCOTIC ANEURYSMS

TB VASCULITIS

SECONDARY IMMUNE MEDIATED VASCULITIS

FUNGAL VASCULITIS

ANGIOCENTRIC ANGIOINVASIVE

SECONDARY IMMUNE MEDIATED

SYPHILITIC VASCULITIS

IMMUNE MEDIATED

Host vs graft disease

ACUTE REJECTION

Graft vs host disease

SMALL VESSEL DISEASE:
    PULMONARY, HEPATIC

COMPLICATIONS

LOCAL
perivascular inflammation
aneurysm formation

DISTAL
thrombosis, distal infarcts

HEALING PHASE COMPLICATIONS
scarring, fibrosis, disorganization

IMAGING (general comments)

in general, imaging findings are either of
    involved vessels (these need to be
    sufficiently large to be visible) or of end
    organ damage (usually infarcts)

CXR/CT

pulmonary infarcts
findings vary from no findings to cavitating
    masses

CT/MR

show distribution and size of masses in
    Wegener's granulomatosis

CT angio/MR angio

in general, useful only in large vessel
    vasculitis (e.g. Takayasu's arteritis)
may show segmental infarcts in
    parenchymal organs

Angio

large or small artery stenoses, occlusions or
    aneurysms

NUC MED (V/Q)

unmatched perfusion defects
classic differential for PE

4.19 VASCULITIS – LARGE ARTERIES

4.19.1 TAKAYASU'S ARTERITIS

CLINICAL

granulomatous arteritis of aorta and its
    large branches (stenosis dominant)
    affecting younger patients
female > male, commoner in Asia
early: mild inflammatory symptoms
established: 'pulseless disease' with visual
    and cerebral disturbances
NO LAB MARKERS

IMAGING

Angio

focal and multifocal orificial stenoses of
    aorta and major aortic branches
    (uncommonly, these have dystrophic
    calcification)
smooth and circumferential, short or long
    segment
brachiocephalic, common carotid,
    subclavian origins
occasionally aorta itself
usually not cerebral circulation
aneurysms uncommon

4.21.2 GIANT CELL (TEMPORAL) ARTERITIS

CLINICAL

granulomatous aortocranial arteritis of large
    arteries
commonest primary vasculitis
older patient with visual disturbance
    progressing to blindness
temporal artery and scalp tenderness (may
    necrose) and headache
jaw claudication (may have tongue necrosis)
markedly elevated ESR, may have anemia
overlap with polymyalgia rheumatica
good response to steroids
NO LAB MARKERS
requires biopsy of sufficient length, as
    lesions are discontinuous

IMAGING

Angio

multifocal large vessel stenoses especially at branchpoints

distribution: aorta (giant cell aortitis), temporal arteries, ophthalmic arteries, external carotid branches

4.20 VASCULITIS – MUSCULAR ARTERIES

4.20.1 CLASSICAL POLYARTERITIS NODOSA (PAN)

EPIDEMIOLOGY

young adults, male > female

1/3 hepatitis B (HBV) serology positive, 5% hepatitis C (HCV) serology positive

classical PAN not associated with P-ANCA (P-antineutrophil cytoplasmic antibody)

CLINICAL

relapsing and remitting cardiovisceral neutrophilic muscular artery arteritis

forms small aneurysms at branch points; metachronous lesions

symptoms are secondary to endorgan ischemia

NO GLOMERULONEPHRITIS OR PULMONARY ANGIITIS by definition

often confused with microscopic PAN variant (which is more common); an overlap syndrome also exists

Mnemonic: GLICK

50%   G-UT
ischemia, infarcts, GIT bleeding, abdominal pain, bowel perforations

65%   LI-VER
ischemia, infarcts, hepatitis B

75%   C-ARDIAC
coronary arteritis, ischemia, infarcts, death

85%   K-IDNEY
ischemic nephropathy, infarcts, hypertension, renal failure

also peripheral neuropathy

Lab markers

HBV, HCV serology
elevated ESR

IMAGING

Angio

microaneurysms (up to 10 mm) at branchpoints in splanchnic beds

multifocal stenoses

branch or main visceral artery occlusion (50%)

4.20.2 KAWASAKI'S DISEASE

= 'mucocutaneous lymph node syndrome'

CLINICAL

childhood coronary neutrophilic arteritis WITH

fever unresponsive to antibiotics

trunkal rash, palm + sole erythema and desquamation

oral and conjunctival erythema and erosions

acute non suppurative cervical lymphadenopathy

2% incidence of sudden death (myocardial infarction or coronary aneurysm rupture)

Lab marker

antiendothelial cell antibodies

ANGIO

coronary aneurysms and occlusions in a child

4.21 VASCULITIS – ARTERIOLOVENULAR

4.21.1 MICROSCOPIC VARIANT OF POLYARTERITIS NODOSA (PAN)

neutrophilic angiitis of small arteries with infarcts and necrosis

more common than classic PAN

mimics Wegener's granulomatosis

pulmonary vasculitis

glomerulonephritis

may involve visceral territories of classic PAN

Lab marker

P-ANCA

4.21.2 WEGENER'S GRANULOMATOSIS

see its own entry

4.22 VASCULITIS – MICROSCOPIC VESSELS

4.22.1 LEUKOCYTOCLASTIC VASCULITIS

microscopic neutrophilic vasculitis with leukocytoclasis and petechial hemorrhages

GI bleeds, hematuria and hemoptysis with palpable purpura and neurological symptoms

4.22.2 HENOCH–SCHÖNLEIN PURPURA

see Ch 16 hematology

4.23 VASCULITIS – OTHER

4.23.1 BUERGER'S DISEASE (thromboangiitis obliterans)

CLINICAL

30–50 year old heavy smokers, male > female

rare in USA, common in Israel, Japan, India

intermittent claudication or painful ischemia, usually below knees

segmental vasculitis of small and medium size arteries, particularly in lower limbs

inflammation involves entire neurovascular bundle including adjacent veins and nerves

stopping smoking may lead to remission

IMAGING

Angio

distribution of occlusions and stenoses restricted to lower limbs, and is multifocal rather than diffuse

no evidence of more widespread disease (i.e. no evidence of atherosclerosis)

4.23.2 RAYNAUD'S PHENOMENON AND DISEASE

DEFINITION

RAYNAUD'S PHENOMENON: intense acral vasospasm followed by reactive hyperemia (white–blue–red disease)

RAYNAUD'S DISEASE: idiopathic Raynaud's phenomenon

ETIOLOGY

Idiopathic (Raynaud's disease)
young females, benign natural history cured by sympathectomy

Vascular causes
CERVICAL RIB
INJURY INCLUDING COLD INJURY
BUERGER'S DISEASE
SYSTEMIC LUPUS ERYTHEMATOSUS
SCLERODERMA

Neurological disease

Vibrating power tools

4.23.3 SYPHILITIC AORTITIS

syphilitic vasculitis of aortic vasa vasorum with slowly progressive dilation and weakening of ascending aortic wall

CLINICAL/IMAGING

rare; 30% have negative syphilis serology
ascending aorta > arch >> descending
'tree bark' intima obscured by atheroma
40% syphilitic saccular aneurysms
30% coronary ostial stenosis
all – eventual aortic root dilation, aortic regurgitation

DIFFERENTIAL: atherosclerotic aneurysm, other causes of aneurysm

4.24 WEGENER'S GRANULOMATOSIS

DEFINITION

necrotizing autoimmune granulomatous vasculitis with local inflammatory destructive masses and arterial downstream infarcts, characteristically upper and lower respiratory tract with glomerulonephritis

CLINICAL

middle aged adults, male > female, white > black
untreated has mortality of 90–100%
ANCA-C associated

Mnemonic: LiNK JEES CC

L-ung (95%)
necrotizing vasculitis
cavitating infarcts
cough, dyspnea, hemoptysis

N-asopharynx and sinuses (90%)
sinusitis, necrosis, masses, destruction, discharge
tracheal and bronchial masses and stenosis
see Ch 12

K-idney (85%)
glomerulonephritis (GN)
arteritis
death of renal failure if untreated

J-oints (60%)
arthralgia

E-ye (60%)
dacryocystitis
uveitis, episcleritis, orbital pseudotumor

E-ar (60%)
blocked auditory tube with otitis media

S-kin (40%)
leukocytoclastic vasculitis with granulomas

C-NS (20%)
cranial nerve mononeuropathies
mononeuritis multiplex

C-ardiac (10%)
coronary vasculitis

IMAGING

CXR/CT (lungs)
multiple pulmonary masses (granulomas and/or infarcts)
may cavitate leaving irregular thick walled cavities
tend to resolve and recur
airspace irregular opacities (pulmonary hemorrhage)
pleural effusions
usually no lymphadenopathy
tracheal or bronchial granulomas may cause diffuse narrowing or focal obstruction

CT/MR (sinonasal)
sinonasal mucosal thickening
sinonasal soft tissue masses or nodules
facial/nasal bone destruction

MR (trachea)
used in assessment of trachea and larynx
destructive soft tissue masses with loss of cartilage
surrounding edema with high T2W signal

16 Hematology

This text follows: WHO Classification of Tumors: Pathology & Genetics, Tumors of Hematopoietic and Lymphoid Tissues, edited by ES Jaffe, NL Harris, H Stein, JW Vardiman, IARC Press, Lyon, 2001 (or J Clin Oncol 1999; 17:3835–3849)

2. GAMUTS

2.1 GENERIC

2.1.1 ANEMIA

Classification and etiological gamut

INCREASED RED CELL LOSS

HEMORRHAGIC ANEMIA

OVERT HEMORRHAGE (e.g. menorrhagia)*

OCCULT HEMORRHAGE (usually GIT)*

HEMOLYTIC ANEMIA (abnormal RBC)*

ACQUIRED

LEAD POISONING*

PAROXYSMAL NOCTURNAL
HEMOGLOBINURIA

RHESUS DISEASE (Ch 22)

CONGENITAL

SPHEROCYTOSIS*

HEMOGLOBINOPATHIES

THALASSEMIA#

SICKLE CELL DISEASE#

OTHER

G6PD (glucose 6 phosphate dehydrogenase)
DEFICIENCY

HEMOLYTIC ANEMIA (normal RBC)*

AUTOANTIBODIES

MALARIA*

HYPERSPLENISM WITH RBC DESTRUCTION*

DRUGS

PARANEOPLASTIC*

MECHANICAL TRAUMA (e.g. prosthetic valve)*

MICROANGIOPATHY (e.g. TTP/HUS)

DECREASED RED CELL PRODUCTION

NUTRITIONAL

B12 AND FOLATE (megaloblastic anemia)*

IRON (microcytic hypochromic anemia)

OTHER

protein, vitamin B6, vitamin C, copper

APLASTIC

HYPOPLASTIC BONE MARROW

CHEMOTHERAPY

CONGENITAL (Fanconi anemia)

OTHER

PURE RED CELL APLASIA

CONGENITAL (Diamond-Blackfan syndrome)

ASSOCIATED WITH SLE#

ASSOCIATED WITH THYMOMA#

BONE MARROW INFILTRATION OR FIBROSIS*

MYELODYSPLASIA*

'ANEMIA OF CHRONIC DISEASE'

RENAL (erythropoietin and other cause)#

HEPATIC#

ENDOCRINE#

CHRONIC INFECTION (e.g. TB)#

AUTOIMMUNE DISEASE (e.g. rheumatoid
arthritis)#

INDOLENT MALIGNANCY (e.g. lymphoma)#

Imaging findings

* MAY HAVE IMAGING FINDINGS

HEMORRHAGE

LABELED RBC GIT LOSS STUDY

ALL HEMOLYTIC ANEMIAS

INCREASED INCIDENCE OF GALLSTONES

BONE MARROW EXPANSION IF
LONGSTANDING AND SEVERE (esp
thalassemias)

SPLENOMEGALY

LEAD POISONING (XR)
dense metaphyseal lines in children

SPHEROCYTOSIS: SPLENOMEGALY

MALARIA: HEPATOSPLENOMEGALY

HYPERSPLENISM: SPLENOMEGALY +/–
portal venous hypertension

MECHANICAL VALVE (CXR)

PARANEOPLASTIC (various)

B12/FOLATE ANEMIA

SUBACUTE COMBINED DEGENERATION OF
THE CORD
(Ch 11)

ATROPHIC GASTRITIS (Ch 06)

BONE MARROW INFILTRATION OR FIBROSIS
altered bone marrow signal on MR
loss of sulfur colloid uptake in bone marrow
see myelofibrosis (Ch 02)
may see dense bones on XR (myelosclerosis)

HAS IMAGING FINDINGS
see separate entry for each entity

2.1.2 COAGULOPATHIES RELEVANT TO PROCEDURES

Normal
in general (in the absence of known
coagulopathies), procedures do not carry
increased risk at APTT <36 s, INR <1.1,
plt >200 (per nl)

in general, normal platelets with platelet
count >75 carries minimal increased risk

Reduced platelet count or platelet dysfunction

DECREASED PRODUCTION

APLASTIC ANEMIA/MYELODYSPLASIA

BONE MARROW INFILTRATION

CHEMOTHERAPY

HIV

INCREASED DESTRUCTION

IMMUNE

AUTOIMMUNE

IDIOPATHIC THROMBOCYTOPENIC PURPURA

SYSTEMIC LUPUS ERYTHEMATOSUS

INFECTIONS

EPSTEIN–BARR VIRUS

CYTOMEGALOVIRUS

MALARIA

NON IMMUNE

DISSEMINATED INTRAVASCULAR
COAGULATION

THROMBOTIC THROMBOCYTOPENIC
PURPURA

HEMOLYTIC UREMIC SYNDROME

HYPERSPLENISM

PLATELET DYSFUNCTION

ASPIRIN AND OTHER ANTIPLATELET
AGENTS

von WILLEBRAND DISEASE

INHERITED FUNCTIONAL DEFECTS

NORMAL BUT TRANSFUSED PLATELETS

Clotting dysfunction

ACQUIRED

THERAPEUTIC

HEPARINIZATION

WARFARINIZATION

ACUTE THROMBOLYTIC THERAPY

CONSUMPTION COAGULOPATHY

HEMORRHAGE WITH MASSIVE
TRANSFUSIONS

DISSEMINATED INTRAVASCULAR
COAGULATION

SYNTHETIC FAILURE

CIRRHOSIS

MALNUTRITION (rare)

CONGENITAL

HEMOPHILIA

FACTOR VIII (hemophilia A)

von WILLEBRAND FACTOR

SECTION 4

FACTOR IX (Christmas disease, hemophilia B)

OTHER RARE FACTOR DEFICIENCIES

2.1.3 NEUTROPENIA

Decreased production

APLASTIC ANEMIA/MYELODYSPLASTIC SYNDROMES/DRUG REACTIONS

MALIGNANT/LEUKEMIC REPLACEMENT
usually with 'leuko-erythroblastic' features

NUTRITIONAL DEFICIENCIES
especially B12/folate – usually macrocytic

CYTOTOXIC THERAPY

ALCOHOL

Increased destruction

OVERWHELMING SEPSIS

SPLENIC SEQUESTRATION

IMMUNE DESTRUCTION

RHEUMATOID ARTHRITIS/FELTY'S SYNDROME

DRUGS (sulfonamides)

IDIOPATHIC

2.1.4 NON NEOPLASTIC LYMPHADENOPATHY

see Ch 14 lymphadenopathy gamut

Acute reactive lymphadenitis

usually in areas draining pyogenic infection (e.g. tonsillitis)

may be associated with viral infection (e.g. mesenteric lymphadenitis in children with abdominal pain)

Chronic lymphadenitis

in areas draining chronically inflamed tissues, or associated with granulomatous inflammation

Lymphadenopathy of autoimmune disease

RHEUMATOID ARTHRITIS

SYSTEMIC LUPUS ERYTHEMATOSUS

Foreign body histiocytosis

nodes draining source of inert foreign material, e.g. carbon

Sarcoidosis

Castleman's disease

Specific infections

INFECTIOUS MONONUCLEOSIS (EBV infection)

TUBERCULOUS LYMPHADENOPATHY

NON TUBERCULOUS MYCOBACTERIA

YERSINIA LYMPHADENITIS

TOXOPLASMOSIS (immunocompetent host)

HIV LYMPHADENOPATHY

2.1.5 SPLENOMEGALY

Traumatic rupture, hematoma

Infective

CHRONIC DISEASE
e.g. SUBACUTE BACTERIAL ENDOCARDITIS

VIRAL DISEASE

INFECTIOUS MONONUCLEOSIS

TB

PARASITIC DISEASE

MALARIA

SCHISTOSOMIASIS

KALA-AZAR

HYDATID

Vascular congestive

PORTAL HYPERTENSION

RIGHT HEART FAILURE

SPLENIC VEIN OBSTRUCTION

CYSTIC FIBROSIS

Tumor

LYMPHOMA

LEUKEMIA (esp CML)

MULTIPLE MYELOMA (rarely)

MYELOPROLIFERATIVE DISORDERS

METASTASES (rare)
particularly melanoma

Extramedullary hematopoiesis

MYELOFIBROSIS

THALASSEMIA

NOT SICKLE CELL DISEASE!

AUTOSPLENECTOMY BY INFARCTION

Autoimmune

FELTY'S SYNDROME

SYSTEMIC LUPUS ERYTHEMATOSUS

SARCOIDOSIS

Storage disease

GAUCHER'S DISEASE

AMYLOIDOSIS

NIEMANN–PICK DISEASE

HEMOCHROMATOSIS

MUCOPOLYSACCHARIDOSES, GLYCOGEN AND LIPID STORAGE DISORDERS

Hypersplenism of hemolytic anemia

SPHEROCYTOSIS

THROMBOTIC THROMBOCYTOPENIC PURPURA

2.1.6 THROMBOCYTOPENIA

see coagulopathies

HEMATOLOGICAL CONDITIONS

3. ONCOLOGICAL AND NON ONCOLOGICAL CONDITIONS

3.1 ANGIOFOLLICULAR LYMPH NODE HYPERPLASIA

(AFH, Castleman's disease)

3.1.1 UNICENTRIC (LOCALIZED) AFH

75% HYALINE VASCULAR TYPE: probably a vascular lymphoid hamartoma; total excision curative, radiation often successful

25% PLASMA CELL TYPE: initially reactive polyclonal proliferation associated with HHV-8 infection in HIV; has moderate risk of progression to true clonal lymphoma

IMAGING

CXR

isolated anterior mediastinal mass
less commonly middle or posterior
   mediastinal mass

CT

isolated anterior mediastinal mass or gross
   lymphadenopathy
less commonly middle or posterior
   mediastinum
may be confused with thymoma
can contain calcification
VIVIDLY ENHANCING WITH CONTRAST

MR

lymphadenopathy has high T2W signal and
   enhances vividly with Gd

3.1.2 MULTICENTRIC (GENERALIZED) AFH

dysplastic lymphoproliferative disorder with
   aggressive clinical behavior and a poor
   prognosis
multifocal lymphadenopathy, hepatomegaly,
   splenomegaly
death often due to superimposed infection
associated with POEMS syndrome (Ch 05,
   plasmacytoma)

3.2 DISSEMINATED INTRAVASCULAR COAGULATION (DIC)

DEFINITION

secondary (by definition) abnormal
   activation of platelet and clotting
   cascades leading to microthrombi and
   consumption coagulopathy

ETIOLOGY

Obstetric

AMNIOTIC FLUID EMBOLISM

ECLAMPSIA

FETAL DEATH IN UTERO

Infective

OVERWHELMING SEPSIS (usually Gram
   negative)

Massive injury

TRAUMA

BURNS

PANCREATITIS

Neoplastic

PANCREATIC CARCINOMA

BRONCHOGENIC CARCINOMA

ACUTE LEUKEMIA

CLINICAL

BLEEDING (common)

DIFFUSE HEMORRHAGES

CIRCULATORY COLLAPSE

Thromboembolism

BRAIN (seizures, infarcts)

LUNGS (ARDS)

KIDNEYS (acute renal failure)

LIVER, SPLEEN (infarcts)

OTHER

3.3 EWING'S SARCOMA

see Ch 05

3.4 HODGKIN'S DISEASE (HD)

DEFINITION

histologically defined, clinically distinct B
   cell lymphoma

CLINICAL

HD is less common than NHL (3/100 000)
bimodal peaks: young adults (usually lower
   grade and stage, male > female), older
   adults (higher grade and stage)
classically spreads via lymphatics to
   contiguous nodal regions

Presentation

LYMPHADENOPATHY
painless, tender, or pain with alcohol

EXTRANODAL HD
organ enlargement, hepatosplenomegaly

CONSTITUTIONAL
fever, loss of weight, malaise, anemia,
   pruritus

SUSCEPTIBILITY TO OPPORTUNISTIC
   INFECTIONS
viral, fungal and mycobacterial, especially
   VZV

COMPARISON WITH NHL
HD: single axial nodal group, ordered
   spread, more commonly upper torso
   presentations
NHL: multiple peripheral nodal groups,
   spreads by dissemination, mesentery
   involved, MALT (mucosa associated
   lymphoid tissue) and extranodal disease
   common

Staging

essential workup: body CT, bone marrow
   aspirate; gallium scan; other: PET scan
   (replacing gallium); excisional biopsy to
   establish diagnosis (FNA/core biopsy can
   be misleading)

ANN ARBOR STAGING SYSTEM
I   single nodal group
I_E single extranodal focus
II   2 or more nodal groups, all on the same
    side of diaphragm
II_E extranodal site and nodes, all on the
    same side of diaphragm
III nodal groups on both sides of diaphragm
III_E extranodal and nodal disease on both
    sides of diaphragm
III_S involves spleen
IV disseminated or diffuse
A: no constitutional symptoms, B: fever,
   night sweats, weight loss >10% over
   6 months

Complications

immune suppression, infections
complications of treatment (short and long-
   term: radiation fibrosis, cardiac disease
   from radiation therapy and
   chemotherapy, infertility, …)
MAY RELAPSE (often contiguous nodal
   groups, more common in those treated
   with radiation therapy alone)

SECOND MALIGNANCY relatively frequent (may occur late; often a NHL) and includes breast carcinoma, thyroid carcinoma, NHL, AML, bone sarcomas within radiation field, cerebral tumors

MACRO

discretely enlarged rubbery nodular lymph nodes
spleen: enlarged, nodular masses
direct spread of lymphomatous tissue from nodes: lungs, spine, retroperitoneum
bone marrow: ivory vertebra (classic but uncommon)

MICRO

Reed–Sternberg (RS) cell

neoplastic clonal cell of HD; B cell lineage in most cases
large cell with bilobed nucleus with large prominent eosinophilic nucleoli inside a clear zone and a reddish blue cytoplasm
variants: popcorn cell, lacunar cell
Reed–Sternberg cells or variants are required for diagnosis of HD

Lymphocyte predominant (lymphocyte rich) (6%)

male > female
few RS cells; infiltrate of mature reactive lymphocytes and macrophages
excellent prognosis

Mixed cellularity (~20%)

male > female
many RS cells, heterogeneous reactive infiltrate (macrophages, lymphocytes, eosinophils, plasma cells)
intermediate prognosis

Lymphocyte depleted (4%)

abundant pleomorphic RS cells, few reactive lymphocytes
older males with poor prognosis

Nodular sclerosing (~70%)

female > male, young adults
few classic RS cells; abundant lacunar cells
variable reactive cells (nodular sclerosing HD subtyped depending on predominance or depletion of reactive cells)
collagen bands across lymph node
most common histology in those with massive mediastinal masses

IMAGING

XR (skeletal)

90% lytic destruction or mixed
10% purely sclerotic (e.g. ivory vertebra)
lesions axial (spine, pelvis, ribs, sternum)
spread hematogenous or from lymph nodes in continuity

CXR

mediastinal or supraclavicular mass
extension of hilar soft tissue into lung (fuzzy edge)

US

solid hypoechoic lymphadenopathy
liver involvement: heterogeneous echotexture or frank masses
spleen involvement: usually discrete foci (echogenic or hypoechoic); 'reactive' splenomegaly without discrete deposits common

CT

soft tissue density enlarged lymph nodes
jugular, posterior cervical, supraclavicular, paratracheal, anterior mediastinal, hilar; celiac, paraaortic, iliac, inguinal (lower torso less common, particularly isolated)
generally no or mild contrast enhancement
usually no necrosis
nodes may coalesce into confluent masses
nodal mass may invade/compress adjacent organs (particularly lung and SVC)
diffuse splenic enlargement vs discrete masses

MR

lymphadenopathy with same morphology as CT
nodes similar to muscle on T1W, high on T2W and have mild contrast enhancement
bone marrow involvement: discrete soft tissue mass or diffuse bone marrow replacement (low on T1W, intermediate or high on T2W; may show mild Gd enhancement)

NUC MED (MDP)

involved bone: usually increased delayed phase uptake (reactive bone formation)

NUC MED (Ga)

HD is virtually always gallium avid
Ga (with SPECT) is an excellent staging and monitoring modality (particularly for assessment of post treatment residual masses, which is a common problem especially if disease initially bulky)
involved lymph nodes show markedly elevated Ga uptake
spleen or liver involvement may manifest as focal inhomogeneity or focally elevated uptake
bone marrow involvement shows focally elevated Ga uptake over and above that of neighboring bones

NORMAL GALLIUM UPTAKE PATTERN

liver and spleen (spleen intensity same or just less than liver)
bone (Ga is a weak bone tracing agent)
kidneys and urine (progressively decreasing from 3 to 5 to 7 days); testes and scrotum
colon (probably mucosal, hence clearance probably depends on mucosal shedding of Ga containing cells), with differing position and Ga distribution on different imaging occasions
salivary glands and lacrimal glands
faintly blood pool and soft tissue (so that mediastinal structures are higher activity than lung)
low grade (<< liver) hilar nodal uptake may be present in normals especially smokers or patients with intercurrent infections

POST TREATMENT GALLIUM UPTAKE PATTERN

bone marrow activation: increased diffuse skeletal uptake with prominence of proximal appendicular skeleton
pneumonitis: variable grade diffuse lung uptake (less than mediastinum, same, more than mediastinum, gross); may have low grade bilateral 'reactive' hilar nodal uptake
NB gross bilateral lung parenchymal uptake is very likely to indicate pneumocystis pneumonia!
effect of radiation: decreased bone marrow and salivary Ga uptake (salivary uptake may eventually rebound)

DIFFERENTIALS OF INCREASED GALLIUM UPTAKE

SARCOIDOSIS

INFECTION

NON HODGKIN'S LYMPHOMA

THYMIC HYPERPLASIA IN YOUNG PATIENTS

PET (FDG)

HD is very FDG avid
reduction in FDG uptake is an excellent measure of metabolic response to treatment
FDG particularly useful in assessment of post therapy residual masses

3.5 IRON DEFICIENCY ANEMIA

DEFINITION

commonest form of anemia, usually due to excess loss of iron, with a microcytic hypochromic blood film

ETIOLOGY

Inadequate intake
poor intake is uncommon unless strict vegetarian

Malabsorption
gastrectomy, achlorhydria, loss of proximal small bowel
malabsorption states, celiac disease

Excess loss

MENSTRUAL

OCCULT

GASTROINTESTINAL

GENITOURINARY
especially paroxysmal nocturnal hemoglobinuria

NASOPHARYNGEAL
especially Osler–Weber–Rendu syndrome

HEMODIALYSIS RELATED

IATROGENIC FROM REPEATED VENESECTIONS

3.6 LANGERHANS CELL HISTIOCYTOSIS

a group of clonal disorders of Langerhans cell histiocytes (antigen presenting cells)
see Ch 05 musculoskeletal tumors, Ch 11 CNS, Ch 13 lungs

3.7 LEUKEMIA

GROUP DEFINITION

malignant white blood cell line neoplasms with monoclonal expansion, differentiation block, diffuse bone marrow replacement and 'spillover' into peripheral blood

GROUP PATHOGENESIS

may evolve from myeloproliferative or myelodysplastic disease
underlying genomic events (mutations, translocations, oncogene activation and amplification, tumor suppressor gene deletions)
abnormal clonal proliferation + maturation block

CLONAL GROWTH RATE LOW, GROWTH FRACTION HIGH LEADING TO:
1. BM flooding and replacement
2. organ infiltration
3. hyperviscosity/leukostasis due to leukemic cells (more common in acute leukemias with larger more adhesive cells)
4. secondary anemia, infections and hemorrhage

3.7.1 ACUTE LYMPHOBLASTIC LEUKEMIA (ALL)

WHO CLASSIFICATION

acute lymphoblastic leukemia and lymphoblastic lymphoma are classified as a single disease entity with different presentations (all termed lymphoblastic leukemia)
morphological grade and cytogenetic abnormalities have prognostic significance

CLINICAL PRESENTATION

80% of all childhood leukemia, male > female
weight loss, infections, thrombocytopenia, anemia, hyperviscosity, bone pain, CNS involvement, organ infiltration (mediastinal mass particularly in T cell disease)
in children, remission rate >90% and 75% cured with treatment; poorer in adults

3.7.2 ACUTE MYELOID LEUKEMIA (AML)

WHO CLASSIFICATION

defined as bone marrow blast count >20%

WITH RECURRENT CYTOGENETIC TRANSLOCATIONS
WITH MULTILINEAGE DYSPLASIA
THERAPY RELATED

CLINICAL

20% of childhood leukemia
most common adult acute leukemia (median age 60–65 years)
weight loss, infections, thrombocytopenia, anemia, hyperviscosity, bone pain, organ infiltration; chloromas (leukemic masses) may occur
60% remission rate, 20% cure rate (younger > older)

3.7.3 CHRONIC MYELOID (MYELOGENOUS) LEUKEMIA (CML)

WHO CLASSIFICATION

classified as a myeloproliferative disorder; related conditions are chronic neutrophilic leukemia, polycythemia rubra vera and idiopathic myelofibrosis

CLINICAL

classically occurs in adults, carries the Philadelphia chromosome in more than 90%
massive splenomegaly
hepatomegaly
bony pain with sternal tenderness
loss of weight and fatigue
median survival 5–7 years; death occurs from blast transformation, rarely from complications of treatment beforehand

3.7.4 CHRONIC LYMPHOCYTIC LEUKEMIA (CLL)

WHO CLASSIFICATION

classified as one disease with B cell small lymphocytic lymphoma, with different clinical presentations (extranodal diffuse in 'CLL', nodal in 'SLL')

CLINICAL

50–70 years old, male:female 2:1

commonest form of leukemia in Western countries

hepatosplenomegaly ('CLL')

splenomegaly usually less marked than in CML

gross lymphadenopathy ('SLL')

fatigue, infections

autoimmune phenomena (e.g. hemolytic anemia, ITP)

indolent disease with variable survival depending on extent of involvement and any associated anemia

IMAGING (group)

Skeletal XR

CHILD: metaphyseal lucent lines, permeative destruction, focal lytic lesions (chloromas), periosteal reaction; sclerosis rare but possible

ADULT: osteopenia and focal lytic lesions (acute > chronic)

Body CT/MR

hepatomegaly, possibly with heterogeneous density/signal pattern

variable splenomegaly, splenic infarcts, heterogeneous density/signal pattern (splenomegaly massive in CML)

lymphadenopathy in CLL (merges into lymphoma)

bilaterally diffusely enlarged kidneys, increased T2W signal, may be abnormal density on CT

NUC MED

MDP

diffusely increased marrow space uptake in tissue and delayed phase, may also be mildly hypervascular on flow phase

often symmetrical; follows red marrow locations (e.g. 'hot spine and knees')

COLLOID

photopenic areas where normal marrow replaced by leukemia

Bone marrow MR

'edema' pattern of diffuse low T1W high T2W signal

CNS MR

leptomeningeal involvement with nodularity and abnormally extensive or nodular contrast enhancement (ALL)

perivascular involvement (contrast enhancement, abnormal soft tissue)

dural involvement uncommon

---

parenchymal involvement uncommon, appearance similar to primary CNS lymphoma

US

hepatomegaly, altered liver echotexture

hypoechoic splenomegaly, splenic infarcts

bilateral diffuse kidney enlargement with diffuse hypoechogenicity and loss of corticomedullary differentiation

testis: diffuse hypoechoic enlargement

3.8 MASTOCYTOSIS

rare proliferative disorder of mast cells with focal, multifocal (skin, gut, bone marrow) or generalized deposits

3.9 MEGALOBLASTIC ANEMIA

DEFINITION

anemia (+/– leukopenia) secondary to ineffective DNA synthesis characterized by arrest in cell maturation, high MCV, low PCV

ETIOLOGY

B12 deficiency

B12 DIETARY DEFICIENCY

VEGANS (takes years)

INTRINSIC FACTOR (IF) DEFICIENCY

PERNICIOUS ANEMIA

ASSOCIATIONS WITH: Anglo-Saxon, elderly; other thyrogastric cluster autoimmune disease

CHRONIC ATROPHIC GASTRITIS

GASTRECTOMY

IF AND B12 LOSS

TERMINAL ILEAL RESECTION, CROHN'S DISEASE

BLIND LOOP SYNDROMES

MALABSORPTION STATES

SCHILLING'S TEST (NUC MED)

differentiation of malabsorption vs B12 vs IF deficiency

Folate deficiency

ABSOLUTE

DIETARY

ALCOHOLISM

RELATIVE

PREGNANCY

ANTIMETABOLITE CHEMOTHERAPY

3.10 MYELOFIBROSIS

DEFINITION

myeloproliferative disorder of megakaryocytes leading to bone marrow fibrosis and extramedullary hematopoiesis

CLINICAL

anemia

massive hepatosplenomegaly (extramedullary hematopoiesis)

IMAGING

XR

diffuse osteosclerosis ('myelosclerosis' rather than 'myelofibrosis') in red marrow bearing skeleton (axial skeleton)

splenomegaly, hepatomegaly, less commonly lymphadenopathy

MR

abnormal bone marrow dark on both T1W and T2W sequences

can lead to other extramedullary sites, e.g. ascites, effusions

3.11 NON HODGKIN'S LYMPHOMA (NHL)

ORBITAL LYMPHOMA (Ch 12)

PRIMARY CNS LYMPHOMA (Ch 11)

PRIMARY BONE LYMPHOMA (Ch 05)

DEFINITION

neoplastic lymphoid proliferation without Reed–Sternberg cells

EPIDEMIOLOGY

approx 10/100 000/year, male:female 1.4:1

NHL is more common than HD

PREVALENCE PATTERNS

Children

~40% precursor T lymphoblastic lymphoma/leukemia (high grade)
~30% Burkitt's lymphoma (high grade)
diffuse large B cell lymphoma (high grade)

Adults

small cell B lymphocytic lymphoma/CLL (low grade)
~30% follicular lymphoma (B cell) (low grade)
~40% diffuse large B cell lymphoma (high grade)
other lymphomas

HIV associated lymphoma

Burkitt's lymphoma (EBV)
diffuse large B cell lymphoma (EBV)
primary GIT and CNS lymphomas
'body-cavity-based' associated with HHV-8
prognosis uniformly poor

BEHAVIOR (NHL as a group)

Growth patterns

LOW GRADE LYMPHOMAS

SMALL LYMPHOCYTIC LYMPHOMA (B)
FOLLICULAR LYMPHOMA (B)
MANTLE CELL LYMPHOMA (B)
MALT LYMPHOMA (B)

low grade lymphoma behavior: indolent untreated; treatment induces remissions but does not cure; eventually dedifferentiates to higher grade in some (blast transformation)
survival curve continues to decline gradually with low grade lymphoma (deaths from complications of recurrence, e.g. infection and secondary to blast transformation)

HIGH GRADE LYMPHOMAS

PRECURSOR B CELL LYMPHOBLASTIC LYMPHOMA/LEUKEMIA
DIFFUSE LARGE B CELL LYMPHOMA
BURKITT'S LYMPHOMA (B)
MYCOSIS FUNGOIDES (T)
ANGIOIMMUNOBLASTIC LYMPHOMA (T)
ANAPLASTIC LARGE CELL LYMPHOMA (T)
ADULT HTLV LYMPHOMA/LEUKEMIA (T)
PRECURSOR T CELL LYMPHOBLASTIC LYMPHOMA/LEUKEMIA
ENTEROPATHY ASSOCIATED LYMPHOMA (T)

high grade lymphoma behavior: fulminant untreated; remission usual; prolonged remission is likely to be a lasting cure

survival curve drops off with high grade lymphoma (initial deaths) but then stays quite flat (lasting cure in a proportion of patients)

CLINICAL PRESENTATION

clinical grouping is by major pattern of presentation: PREDOMINANTLY NODAL, PRIMARY EXTRANODAL and PREDOMINANTLY DISSEMINATED/LEUKEMIC
histologic and cytologic type (which classifies and grades the lymphoma) is important for treatment and prognosis and requires a generous biopsy

Predominantly nodal lymphoma

LYMPHADENOPATHY
HEPATOSPLENOMEGALY
BONE MARROW INFILTRATION
HYPERVISCOSITY

Primary extranodal lymphoma

local mass effects
skin lesions (cutaneous T lymphoma)
GIT: mass which ulcerates, perforates, obstructs, intussuscepts, bleeds

Predominantly disseminated/leukemic

BONE MARROW INFILTRATION
HEPATOSPLENOMEGALY
DIFFUSE ORGAN INFILTRATION

Staging

uses the Ann Arbor system (see Hodgkin's disease)
less prognostically relevant than in Hodgkin's disease as in most presentations the lymphoma has already disseminated

LYMPHOMA TYPES MORE PREVALENT WITH SPECIFIC MACRO PATTERNS

Infiltrative

MASSIVE NODES

B cell small lymphocytic lymphoma
B cell follicular lymphoma

HEPATOSPLENOMEGALY

B cell small lymphocytic lymphoma
B cell follicular lymphoma
B cell mantle lymphoma
HTLV T cell lymphoma leukemia

Focal mass

CNS (parenchymal focal)

B cell diffuse large lymphoma and higher grades

GIT

sporadic (Western) type Burkitt's lymphoma (child; HIV associated)
MALT lymphoma
enteropathy associated T cell lymphoma
classic but rare 'lymphomatous polyposis' of mantle cell NHL

RETROPERITONEUM

B cell diffuse large lymphoma and higher grades
sporadic (Western) type Burkitt's lymphoma

MEDIASTINUM

precursor T cell lymphoblastic lymphoma (classically teenage to young adult males)
primary mediastinal B cell NHL with sclerosis (classically young adult women)

PHARYNX/WALDEYER

B cell diffuse large lymphoma and higher grades

FACE

salivary (Sjögren's syndrome associated): diffuse lymphoma
thyroid (Hashimoto's disease associated)
mandible, maxilla – endemic (African) type Burkitt's lymphoma
orbital – MALT

SKIN

cutaneous T lymphomas

3.11.1 B CELL SMALL LYMPHOCYTIC LYMPHOMA (low grade)

same disease as chronic lymphocytic leukemia (CLL) with different (nodal) presentation
common (in combination with CLL); 60–70 year olds
generalized lymphadenopathy ('SLL' features)
bone marrow infiltration, hepatosplenomegaly, elevated peripheral lymphocyte counts ('CLL' features)
indolent, but ultimately resistant to treatment with low cure rates

3.11.2 B CELL FOLLICULAR LYMPHOMA (low grade)

commonest single form of NHL (~30%)
60–65 years old, male > female

usually generalized lymphadenopathy (localized in ~25%)

bone marrow involvement early (75% at presentation)

extranodal disease rare, unless histologic transformation has developed

usually a good initial response to treatment but with subsequent relapsing–remitting course

3.11.3 MANTLE CELL LYMPHOMA (B CELL) (low grade)

50–70 years old, male > female

focal or generalized lymphadenopathy, primary splenic lymphoma, primary GIT lymphoma; bone marrow usually involved, may have leukemic manifestations

3.11.4 MALT TYPE B CELL LYMPHOMA (low grade)

FULL WHO TERM: EXTRANODAL MARGINAL ZONE B CELL LYMPHOMA OF MUCOSA-ASSOCIATED LYMPHOID TISSUE

Gastric MALT lymphoma

associated with Helicobacter pylori

originates from stimulated polyclonal MALT proliferation

recapitulates behavior of MALT lymphocytes; tends to invade epithelium and to form lymphoepithelial lesions

neoplastic clone partly immune driven (may respond to Helicobacter pylori eradication)

disseminates late and may be cured by locoregional treatment

Small bowel MALT lymphoma

similar presentation to gastric MALT lymphoma

focal mucosal mass, obstructs, intussuscepts, perforates

commonest in terminal ileum (arising in Peyer's patches)

3.11.5 PRECURSOR B CELL LYMPHOBLASTIC LYMPHOMA/LEUKEMIA

see acute lymphoblastic leukemia

3.11.6 DIFFUSE LARGE B CELL LYMPHOMA (high grade)

30–40% or so of adult NHL

usually regional lymphadenopathy or extranodal masses

bone marrow and spleen involved at presentation in <30% of cases

3.11.7 BURKITT'S LYMPHOMA (B CELL) (high grade)

sheets of small round blue cells; reactive macrophages phagocytosing dead cell debris form pale 'stars' in a blue 'sky' ('starry sky' appearance)

Endemic form

African children; Epstein–Barr virus associated (EBV genome present in clonal cells)

presents with large facial masses with facial bone/jaw destruction

other presentations: retroperitoneal/ileocecal, renal, gonadal mass

Sporadic form

retroperitoneal, renal, GIT masses, or disseminated

usual form in Western countries

Immunodeficiency associated

EBV genome present in clone

body-cavity-based NHL related to HHV-8

3.11.8 MYCOSIS FUNGOIDES/ SEZARY SYNDROME (T CELL) (high grade)

cutaneous T cell lymphoma with infiltration of dermis and then of epidermis

NOT A MYCOSIS! NO FUNGUS!

SEZARY'S SYNDROME: cutaneous cerebriform T cell lymphoma and cerebriform T cell leukemia

3.11.9 ANGIOIMMUNOBLASTIC T CELL LYMPHOMA (high grade)

common in Japan

generalized lymphadenopathy, hepatosplenomegaly and skin involvement

3.11.10 ANAPLASTIC LARGE CELL LYMPHOMA (T CELL) (high grade)

aggressive tumor of children and young adults, often with multifocal skin involvement

3.11.11 ADULT HTLV LYMPHOMA/LEUKEMIA (high grade)

associated with HTLV-1 infection (common in Japan and Asia and Caribbean)

generalized lymphadenopathy, hepatosplenomegaly, hypercalcemia, skin lesions, lytic bone lesions

rapidly fatal

3.11.12 PRECURSOR T LYMPHOBLASTIC LYMPHOMA/LEUKEMIA (high grade)

considered the same disease as T cell acute lymphoblastic leukemia ('ALL') in the WHO classification

40% of childhood NHL

occurs <20–25 years, rare in adults

male:female 2:1

presents with lymphadenopathy; ¾ have a mediastinal mass centered on the thymus

3.11.13 ENTEROPATHY ASSOCIATED T CELL LYMPHOMA (high grade)

complicates long-standing poorly controlled celiac disease; poor prognosis

multifocal mucosal masses, widely disseminated within GI tract at time of diagnosis, later systemic dissemination later

IMAGING OF LYMPHOMA

IMAGING (nodal mass)

US

hypoechoic enlarged mass with loss of internal architecture

variably hypervascular

? local infiltration beyond capsule

CT

size criterion of lymphadenopathy: transverse diameter of node >10 mm (neither sensitive nor specific)

soft tissue or lower density lymphadenopathy

confluent nodal masses

mild contrast enhancement

central low density implies necrosis (high grade)

mesenteric nodal masses enclose the vascular pedicle ('mesenteric sandwich')

anterior mediastinal mass

retroperitoneal mass may be centered on paraaortic nodes, root of mesentery, or elsewhere

following treatment small nodes or residual tissue are common: structural diagnostic problem of 'sterilized' lymphoma vs residual active disease

MR

signal usually intermediate or low on T1W and high on T2W sequences

NUC MED

GALLIUM

most NHL takes up gallium (large cell > follicular > small cell); but sensitivity in low grade NHL is <60%

low grade NHL may not take up Ga (use PET), and metabolic response is difficult to differentiate from non avid disease without a baseline

low intensity extranodal lymphoma difficult to differentiate from normal (see Hodgkin's disease)

in children, thymic rebound vs residual/ recurrent lymphoma is difficult

THALLIUM

in general, follows same rules as PET but unsatisfactory with deeper organs because of attenuation

PET (FDG)

will become the functional imaging of choice in NHL

NHL is FDG avid (large cell >95%, low-grade lymphoma 80–90%)

differentiation of extranodal lymphoma (especially colorectal) and physiologic or reactive uptake may be difficult, and depends on non uniform focal uptake or evolution over time

decrease in FDG uptake is an excellent predictor of metabolic response

better than Ga for thymic rebound (no uptake/low uptake) vs recurrent lymphoma (high grade uptake)

IMAGING (extranodal disease)

Pulmonary (uncommon with NHL, more common with HD)

direct extension from nodes

peribronchial MALT nodules

airspace form (bronchioloalveolar lymphoma)

lymphangitic form (rare)

parenchymal lung masses +/– effusions and pleural thickening

Thymic

main problem is rebound thymic hyperplasia vs recurrence

Hepatosplenorenal

DIFFUSE INVOLVEMENT (most common in low grade NHL)

altered echotexture, MR signal or density

nodular pattern

FOCAL MASS (more common in large cell NHL)

usually hypoechoic (may be hyperechoic), low density, high T2W signal

DIRECT INVASION FROM PORTAL NODES

Stomach

FLUORO

DIFFUSE

linitis plastica pattern

thickened mucosal fold pattern

may have loss of peristalsis, dilation, ulceration

FOCAL

less common

mimics carcinoma

CT

non specific diffuse or focal gastric wall thickening; may have nodular surface

appearance overlaps that of carcinoma

NUC MED (Ga)

often Ga avid

focal, intense fixed uptake in position of gastric wall

PET (FDG)

FDG avid

differential is normal muscle FDG uptake (see carcinoma)

Bowel (SB > LB)

STOMACH > SB (terminal ileum > other) > LB

FLUORO

mucosal thickening, polypoid masses, ulceration

loss of normal peristalsis

aneurysmal dilation

intussusception, obstruction

strictures, fistulas

CT

focal or multifocal bowel wall thickening

aneurysmal bowel dilation

extramucosal lymphoid mass, may encase adjacent loops

ascites, omental disease, mesentery base masses

PET (FDG)

lymphoma is FDG avid

focal or multifocal abnormally elevated FDG uptake centered on bowel

Bone

NHL: primary bone lymphoma vs secondary lymphoma

lytic focal or diffuse areas, commonly in the axial skeleton

endemic type Burkitt's lymphoma: 50% have mandible or maxillary lesions with floating teeth

CNS

PRIMARY CNS (Ch 11)

SECONDARY NHL (in general, late in natural history)

leptomeningeal involvement with nodularity and abnormally extensive or nodular contrast enhancement

perivascular involvement (contrast enhancement, abnormal soft tissue)

dural involvement uncommon

parenchymal involvement uncommon, appearance similar to primary CNS lymphoma

Head and neck

Waldeyer's ring enlargement (common); differential is tonsillar SCC

orbital lymphoma (Ch 12)

paranasal sinuses: mass

salivary mass (Sjögren's syndrome)

thyroid mass (Hashimoto's thyroiditis)

Testis

diffuse involvement with enlargement and abnormal echotexture

focal hypoechoic mass (differential is of hematoma or primary testicular neoplasm)

may be bilateral in 5–15%

Renal

virtually all renal lymphoma is secondary and not primary renal; NHL > HD may directly invade from adjacent lymphadenopathy along renal pedicle

hypoechoic, hypovascular mass; solitary ~20%

bilateral ~80% (multiple masses, diffuse infiltration or perinephric mass)

3.12 PLASMACYTOMA, MULTIPLE MYELOMA

see Ch 05

3.13 POLYCYTHEMIA RUBRA VERA

myeloproliferative disease with excessive production of mature red blood cells (7–10 per fl)

median age ~60 years

red or cyanosed skin ('rubra')

blood hyperviscosity with visual disturbances, thrombotic complications and thrombotic strokes

splenomegaly, hepatomegaly

tendency to evolve to other myeloproliferative conditions

DIFFERENTIAL DIAGNOSIS

Secondary polycythemia
hypoxia of COAD
heavy smokers
congenital heart disease
altitude polycythemia

Ectopic erythropoietin secretion

Hemoconcentration
Cr-51 red cell labeled dilution study determines red cell and plasma volume (differentiation of polycythemia from hemoconcentration)

3.14 PURPURAS

3.14.1 IDIOPATHIC THROMBOCYTOPENIC PURPURA

idiopathic (by definition) platelet destruction by autoimmune antibodies

adult females, abrupt or insidious onset

diffuse petechial bleeds

must rule out HIV, SLE, underlying lymphoproliferative disorder, drug effect, post viral, etc

3.14.2 THROMBOTIC THROMBOCYTOPENIC PURPURA AND HEMOLYTIC UREMIC SYNDROME

DEFINITION

idiopathic widespread platelet thrombosis of the microcirculation without activation of the clotting cascade, with multifocal ischemic damage and fragmentation hemolysis

CLINICAL

Thrombotic thrombocytopenic purpura
adult females > males, usually previously well

present with the classic pentad of fever, thrombocytopenia, hemolytic anemia, neurological deficits and renal failure, although many will not have the 'full hand'

Hemolytic uremic syndrome
pediatric disorder with purpura, hemolysis and acute renal failure

often preceded by E coli O157 infection

3.14.3 HENOCH–SCHÖNLEIN PURPURA

childhood (or adulthood) small vessel vasculitis characterized by local petechial hemorrhages

follows upper respiratory infections

purpura, arthralgia, GIT mucosal bleeds, abdominal pain

hematuria, nephrotic syndrome (in 1/3)

3.15 SICKLE CELL DISEASE

DEFINITION

point hemoglobin (Hb) mutation predisposing to sickling, with predictable effects of anemia and small vessel thrombotic crises with infarction

EPIDEMIOLOGY

African (selection pressure of malaria); endemic malarial areas – 30% heterozygotes; US blacks – 10% heterozygotes

Mediterranean – less prevalent

ETIOPATHOGENESIS

beta chain mutation (HbS)

(HbS confers resistance against infection with Plasmodium falciparum)

heterozygote: sickle cell trait

homozygote: sickle cell disease

HbS forms rigid insoluble polymers at low O_2 tension and low pH

this produces deformed sickle cells which cause microvascular infarcts, and reduced lifespan of abnormal cells leads to anemia

sickling depends on proportion of HbS: silent in TRAIT and less severe in sickle thalassemia (lesser MCHC)

CLINICAL

Trait
mild, often asymptomatic

sickling crises and avascular necrosis rare

renal papillary necrosis, liver and splenic infarcts may occur

Disease manifestations

1. MICROINFARCTS (capillary occlusion)

bone – avascular necrosis (AVN), bone marrow infarcts

sickle dactylitis: children with acutely swollen painful hands or feet

spleen – congestion, then autosplenectomy

liver – infarcts

kidneys – papillary necrosis, renal failure

brain, retina – infarcts

lungs – pulmonary hypertension

2. SICKLING CRISES

precipitated by intercurrent illness, dehydration, cold (acidemia)

abdominal visceral or bone infarcts (acute chest syndrome) with pain

pulmonary infarcts

stroke-like episodes

acute renal failure

3. SICKLE CELL HEMOLYSIS

hypersplenism then autosplenectomy

hemolytic anemia

bone marrow expansion

iron overload
pigment gallstones

4. APLASTIC CRISES
related to viral infections

5. SUPERIMPOSED SEPSIS
Staphylococcus commonest
Salmonella osteomyelitis classic
Streptococcus pneumoniae meningitis
(children)
systemic septicemia

6. GROWTH DISTURBANCE
failure to thrive
short stature
bone deformities

IMAGING (all modalities)

Multiple AVN
see avascular necrosis entry (Ch 02 general
musculoskeletal conditions) for imaging
findings
metadiaphyseal (may produce growth plate
arrest)
epiphyseal with later articular collapse
sickle cell dactylitis occurs in 20% of
homozygote children
H shaped vertebrae

Bone marrow expansion
mild osteopenia, mild bone marrow
expansion compared to thalassemia

Osteomyelitis
see osteomyelitis entry (Ch 02 general
musculoskeletal conditions)

Hepatomegaly, autosplenectomy, gallstones

Kidneys in acute sickling crisis
swollen kidneys, striated nephrogram on CT
beware: IV contrast may precipitate further
renal deterioration

Chronic renal changes
small scarred kidneys
multifocal renal infarcts
papillary necrosis (see its own entry)
renal iron deposition (on MR)
rarely, sickle cell glomerulonephritis

IMAGING (characteristic findings)

XR
H shaped vertebrae

multiple bone marrow infarcts of various
ages
secondary growth disturbance or articular
collapse

NUC MED

MDP
multiple healing infarcts (increased uptake),
possible acute infarcts (photopenic)
background diffusely increased uptake (bone
marrow expansion)
uptake in splenic infarction

COLLOID
photopenic infarcts – see avascular necrosis
entry in Ch 02 musculoskeletal conditions
absent spleen

MR
multiple infarcts of various ages – see
avascular necrosis entry in Ch 02
musculoskeletal conditions

3.16 THALASSEMIA

DEFINITION

hemoglobinopathy with deficient normal
hemoglobin (Hb) formation and
secondary bone marrow expansion

EPIDEMIOLOGY

beta thalassemia: Europe, Mid East; alpha
thalassemia: Far East
Sickle thalassemia is an uncommon severe
combination of HbS and thalassemia

ETIOPATHOGENESIS

Beta thalassemia
absent or abnormal Hb beta chain gene
b/- thalassemia minor; -/- thalassemia major

Alpha thalassemia
absent or abnormal Hb alpha chain gene
aa/a- asymptomatic; a-/a- or aa/--
thalassemia minor; a-/-- thalassemia
major

CLINICAL (thalassemia major)

Anemia
variant Hb with reduced O2 carrying
capacity

reduced RBC survival, raised erythropoietin
levels
hyperdynamic circulation, LV failure
growth disturbance

Bone marrow expansion
ineffective erythropoiesis
osteopenia, bone deformities, abnormal
facies
extramedullary hemopoiesis

Fe overload and hyperbilirubinemia
hemolysis hyperbilirubinemia, pigment
gallstones
Fe overload from increased absorption and
transfusions

HEMOSIDEROSIS
cirrhosis
pancreatic failure, secondary diabetes
mellitus
cardiomyopathy
testicular involvement with gonadal failure

IMAGING (all modalities – thalassemia major)

thalassemia minor has no imaging findings
or mild osteopenia with bone marrow
expansion only
MOST FINDINGS REFLECT BONE MARROW
EXPANSION AND EXTRAMEDULLARY
HEMATOPOIESIS
osteopenia, coarse primary trabeculae, loss
of secondary trabeculae, thinned cortex
red bone marrow expansion in long bones,
conversion of yellow to red marrow and
red marrow in peripheral bones
MR and NUC MED appearance of bone
marrow expansion
long bone deformity (widened
undertubulated diaphyses, expanded
metaphyses)
Erlenmeyer flask deformities (expanded
distal femoral metadiaphyses)
skull diploe expansion ('hair on end'
appearance)
hypoplastic sinuses caused by facial bone
red marrow expansion
extramedullary hematopoiesis (posterior
mediastinal bone marrow masses, liver,
spleen)
cardiomegaly, frank congestive cardiac
failure

Pediatrics

17 | Pediatric musculoskeletal

1. NORMAL

1.1 SKELETAL NORMAL VALUES

Cervical spine
atlantoaxial distance in neutral <5 mm
lateral neck soft tissue <1/2 vertebral body

Hips plain film

BASELINES
Hilgenreiner (Y-Y line)
acetabular roof line
Perkins line (vertical line through outer acetabulum lip)

ACETABULUM
NORMAL ACETABULAR ROOF ANGLE is 28 degrees at birth, 22 degrees at 1 year (2SD is 8 degrees)
medial hip cartilage space symmetry (femoral head cortex to tear drop) is <1 mm

FEMUR
AP: epiphysis inside Perkins line
frog leg: midshaft line points to Y cartilage
neck to shaft angle 150 degrees at birth, 120–130 degrees in adult

Hips – ultrasound

DYNAMIC TESTING
hip does not dislocate or shift out of acetabulum

STATIC MEASUREMENTS
ACETABULAR ANGLES (Graf)
vertical baseline through vertical ilium
acetabular roof line lower margin ilium at Y cartilage to bony acetabular margin
acetabular labrum line from bony acetabular margin to tip of labrum
alpha angle is acetabular roof to baseline (normal: >60 degrees, correlates with plain film)
beta angle is labral line to baseline (normal: <55 degrees)
DEGREE OF COVERAGE
femoral head circle gives femoral head diameter
measure covered and uncovered femoral head from acetabular margin
>60% coverage is normal, <33% abnormal

Gestational age from plain film (time of epiphyseal appearance)
humeral head 36 weeks, first molars 33 weeks, second molars 36 weeks
distal femur 31 weeks, proximal tibia 34 weeks

Foot angles
Lateral projection: talocalcaneal angle 25–45 degrees, calcaneal pitch (long axis of calcaneum to horizontal) 20–30 degrees
AP projection: talocalcaneal angle 15–35 degrees
CT heel: normal calcaneal valgus is 5–10 degrees

Kyphosis/lordosis
Lipmann-Cobb method
NORMAL thoracic kyphosis (T5 to T12): 27 degrees, 90th centile 40 degrees
NORMAL lumbar lordosis (L1 to L5): 40 degrees, 90th centile 54 degrees
NORMAL lumbosacral angle 5 to 21 degrees
Reference: Resnick

1.2 ELBOW OSSIFICATION TIMES AND ALIGNMENT

Mnemonic: CRITOL
average time of appearance on XR:
C-apitellum 1 year
R-adial head 5 years
I-nternal epicondyle 5 years
T-rochlea 10 years
O-lecranon 10 years
L-ateral epicondyle 12 years

Alignment
anterior humeral line passes through 1/3 to 1/2 of capitellum
capitellum on line with radial axis

2. GAMUTS

2.1 GENERIC (all modalities)

2.1.1 BACK PAIN IN CHILDREN

TRAUMA
FRACTURE, DISK PROTRUSION, STRESS FRACTURE
PARS DEFECTS

OSTEOMYELITIS/DISCITIS

NON INFECTIOUS DISCITIS

MALFORMATION/ SPONDYLOLISTHESIS

SCHEUERMANN DISEASE

TUMOR
OSTEOID OSTEOMA, OTHER

SYSTEMIC DISEASE (avascular necrosis, sickle cell disease)

REFERRED PAIN (kidneys and hips)

2.1.2 BONY MALIGNANCY (child)

NEUROBLASTOMA METASTASIS

EWING'S AND BONE PNET (primitive neuroectodermal tumor)

METASTATIC LEUKEMIA

OSTEOSARCOMA

BONE LYMPHOMA

2.1.3 HIP ARTHRITIS WITH EFFUSION (child)

TRANSIENT SYNOVITIS (irritable hip)

SEPTIC ARTHRITIS

PERTHES' DISEASE

LEUKEMIA

JUVENILE CHRONIC ARTHRITIS

SLIPPED UPPER CAPITAL FEMORAL EPIPHYSIS

2.1.4 POROTIC BALLOON JOINT (overgrown epiphyses)

JUVENILE CHRONIC ARTHRITIS

HEMOPHILIA

INFECTION (tuberculosis)

PARALYSIS, PARESIS

2.1.5 PRESACRAL MASS (child)

SACROCOCCYGEAL TERATOMA

NEUROBLASTOMA

ANTERIOR MENINGOCELE

LIPOMA

RECTAL DUPLICATION

ABSCESS

2.2 XR (AND CT)

2.2.1 FOCAL SCLEROSIS (child)

STRESS FRACTURE

CHRONIC OSTEOMYELITIS

OSTEOID OSTEOMA

OSTEOSARCOMA

TRANSIENT SYNOVITIS (irritable hip)

SEPTIC ARTHRITIS

PERTHES' DISEASE

LEUKEMIA

JUVENILE CHRONIC ARTHRITIS

2.2.2 IRREGULAR EPIPHYSES

Solitary

POST TRAUMATIC

POST INFECTIVE

POST AVASCULAR NECROSIS (focal)

HIP: MEYER'S DYSPLASIA (resembles AVN)

Multiple

EXTRINSIC

TORCH INFECTIONS

WARFARIN EMBRYOPATHY

CRETINISM

INTRINSIC

MULTIPLE EPIPHYSEAL DYSPLASIA

CHONDRODYSPLASIA PUNCTATA

TRISOMY 21

2.2.3 METAPHYSEAL BANDS – DENSE

SYSTEMIC ILLNESS (growth arrest lines)

LEAD POISONING

SCURVY

HEALED RICKETS

CRETINISM

HYPERPARATHYROIDISM

CONGENITAL SYPHILIS

2.2.4 METAPHYSEAL LUCENCIES (child)

RICKETS, HYPOPHOSPHATASIA

SCURVY, SYPHILIS

NEUROBLASTOMA, LEUKEMIA METASTASES

CHILD ABUSE

METAPHYSEAL CHONDRODYSPLASIA

2.2.5 OSTEOPENIA – GENERALIZED (child)

Generalized congenital

OSTEOGENESIS IMPERFECTA

MARROW EXPANSION (thalassemia, other)

STORAGE DISORDERS

MUCOPOLYSACCHARIDOSES

MUCOLIPIDOSES

GAUCHER'S DISEASE

NIEMANN–PICK DISEASE

NEUROFIBROMATOSIS 1

Generalized metabolic

RENAL

HYPERPARATHYROIDISM

RICKETS

STEROIDS

Tumor

LEUKEMIA, LYMPHOMA

NEUROBLASTOMA METASTASES

LANGERHANS CELL HISTIOCYTOSIS

2.2.6 PERIOSTEAL REACTION (neonate, infant)

Mnemonic: FRACTURED POTS

Fractured

CHILD ABUSE

OSTEOGENESIS IMPERFECTA

P-hysiological

PHYSIOLOGICAL

CAFFEY'S DISEASE

O-steomyelitis

MULTIFOCAL OSTEOMYELITIS

T-umor

EWINGS, NEUROBLASTOMA, LEUKEMIA

MULTIFOCAL HISTIOCYTOSIS

S-curvy

SCURVY, SYPHILIS, (healing rickets)

OTHER TORCH INFECTIONS

3. PEDIATRIC MUSCULOSKELETAL CONDITIONS

3.1 BLOUNT'S DISEASE

CLINICAL

retarded growth of the medial aspect of the proximal tibial epiphysis possibly due to compression

INFANTILE: usually symmetrical, high prevalence of obesity

LATE ONSET: less common than infantile (6–15 years), usually unilateral

IMAGING

XR

extreme tibia vara

thinning, fragmentation and irregularity of medial aspect of tibial epiphysis

MR

enlargement of epiphyseal cartilage and medial meniscus

the physis narrows medially and fuses prematurely

3.2 CHILD ABUSE

CLINICAL

Cardinal sign

multiple injuries of different ages, injuries out of keeping with age or history

Commonest injuries are

rib fractures from thoracic compression

long bone metaphyseal and diaphyseal fractures from indirect force (twisting, pulling)

closed head injury (subdural hemorrhages and contusions, also retinal detachment) from shaking injury

anal/vaginal injuries, skin burns

IMAGING (XR + MDP + US)

use a combination of (high quality) skeletal radiographic survey and MDP bone scan for bone injuries

combination also allows rough determination of fracture age

periosteal reaction becomes radiographically detectable approximately 1 week post injury; osteoblastic activity shows on MDP at 24 hours or even earlier

Long bones

bucket handle fractures

corner fractures through metaphyseal collar

subperiosteal bleeds

exaggerated callus indicates repetitive injuries

Chest

spine fractures, posterior rib and sternal fractures

Brain + skull

multiple, complex skull fractures

subdural hematomas of different ages

interhemispheric subdural hematoma

cortical contusions, white matter shearing injury

infarcts

retinal hemorrhages and detachment

Abdomen

blunt abdominal injury

Blind areas

XR

skeletal injuries missed radiographically in at least one third of physically abused infants

stress fractures

subperiosteal bleeds

MDP

skull fractures

metaphyseal corner fractures (must have perfect positioning)

3.3 CLEIDOCRANIAL DYSOSTOSIS

see Ch 02

3.4 CONGENITAL SYPHILIS (manifestations)

3.4.1 CONGENITAL

IMAGING

XR

SKELETAL LYTIC LESIONS

lytic lesions in flat bones

lucent metaphyseal bands

widened growth plates

spared Jeantet Laval collar (collar of subperiosteal bone around a growth plate)

Wimberger sign (lysis medial tibial metaphysis)

SKELETAL REACTIVE LESIONS

periosteal reactions

3.4.2 ADULT (syphilis and yaws)

IMAGING

XR

diffuse fibrosis, extensive sclerosis

irregular areas of destruction

3.5 DEVELOPMENTAL HIP DYSPLASIA

DEFINITION

a spectrum of congenital hip abnormalities ranging from ligamentous laxity to complete hip dislocation; DDH: developmentally dysplastic hip

EPIDEMIOLOGY

incidence of overt hip dislocation in Caucasians is 1.5–1.7 per 1000 live births

Risk factors for DDH

first born female (female:male = 5:1)

breech presentation

positive family history

spina bifida, cerebral palsy, other neuromuscular disease

PATHOGENESIS

abnormal ligamentous laxity accentuated by high maternal estrogen, hereditary factors and abnormal positioning in utero

if untreated, progresses to disordered acetabular development producing a dysplastic acetabulum, and a partial or full dislocation

IMAGING – PLAIN FILM

see skeletal normal values (hips plain film)

displaced femoral capital epiphysis (either visible ossification center or its expected position) – lateral to Perkins line, abnormal orientation of femur long axis in frog leg view

increased acetabular roof angle

ACETABULAR ROOF ANGLE INCREASED IN

developmental hip dysplasia

neuromuscular disorders

ACETABULAR ROOF ANGLE DECREASED IN

Down's syndrome

skeletal dysplasias

osteogenesis imperfecta

hypophosphatasia

IMAGING – ULTRASOUND

ultrasound should preferably be done after 2 weeks of age

Dynamic hip testing

TECHNIQUE

scanning from posterolateral aspect of the hip

hip raised from neutral position to a flexed position

with the hip flexed, the femur is moved through a range of abduction and adduction

stress views are taken in the adducted position (i.e. ultrasound equivalent of Barlow's and Ortolani's tests)

FINDINGS

the normal hip remains entirely enlocated during motion

the lax hip has a normal position at rest but shows abnormal movement with stress

the subluxed hip is displaced at rest and is loose but not dislocatable (SUBLUXATION: the femoral head is at least partly covered by the acetabulum)

the dislocatable hip can be returned to the acetabulum with traction and abduction the dislocated hip is displaced at rest and can not be reduced (DISLOCATION: no contact or coverage of femoral head by the acetabulum)

Static assessment

DEGREE OF COVERAGE (commonest parameter)

measure from acetabular margin
>60% normal, <33% abnormal

ACETABULAR ANGLES (Graf angles)

normal is alpha <60 degrees (correlates with plain film), beta <55 degrees
as alpha angle decreases, the hip dysplasia grade increases

3.6 DISCOID MENISCUS

see Ch 04

3.7 DOWN'S SYNDROME
(postnatal manifestations)

also see Ch 22 obstetrics, trisomy 21

Chest

11 ribs, multiple sternal ossification centers
atrial septal defect, ventricular septal defect, atrioventricular septal defect, patent ductus arteriosus, aberrant right subclavian artery

Abdo

duodenal atresia, esophageal atresia, tracheoesophageal fistula
anorectal anomalies, Hirschsprung's disease

Pelvis

wide iliac wings, flat acetabular angles ('elephant ears')

Hands

clinodactyly, simian crease

Spine

atlantoaxial instability (25%)
anterior scalloping
short stature

Skull/face

brachycephalic microcephaly, hypotelorism
persistent metopic suture after age 10 years
hypoplastic sinuses and facial bones

3.8 DYSOSTOSIS MULTIPLEX

DEFINITION

spectrum of skeletal radiological signs (fully or partly expressed) present in genetic disorders of metabolism and accumulation of complex structural carbohydrates

CLASSIFICATION

Mucopolysaccharidoses (MPS)

Hurler's syndrome (MPS type I): autosomal recessive
Hunter's syndrome (MPS type II): X-linked
Morquio's syndrome (MPS type IV): autosomal recessive

Mucolipidoses

Note: glycogen storage diseases (glycogenoses)

do not produce characteristic dysostosis multiplex signs; may have non specific skeletal abnormalities secondary to bone marrow packing, visceromegaly and abnormal muscle

IMAGING MANIFESTATIONS (group)

Plain XR

abnormal bone texture
widening of diaphyses
large skull with thickened calvarium, J shaped sella
overconstriction ('pointing') of proximal ends of metacarpals; distal ulna and radius tilted towards each other
anterior beaking of vertebral bodies (on lateral view)

IMAGING (Hurler's/Hunter's)

macrocephaly, thick vault, J shaped sella
ovoid vertebrae, inferior beak
odontoid hypoplasia, thoracolumbar (L1 or L2) kyphosis
flared iliac wings, coxa valga, small epiphyses
thin long bone cortex, coarse trabeculae, abnormal modeling; proximally overconstricted metacarpals

short stature, coarse facies, corneal opacities, mental retardation, hepatosplenomegaly

IMAGING (Morquio's)

absent odontoid, C1–C2 instability, platyspondyly, central beak, thoracolumbar kyphosis
flared iliac wings, coxa valga, absent epiphyses
genu valgum, abnormal epiphyses, proximally overconstricted metacarpals
short stature, normal intelligence

3.9 EWING'S SARCOMA

see Ch 05

3.10 FOOT CONGENITAL DISORDERS

GROUP DEFINITIONS AND TERMINOLOGY

Talipes

general term for any congenital foot deformity

Pes

general term for any acquired foot deformity

Varus

distal part angulated inwards to midline (e.g. hindfoot on talus)

Valgus

distal part angulated outwards away from midline (e.g. hindfoot on talus)

3.10.1 TALIPES EQUINOVARUS
('clubfoot')

ETIOLOGY

congenital (most common)
teratologic (meningocele, arthrogryposis)
syndromic (diastrophic dysplasia, tibial hemimelia)

CLINICAL AND IMAGING

ankle equinus (plantarflexed), hindfoot varus, forefoot varus

post treatment appearance: normal, rocker bottom foot, flat top talus (talar dome avascular necrosis/collapse)
talocalcaneal angle decreased, calcaneal pitch (angle between calcaneum long axis and horizontal) decreased

3.10.2 TALIPES CALCANEOVALGUS

ankle dorsiflexed, hindfoot valgus, forefoot planus

3.10.3 FLEXIBLE FLATFOOT

ankle normal, hindfoot valgus, forefoot planus
talocalcaneal angle increased

3.10.4 RIGID FLATFOOT

painful stiff flat foot in older child
talocalcaneal coalition, calcaneonavicular coalition, other coalitions (see tarsal coalition)
also associated with rheumatoid arthritis and prior osteochondral fractures

3.10.5 VERTICAL TALUS

ankle equinus, hindfoot valgus, talonavicular dislocation
talocalcaneal angle increased

3.10.6 PES CAVUS

ETIOLOGY

neuromuscular atrophy
peroneal muscular atrophy
arthrogryposis: congenital muscular atrophy and fibrosis, joint contractures
(differential diagnosis is talipes equinovarus)

3.11 FRACTURES IN CHILD: CLASSIFICATION

DIAMETAPHYSEAL TYPES

3.11.1 PLASTIC BOWING

3.11.2 BUCKLE (TORUS)

3.11.3 GREENSTICK

3.11.4 COMPLETE

SALTER–HARRIS (SH) TYPES

passes through hypertrophied cartilage zone

3.11.5 SHI   THROUGH GROWTH PLATE

3.11.6 SHII   METAPHYSEAL CORNER, GROWTH PLATE

3.11.7 SHIII   GROWTH PLATE, EPIPHYSEAL CORNER

3.11.8 SHIV   OBLIQUE, A CORNER OF EACH

3.11.9 SHV   CRUSHED GROWTH PLATE

PROGNOSTICATORS

Fracture remodels well if

>2 years of growing remaining before epiphyseal closure age
fracture at bone end
fracture in plane of joint movement

Fracture remodels poorly if

displaced intraarticular fracture
midshaft fracture
perpendicular to plane of joint movement
rotational deformity or severe angulation
SH IV

3.12 HEMOPHILIA

see Ch 02

3.13 INFANTILE CORTICAL HYPEROSTOSIS (Caffey's disease)

self limiting infantile (<6 months of age) cortical hyperostosis of uncertain etiology
soft tissue swelling, underlying bony cortical thickening fever, irritability
mandible, ribs (most common)
other: clavicle, humerus, upper limb and lower limb long bones

IMAGING

XR
early: smooth linear periosteal reaction with laminated new bone formation
later: thick benign 'casting' periosteal new bone producing marked cortical hyperostosis

3.14 JUVENILE CHRONIC ARTHRITIS (JCA)

see Ch 03

3.15 LANGERHANS CELL HISTIOCYTOSIS

see Ch 05

3.16 OSTEOGENESIS IMPERFECTA

DEFINITION

heterogeneous group of autosomal recessive and autosomal dominant conditions with abnormal collagen and fragile bone

CLINICAL

may have blue sclerae and deafness

Osteogenesis imperfecta congenita
manifest at birth
autosomal dominant
'thick bone type'

Osteogenesis imperfecta tarda
usually not manifest at birth
recessive or dominant
'thin bone type'

IMAGING

XR
variable degrees of osteopenia, multiple fractures with hypertrophic callus, bowing deformities, gracile bones, calcific popcorn metaphyses
dentinogenesis imperfecta
large skull fontanelles, Wormian bones, basilar invagination
codfish vertebrae
trident pelvis with severe protrusio acetabuli

3.17 OSTEOMYELITIS

see Ch 02

3.18 OSTEOSARCOMA

see Ch 05

3.19 PERTHES' DISEASE

DEFINITION

idiopathic avascular necrosis of capital
femoral epiphysis

CLINICAL

4–10 years old, boys > girls
bilateral in ~15%
younger age than slipped upper femoral
epiphysis
present with pain, limp, limitation of
movement

IMAGING

XR

in general, XR changes are late compared to
NUC MED or MR

EARLY

widened joint space due to effusion or wider
cartilage
subchondral fissure fracture
increased bone density

INTERMEDIATE

granular/fragmented/sclerotic epiphysis
irregular growth plate
sclerotic metaphysis +/– cysts

LATE

full resolution, restoration of normality or
coxa plana (flattening of upper femoral
contour, 'mushroom' femoral head)
secondary degenerative changes

PLAIN FILM DIFFERENTIAL

AVN OF KNOWN CAUSE

SICKLE CELL DISEASE

INFECTION

STEROIDS

TRAUMA

MEYER'S FEMORAL HEAD DYSPLASIA

NUC MED

MDP

EARLY

corresponding tissue phase photopenic
defect and delayed phase photopenic
defect

!use pinhole views to compare the sides
extent of photopenia and its location affects
prognosis
LATE
photopenic defect in active ring or irregular
hot areas
possibly restoration of normality

MR

see avascular necrosis Ch 02
by definition, changes are epiphyseal
MR done in particular for evaluation of
articular cartilage and degree of femoral
head coverage

3.20 RHABDO-MYOSARCOMA

see Ch 05

3.21 RICKETS

see Ch 02

3.22 RUBELLA AND CMV
(congenital)

IMAGING (XR)

vertical striations ('celery stalking')
especially around knees
narrow sclerotic medullary cavity
delayed maturation
heals by 6 months

3.23 SCHEUERMANN DISEASE

see Ch 02

3.24 SCOLIOSIS

DEFINITION

abnormal non positional lateral curvature of
spine

ETIOLOGY

Idiopathic (most)

beware cardiac anomalies

INFANTILE (<4 years old)
male > female

JUVENILE (4–10 years old)
female > male

ADOLESCENT (>10 years old)
female >> male
usually thoracic, convex to right

Bony anomaly

HEMIVERTEBRAE
FUSIONS, KLIPPEL–FEIL SYNDROME

Neuromuscular

CEREBRAL PALSY
SPINA BIFIDA
TETHERED CORD
SYRINX
POLIO
MUSCULAR ATROPHIES AND DYSTROPHIES

Syndromic

NEUROFIBROMATOSIS 1
ARTHROGRYPOSIS
MARFAN'S SYNDROME
CYSTINURIA
CHONDRODYSPLASIAS
SPONDYLODYSPLASIAS
POST RADIOTHERAPY

ASSESSMENT

(Lipmann-Cobb method)

extend line along outer endplates of the last
involved segments, measure angle
can use pedicles if endplate indistinct
error in the order of 4 degrees expected

Direction

NAMED BY CONVEXITY
*ambiguity avoided if direction of convexity
stated explicitly*

Primary curve vs secondary curve

PRIMARY CURVE FIXED
SECONDARY CURVE COMPENSATORY
*can differentiate by films in lateral flexion
to assess fixity of each curve*

Rotatory component

in general bodies rotate towards convexity,
pedicles towards concavity
can assess from pedicle symmetry or derive
exact angle from CT

Balance

LATERAL BALANCE: T1 OVER S1 in neutral
standing posture

Leg length discrepancy

3.25 SCURVY

DEFINITION

vitamin C deficiency leading to failure of osteoid formation but preserved calcified cartilage, and fragile vessel walls prone to petechial and soft tissue bleeding

3.25.1 CHILDHOOD SCURVY

CLINICAL

clinical manifestations take several months to develop
occurs after 6 months of age
dietary cause (boiled cow's milk)
skin and mucosal petechiae and bleeds
subperiosteal bleeds
'failure to thrive'

IMAGING (XR)

3 metaphyseal findings
white line of Frankel (preserved provisional calcification)
lucent band (no normal ossification) metaphyseal to this
metaphyseal fractures and spurs

Epiphyseal finding
Wimberger ring (preserved provisional calcification)

Periosteal finding
elevation by hemorrhages with periosteal reaction

XR differential
CHILD ABUSE
SYPHILIS
LEUKEMIA
TREATED RICKETS

3.25.2 ADULT SCURVY

ongoing bone resorption with reduced new osteoid producing osteopenia
abnormal vessel walls – soft tissue and cutaneous hemorrhages

3.26 SLIPPED UPPER FEMORAL EPIPHYSIS

CLINICAL

shearing displacement of upper femoral epiphysis along growth plate (analogous to Salter–Harris type I fracture)
10–15 year olds, more prevalent in heavy, tall or obese
20% is bilateral
presents with pain (may be referred to knee), limp and limitation of range of motion

IMAGING

XR
displacement of epiphysis is posteriorly then medially
requires two views for diagnosis: AP and lateral (may be frog leg)
displacement of cortical margins of epiphysis and metaphysis relative to each other (in the expected direction) causing a step
AP view: line along upper femoral neck does not intersect epiphysis
widening, blurring of epiphyseal plate
periosteal new bone formation implies chronicity
symmetry is useful, but a potential pitfall in symmetrical bilateral slip

MR
morphology analogous to XR
assesses for avascular necrosis of the epiphysis

NUC MED
diffuse growth plate abnormality on MDP
if gross slip, deformity evident

3.27 SPINAL INFECTION

see Ch 02

3.28 TARSAL COALITION

CLINICAL

1–2% of population, male > female; 50% bilateral
presents in adolescence or early adulthood with foot pain after increased activity
may present with rigid flat foot ('peroneal spastic flat foot')

PATHOLOGY

abnormal fibrous, fibrocartilage, cartilaginous or osseous union with some initial mobility (unless osseous)
secondary degenerative change develops at the coalition or away from it because of altered biomechanics
commonest location (often asymptomatic) is calcaneonavicular; next commonest (usually symptomatic) is talocalcaneal at the sustentaculum tali; these two comprise 90% of tarsal coalitions

IMAGING

XR

CALCANEONAVICULAR COALITION (use 45 degree oblique view)
'anteater sign' of anterior dorsal calcaneus
abnormal calcaneonavicular articulation
frank bony bridge
elongated anterior process of the calcaneum

TALOCALCANEAL COALITION
most commonly involves middle calcaneal facet at the level of the sustentaculum tali
nil on XR
narrowed talocalcaneal joints
talar beak (periosteal elevation and ossification on dorsum of talus secondary to subtalar joint traction)

NUC MED
increased MDP uptake at the site of the fibrous joint (not invariable) or in hindfoot more diffusely

CT (direct coronal and direct axial scans, compare sides)
frank bony union with trabecular continuity
or
abnormal irregular sclerotic joint with thin soft tissue density core and secondary degenerative changes
coronal CT demonstrates the downward slope of sustentaculum or other articular surfaces oriented in the axial plane

MR
characterizes joint as fibrous tissue, cartilaginous tissue or bone
bone marrow edema is frequently present along the fused articulation

18 Pediatric gastrointestinal

1. NORMAL

1.1 APPENDIX

normal is <6 mm diameter, compressible, seen in 5%

1.2 DUODENOJEJUNAL FLEXURE POSITION

above or at transpyloric plane to left of spine duodenal cap = 1/2 way between curvatures (need perfect AP positioning)

1.3 NEONATAL GIT GAS

present in stomach at birth, small bowel at 6 hours, rectum at 24 hours

1.4 PYLORUS

transverse diameter <8 mm, length <15 mm, single wall muscle thickness <3 mm

1.5 RECTOSIGMOID INDEX (AP view)

rectum:sigmoid transverse size ratio is 0.9 or above

2. GAMUTS

2.1 NEONATE GIT GAMUTS

2.1.1 NEONATE WITH ABDOMINAL MASS

Renal

HYDRONEPHROSIS

MULTICYSTIC DYSPLASTIC KIDNEY – POLYCYSTIC KIDNEY DISEASE SPECTRUM

ECTOPIC KIDNEY

RENAL VEIN THROMBOSIS
associated with nephrotic syndrome and dehydration

TUMOR

Gynecologocal

OVARIAN CYSTIC FOLLICLE

HYDROMETROCOLPOS

Adrenal

HEMATOMA

TUMOR

Bowel

OBSTRUCTION, MECONIUM ILEUS, VOLVULUS

DUPLICATION CYST, MESENTERIC CYST

Liver

HEMATOMA (trauma)

CHOLEDOCHAL CYST

HEMANGIOENDOTHELIOMA

2.1.2 NEONATE WITH BOWEL OBSTRUCTION

Differential is ileus

Duodenal

ATRESIA SPECTRUM

ATRESIA

STENOSIS

DIAPHRAGM

ANNULAR PANCREAS

PREPYLORIC PORTAL VEIN

High non duodenal

MALROTATION

LADD BANDS

VOLVULUS

JEJUNAL ATRESIA

CYST/MASS

Low

INGUINAL HERNIA

MECONIUM ILEUS/MECONIUM PLUG

HIRSCHSPRUNG'S/ILEAL ATRESIA

SMALL (HYPOPLASTIC) LEFT COLON

Anorectal

ATRESIA (+/– fistula)

Hypertrophic pyloric stenosis is not neonatal (6–8 weeks of age)

2.1.3 NEONATE WITH GIT BLEEDING

NECROTIZING ENTEROCOLITIS VS

SWALLOWED MATERNAL BLOOD

2.2 CHILD GIT GAMUTS

2.2.1 CHILD WITH ABDO CALCIFICATION

see Ch 19

2.2.2 CHILD WITH ABDO MASS

Blastoma

NEPHROBLASTOMA

NEUROBLASTOMA

HEPATOBLASTOMA

Non blastoma

HYDRONEPHROSIS

APPENDIX ABSCESS

INTUSSUSCEPTION

CHOLEDOCHAL CYST

OMPHALOMESENTERIC CYST

2.2.3 CHILD WITH BOWEL OBSTRUCTION

MNEMONIC: AIM

A-PPENDIX AND A-DHESIONS

I-NTUSSUSCEPTION AND I-NGUINAL HERNIA

M-ALROTATION, M-ECKEL'S, M-ASS

2.2.4 CHILD WITH BOWEL PERFORATION

Gastric

STRESS ULCERS

SB

NECROTIZING ENTEROCOLITIS IN NEONATE

LOW OBSTRUCTION

MECKEL'S DIVERTICULUM

LB

APPENDIX

HIRSCHSPRUNG'S WITH TOXIC MEGACOLON

Iatrogenic

2.2.5 CHILD WITH GIT BLEEDING

Esophageal

REFLUX

FOREIGN BODY

VARICES

Gastric

ACUTE HEMORRHAGIC GASTRITIS

STRESS ULCERS

SB

NECROTIC BOWEL

INFARCT

VOLVULUS

MECKEL'S DIVERTICULUM

ENTERITIS

DUODENAL ULCER

LB

INTUSSUSCEPTION

COLITIS

POLYP

INFLAMMATORY BOWEL DISEASE

Anorectal

FISSURE

CHILD ABUSE

2.2.6 FREE INTRAPERITONEAL FLUID

see Ch 06

2.3 LIVER GAMUTS

2.3.1 NEONATAL JAUNDICE

Non cholestatic

PHYSIOLOGIC

HEMOLYTIC

Cholestatic

FOCAL COMPRESSION OR MASS

BILIARY DILATION SPECTRUM
see its own entry
CHOLEDOCHAL CYST
CAROLI'S DISEASE
POLYCYSTIC KIDNEY DISEASE
CONGENITAL HEPATIC BILIARY FIBROSIS

BILIARY ATRESIA SPECTRUM
see its own entry
EXTRAHEPATIC BILIARY ATRESIA
INTRAHEPATIC BILIARY ATRESIA

NEONATAL HEPATITIS

Investigations

US
diagnoses focal lesion, biliary dilation

HIDA SCAN
UPTAKE AND EXCRETION
neonatal hepatitis likely (differential is normal)
UPTAKE NO EXCRETION
biliary atresia spectrum
do cholangiography
POOR UPTAKE
probably neonatal hepatitis
?phenobarbital induction, repeat

2.3.2 PEDIATRIC FATTY LIVER

CYSTIC FIBROSIS

ALPHA 1 ANTITRYPSIN DEFICIENCY

ACUTE HEPATITIS

HEPATOTOXINS

MALABSORPTION

STORAGE DISEASE, METABOLIC DISEASE

2.3.3 PEDIATRIC GALLSTONES

PIGMENT STONES

METABOLIC DISEASE

MALABSORPTION

2.3.4 PEDIATRIC LIVER MASS

Pseudotumor

SIMPLE CYST

HYDATID

CHOLEDOCHAL CYST

HEMATOMA, TRAUMA

FATTY HEPATOMEGALY

Non tumor

FOCAL NODULAR HYPERPLASIA

Vascular

HEMANGIOMA

HEMANGIOENDOTHELIOMA

ANGIOSARCOMA

Hepatocellular

ADENOMA

HEPATOBLASTOMA

HEPATOCELLULAR CARCINOMA

Biliary tumor

MESENCHYMAL HAMARTOMA

BILIARY ADENOMA

CHOLANGIOCARCINOMA

Mass of non liver tissue origin

GERM CELL TUMOR

RHABDOMYOSARCOMA

NEUROBLASTOMA METASTASIS

PEDIATRIC GIT AND LIVER CONDITIONS

3. GIT CONDITIONS

3.1 ANORECTAL ATRESIA SPECTRUM

CLASSIFICATION

Relation to levator

HIGH

INTERMEDIATE

LOW (transperineal only surgery)

Fistulation (depends on position of atresia)

NIL

TO UTERUS, VAGINA, VULVA

TO BLADDER, URETHRA

TO PERINEUM

ASSOCIATIONS

50% have spinal cord anomalies
40% have bladder and renal malformations
VATER: Vertebral, Anal, Tracheo-
  Esophageal, Renal and Radial
  malformations
SACRAL AGENESIS, CAUDAL REGRESSION

RADIOLOGICAL WORKUP

Aims

DETERMINE LEVEL OF ATRESIA

INVERTOGRAM + MR (US)

ASSESS SPINE AND CORD

PLAIN FILMS + MR

ASSESS BLADDER AND KIDNEYS

ULTRASOUND AND VCUG
  (voiding/micturating cystourethrogram)

ASSESS FISTULATION AND UTERUS

FISTULOGRAM, GENITOGRAM

Invertogram

perfect lateral, not crying, no adherent
  meconium in bowel, anal dimple marker

BASELINES

pubococcygeal line (to sacrococcygeal joint)
line through ischial tuberosity parallel to
  that
halfway line parallel to both = levator line

LOW

= anorectal air caudal to levator line
= <1.5 cm to perineum on US

3.2 APPENDICITIS

see Ch 06

3.3 DUODENAL ATRESIA SPECTRUM

CLINICAL

incidence 1/3500, male = female
associations: Down's syndrome, cardiac
  malformations, malrotation
ATRESIA: short, long, multiple
STENOSIS: short, long
DIAPHRAGM: complete, incomplete,
  'windsock' (incomplete diaphragm
  stretched distally)
ANNULAR PANCREAS

IMAGING

Fluoro

upper GI contrast study demonstrates first
  level of obstruction and morphology

Differential

MALROTATION, VOLVULUS, LADD BANDS
PREPYLORIC PORTAL VEIN
DIFFERENTIAL OF MASS: HEMATOMA,
  DUPLICATION CYST, CHOLEDOCHAL
  CYST

3.4 DUPLICATION CYST

DEFINITION

blind endodermal cyst duplicating bowel

CLINICAL

male = female
85% present <1 year with mass or small
  bowel obstruction
terminal ileum > stomach > proximal small
  bowel
spherical or tubular mesenteric aspect cyst
  with muscular (therefore hypoechoic)
  wall and mucosal (therefore bright) lining

IMAGING

XR

rarely calcify; otherwise bowel obstruction
  or no findings

US

thick walled cystic mass
muscular hypoechoic rim

bright internal mucosal lining (if mucosa
  intact)
may contain clear fluid or debris or clot

CT/MR

cyst wall may enhance in a fashion similar
  to bowel
contents watery or inspissated or
  hemorrhagic (if gastric mucosa) with
  variable density and MR signal

NUC MED (TcO4)

if present, ectopic gastric mucosa parallels
  stomach pertechnetate uptake (similar to
  Meckel's scan)

3.5 ESOPHAGUS DEVELOPMENTAL ANOMALIES

3.5.1 ATRESIA AND TRACHEOESOPHAGEAL FISTULA (TEF)

CLASSIFICATION

ATRESIA, DISTAL TEF 80%

ATRESIA NO TEF 10%

H FISTULA 5%

OTHER FORMS 5%

CLINICAL

antenatal polyhydramnios (>50%)
excessive salivation
coughing, choking and cyanosis with feeding
aspiration pneumonia (saliva, feeds, gastric
  contents reflux)
bowel gas usually present (passes via distal
  fistula)
inability to pass a nasogastric tube into
  stomach

Associations

VATER (Vertebral, Anal, Tracheo-
  Esophageal, Renal and Radial
  malformations)
DOWN'S SYNDROME
CARDIAC MALFORMATIONS

Postop problems

recurrence of stricture

tracheomalacia
abnormal distal motility
reflux

IMAGING

XR
rarely, gasless abdomen (atresia, no TEF)
rarely, distended upper blind esophageal
    pouch outlined by air
commonly, nasogastric tube curled in
    esophageal pouch
secondary aspiration pneumonia

Fluoro
use cautiously because of aspiration risk
use non-ionic, isosmolar IV contrast in
    preference
blind esophageal pouch (outlined via
    nasogastric tube) with or without a
    fistula
supine contrast study via nasogastric tube
    that is slowly withdrawn best chance of
    showing a 'H' fistula

MR
coronal and sagittal studies may show
    anatomy layout

3.5.2 DUPLICATION CYST

PATHOLOGY

duplication cyst in isolation vs cyst with
    neurenteric fistula
lining: bronchial/squamous/cuboidal
    epithelia

IMAGING

CT/MR
duplication cyst in isolation: usually
    mediastinal mass (asymptomatic or with
    mass effect)
neurenteric fistula: may have evidence of
    hemivertebrae and other structural
    vertebral anomalies

3.5.3 ECTOPIC GASTRIC MUCOSA

PATHOLOGY

usually asymptomatic patches

IMAGING

Fluoro
usually no findings OR
areas of minimal contour depression on
    barium swallow

3.5.4 NEURENTERIC CYST OR FISTULA

PATHOLOGY

failure of closure or remnant cyst of
    embryonal neurenteric canal
posterior mediastinal enteric cyst in
    association with vertebral or neural
    abnormalities

Skeletal
spina bifida, hemivertebrae, scoliosis, bony
    cleft

Neural
tethered cord, fistulous track, intradural
    extension of cyst

IMAGING

combination of posterior mediastinal cyst
    and vertebral or spinal cord anomalies,
    often cranial to the cyst

3.6 HENOCH–SCHÖNLEIN PURPURA

see Ch 16 purpuras

3.7 HYPERTROPHIC PYLORIC STENOSIS

CLINICAL

male:female 4:1
associations: Turner's syndrome, trisomy 18,
    congenital rubella, tracheoesophageal
    fistula, first born male child
presents with non bilious vomiting
    developing after birth, palpable
    epigastric 'olive'
benign self limiting course if treated
    conservatively; surgical treatment is
    muscle coat split ('pyloromyotomy')

Differential

PYLOROSPASM
structurally normal
associated with dehydration, sepsis, ulcer,
    idiopathic

MALROTATION WITH VOLVULUS
bilious vomiting more likely

IMAGING

US
NORMAL is diameter <8 mm, muscle
    thickness <3 mm, length <15 mm
use sugary water rather than milk or
    formula (causes a 'snowstorm')
STENOSIS: vigorous peristalsis and failure to
    open over time with abnormal
    measurements

Fluoro
non distensible aperistaltic pylorus with
    elongated canal and thick muscle
SIGNS: caterpillar (peristalsis), beak
    (proximal mouth of stenosis), teat
    (proximal shoulder), diamond and double
    track (pyloric mucosal folding),
    mushroom (distal shoulders)

AXR
often normal
dilated stomach with peristaltic waves and
    bulging pylorus

3.8 INTUSSUSCEPTION

EPIDEMIOLOGY

male:female 2:1
50% <1 year old, 75% <2 years old
if >3 years old always look for pathological
    lead point

ETIOLOGY

Location
90% ILEOCOLIC
ILEOILEAL
COLOCOLIC (rare)

(90%) Idiopathic
Peyer's patch hypertrophy

Pathological intussusception
EMBRYONAL
MECKEL'S

DUPLICATION

INFECTIVE
INFLAMMATORY MASS
HENOCH–SCHÖNLEIN PURPURA

NEOPLASTIC
POLYP
LYMPHOMA
CANCER

CLINICAL

lead point dragged distally into bowel lumen by peristalsis, with its bowel forming an inner doubly folded 'teat' (intussusceptum) encased by dilated single walled distal bowel (intussuscipiens)
abdominal pain, vomiting, diarrhea (bloody diarrhea late), may have palpable mass
eventual complete constipation, and eventually perforation with peritonitis

IMAGING

AXR

empty large bowel, eventual small bowel obstruction
possible soft tissue mass at transition zone (most commonly right iliac fossa); mass rarely has a crescent of gas or fat
normal AXR does not exclude

Barium

classic 'coiled spring' appearance with barium tracking between intussusceptum (inner bowel) and intussuscipiens (receiving bowel)
for reduction see below

US

concentrically layered mass with crescent of echogenic fat (US crescent sign) rarely a complete circle of fat
can usually identify transverse and longitudinal orientations
may see peristalsis into the intussusception
may see gut wall signature in outer and inner bowel; more commonly too edematous to discern
color flow confirms (at least arterial) vascular integrity

CT

focal mass at transition point with crescent of mesenteric fat separating inner soft tissue mass from outer bowel
may see mesenteric edema and distortion of mesenteric vessels

Reduction

PREPARATION

resuscitate and rehydrate
surgeon on standby
no heavy sedation (need child to Valsalva)

ABSOLUTE CONTRAINDICATION

perforation or peritonitis

COMPLICATION RATE

perforation rate 1/250 (IV cannula on hand)

HYDROSTATIC

3 times, 3 minutes, 3 feet (classic method)

PNEUMATIC

diagnostic phase at 60 mmHg
reduction phase 80 mmHg to 120 mmHg
requires dedicated equipment
ADVANTAGES: control of pressure; higher success rate (?); less fecal contamination if perforates

FOLLOWUP

must exclude mass as a lead point
recurs in 10%

3.9 MALROTATION SPECTRUM

CLASSIFICATION

! duodenal and cecal rotation are partly independent

Non rotation (SB in left abdomen, LB in right abdomen)

Incomplete rotation

Non fixation (position normal, too mobile)

Reverse rotation (full or partial)

Malrotation is obligatorily present in
OMPHALOCELE
GASTROSCHISIS
DIAPHRAGMATIC HERNIA
HETEROTAXY SPECTRUM

Associated abnormality: Ladd bands

abnormal fibrous attachments of malrotated bowel that cross duodenum and may obstruct the deeper bowel loop

CLINICAL PRESENTATION

Acute

SMALL BOWEL OBSTRUCTION

bilious vomiting
double or triple bubble on AXR
CAUSES: volvulus, Ladd bands, hernia, intraluminal web

ISCHEMIC BOWEL

volvulus with gangrene (venous infarction first)
multiple dilated closed loops

Chronic

lymphatic stasis
intermittent torsion
pain, malabsorption, partial small bowel obstruction

IMAGING

AXR

normal OR
small bowel obstruction (usually high, with a double or triple bubble)

Fluoro

principal study
need perfect positioning and small aliquots of contrast to avoid flooding
DEFINED as absence of a normally positioned duodenojejunal flexure in two views (see normal)
commonest is zigzagging continuation of second or third parts of duodenum
if complete obstruction from volvulus, may show a 'twist'
PITFALL: redundant duodenal loop with normal duodenojejunal flexure

US

malposition of superior mesenteric vein relative to superior mesenteric artery

CT

shows transition zone
shows enhancement of bowel wall (normal consistent with viability or abnormal delayed consistent with infarction/venous infarction or none consistent with established gangrene)
shows intramural gas
signs of malrotation: malpositioned superior mesenteric vein relative to superior mesenteric artery (usually in front of or to left)
abnormal course of duodenum

3.10 MECKEL'S DIVERTICULUM

CLINICAL

persistent remnant of omphalomesenteric duct forming a blind ending pouch arising from antimesenteric border of small bowel

2% of population, but only 2% symptomatic; within 2 ft of ileocecal valve

commonest complications are hemorrhage (from ectopic gastric mucosa producing acid), intussusception, and small bowel obstruction

IMAGING

Fluoro
rarely may show on contrast studies

NUC MED (TcO4)
ectopic gastric mucosa in Meckel's diverticulum follows behavior of orthotopic gastric mucosa

commonest location is right iliac fossa

most if not all detectable Meckel's diverticula show by 30 min

FALSE POSITIVES
urinary activity (renal pelves, ureters, bladder diverticula)

blood pool activity including hemangiomas

duplication cyst with gastric mucosa

spontaneously or therapeutically reduced volvulus or intussusception

post instrumentation

FALSE NEGATIVES
Meckel's diverticulum without gastric mucosa

(theoretically) Meckel's diverticulum next to bladder

3.11 MECONIUMS

3.11.1 MECONIUM ILEUS

see under neonatal LBO

3.11.2 MECONIUM PERITONITIS

see Ch 22

peritoneal calcification in neonate; sequel of any intrauterine bowel perforation

association with bowel atresia (bowel proximal to atresia decompresses by perforation)

FOCAL vs GENERALIZED

3.11.3 MECONIUM PLUG SYNDROME

see under neonatal LBO

3.11.4 MECONIUM ILEUS EQUIVALENT

ileal or cecal obstruction by tenacious feces in an older cystic fibrosis patient

3.12 NECROTIZING ENTEROCOLITIS

DEFINITION

neonatal bowel ischemia with secondary bacterial invasion producing significant morbidity

EPIDEMIOLOGY

80% occurs in premature neonates

Risk factors multifactorial
hypoxia/ischemia
sepsis
enteric formula feeds

PATHOGENESIS

mucosal ischemia, edema, necrosis

bacterial invasion, mural gangrene, perforation

pneumatosis intestinalis, portal venous gas

CLINICAL

usually sick premature neonate of 3–7 days of age

abdominal distension, bloody stools, small or large bowel obstruction

sepsis, cardiovascular collapse, metabolic acidosis, DIC

LATE: strictures and short gut syndrome

IMAGING

AXR
right iliac fossa bowel dilation
subserosal linear pneumatosis
submucosal bubbly pneumatosis
portal venous gas
perforation, free intraperitoneal air

3.13 NEONATAL LARGE BOWEL OBSTRUCTION

3.13.1 HIRSCHSPRUNG'S DISEASE

CLINICAL

1/5000–1/8000

RISK FACTORS: family history, Down's syndrome, other neuromuscular abnormalities

80% present with large bowel obstruction under 6 weeks of age

80% have short segment involvement, male:female 4:1

15% have long segment involvement (female > male)

5% involve total colon

ultra short segment Hirschsprung's disease is controversial

PATHOGENESIS/ MORPHOLOGY

failure of neural crest cell migration into a bowel segment

no submucosal or myenteric neural plexi, and hypertrophied parasympathetic nerve endings in wall of abnormal bowel

hypertrophy of proximal normal bowel

IMAGING

AXR
abnormally distended proximal bowel often filled with mottled feces

Fluoro (enema)
narrow rectum with larger proximal bowel

abnormal rectosigmoid index (AP view, transverse diameter of rectum:sigmoid <0.9)

abnormal disorganized contractions in
abnormal segment
transition zone (funnel shaped in older child)
aperistalsis or spasm in abnormal segment

Differential diagnosis

NEONATE
hypoplastic left colon
meconium plug syndrome
functional large bowel obstruction
stricture (traumatic or ischemic)

OLDER CHILD
functional megacolon (normal rectosigmoid
index, levator sling impression with
sharp shoulders)
Chagas disease
stricture

3.13.2 MECONIUM PLUG SYNDROME

CLINICAL

neonatal colonic inertia
presents with large bowel obstruction at
2–3 days of age
must consider underlying Hirschsprung's
disease or cystic fibrosis

IMAGING

intact colon
no transition zone demonstrated
meconium plug

3.13.3 HYPOPLASTIC LEFT COLON SYNDROME

CLINICAL

functional left colon immaturity
presents with large bowel obstruction at
2–3 days of age
maternal diabetes mellitus

IMAGING

normal rectum, normal rectosigmoid index
small left colon, transition at splenic flexure

3.13.4 PREMATURE INFANT FUNCTIONAL LARGE BOWEL OBSTRUCTION

CLINICAL

immature colon in premature infant
presents with large bowel obstruction at 2–3
days of age

IMAGING

intact but unused colon
no transition zone
no ileal atresia

Differential
meconium ileus
Hirschsprung's disease

3.13.5 MECONIUM ILEUS

CLINICAL

common neonatal presentation of cystic
fibrosis
presents with bowel obstruction at 2–3 days
of age and either failure to pass
meconium or abnormal sticky meconium
differential is meconium ileus vs atresia vs
total colon Hirschsprung's disease

IMAGING

AXR
mottled density in right iliac fossa, multiple
dilated small bowel loops, no air–fluid
levels, eventual small bowel obstruction

Fluoro (enema)
microcolon, meconium impaction in ileum
+/– meconium peritonitis, ileal atresia

3.14 POLYPS (juvenile)

see Ch 06 polyps and polyposis syndromes

3.15 REFLUX ESOPHAGITIS

see Ch 06

3.16 SMALL BOWEL CONGENITAL DISEASE

3.16.1 DUODENAL ATRESIA SPECTRUM (dysembryogenesis)

see its own entry

3.16.2 MALROTATION SPECTRUM

see its own entry

3.16.3 MECKEL'S DIVERTICULUM

see its own entry

3.16.4 DUPLICATION CYST

see its own entry

3.16.5 MESENTERIC CYST

see mesenteric cyst in Ch 06

3.16.6 ILEOJEJUNAL ATRESIA (vascular accident)

interruption in small bowel continuity of
variable severity
postulated intrauterine ischemia leading to
focal ischemic atresia
spectrum varies from stenosis to fibrous
band to complete absence of segment of
bowel
atresia may be unifocal or multifocal
proximal bowel dilates, distal bowel remains
small caliber and unused

4. LIVER CONDITIONS

4.1 ALPHA 1 ANTITRYPSIN (alpha 1 AT) DEFICIENCY

CLINICAL

abnormal Pi (protease inhibitor) gene
Europeans: 3% heterozygotes, 1/7000
homozygotes (10% alpha 1 AT activity)

Lung disease
see Ch 13 lungs

Liver disease (20% of homozygotes)
neonatal or childhood hepatitis, cholestasis
childhood, adolescent cirrhosis
hepatocellular carcinoma in 3%

4.2 BILIARY ATRESIA SPECTRUM

4.2.1 EXTRAHEPATIC BILIARY ATRESIA

antenatal/perinatal sclerosing cholangitis
with loss of patency but no proximal
dilation
10% have major bile ducts present;
treatment is by roux en Y loop
90% have no major bile ducts present;
treatment is by Kasai procedure
(anastomosis of a bowel loop to dissected
porta hepatis)

4.2.2 INTRAHEPATIC BILIARY ATRESIA

ETIOLOGY

CYSTIC FIBROSIS
ALPHA 1 ANTITRYPSIN DEFICIENCY (20%
of all neonatal jaundice!)
TRISOMY 21

CLINICAL

cholestasis; inflamed edematous portal
tracts with no bile ducts
prognosis poor without liver transplantation

IMAGING (group)
US

presence of normal bile ducts rules out
atresia with a good degree of confidence
gallbladder may be present with bile duct
atresia
failure to identify biliary tree suggestive but
not absolutely conclusive
combination of US and HIDA more powerful
than either alone

MR
MRCP generally used for problem solving
and may demonstrate level of atresia and
relationship to portal vein and hepatic
artery
useful overview in dysmorphic or ambiguous
liver and biliary tree

NUC MED (IDA)
NORMAL CHILDREN: liver is shown by 5 min,
biliary tree by 10 min, gut by
10–15 min, gallbladder by 30 min
(assuming child has fasted)
DISIDA currently the preferred isotope;
intermittent delayed imaging done to
24 hours; there is never any vicarious
bowel excretion
low biliary atresia: good hepatocellular
uptake, delayed excretion into biliary
tree that never reaches bowel
high biliary atresia: good hepatocellular
uptake, no excretion
cardinal sign of atresia: failure of biliary tree
demonstration and failure of tracer
passage into bowel
ancillary findings: increased renal and
urinary tracer activity (renal excretion)
presence of tracer in bowel rules out atresia
or high grade obstruction
major differential is intracellular cholestasis
hepatocellular dysfunction has poor tracer
uptake by liver; in general, at least some
tracer reaches bowel by 24 hours
if there is very poor tracer uptake by liver
the test is inconclusive and may
occasionally need barbiturate induction

Combination US and DISIDA
if CBD and gallbladder found on US, then
even a little extrarenal abdominal IDA
activity represents bowel and confirms
patency
if US can not find bile ducts but IDA shows
clear bowel activity, then atresia is
excluded
if US shows a gallbladder but IDA has good
liver uptake and no excretion, IDA is
right (i.e. gallbladder with bile duct
atresia is likely)

4.3 BILIARY DILATION SPECTRUM

*also see tubular cystic disease spectrum in
Ch 19*

4.3.1 CHOLEDOCHAL CYST

see its own entry

4.3.2 CAROLI'S DISEASE

see its own entry

4.3.3 POLYCYSTIC KIDNEY DISEASE (PCKD)

Infantile PCKD

Juvenile PCKD (nephronophthisis)

4.3.4 CONGENITAL HEPATIC BILIARY FIBROSIS

irregular dilated ducts
periportal fibrosis, bridging fibrous septa

4.3.5 COMPLICATIONS OF ALL FORMS OF BILIARY DILATION

ASCENDING CHOLANGITIS
STONES AND STRICTURES
SECONDARY BILIARY CIRRHOSIS
PORTAL HYPERTENSION AND VARICES
CHOLANGIOCARCINOMA

4.4 CAROLI'S DISEASE

CLINICAL

multifocal segmental cystic dilation of major
intrahepatic bile ducts without distal
obstruction
occasionally presents in infancy; usually
childhood to 30's
ductal stones
recurrent cholangitis, liver abscesses
elevated risk of cholangiocarcinoma

Associations
medullary sponge kidney (80%)
infantile polycystic kidney disease
renal tubular acidosis
rarely choledochal cyst or hepatic fibrosis

IMAGING
US
multiple cysts, intracystic stones, cysts may
or may not visibly link to biliary tree

CT

hypodense cysts typically around portal
veins

CTIVC (CT intravenous cholangiography)

proves that cysts communicate with the
biliary tree

ERCP/MRCP

saccular dilations from bile ducts

4.5 CHOLEDOCHAL CYST

CLINICAL

abnormal dilation of the biliary tree without
current distal obstruction
female > male; age at diagnosis 30% <1
year, 50% 1–10 years old
presents with R upper quadrant pain,
jaundice, occasionally a mass
CONGENITAL: associated with CBD atresias
and stenoses
ACQUIRED: pancreatitis, stones, cirrhosis
COMPLICATIONS: cholangitis, stones and
strictures, secondary biliary cirrhosis,
cholangiocarcinoma

MACRO CLASSIFICATION

I 'aneurysm'

fusiform aneurysmal dilation of CBD

II 'diverticulum'

focal diverticulum off the CBD

III 'choledochocele'

distal CBD dilation with possible protrusion
into duodenum

IV Caroli's disease
(multifocal dilation)
see separate entry

IMAGING

US

abnormal cystic structure replacing or
displacing CBD
may or may not demonstrate continuity with
biliary tree
wall may be thickened (inflammation; settled
debris)

content may have echogenic mobile debris
or stones
location variable (see macro classification)

NUC MED (IDA)

may show delay in tracer passage
may show abnormal expansion of biliary tree
may be totally normal

CT

CTIVC useful in demonstrating morphology
and proving continuity of cyst with biliary
tree; can show intraluminal filling defects
(stones, clot)

MR

MRCP acts as a preoperative roadmap, and
also demonstrates intraluminal filling
defects

ERCP

demonstrates morphology and continuity
with biliary tree

4.6 HEMANGIO-ENDOTHELIOMA

CLINICAL

neonatal hepatic vascular malformation/
tumor
neonate or infant with high output cardiac
failure, liver mass, normal
alphafetoprotein
cutaneous hemangiomas in 50%

IMAGING

US

multifocal or diffuse areas of mixed
echogenicity; may see shunt flow

MR/CT

as for hemangioma

IDA

high in blood pool phase, cold defect in
static phase

Angio

multiple lakes in capillary phase
enlarged hepatic artery +/– arteriovenous
shunts

4.7 HEPATOBLASTOMA

CLINICAL

malignant embryonal liver cell tumor
male > female, occurs <3 years
failure to thrive, liver mass, massively raised
alphafetoprotein
EPITHELIAL TYPE: fetal large hepatocytes
in two cell thick plates, embryonic
hepatocytes in rosettes, acini, mitoses
MIXED EPITHELIAL AND MESENCHYMAL
TYPE: also a primitive mesenchymal
component

IMAGING

AXR

hepatomegaly, may show calcification

US

heterogeneous vascular mass, often
hypoechoic
may show arterial flow on Doppler
may show venous invasion

CT

hypodense mass with vivid arterial phase
enhancement
less enhancing than liver in portal venous
phase
may have venous invasion
may have areas of hemorrhage or
calcification

MR

non specific mass, low T1W, high T2W
signal, arterial phase enhancement with
Gd
may have intratumoral hemorrhage
best demonstration of portal and hepatic
vein invasion

Angio

mass with tumor neovascularity
allows preoperative embolization

4.8 LIVER TUMOR OVERVIEW

see Ch 07

4.9 NEONATAL HEPATITIS

DEFINITION

neonatal cholestatic liver disease with patent biliary tree

ETIOLOGY

Idiopathic

Infective
hepatitis B virus
herpes simplex virus
toxoplasmosis

Metabolic
alpha 1 antitrypsin deficiency (20% of neonatal jaundice)
cystic fibrosis
storage diseases
liver enzyme absence

IMAGING

also see biliary atresia spectrum (principal differential)

XR
no findings or possibly hepatomegaly

US
may be normal, in particular, biliary tree present
may have diffusely decreased echogenicity
absence of biliary tree suggests atresia but is not diagnostic

NUC MED (IDA)
see comments on DISIDA in biliary atresia spectrum
main role is confirmation of anatomical patency of biliary tree
presence of tracer in bowel rules out atresia or total obstruction
commonly poor liver uptake with eventual excretion into bowel
normal study supports neonatal hepatitis
if liver uptake very poor, study indeterminate

4.10 WILSON'S DISEASE

see Ch 07

19 Pediatric urogenital

1. NORMAL

1.1 ABBREVIATIONS

MCU: micturating cystourethrogram
PUJ: pelviureteric junction
VUJ: vesicoureteric junction
VCUG: voiding cystourethrogram
UTI: urinary tract infection

1.2 DTPA – MAG3 NORMAL VALUES

(source: Royal Children's Hospital, Melbourne)
Lasix (furosemide) dose 1mg/kg up to 20 mg
normal washout T 1/2 post Lasix is <12 min with MAG3, <15 min with DTPA
normal retention at 30 min post Lasix is <30% MAG3, <40% DTPA
limit of normal split renal mass is 45% to 55% (no depth correction)

1.3 GFR

1/3 adult at birth, 2/3 adult by 6 months, normal adult by 1 year (assuming normal adult GFR is ~120 ml/min)
maximum angiographic contrast dose (300 strength) is 4 ml/kg

1.4 KIDNEY SIZE

SIZE (cm)	AGE (y)	RANGE
5	0	+/– 3/4 cm
6	1	
7	3	
8	6	
9	9F, 12M	+/– 1 cm

1.5 OVARY and UTERUS

see Ch 23

2. GAMUTS

2.1 RENAL GAMUTS

2.1.1 ABDOMINAL CALCIFICATION IN A CHILD

Renal

MEDULLARY NEPHROCALCINOSIS
NEPHROLITHIASIS
NEPHROBLASTOMA
OXALOSIS
RENAL TB
SEQUELAE OF ACUTE CORTICAL NECROSIS

Adrenal

HEMORRHAGE
TB
NEUROBLASTOMA

Hepatic

HEMANGIOMA
HEPATOBLASTOMA
GRANULOMATOUS DISEASE (e.g. healed TB focus)
CALCIFIED HEMATOMA

Gallbladder

STONES

Gynecological

TERATOMA

Gut

MESENTERIC CYST
DUPLICATION CYST

Appendicolith

Peritoneal

MECONIUM PERITONITIS
TB

Vascular

THROMBUS (VV > AA)

2.1.2 ADRENAL MASS IN A CHILD

HEMATOMA
NEUROBLASTOMA
TB
PHEOCHROMOCYTOMA
MYELOLIPOMA
ADENOMA, CARCINOMA
METASTASIS

2.1.3 CYSTIC RENAL DISEASE IN A CHILD

EXCLUDE HYDRONEPHROSIS, OBSTRUCTED CALYX OR CALYCEAL DIVERTICULUM
MULTICYSTIC DYSPLASTIC KIDNEY
AUTOSOMAL RECESSIVE POLYCYSTIC KIDNEY DISEASE
AUTOSOMAL DOMINANT POLYCYSTIC KIDNEY DISEASE
JUVENILE NEPHRONOPHTHISIS
GLOMERULOCYSTIC DISEASE
CYSTIC DYSPLASIAS ASSOCIATED WITH SYNDROMES

2.1.4 ENLARGED KIDNEY IN A CHILD (unilateral)

HYDRONEPHROSIS IN A CHILD (see its own gamut)
RENAL MASS IN A CHILD (see its own gamut)
PYELONEPHRITIS
RENAL VEIN THROMBOSIS
TRAUMATIC HEMATOMA
DUPLICATION OR CROSSED FUSED RENAL ECTOPIA
COMPENSATORY HYPERTROPHY OR SOLITARY KIDNEY

2.1.5 ENLARGED KIDNEYS IN A CHILD (bilateral)

Bilateral only causes

GLOMERULONEPHRITIS
AUTOSOMAL RECESSIVE POLYCYSTIC KIDNEY DISEASE
AUTOSOMAL DOMINANT POLYCYSTIC KIDNEY DISEASE
NEPHROBLASTOMATOSIS
LEUKEMIA, LYMPHOMA, BILATERAL TUMOR INFILTRATION
BECKWITH–WIEDEMANN SYNDROME

Unilateral cause present bilaterally

BILATERAL PYELONEPHRITIS

BILATERAL RENAL VEIN THROMBOSIS

BILATERAL DUPLICATION

BILATERAL WILMS'

2.1.6 FOCAL KIDNEY DEFECT

see Ch 08

2.1.7 HYDRONEPHROSIS IN A CHILD

NEED TO DIFFERENTIATE HYDRONEPHROSIS FROM MULTICYSTIC DYSPLASTIC KIDNEY

PELVIURETERIC JUNCTION (PUJ, UPJ) OBSTRUCTION

REFLUX NEPHROPATHY
commonest is without a duplex, but also the lower moiety of a duplex inserts orthotopically and tends to reflux

VESICOURETERIC JUNCTION (VUJ, UVJ) OBSTRUCTION

ECTOPIC URETEROCELE WITH OBSTRUCTION
upper moiety of a duplex inserts low and tends to obstruct

NEUROPATHIC BLADDER WITH REFLUX

POSTERIOR URETHRAL VALVES WITH REFLUX

PRIMARY MEGAURETER/ MEGACALYCOSIS

EXTERNAL COMPRESSION
usually tumor

LUMINAL OBSTRUCTION
usually sloughed papilla – rare

2.1.8 RENAL MASS IN A CHILD

Unifocal/isolated

WILMS' TUMOR (nephroblastoma)

TUMORS SIMULATING NEPHROBLASTOMA

CONGENITAL MESOBLASTIC NEPHROMA

MULTILOCULAR CYSTIC NEPHROMA

RHABDOID TUMOR

CLEAR CELL SARCOMA

CYST

PYELONEPHRITIS/LOBAR NEPHRONIA/ABSCESS

RENAL CELL CARCINOMA

ANGIOMYOLIPOMA

MESENCHYMAL MASS (lipoma, fibroma)

PSEUDOTUMOR (prominent parenchyma)

Multifocal/bilateral

CYSTS

NEPHROBLASTOMATOSIS

BILATERAL PYELONEPHRITIS/LOBAR NEPHRONIA

LYMPHOMA, METASTASES

INFARCTS

2.1.9 SMALL BUMPY KIDNEY IN A CHILD

REFLUX SCARS

INFARCTS

TRAUMA

TB

DYSPLASIA

2.1.10 SMALL SMOOTH KIDNEY IN A CHILD (one or both)

Unilateral

MULTICYSTIC DYSPLASTIC KIDNEY

OTHER DYSPLASIA

OBSTRUCTIVE ATROPHY

INFARCT

LATE SEQUEL OF RENAL VEIN THROMBOSIS

WHOLE KIDNEY HYPOPLASIA OR APLASIA

Bilateral

CHRONIC GLOMERULONEPHRITIS AND VARIANTS

MEDULLARY CYSTIC DISEASE

VASCULITIS

UNILATERAL CAUSE PRESENT BILATERALLY

3. PEDIATRIC UROGENITAL CONDITIONS

3.1 BLADDER–URETHRA MALFORMATION SPECTRUM

3.1.1 CONGENITAL DIVERTICULUM

3.1.1.1 Primary diverticulum (three layer)

GENERAL
complications: stasis, stone, infection

AT VUJ = HUTCH DIVERTICULUM
COMPLICATIONS: vesicoureteric reflux, ureteric obstruction

AT INTERNAL SPHINCTER

3.1.1.2 Secondary diverticulum (no muscle layer)
mechanical outflow obstruction or dyssynergic bladder with subsequent outpouching of mucosa through muscle

3.1.2 EXTROPHY

failure of midline mesodermal fusion with bladder mucosa open to skin surface
association: anorectal and vaginal malformations, spinal dysraphism
widened symphysis pubis (>1 cm)

3.1.3 DUPLICATION, SEPTATION

3.1.4 OUTFLOW OBSTRUCTION

3.1.4.1 Urethral valves

CLINICAL
commonest cause of bladder outlet obstruction in boys
large bladder residual, poor stream, overflow dribbling, reflux hydronephrosis, UTI

IMAGING

VOIDING CYSTOURETHROGRAM

location usually just distal to verumontanum (distal prostatic urethra)

transition zone with dilated urethra above, narrow below

membrane outline may be visible

bulging valve membrane may form a rounded 'windsock'

reflux and bladder diverticula common

US

hydronephrosis, dilated ureters

thickened bladder wall with diverticula

3.1.4.2 Anterior urethral diverticulum

rounded ventral outpouching from penile urethra that swells with voiding

may present with 'balloon valve' obstruction

3.1.4.3 Ureterocele

see under ureteric malformation spectrum

3.1.4.4 Dyssynergia

3.1.5 CONGENITAL NEUROPATHIC BLADDER

3.2 BECKWITH–WIEDEMANN SYNDROME

('exomphalos-macroglossia-gigantism' or 'visceromegaly-hemihypertrophy' syndrome)

hemihypertrophy or generalized hypertrophy and macroglossia

omphalocele

large kidneys with renal medullary dysplasia

increased incidence of Wilms' tumor (nephroblastoma)

hepatomegaly (increased incidence of hepatoblastoma)

fetal adrenocortical cytomegaly

3.3 BENIGN RENAL TUMORS SIMULATING NEPHROBLASTOMA

3.3.1 CONGENITAL MESOBLASTIC NEPHROMA

CLINICAL

neonatal tumor, male > female

benign but locally invasive

gray-white whorled mass in medulla

spindle cell histology with trapped nephrons

IMAGING

US

hyperechoic or mixed echogenicity intrarenal mass

CT

hypodense mass with mild enhancement and possibly calcification

NUC MED (DTPA/MAG3)

may have enough functional nephrons to trap tracer

3.3.2 MULTILOCULAR CYSTIC NEPHROMA

children: male > female, adults: female > male

encapsulated multicystic tumor with septa separating fluid filled locules

flat or columnar cyst lining, fibroblastic stroma, foci of blastema, nephroblastoma, renal cell carcinoma in septa

3.4 CHILD URINARY TRACT INFECTION (UTI)

CLINICAL

Anatomy

NORMAL

OBSTRUCTION (PUJ > VUJ > POSTERIOR URETHRAL VALVES)

VESICOURETERIC REFLUX

Late sequels

RENAL SCARRING

HYPERTENSION, PREECLAMPSIA

REFLUX NEPHROPATHY, CHRONIC RENAL FAILURE

IMAGING

US

first line investigation

main role is to exclude underlying structural abnormality (hydronephrosis, duplication, ureterocele, bladder diverticulum)

ACUTE PYELONEPHRITIS ('acute lobar nephronia')

US has ~25% sensitivity for pyelonephritis

segment of abnormal reduced echogenicity (edema) or a swollen hypoechoic kidney

segment of reduced color/power Doppler perfusion

SCAR

scars develop over months

scar: focal deficiency of cortex, usually opposite upper or lower pole calyx (compound calyx)

DTPA/MAG3

assessment of overall renal function and side to side function split

may show scars (photopenic defects)

Lasix washout quantifies degree of holdup in hydronephrosis (and allows quantitation for upper and lower moieties)

VCUG/MCU

detects reflux (not 100% sensitive) and quantifies it

detects and quantifies bladder outflow obstruction

determines layout of refluxing moieties

may detect ureteroceles (as filling defects)

WHO TO INVESTIGATE

any male child with UTI

any female child <6 years with UTI

any female child >6 years with febrile UTI or recurrent UTI

any newborn with prenatal hydronephrosis

TECHNIQUE (radiographic VCUG/MCU)

sterile catheterization

slow gravity feed of contrast

frequent but very short bursts of screening

early filling shot (for filling defects, ureteroceles)

early oblique shots (for ?low grade reflux)

voiding shot (AP for girls, steep oblique for boys) for ?outflow obstruction (e.g. valves)

renal area shot for ?small amount of reflux

if reflux to renal pelvis – delayed 10 min shot for ?drainage

TERMINOLOGY

low pressure reflux: passage of contrast into ureter with filing

high pressure reflux: contrast passing into ureter with voiding

Radionuclide VCUG

followup of reflux

more sensitive in detection of reflux than radiographic VCUG but does not provide anatomical detail

indirect VCUG is possible in older cooperative children (IV injection of MAG3 or DTPA with lasix; once upper systems washout, void in front of gamma camera)

DMSA

labels functioning renal tissue and detects scars better than ultrasound (use SPECT as well as planar imaging)

allows side to side renal mass quantitation

scar is a focal photopenic area, commonly at upper or lower pole

whole kidney may be small and scarred

can not differentiate acute segmental pyelonephritis ('lobar nephronia') from scar – requires delayed followup imaging

very sensitive in detecting acute lobar nephronia (same signs as scar) but role in acute UTI not established

Long term followup

proven reflux treated with maintenance antibiotics or strict urine monitoring until child can reliably report symptoms of UTI

age cutoff after which development of new scars is unlikely is 5 years (controversial)

BP monitoring in reflux or pyelonephritis

delayed imaging looking for development of scars: DMSA at 12 months or US at 24 months

3.5 FEMALE GENITAL MALFORMATION SPECTRUM

3.5.1 MULLERIAN DEVELOPMENTAL ANOMALIES (Ch 23)

3.5.2 HEMATOCOLPOS (Ch 23)

3.5.3 VAGINAL ATRESIA AND COMPLEX MALFORMATIONS

vaginal atresia is often associated with complex cloacal malformations (urethrovaginal, rectovaginal, rectovesical, cloacal fistulas)

often presents with hydrometra (uterine dilation) as neonate

IMAGING

US

may show dilated uterus

MR

shows presence and gross location of organs

Contrast studies

required for mapping out fistulas

3.6 INFUNDIBULOPELVIC DYSPLASIA SPECTRUM

3.6.1 MULTICYSTIC DYSPLASTIC KIDNEY

CLINICAL

second commonest neonatal abdominal mass (after hydronephrosis)

male > female, L > R

25% have contralateral PUJ obstruction

sporadic and non heritable

cystic mass formed by metanephric blastema secondary to failure of induction; no communication with any collecting element

IMAGING

US/CT/MR

multicystic mass of variable size in renal bed

no normal kidney

no evidence of invasion or local aggressive behavior

no distant metastases

NUC MED (DTPA/MAG3/DMSA)

no tracer uptake during normal acquisition

small islands of renal tissue may be present, and tracer may trap in the mass or cysts on delayed (4 or 24 hour) images

3.6.2 PELVIURETERIC JUNCTION OBSTRUCTION

CLINICAL

presents at virtually any age and depends on degree of obstruction

commonest neonatal abdominal mass

child: UTI, mass, poor renal function, loin pain

adolescent: trauma, loin pain, UTI

adult: loin pain similar to renal colic

may be bilateral

more common in horseshoe kidney

PUJ has segmental muscular hypoplasia, disorganization, absent longitudinal coat

some 15% are due to aberrant lower pole renal artery – may show small segment of proximal ureter

IMAGING

IVU

least severe: baggy pelvis, rounded shape, abnormal PUJ with intermittent trickle of urine

moderate: delayed nephrogram, delayed pyelogram, dilated baggy pelvis

most severe: negative pyelogram, shell nephrogram, crescent sign (opacified excretory ducts reoriented circumferential to very dilated calyces)

VCUG/MCU

excludes reflux

US (done first)

dilated pelvis and calyces with no identifiable ureter and no ureterectasis

secondarily enlarged kidney with variably thin parenchyma

CT/MR

combination of similar findings to US and IVU depending on scanning protocol

NUC MED (DTPA/MAG3)

delayed parenchymal transit

delayed opacification of pelvis

delayed kidney washout with Lasix

dilated collecting system

reduced renal functional mass

3.6.3 FRALEY SYNDROME

upper pole renal artery crossing and obstructing upper pole calyx

3.6.4 CYSTIC RENAL DYSPLASIA

process similar to multicystic dysplastic kidney but some renal pelvis is present

late fetal ureteric atresia/obstruction; multiple cysts opening to hydronephrosis

3.6.5 CALYCEAL DIVERTICULUM

see Ch 08

3.6.6 MEGACALYCOSIS

CLINICAL

failure of medullary pyramid formation
rare, male > female, 20% bilateral
associated with megaureter
large kidneys, fetal lobulation, many
  facetted calyces with flat papillae
stable but slightly reduced renal function

IMAGING

involves some or all calyces on the affected
  side

IVP

absent normal papillary impressions
large multifaceted calyces
normal otherwise, in particular normal
  parenchymal width, and no holdup

VCUG/MCU

no reflux

US/CT

large calyces, attenuated medulla/pyramids
normal cortex

3.7 MALIGNANT RENAL TUMORS SIMULATING NEPHROBLASTOMA

3.7.1 CLEAR CELL SARCOMA

male > female, 3–5 years
polygonal cells with large nuclei
early metastases to bone
poor prognosis (50% mortality)

3.7.2 RHABDOID TUMOR

peak incidence at 1 year
eosinophilic rhabdomyoblast like cells
early metastases to brain
poor prognosis (90% mortality)

3.8 NEPHROBLASTOMA (WILMS' TUMOR)

DEFINITION

embryonal tumor of metanephric
  mesenchyme

EPIDEMIOLOGY

most common pediatric renal neoplasm
peak incidence is at 3–4 years
male = female, geographically stable
10% bilateral (all heritable), 1/3 of these is
  synchronous and 2/3 metachronous
2/3 of Wilms' is sporadic, 1/3 is familial
  (germ line mutation)

ETIOLOGY

Precursor condition: nephroblastomatosis

presence of metanephric blastema beyond
  36 weeks of gestation
macroscopic masses or microscopic nests
<1% of neonates, usually regresses
seen in 20% of Wilms'

IMAGING

US/CT
multiple subcapsular masses without
  hemorrhage, necrosis or calcification
mixed echogenicity on US and hypodense on
  CT
usually bilateral
kidneys enlarged

Syndromes with nephroblastoma

11p13 deletion: WAGR syndrome
W-ilms'
A-niridia
G-enital abnormalities
R-etardation

11p13 mutation: Denys Drash
  syndrome
streak gonads (male
  pseudohermaphroditism)
nephropathy and Wilms'

11p15 mutation: Beckwith–Wiedemann
  syndrome

CLINICAL

abdominal mass, pain, fever, hematuria
10% present with metastases

Staging (surgical postoperative)
I   IN KIDNEY, RESECTED
II BEYOND KIDNEY, RESECTED
III RESIDUAL MASS AFTER RESECTION
IV DISTANT METASTASES
V   BILATERAL

Spread

LYMPHATIC

VENOUS DIRECT

DISTANT HEMATOGENOUS
lung (20% at diagnosis)
liver
bones (clear cell sarcoma)
brain (rhabdoid tumor)

MICRO

90% triphasic histology (favorable) – 90% survival
BLASTEMAL: small round blue cells;
  TUBULOGLOMERULAR: primitive forms;
  STROMAL: spindle cells; also ectopic
  epithelium, striated muscle, cartilage,
  bone

10% anaplastic (unfavorable)

IMAGING

CT/MR/US
renal mass
solid, with echogenicity similar to liver
hypodense, with heterogeneous contrast
  enhancement
intermediate T1W signal, high T2W signal
margin well defined (may have
  pseudocapsule)
15% calcify
hemorrhage, necrosis, cystic change
  common
renal vein and IVC invasion common
necrotic nodal metastases, distant
  metastases
no vessel encasement and no retroaortic
  mass (features of neuroblastoma)

3.9 NEUROBLASTOMA

DEFINITION

pediatric malignant tumor of neural crest neuroblasts with a wide range of behavior and prognosis

EPIDEMIOLOGY

subclinical in situ disease very common (may be as common as 1/40) and most usually regresses

third commonest childhood tumor (after lymphoma and CNS)

90% <5 years, 50% <1 year old

familial predisposition in ?20%

ETIOLOGY

chromosome 1p deletion with loss of tumor suppressor gene

N-myc oncogene amplification, DNA aneuploidy

CLINICAL

abdominal mass, pain, fever, weight loss, skin masses, bone pain

VIP secretion – hypokalemic diarrhea

vanillylmandelic acid and homovanillic acid in urine

Prognostic factors

AGE (the younger the better)

GRADE (well differentiated better)

STAGE (low or IVs better)

ADVERSE CYTOLOGY: N-myc amplifications, 1p deletions, DNA polyploidy

FAVORABLE CYTOLOGY: nerve growth factor receptors, high VMA:HMA ratio

95% 5 year survival for stages I, II, IVs under 1 year (with treatment)

10% 5 year survival for stages III, IV over 1 year (with treatment)

MACRO

fleshy gray–yellow mass with calcification, hemorrhage, necrosis, cystic change

Location

ADRENAL MEDULLA (30% OVERALL)

POSTERIOR MEDIASTINUM

PARASPINAL RETROPERITONEUM

NECK OR SKULL BASE

CEREBRAL – rare, early CSF spread, poor prognosis

head and neck, skin, legs – all rare

Spread and staging

EXTENSIVE LOCAL SPREAD

encases vessels, extends BEHIND aorta

enters spinal canal and extends up and down

LOCAL LYMPH NODES

EARLY HEMATOGENOUS SPREAD (70% at diagnosis)

liver, bone marrow, bone cortex, skin, other

STAGING (Evans stage)

I   confined to organ of origin (OOO)

II outside of OOO, +/– nodes but not across midline

III across midline or contralateral nodes (>50% of cases)

IV distant metastases

IVs stage I or II, metastases only to liver, bone marrow, skin; age <1 year, favorable histology

MICRO

POORLY DIFFERENTIATED: sheets of round blue cells with large nuclei

MODERATELY DIFFERENTIATED

WELL DIFFERENTIATED: neuroblasts with neurofilaments and secretory granules

commonly mixed; may mature spontaneously

IMAGING

AXR

large abdominal mass, 50% or so have visible calcification

may show vertebral destruction or interpedicular widening (invasion)

US

extrarenal heterogeneous mass with calcification, hemorrhage, necrosis, cysts

CT

hypodense mass

85% have visible calcification

central necrosis, vivid peripheral enhancement

encases vessels, crosses midline, extends behind aorta, enters spinal canal

direct demonstration of bony cortical metastases

MR

low T1W signal, high T2W signal, vivid contrast enhancement

extends paraspinally, invades spinal canal, encases vessels, crosses behind aorta

direct demonstration of bone marrow metastases

NUC MED (MDP)

bone cortex metastases

60% of primary tumors take up MDP

NUC MED (MIBG)

100% of primary tumors take up MIBG

Imaging differential

NEUROBLASTOMA RELATIVE

GANGLIONEUROBLASTOMA

GANGLIONEUROMA

(less hemorrhage and necrosis, coarser calcification)

UNRELATED ADRENAL MASS

PHEOCHROMOCYTOMA

MYELOLIPOMA

CORTICAL ADENOMA, CARCINOMA

ADRENAL HEMORRHAGE

usually neonatal

shrinks over time

anechoic, liquid, blood products, no contrast enhancement (except rim)

3.10 NEURAL CREST TUMORS (not neuroblastoma)

3.10.1 GANGLIONEUROMA

benign tumor of neural crest origin composed of well differentiated neuroblasts and neural crest cells

may derive from maturing neuroblastoma

child – paraspinal; adult (30–50 years old) – adrenal

usually silent, rarely secretes catecholamines or VIP

may atrophy or calcify

3.10.2 GANGLIO-NEUROBLASTOMA

tumor intermediate between neuroblastoma and ganglioneuroma

<10 year old child, natural history unpredictable

encapsulated or not, may invade spinal canal with mass effect, may invade bone in continuity

3.11 PRUNE BELLY (EAGLE–BARRETT) SYNDROME

postulated in utero bladder outlet obstruction that subsequently resolves, and anterior abdominal wall atrophy secondary to urinary tract dilation; male >> female

hypoplasia or aplasia of anterior abdominal wall muscle with thin wrinkled flabby anterior abdominal wall (prune like)

dilated hypotonic bladder and ureters, dilated posterior urethra

associated other malformations

3.12 PYELONEPHRITIS

see Ch 08

3.13 TUBULAR DYSPLASIA SPECTRUM

3.13.1 SIMPLE CYST

see Ch 08

3.13.2 PARAPELVIC CYST

see Ch 08

3.13.3 INFANTILE POLYCYSTIC KIDNEY DISEASE

CLINICAL

autosomal recessive
1/6000–1/14 000
female:male 2:1, fatal
bilateral renal enlargement and renal failure
multiple small cysts formed of collecting ducts

IMAGING

bilateral large spongy kidneys
bright on US (thin shell of normal echogenicity capsule may be present)
streaky on IVP/CT

3.13.4 RENAL TUBULAR ECTASIA AND CONGENITAL BILIARY FIBROSIS

CLINICAL

autosomal dominant, autosomal recessive forms

kidneys: medullary tubular ectasia and cysts

liver: portal fibrosis, portal hypertension, biliary dilation, varices

severity of cirrhosis and extent of renal disease are inversely related

IMAGING

enlarged kidneys with increased medullary echogenicity and loss of corticomedullary differentiation

for cirrhosis and portal hypertension see Ch 07

3.13.5 MEDULLARY CYSTIC DISEASE (AD) AND JUVENILE NEPHRONOPHTHISIS (AR)

adolescents with chronic renal failure

microscopic cysts at corticomedullary junction (may be visible in medullary cystic disease)

small echogenic kidneys with little parenchyma

3.13.6 ADULT POLYCYSTIC KIDNEY DISEASE

see Ch 08

3.13.7 MEDULLARY SPONGE KIDNEY

rare disorder in children
see Ch 08

3.14 URACHAL ABNORMALITIES

3.14.1 PERSISTENT URACHUS SPECTRUM

urachus is a remnant of the allantoic duct (extension of bladder apex into umbilical cord)

3.14.1.1 Urachal cyst
incomplete obliteration of urachus with resultant midline epithelial cyst between bladder and umbilicus

3.14.1.2 Urachal fistula
patent channel from bladder to umbilicus, usually presents in a neonate with non healing inflamed umbilicus dripping urine

3.14.1.3 Urachal diverticulum
closed elongated extension of bladder towards umbilicus

3.14.1.4 Urachal sinus
persistent distal urachus opening at umbilicus but without connection to bladder

3.14.2 URACHAL CARCINOMA

carcinoma of urachal remnant, therefore midline somewhere between bladder and umbilicus

usually a mucinous adenocarcinoma with tendency for local recurrence

3.15 URETERIC MALFORMATION SPECTRUM

3.15.1 CONGENITAL MEGAURETER

CLINICAL

aperistalsis in distal ureter causing relative obstruction and proximal dilation

male:female 4:1, bilateral in 20%
associated with PUJ obstruction or
vesicoureteric reflux

IMAGING

first exclude other causes of hydroureter

IVP

bulbous ureter above aperistaltic segment
with funneling; no peristalsis in distal
segment

Retrograde pyelogram

NO OBSTRUCTION

3.15.2 DUPLEX KIDNEY +/– URETEROCELE

CLINICAL

very common
usually asymptomatic

Asymptomatic duplex

degree of duplex varies from a deeply
divided pelvis through 'Y' ureter to
complete duplex

Symptomatic duplex

OBSTRUCTION
REFLUX
ECTOPIC INSERTION
URETEROCELE

Weigert-Meyer rule

ECTOPIC URETER

upper moiety, crosses other ureter in 3
locations, has the lower and medial
ureteric orifice with/without ureterocele,
tends to obstruct

ORTHOTOPIC URETER

lower moiety (drooping lily appearance), has
the upper lateral (patulous) orifice, tends
to reflux

IMAGING

IVP

demonstration of each moiety depends on
amount of remaining renal function and
degree of obstruction
same rules apply as in single kidney
upper moiety usually smaller

lower moiety has a 'drooping lily'
configuration with all calyces pointing
down or laterally and down
suspicion of non functioning non
demonstrated moiety depends on calyceal
count and/or comparison with other side
may show ureterocele as 'cobra head'

MCU/VCUG

reflux commonly occurs into lower pole
moiety only
drooping lily shape and fewer calyces than
other side or than expected

US/MR

deep separating septum (too deep for a
column of Bertin)
may see two separate collecting systems
(depends on degree of dilation)

CT

as septum is mostly horizontal, duplex may
be missed on axial CT
may show two ureters, differential dilation
or enhancement, etc

NUC MED (DTPA/MAG3)

if neither moiety obstructed, usually can not
diagnose
if one moiety is obstructed, the upper and
lower pole difference can be identified
and behaves similarly to a single kidney

3.15.3 ECTOPIC URETER +/– URETEROCELE

female:male 4:1
often a duplex above, one moiety empties
into the ureterocele

FEMALE

duplex likely
ectopic orifice lies along the course of the
Wolffian duct: bladder, urethra, vagina,
less commonly uterus, rectum
often incontinent

MALE

position of ectopic orifice: bladder, posterior
urethra, ejaculatory ducts, vas deferens,
rectum
usually continent

3.16 URETEROCELE

DEFINITION

herniation of dilated sac-like distal ureter
and its orifice into the bladder

3.16.1 ECTOPIC URETEROCELE

CLINICAL

'infantile' type
belongs to upper moiety of a duplex (usually
dilated and non functional)
usually obstructed
often lies medially and inferiorly, and may
enter urethra
may cause bladder outlet obstruction or
obstruction of other ureteric orifices

IMAGING

IVP

non functional upper moiety
rounded bladder filling defect

MCU/VCUG

rounded filling defect

US/CT/MR

dilated thin walled non functioning or very
poorly functioning upper pole moiety
dilated tortuous ureter opening into a fluid
filled cystic thin walled mass within
bladder (may be quite distal)

3.16.2 SIMPLE URETEROCELE

CLINICAL

'adult' type
orthotopic position
duplex incidence not increased above
baseline
may or may not have significant obstruction

IMAGING

IVP/CT

'cobra head' produced by contrast in the
ureterocele and contrast in the bladder
outlining ureterocele wall

MCU/VCUG

rounded filling defect, often at lateral corner
of trigone

US/MR

rounded fluid filled thin walled cystic mass

3.16.3 PSEUDOURETEROCELE

INFECTIVE OR INFLAMMATORY DISTAL
  URETERIC STRICTURE
NEOPLASTIC DISTAL URETERIC
  STRICTURE
has a thick irregular wall, especially if
  neoplastic

3.17 VESICOURETERIC REFLUX (VUR)

ETIOLOGY

Primary
anatomicaly normal but incompetent VUJ –
  may mature and stop refluxing
  spontaneously in low grade
in duplex systems the lower moiety usually
  inserts orthotopically but refluxes – less
  likely to mature

Secondary
Hutch diverticulum, neuropathic bladder,
  outflow obstruction

GRADING

I   to lower ureter
II   to calyces
III forniceal dilation
IV   calyceal dilation
V   gross dilation of collecting system
LOW PRESSURE (during FILLING)
HIGH PRESSURE (during VOIDING)
?intrarenal reflux present

COMPLICATIONS

Ascending pyelonephritis
REQUIRES
bladder infection
VUR
bacterial seeding by intrarenal reflux

INTRARENAL REFLUX
occurs at compound papillae as excretory
  duct openings do not open obliquely
  (hence no valve effect with pressure)
reflux pyelonephritis more prevalent at
  upper and lower renal poles (which have
  compound papillae)

MAY PROGRESS TO REFLUX
NEPHROPATHY

Backpressure effect
obstructive uropathy if high grade reflux

CLINICAL

FETAL HYDRONEPHROSIS
UTI/PYELONEPHRITIS
INCIDENTALLY FOUND RENAL SCARS
LATE PRESENTATION WITH REFLUX
  NEPHROPATHY: HYPERTENSION,
  PREECLAMPSIA OR RENAL FAILURE
conservative treatment of low grade reflux is
  to prevent ascending infections
  (maintenance antibiotics till ~5 years old,
  meticulous urine monitoring)
higher grade reflux or recurrent
  pyelonephritis treated with ureteric
  reimplantation

IMAGING

see UTI

3.18 WHOLE KIDNEY MALFORMATION SPECTRUM

3.18.1 AGENESIS

unilateral 1/1000
bilateral (Potter sequence) 1/3000–1/10 000,
  1% recur

3.18.2 HYPOPLASIA

small kidney, <6 pyramids; includes
  unipapillary kidney

3.18.3 ECTOPIA

0.2%
MOST COMMON IS PELVIC KIDNEY

3.18.4 FUSION

HORSESHOE (1/500)
CROSSED FUSED RENAL ECTOPIA

3.18.5 MALROTATION

3.18.6 DUPLICATION

BIFID PELVIS
Y URETER
DUPLEX WITH NORMAL ORIFICES
DUPLEX, ONE ORIFICE ECTOPIC

20 Pediatric CNS

SECTION 5

1. NORMAL

1.1 MYELINATION

GERMINAL MATRIX IS PRESENT BETWEEN 7–34 WEEKS' GESTATION
NEURONAL MIGRATION OCCURS BETWEEN 8–20 WEEKS' GESTATION
MYELINATION OCCURS BETWEEN 24 WEEKS' GESTATION and 18 MONTHS

Rules of myelination

CAUDAL TO CRANIAL
brainstem then basal ganglia then cerebellum then cerebrum

DORSAL TO VENTRAL

CENTRAL TO PERIPHERAL

SENSORY FIRST, THEN MOTOR

PREMATURE INFANTS MYELINATE AT THE SAME RATE AS IN UTERO (no acceleration of maturation after birth)

White matter on MR

premyelinated white matter is high signal on T2W and low signal on T1W compared with gray matter (myelinated or not)
myelinated white matter is high signal on T1W and low signal on T2W compared with gray matter (myelinated or not)
partly myelinated white matter can be isointense to gray matter

Myelination timetable

approximate milestones only

TERM
dorsal medulla, dorsal midbrain, inferior and superior cerebellar peduncles
ventrolateral thalamus, posterior limb of internal capsule

1 MONTH
middle cerebellar peduncles, cerebral peduncles, ventral lateral thalami and somatosensory radiations (posterior limb of internal capsule), corticospinal tracts, optic nerves and tracts, precentral gyrus, post central gyrus

3 MONTHS
ventral brainstem, cerebellar hemisphere white matter, anterior limb of internal capsule, optic radiations, splenium of corpus callosum, occipital and white matter and white matter deep to somatosensory and primary motor cortex

6 MONTHS
genu of corpus callosum
centrum semiovale

1.2 NORMAL SINUS DEVELOPMENT

Bone marrow
red marrow then
yellow marrow then
opacified sinus then
aerated sinus

PITFALL TO BEWARE
calling normal red marrow tumor replacement or normal yellow marrow cholesterol granuloma

Sphenoid
at superior concha at birth, presphenoid part of sphenoid bone at 3–4 years, post sphenoid part of sphenoid bone at puberty
may extend far laterally to pneumatize greater sphenoid wings

Ethmoid
rudimentary at birth, develops gradually to puberty

Frontal
absent at birth, aerated by 6 years, full size at puberty
may extend far laterally to pneumatize orbital roofs

Maxillary
absent at birth, enlarges with tooth eruption (see tooth eruption timetable)

Mastoid
absent at birth, full size by 2 years

Generally
opacified sinuses normal <1 year old
between 1 and 3 years opacification is variable

1.3 NORMAL VALUES

Tip of conus
lowest allowed is mid L3 at birth, L2/3 at 5 years, mid L2 at 12 years; lowest allowed tip of theca is S2

Cord diameter
neonate: cervical 5 mm, thoracic 4 mm, lumbar 5 mm +/– 0.5 mm

Tonsils at foramen
normal is less than 5 mm through foramen magnum

2. GAMUTS

2.1 GENERIC (all modalities)

2.1.1 COTTON WOOL BRAIN ON US

HEMORRHAGE (positive mass effect)

EDEMA, ISCHEMIA

INFARCT, PERIVENTRICULAR LEUKOMALACIA

INFECTION, HERPES SIMPLEX VIRUS ENCEPHALITIS

CALCIFICATION OCCURS IN
TORCH INFECTIONS
CYTOMEGALOVIRUS (especially if calcifications thalamic linear)

2.1.2 INTRACRANIAL CALCIFICATION

see Ch 10

2.1.3 INTRACRANIAL CYSTIC SPACE (child)

Probably extraaxial

PORENCEPHALIC CYST

ARACHNOID CYST

MEGACISTERNA MAGNA

POSTERIOR FOSSA EXTRAAXIAL CYST
(SPECIFIC INSTANCE OF ARACHNOID CYST)

SUBDURAL HYGROMA/EMPYEMA

EPIDERMOID/DERMOID

Probably intraaxial

HOLOPROSENCEPHALY SPECTRUM

DANDY–WALKER MALFORMATION

CYSTIC NEOPLASM

CYSTIC ABSCESS

COLLOID CYST OF THE THIRD
VENTRICLE

Vascular structure, not a cyst: aneurysmal vein of Galen
(Ch 11)

Tumor with cystic spaces: craniopharyngioma

2.1.4 MACROCEPHALY

By definition head circumference >98th centile

Megalencephaly

FAMILIAL

NEUROFIBROMATOSIS 1 AND 2,
TUBEROUS SCLEROSIS

STORAGE, MYELIN AND METABOLIC
DISEASE

Collection

BRAIN ATROPHY, RESIDUAL SPACE

EXTRAVENTRICULAR
HYDROCEPHALUS

CSF HYGROMA

SUBDURAL HYGROMA

SUBDURAL EMPYEMA

DIFFERENTIAL

NORMAL SUBARACHNOID SPACE <2 years

Mass

Hydrocephalus

HYDROCEPHALUS VS ATROPHY

HYDROCEPHALUS VS LARGE
SUBARACHNOID SPACE

ASSESS

DYNAMIC SIGNS

SYMMETRY

SUPPORTING SIGNS OR CAUSE

Arachnoid cyst

DIFFERENTIAL IS PORENCEPHALY

Dynamic signs of increased intracranial pressure
see hydrocephalus

2.1.5 ORBIT–GLOBE

Retinoblastoma and mimics
see entries in conditions section

RETINOBLASTOMA

PERSISTENT HYPERPLASTIC
PRIMARY VITREOUS

RETROLENTAL FIBROPLASIA

COATS' DISEASE

TOXOCARA ENDOPHTHALMITIS

HEMATOMA, RETINAL DETACHMENT

Congenital whole eye abnormalities

MICROPHTHALMIA

COLOBOMA, PROTRUDED VITREOUS

MACROPHTHALMIA, JUVENILE
GLAUCOMA

2.1.6 ORBIT–CONAL/ EXTRACONAL MASSES

MNEMONIC: MORBID ORBIT

M-ETASTASIS (neuroblastoma,
melanoma)

O-PTIC NERVE GLIOMA
very strong association with NF1

R-HABDOMYOSARCOMA
may mimic abscess

B-LOOD FILLED HEMANGIOMA

I-NFECTION AND ABSCESS

D-ERMOID

2.1.7 SKULL GAMUTS

see Ch 10

2.1.8 T1W HIGH SIGNAL

see Ch 10

2.1.9 T2W LOW SIGNAL

see Ch 10

2.2 TUMOR GAMUTS

also see Ch 10, tumor gamuts

2.2.1 TUMORS COMMON IN CHILDREN

Infratentorial

MEDULLOBLASTOMA (PNET)

cerebellar vermis

PONTINE ASTROCYTOMA

JUVENILE PILOCYTIC ASTROCYTOMA

cerebellar hemispheres

EPENDYMOMA

fourth ventricle

Pineal

GERM CELL TUMORS

PINEOBLASTOMA (PNET)

Sellar/parasellar

CRANIOPHARYNGIOMA

GERM CELL TUMORS

HYPOTHALAMIC HAMARTOMA

LANGERHANS CELL HISTIOCYTOSIS

METASTASES

PARTICULARLY NEUROBLASTOMA,
RETINOBLASTOMA

Supratentorial

ASTROCYTOMA

PLEOMORPHIC
XANTHOASTROCYTOMA

NEURAL AND NEUROGLIAL TUMORS

GANGLIOGLIOMA/GANGLIOCYTOMA

DNET

CHOROID PLEXUS PAPILLOMA

SUPRATENTORIAL PNET =
CEREBRAL NEUROBLASTOMA

Optic nerve

OPTIC NERVE GLIOMA (NF1)

Neurofibromatosis 1 (NF1) tumors
see NF1 in Ch 11

Neurofibromatosis 2 (NF2) tumors
see NF2 in Ch 11

Tuberous sclerosis tubers and subependymal giant cell astrocytomas
see tuberous sclerosis in Ch 11

Extraaxial

CHORDOMA

LIPOMA

DERMOID, EPIDERMOID

CRANIOPHARYNGIOMA (see sellar group)

PEDIATRIC CNS AND HEAD AND NECK CONDITIONS

3. GENERAL CONDITIONS

3.1 ARACHNOID CYST

see Ch 11

3.2 ATROPHY

DEFINITION

reduction in amount of gray matter and/or white matter through destruction or dysgenesis
differential of hydrocephalus

CLINICAL: KEY HISTORY

static neurological deficit
head size stable or decreasing
history of appropriate insult or injury

IMAGING

Symmetrical atrophy

gray matter, subcortical and deep white matter all involved
diffuse volume loss, colpocephaly

Asymmetrical atrophy

preferential loss of periventricular and deep white matter
periventricular leukomalacia

Pitfall

white matter gliosis in atrophy may look like transependymal edema in hydrocephalus

3.3 CEPHALOCELES

DEFINITION

herniation of subarachnoid space and/or brain tissue through a dural and skull defect

Meningocele

contains leptomeninges and CSF only

Encephalocele

contains brain tissue

EPIDEMIOLOGY

usually not syndromic
overall incidence approximately 1–3 per 10 000
occipital cephaloceles most common form in Europeans
anterior cephaloceles most common form in Asians

CLINICAL/MACRO

midline occipital sac or midline facial/nasal mass, associated facial malformations, hypertelorism; microcephaly depending on amount of herniated brain
neurological deficit depends on severity and degree of associated abnormal function

Occipital

midline posterior, often contains dysplastic cerebellum
association with neural tube closure malformations

Anterior

persistence of frontonasal diverticulum with herniation of CNS along its track
named after suture through which it herniates
may be occult depending on location of suture

may be associated with facial or optic system or corpus callosum malformations

FRONTOETHMOIDAL
frontal and nasal bones

NASOETHMOIDAL
distal to nasal bones

NASOORBITAL
frontal process of maxilla and lacrimal bone

NASOPHARYNGEAL
rare base of skull cephaloceles
bone defect with hernial sac containing basal brain structures
may be asymptomatic

Parietal

non midline ('non anatomical') cephalocele
may be due to amniotic bands
association with other CNS malformations

Nasal dermoid with/without track

track of frontonasal diverticulum runs from foramen cecum (at base of crista galli) to nasal structures
may or may not be in communication with CNS
may or may not have a dermal sinus track
may develop a dermoid (nasal dermoid) along the track

IMAGING

CT
CSF or mass protruding through bony defect

MR
cranial defect with a skin covered sac that contains CSF and a variable amount of brain tissue which often has abnormal signal (gliosis, high on T2W)
sac may contain dysplastic neuronal tissue
blood supply of herniated brain often abnormal
ventricles may herniate as well (and may trap)

NASAL DERMOID
midline high T1W signal mass in nasal septum with/without track to anterior cranial fossa

3.4 CHILD ABUSE

see Ch 17

3.5 CHOROID PLEXUS TUMORS

see Ch 11

3.6 COMPLEX PARTIAL SEIZURES (CPS)

see Ch 11

3.7 CRANIO-PHARYNGIOMA

see Ch 11

3.8 CRANIOSYNOSTOSIS

DEFINITION

premature skull suture fusion (under 1 year of age)

CLINICAL

sagittal > coronal > lambdoid sutures
if late or mild, exaggerated skull shape only
if more severe, grossly abnormal skull shape
if more than one suture, compression of neural structures may be significant

Cloverleaf skull

fusion of all sutures with bulging of parietal bones and of fontanelles; associated with craniolacunia and exophthalmos

IMAGING

XR/CT

sclerosis around sutures
sharp suture margins, then narrowing and bridging
late deformity
scaphocephaly (sagittal synostosis)
turricephaly (bilateral coronal synostosis), harlequin orbit (bony superior orbital rim pulled up–unilateral coronal synostosis)
plagiocephaly (unilateral lambdoid synostosis)

3.9 CRETINISM

DEFINITION

syndrome caused by uncorrected congenital deficiency of thyroid hormone (usually due to thyroid agenesis)

IMAGING

CXR

cardiomegaly, pericardial effusion
congestive cardiac failure

XR (skull)

delayed fontanelle closure
Wormian bones
large sella (cherry sella)
brachycephaly, delayed appearance of vascular markings
delayed diploic differentiation
late development of paranasal sinuses and mastoid air cells

XR (peripheral skeletal)

irregular stippled fragmented late epiphyses
dense metaphyseal bands
short retarded shafts
kyphosis, flattened + bullet vertebrae

US

no thyroid gland (thyroid agenesis)
thyroid gland (metabolic thyroid dysfunction)

NUC MED (TcO4, I)

no evidence of thyroid tracer accumulation anywhere (stomach, colon, salivary, renal and urinary activity is physiological)

3.10 EPENDYMOMA

see Ch 11

3.11 FACIAL DYSMORPHIC SYNDROMES

3.11.1 CLEIDOCRANIAL DYSOSTOSIS

see Ch 02

3.11.2 CROUZON SYNDROME (craniofacial dysostosis)

ocular hypertelorism
maxillary hypoplasia
parrot beak nose
craniostenosis
middle ear deformities

3.11.3 FIBROUS DYSPLASIA (facial)

usually monostotic (associated with NF1) – often temporal bone or base of skull
polyostotic (syndromic): cherubism (mandible, maxilla); leontiasis ossia (all facial bones)
expanding radiolucent mass, does not cross sutures
progressive sclerosis with coalescence
groundglass density on plain film
generalized expansion (groundglass, lucency, sclerosis)
non aeration of sinuses, possibly non eruption of teeth
static in adult life

3.11.4 GARDNER'S SYNDROME

see full entry in GIT chapter
familial polyposis coli with additional features
facial bones: multiple osteomas

3.11.5 GORLIN–GOLTZ SYNDROME (basal cell nevus)

see Ch 11

3.11.6 PIERRE–ROBIN'S SYNDROME

mandibular hypoplasia

3.11.7 TREACHER-COLLINS SYNDROME (mandibulo–facial dysostosis)

antimongoloid palpebral slant
underdeveloped zygomatic arches
hypoplastic maxilla and mandible
underdeveloped middle ear and ossicles
deformed external ears

3.12 GERM CELL TUMORS

see Ch 11

3.13 GERMINAL MATRIX HEMORRHAGE

DEFINITION

spontaneous hemorrhage into active germinal matrix with complications from disruption to brain parenchyma and secondary hydrocephalus

Germinal matrix

vascular subependymal zone of neuroblast and spongioblast proliferation, with the cells then migrating into forming cortex

normally present at least until 34–36 weeks of gestation

has an endarterial supply by deep central arteries and perforating branches

active in premature neonates, absent in term neonates

CLINICAL

occurs in premature neonates <32 weeks' gestation and <1500 g usually in the first few days of extrauterine life

compete resorption (if small or mild)

prognosis good for grades I and II, poor for grades III and IV

Grading

I   germinal matrix only (definitely so if hematoma lies anterior to caudothalamic groove)

II intraventricular hemorrhage, no ventricular dilation

III intraventricular hemorrhage, ventricular dilation

IV intraparenchymal extension

Complications of parenchymal involvement

cystic encephalomalacia, porencephaly motor palsies, intellectual impairment

Complications of intraventricular hemorrhage

obstructive hydrocephalus

communicating hydrocephalus

complications of shunting

IMAGING

US

GRADE I/II

expanded choroid plexus

hyperechoic mass in caudothalamic groove involving choroid plexus

GRADE II/III

hyperechoic hematoma extending into lateral ventricle

extension of hyperechoic hematoma into third or fourth ventricles

GRADE III

expansion of ventricles (blood or hydrocephalus)

GRADE IV

hematoma extending into periventricular white matter (acutely hyperechoic, slowly decreasing echogenicity with time)

LATE COMPLICATION

cystic encephalomalacia: cavitation of periventricular brain with small and large CSF filled spaces

CT

high density curved mass in lateral aspect of lateral ventricle (caudothalamic groove)

intraventricular free blood, subarachnoid free blood

intraparenchymal extension

3.14 GLOBAL HYPOXIC ENCEPHALOMALACIA
(manifestations)

IMAGING

US

diffuse increase in brain parenchymal echogenicity (generalized edema)

CT

loss of gray–white interface

loss of cortical density, often with preservation of deep gray matter density on CT ('CT density reversal sign')

MR

high T2W white matter signal, myelination delay

high T2W gray matter signal – cortex or deep gray

eventual cystic encephalomalacia or diffuse atrophy

3.15 GRAY AND WHITE MATTER DEGENERATIONS

see Ch 11

3.16 GRAY MATTER DEGENERATIONS

see Ch 11

3.17 HYDROCEPHALUS

also see hydrocephalus gamut in Ch 10

DEFINITION

dilation of ventricles from excessive CSF accumulation

EPIDEMIOLOGY

infantile hydrocephalus: 4/1000 births; usually related to malformations, less commonly intraventricular hemorrhage

ETIOPATHOGENESIS

Obstructive hydrocephalus

obstruction to CSF flow within the ventricular system, most commonly at the aqueduct

CAUSES
MASS
STENOSIS
MALFORMATION

LOCATIONS
FORAMEN OF MONRO
COLLOID CYST, TUBER (of tuberous sclerosis), GIANT CELL ASTROCYTOMA, SELLAR MASS

THIRD VENTRICLE AND AQUEDUCT
PINEAL MASS, GALENIC AV MALFORMATION, AQUEDUCT STENOSIS

FOURTH VENTRICLE

CHIARI SPECTRUM, DANDY–WALKER SPECTRUM, ARACHNOID CYST

Communicating hydrocephalus

obstruction to CSF flow outside the ventricular system (often at tentorial notch); or obstruction to CSF absorption (usually at arachnoid granulations)

CAUSES

MENINGITIS
HEMORRHAGE, TRAUMA
CARCINOMATOUS
VENOUS THROMBOSIS
IDIOPATHIC

LOCATIONS

TENTORIAL HIATUS
ADHESIONS (POST MENINGITIS OR MALIGNANT)
ARACHNOID GRANULATIONS
OBSTRUCTION (NEOPLASTIC, INFECTIVE, OR POST HEMORRHAGE)
DURAL SINUSES
THROMBOSIS

OVERPRODUCTION OF CSF (rare)

CHOROID PLEXUS PAPILLOMA

Normal pressure hydrocephalus

defined as hydrocephalus with normal lumbar CSF pressure

a condition of older adults – see entry in Ch 11

CLINICAL

Adult and child after sutural fusion

headaches, nausea and vomiting, memory loss, ataxia, papilloedema, decreasing conscious state

may progress relatively fast (acute presentation, rapid deterioration of conscious state) or more slowly

Child (before sutural fusion)

increasing head size; neurological deficits; failure of normal development

IMAGING

XR

SIGNS OF RAISED INTRACRANIAL PRESSURE: increased convolutional markings, sellar/clinoid erosion (all rare)
sutural diastasis in a child

CT/MR

look for evidence of causative mass or meningitis

SIGNS OF HYDROCEPHALUS

progressive dilation of ventricles
dilation of temporal horns, inferior recesses of third ventricle; lamina terminalis
bowing of corpus callosum upwards; fenestration of septum pellucidum
transependymal edema (high T2W and low T1W signal or low density surrounding the lateral ventricles)

OBSTRUCTIVE HYDROCEPHALUS

asymmetrical dilation of ventricles upstream of obstruction with normal size ventricles downstream of obstruction

COMMUNICATING HYDROCEPHALUS

fourth ventricle may dilate less than third and lateral ventricles

NON TUMORAL AQUEDUCT OBSTRUCTION

failure of CSF flow void or abnormal morphology of aqueduct on MR

DIFFERENTIAL: ATROPHY (see in gamuts)

NUC MED (radionuclide cisternography)

In or Tc DTPA with lumbar puncture injection

NORMAL

basal cisterns by 1 hour, Sylvian fissure by 2–6 hours, cerebral convexities by 12 hours, vertex/superior sagittal sinus by 24 hours
no ventricular reflux

COMMUNICATING HYDROCEPHALUS

ventricular reflux, prolonged delayed clearance
clearance without migration to vertex may occur transependymally
transient ventricular reflux is less significant

NON COMMUNICATING HYDROCEPHALUS

study may be normal, or
delayed migration, but no ventricular reflux (differential is normal aging adult, cerebral atrophy)

SHUNT PATENCY STUDIES

injection of radionuclide into shunt valve reservoir, with activity outlining peritoneal cavity confirming patency

Communicating hydrocephalus vs atrophy

DYNAMIC SIGNS

CHILD
sutural diastasis
ADULT
convolutional markings
sellar, clinoid erosion
transependymal edema

NUC MED VENTRICULOGRAPHY

intraventricular reflux with delayed clearance: hydrocephalus
normal pattern: atrophy
delay in clearance, no reflux: probably atrophy
delay in clearance, transient reflux: probably hydrocephalus
BUT obstructive hydrocephalus has no ventricular reflux

MORPHOLOGY

VENTRICLES AND CISTERNS
    VENTRICLE AND CISTERN DISTENSION ASYMMETRICAL (INCLUDING THIRD AND FOURTH VENTRICLES)
no white matter loss – hydrocephalus
gray matter and white matter loss – probably atrophy
    VENTRICLE AND CISTERN DISTENSION SYMMETRICAL
no white matter loss–probably hydrocephalus
gray matter and white matter loss – atrophy
    SIGNS RELATIVELY SPECIFIC TO HYDROCEPHALUS
temporal horn dilation (little atrophy occurs here)
bowing of corpus callosum and fenestration of septum pellucidum
bowing of lamina terminalis and recesses of third ventricle

SUPPORTING SIGNS

TUMOR OR MASS
LESION LOCATION APPROPRIATE FOR HYDROCEPHALUS
APPROPRIATE HISTORY
INCREASING SERIAL HEAD SIZE

PROOF

SERIAL CT, SERIAL HEAD CIRCUMFERENCE
INTRACRANIAL PRESSURE MONITOR

3.18 HYPOTHALAMIC HAMARTOMA

CLINICAL

non neoplastic mass of mature neurons and glia in tuber cinereum

presents with childhood gelastic (laughing)
seizures, precocious puberty, behavioral
change

IMAGING

CT

isodense suprasellar mass
no calcification

MR

mass descending from hypothalamus
isointense to gray matter on T1W and PD;
higher signal on T2W
no contrast enhancement

3.19 LANGERHANS CELL HISTIOCYTOSIS

see Ch 05 musculoskeletal tumors, Ch 11
CNS, Ch 13 lungs

3.20 LEUKO-DYSTROPHIES

see Ch 11

3.21 MEDULLO-BLASTOMA

DEFINITION

malignant embryonal small round blue cell
posterior fossa tumor with tendency to
extensive CSF spread

CLINICAL

second commonest childhood tumor, male >
female
uncommon in young adults, and may be in
lateral cerebellum
presents with cerebellar signs and raised
intracranial pressure from fourth
ventricle obstruction
1/3 of patients have CSF drop metastases at
presentation
rarely, metastases found outside the CNS
prognosis poor overall, but better with
complete resection
occasionally residual medulloblastoma may
mature to ganglionic type tumors

MACRO

gray friable mass arising from roof of fourth
ventricle and expanding it
hemorrhage and necrosis common;
calcification common

MICRO

chromosome 17p genetic losses
postulated origin is from the external
granular layer cell
small round blue cells in sheets, highly
mitotic, invasive
UNDIFFERENTIATED TYPE, NEURONAL
LINE, GLIAL LINE

IMAGING

CT

posterior fossa dense intraaxial mass
1/3 calcifies
vividly enhances with contrast
hydrocephalus above
5% have sclerotic metastases to bone

MR

intraventricular midline mass
low T1W and low T2W and variable PD
signal (occasionally high T2W signal)
cystic change, possibly hemorrhage and
necrosis
vividly enhances with contrast

DROP METASTASES COMMON (leptomeningeal deposits)

1/3 of patients at first presentation
1/3 of patients with recurrence
soft tissue masses in basal cisterns, fissures,
spinal subarachnoid space
contrast enhancing; may form a continuous
rind of tumor
secondary hydrocephalus

IMAGE ENTIRE NEURAXIS

PET (FDG)

increased FDG uptake

3.22 MITOCHONDRIAL ENCEPHALOPATHIES

see Ch 11

3.23 PERIVENTRICULAR LEUKOMALACIA

CLINICAL

hypoxia or infarction in deep arterial
distribution
occurs particularly in premature neonates
white matter (WM) involved more than gray
matter, post trigonal WM, WM deep to
frontal horns

IMAGING

US

early: 'cotton wool brain': areas of increased
US echogenicity particularly lateral and
superolateral to lateral ventricles but
may be more extensive
late: cavitation of infarcted areas, cystic
encephalomalacia, white matter atrophy

CT

areas of low density with eventual cavitation
and secondary enlargement of ventricles

MR

areas of high T2W signal, possibly with
secondary hemorrhagic signal
eventual white matter atrophy with reduced
white matter mass and secondarily
enlarged ventricles – may be symmetrical
or asymmetrical

3.24 PINEAL CELL LINE TUMORS

see Ch 11

3.25 PORENCEPHALY

DEFINITION

acquired cystic space replacing normal
brain (usually cerebral) parenchyma;
commonly prenatal (and therefore
congenital) but may be postnatal

ETIOLOGY

INFARCT
INTRAPARENCHYMAL HEMORRHAGE
TRAUMATIC ENCEPHALOMALACIA
INFECTIVE ENCEPHALOMALACIA,
    ATROPHY

PATHOGENESIS

gross focal parenchymal necrosis producing
    cystic encephalomalacia ('porencephalic
    cyst')
usually in full communication with CSF
    cisterns and ventricles
may occasionally seal off, and then behaves
    similarly to arachnoid cyst
if the encephalomalacia occurs in first
    trimester, the falx is displaced to the side
    of the encephalomalacia and the
    hemicranium is small
with later encephalomalacia the falx
    attachment does not migrate and the
    skull is less asymmetrical

IMAGING

CT/MR

area of absent brain parenchyma containing
    CSF
communication with CSF cisterns and/or
    ventricles usually obvious, but can be
    proven with subarachnoid contrast
no mass effect (unless becomes sealed off)
no contrast enhancement
lined by both gray and white matter
    depending on the margin of the
    encephalomalacia (differential:
    schizencephalic cleft, which is lined by
    dysmorphic gray matter)
associated falx or skull abnormalities

3.26 PRIMITIVE NEUROECTODERMAL TUMORS (PNET)

DEFINITION

a unifying grouping of aggressive small blue
    round cell embryonal tumors of
    neuroectodermal lineage

CLASSIFICATION

MNEMONIC: PNETEM
P-INEOBLASTOMA

N-EUROBLASTOMA, RHABDOID TUMOR
E-PENDYMOBLASTOMA
RE-T-INOBLASTOMA
MEDULLO-E-PITHELIOMA
M-EDULLOBLASTOMA

3.26.1 NEUROBLASTOMA

see Ch 19

3.26.2 PINEOBLASTOMA

see Ch 11

3.26.3 MEDULLOBLASTOMA

see its own entry

3.26.4 RETINOBLASTOMA

see its own entry

3.26.5 SUPRATENTORIAL PNET = CEREBRAL NEUROBLASTOMA

CLINICAL

rare aggressive deep cerebral tumor
large mass with areas of hemorrhage and
    necrosis, CSF spread and dystrophic
    calcification

IMAGING

CT/MR

heterogeneous necrotic cystic mass with
    contrast enhancement and calcification

3.27 RETINOBLASTOMA

DEFINITION

malignant primitive embryonal retinal tumor

EPIDEMIOLOGY

uncommon; presents <2 years, often
    <3 months
90% sporadic (of this 80% is monocular non
    heritable)

10% familial (all heritable)

bilateral retinoblastoma

trilateral retinoblastoma (bilateral
    retinoblastoma and pineal tumor)
osteosarcomas
soft tissue sarcomas

ETIOLOGY

chromosome 13q14 (Rb gene) mutation
    (tumor suppressor gene, autosomal
    recessive mutation)
heritable: germ line has an autosomal
    recessive mutant gene and one somatic
    mutation is superimposed
non heritable: two somatic mutations

CLINICAL

leukokoria, strabismus, orbital mass, painful
    eye, decreasing vision, metastases

Spread

orbit in continuity
CNS via optic nerve
local lymph nodes (via orbit)
uveal tract and hematogenous to bone

MORPHOLOGY

starts in retina, grows between retina and
    vitreous and between retina and uveal
    tract (dumbbell); 95% CALCIFY
small round blue cells forming primitive
    rosettes with rudimentary photoreceptors
    in lumen

IMAGING

CT

95% calcify
dumbbell dense mass with variable
    enhancement

MR

low T2W high T1W mass compared with
    vitreous
dumbbell shape
shows extension along optic nerve

3.28 RETINOBLASTOMA MIMICS

3.28.1 PERSISTENT HYPERPLASTIC PRIMARY VITREOUS

CLINICAL

microphthalmia, small irregular lens

IMAGING

CT

dense mass, enhances with contrast, may
follow Cloquet's canal
NO CALCIFICATION

3.28.2 RETROLENTAL FIBROPLASIA

CLINICAL

history of prematurity and oxygen therapy

IMAGING

CT

bilateral dense masses, enhance with
contrast
NO CALCIFICATION

3.28.3 COATS' DISEASE

CLINICAL

tends to affect 6–8 year old males
congenital telangiectasia and exudate
subsequent retinal detachment with dense
mass

IMAGING

NO CALCIFICATION

3.28.4 TOXOCARA ENOPHTHALMITIS

IMAGING

diffusely dense vitreous with focal nodules
NO CALCIFICATION, no enhancement

3.28.5 HEMATOMA, RETINAL DETACHMENT

CLINICAL

history of trauma

IMAGING

hematoma mass does not enhance
NO CALCIFICATION

3.29 SCHIZENCEPHALY

see migration and sulcation anomalies in 4.9

3.30 SEIZURE CLASSIFICATION

see Ch 11

3.31 SINONASAL MALFORMATIONS

3.31.1 CHOANAL ATRESIA

CLINICAL

failure of orochoanal membrane to involute
bony or membranous occlusion of posterior
one or both nares
unilateral presents with recurrent infections
of one nasal passage
bilateral presents early with respiratory
distress most marked when feeding, and
failure to pass nasogastric tube

IMAGING

Fluoro

pooling of contrast in posterior nasal
passage with no progress to nasopharynx

CT

bony or fibrous choanal septum, usually
with tapering of posterior nares

3.31.2 NASAL GLIOMA

CLINICAL

extracranial rest of benign glial tissue

IMAGING

non aggressive soft tissue mass in roof of
nose or nasal septum

by definition, no connection to brain tissue
and no CSF extension

3.31.3 CEPHALOCELES

see its own entry

3.31.4 DERMOID, EPIDERMOID

CLINICAL

rest of enclosed ectodermal tissue along
course of foramen cecum
variable presentation spectrum from midline
nasal dimple to mass with hypertelorism

IMAGING

same features as dermoid or epidermoid
elsewhere
position midline between nasal septum and
crista galli

3.32 SPINAL MALFORMATIONS

3.32.1 OPEN DYSRAPHISM

Chiari II/myelomeningocele
90% myelomeningocele to 10% meningocele
70% low (lumbar > thoracic > sacral), rest
high (cervical, occipital)

NEURAXIS CHANGES

SPINE

   PRIMITIVE PLACODE

   TETHERED CORD, LIPOMA

   DISTORTED CAUDA

HEAD

   CHIARI II MALFORMATION

   SYRINGOMYELIA

DISTAL

   CLUBFOOT

   DYSPLASTIC HIPS

   NEUROPATHIC BLADDER

VERTEBRAL CHANGES

   PROGRESSIVE KYPHUS

   HEMIVERTEBRAE, FUSIONS

   CAUDAL HYPOPLASIA

VISCERAL CHANGES

   25% VESICOURETERIC REFLUX

OTHER UROGENITAL MALFORMATIONS

RECTAL AGENESIS

CARDIAC MALFORMATIONS

Complications in repaired spina bifida

NEURAL

TIGHT CRANIOCERVICAL JUNCTION

HYDROCEPHALUS

TRAPPED FOURTH VENTRICLE

SHUNT BLOCK

SYRINX

TETHERED CORD (DIAGNOSIS OF EXCLUSION)

UROLOGICAL

INCONTINENCE

VESICOURETERIC REFLUX

NEUROPATHIC BLADDER

INFECTIONS

ORTHOPEDIC

HIP DYSPLASIA

FOOT AND LEG DEFORMITIES

UNBALANCED SCOLIOSIS

3.32.2 OCCULT DYSRAPHISM

Meningocele

NB lateral meningoceles is part of NF1

Spinal lipoma spectrum

LIPOMYELOMENINGOCELE

FILUM FIBROLIPOMA

SUBPIAL LIPOMA

Diastematomyelia

1/3 bony, 2/3 cartilaginous or fibrous

3.32.3 CAUDAL REGRESSION SPECTRUM

DEFINITION

variably extensive non hereditary defect in development of caudal structures; related to maternal diabetes

CLINICAL

Skeletal deficit grading

STABLE

I   partial unilateral sacral agenesis

II partial bilateral sacral agenesis

UNSTABLE

III total sacral +/– lumbar agenesis, iliolumbar joints

IV total sacral +/– lumbar agenesis, ilioilial joint

Neural deficit

motor is level of absent vertebral structures +/– 1

sensory is lower

commonest is hip dysplasias and clubfoot neuropathic bladder

Associated visceral malformations

ANORECTAL

UROGENITAL

3.32.4 ANTERIOR MENINGOCELE

rare, female > male

sickle shaped sacral defect with meningeal sac

rectal malformations and strictures

3.32.5 SPLIT NOTOCHORD SPECTRUM

Neurenteric fistula

Neurenteric cyst

3.32.6 SYRINGOMYELIA

see Ch 11

3.32.7 TETHERED CORD SYNDROME

NORMAL CORD LEVEL

conus lower limit mid L3 at birth, L2/3 at 5 years, mid L2 at 12 years

CLASSIFICATION

Repaired spina bifida

No previous surgery

NB cutaneous stigmata in 50% overall

LIPOMA 70%

TIGHT FILUM

DIASTEMATOMYELIA

MYELOMENINGOCELE

3.33 TORCH INFECTIONS

GROUP DEFINITION

intrauterine (or perinatal, for HSV) infections producing multisystem congenital abnormalities, with neurological abnormalities dominant

T-OXOPLASMOSIS

O-THER (LISTERIA, SYPHILIS)

R-UBELLA

C-YTOMEGALOVIRUS (CMV)

H-ERPES SIMPLEX VIRUS (HSV)

H-UMAN IMMUNODEFICIENCY VIRUS (HIV)

CLINICAL PATTERNS

Overall pattern common to all TORCH infections

HEAD

MICROCEPHALY WITH CALCIFICATION

PORENCEPHALY

HYDROCEPHALUS WITH AQUEDUCT OBSTRUCTION

INTELLECTUAL DEFECTS, DEVELOPMENTAL DELAY

OTHER

CARDIAC, OCULAR, INNER EAR MALFORMATIONS

HEMATOPOIETIC AND LUNG INFECTION

Specific findings

MIGRATION ANOMALIES: CMV

WIDESPREAD CALCIFICATION: TOXOPLASMOSIS

3.33.1 TOXOPLASMOSIS

Neural

WIDESPREAD CALCIFICATIONS

microcephaly, porencephaly, periventricular leukomalacia

chorioretinitis

no migration anomalies

ependymitis, aqueduct obstruction

Extraneural

hepatosplenomegaly, anemia, pneumonia

3.33.2 RUBELLA

Neural

INCONSPICUOUS PUNCTATE
    CALCIFICATIONS
microcephaly, diffuse atrophy
chorioretinitis
inner ear lesions

Extraneural

congenital cardiac defects,
    hepatosplenomegaly, anemia, pneumonia

3.33.3 CMV

Neural

CENTRAL PERIVENTRICULAR
    CALCIFICATIONS
microcephaly, porencephaly, periventricular
    leukomalacia
chorioretinitis
migration anomalies (heterotopic gray,
    gyration and sulcation anomalies)

Extraneural

cardiac, hepatosplenomegaly, anemia

3.33.4 HSV2 (perinatal infection)

Neural

PUNCTATE PARENCHYMAL CALCIFICATION
multicystic encephalomalacia
microvascular thrombosis

Extraneural

pneumonia

3.33.5 HIV

DELAYED (>1 year old) BASAL GANGLIA
    CALCIFICATION

3.34 VASCULAR MALFORMATION SPECTRUM

see Ch 11

4. SYNDROMES

4.1 ATAXIA TELANGIECTASIA

see Ch 11

4.2 BASAL CELL NEVUS SYNDROME (Gorlin–Goltz)

see Ch 11

4.3 CHIARI I

not related to Chiari II

CLINICAL

most commonly asymptomatic
central cord syndrome 50%
foramen magnum compressive myelopathy
    25%

IMAGING

Brain

tonsillar ectopia >5 mm below plane from
    tip of clivus to posterior margin of
    foramen magnum
2/3 have tonsils at C1, 1/4 at C2
non specific hydrocephalus 20–50%
hydromyelia 75%

Spine

basilar invagination 25–50%
Klippel–Feil syndrome 10%
RARE: spina bifida occulta, atlantooccipital
    assimilation

4.4 CHIARI II

PATHOGENESIS

decompression of fourth ventricle through
    open spina bifida, abnormal induction of
    posterior fossa mesenchyme

IMAGING

Skull

lacunar skull (craniolacunia, luckenschadel)
small posterior fossa, low torcula
scalloped clivus + temporal bones
gaping foramen magnum
incomplete C1 ring 90%

Posterior fossa

inferiorly displaced tonsils + vermis
inferiorly displaced medulla and fourth
    ventricle
inferiorly displaced choroid plexus
medullary kink

creeping and towering cerebellum
transincisural upwards cerebellar herniation
beaked tectum
hourglass fourth ventricle
aqueduct frequently occluded from external
    compression or stretching, less
    commonly stenotic or atretic or forked

Cerebrum

hydrocephalus in over 90%
hypoplastic falx, interdigitating gyri,
    stenogyria
callosal atrophy
inferiorly pointing lateral ventricles
massa intermedia, Meynert's commissure
migration anomalies

Spine

myelomeningocele 100%
syrinx
diastematomyelia 10%

4.5 CHIARI III

Chiari II with a low occipital/high cervical
    cephalocele

4.6 CHIARI IV

not related to Chiari I or Chiari II/III
severe vermian, cerebellar and brainstem
    hypoplasia

4.7 CORPUS CALLOSUM AGENESIS

4.7.1 COMPLETE AGENESIS

ASSOCIATIONS

LIPOMA (50%)
AZYGOS ANTERIOR CEREBRAL ARTERY
CHIARI II, CEPHALOCELES
DANDY–WALKER
HOLOPROSENCEPHALY SPECTRUM
MIGRATION DISORDERS
MIDLINE FACIAL ANOMALIES, COLOBOMAS

MORPHOLOGY

absent corpus callosum and cingulate gyri
spoke like gyral pattern
parallel lateral ventricles indented by
    medially placed bundles of Probst (neural
    tracts that would have normally formed

the corpus callosum running sagittally along the hemisphere)

high riding third ventricle open to interhemispheric fissure

4.7.2 PARTIAL AGENESIS

ASSOCIATIONS

LIPOMA ONLY
HOLOPROSENCEPHALY SPECTRUM

4.8 HOLOPROS-ENCEPHALY SPECTRUM

4.8.1 ALOBAR

monoventricle, fused thalami, no falx or corpus callosum

cyclopia, facial clefts, fusions, hypotelorism

4.8.2 SEMILOBAR

rudimentary occipital horns, part falx, corpus callosum

partly fused thalami, fused frontal lobes, azygos anterior cerebral artery

4.8.3 LOBAR

well formed ventricle bodies + posterior horns, box like anterior horns, no septum pellucidum, fused inferior frontal lobes; falx, corpus callosum present; hypoplastic optic tracts

4.8.4 SEPTOOPTIC DYSPLASIA

hypoplastic optic nerves and tracts, absent septum pellucidum

4.8.5 ARHINENCEPHALY

absent olfactory bulbs and tracts

4.9 MIGRATION AND SULCATION ANOMALIES, CORTICAL DYSMORPHISM

4.9.1 HETEROTOPIC GRAY MATTER

DEFINITION

islands of arrested migrating neurons; therefore occurs anywhere from subependymal to subcortical areas, often bilateral and symmetrical

CLASSIFICATION

4.9.1.1 Band heterotopia

gray matter lamina of variable thickness placed in deep hemispheric white matter between cortex and ventricle

4.9.1.2 Nodular heterotopia

commonest form of gray matter heterotopia

SUBEPENDYMAL

'bumpy' gray matter foci along lateral margins of lateral ventricles

DEEP

intermediate location

SUBCORTICAL

peripheral location, but identifiable separately from the cortex

DIFFERENTIAL

tubers of tuberous sclerosis (different appearance)

low grade neural or neuroglial tumor (gangliocytoma, DNET)

heterotopic gray matter has the MR characteristics of gray matter elsewhere and does not enhance; low grade neural/neuroglial tumors do not enhance, but have higher T2W/PD signal

4.9.2 SCHIZENCEPHALY

DEFINITION AND MORPHOLOGY

cerebral transcortical cleft of variable width lined by dysplastic gray matter (usually polymicrogyric)

frequently bilateral and may be symmetrical

other migration and sulcation anomalies frequently associated

CLASSIFICATION

4.9.2.1 Closed lip

walls of the cleft touch with no visible CSF space between them (double layer of cortex)

ventricular 'dimple' or 'nipple' of cortex projecting into the ventricular CSF

4.9.2.2 Open lip

cleft contains CSF extending from ventricle to convexity

DIFFERENTIAL

porencephalic cyst: not lined by dysmorphic gray matter

4.9.3 LISSENCEPHALY
(agyria–pachygyria)

severe global cortical dysmorphism with absence of sulcation

global absence of sulcation: lissencephaly, agyria

abnormally small number of gyri/sulci: pachygyria

thickened abnormal cortex, smooth cortical surface, abnormal and shallow Sylvian fissures (agyria)

few flat gyri, shallow sulci (pachygyria)

changes usually symmetrically bilateral

4.9.4 POLYMICROGYRIA SPECTRUM

cortical dysmorphism association with cytomegalovirus

focally abnormal thick cortex with focally absent or very small gyri and sulci

may have associated vascular malformations

may have abnormally high T2W or FLAIR signal

4.9.5 HEMIMEGALENCEPHALY SPECTRUM

hamartomatous malformation and enlargement of one cerebral hemisphere with thickened often pachygyric cortex and enlarged ventricle; migration anomalies and heterotopic gray present

4.9.6 FOCAL CORTICAL DYSMORPHISM

some types associated with intrauterine cytomegalovirus infection

focal abnormal gyration and sulcation

focal polymicrogyria

focal clefts (not transcortical)

may have ipsilateral thalamic and cerebral peduncle hypoplasia

4.10 NEURO-FIBROMATOSIS 1 (NF1)

see Ch 11

4.11 NEURO-FIBROMATOSIS 2 (NF2)

see Ch 11

4.12 OSLER–WEBER–RENDU SYNDROME

(hereditary hemorrhagic telangiectasia)

see Ch 15

4.13 POSTERIOR FOSSA MALFORMATIONS AND MASSES

4.13.1 DANDY–WALKER MALFORMATION

cystic dilation secondary to intrauterine obstruction of fourth ventricle outlets

vermian and cerebellar hypoplasia, hugely dilated fourth ventricle, torculolambdoid inversion with elevation of transverse sinuses, hydrocephalus above the fourth ventricle
associations: corpus callosum agenesis 30%, migration disorders 10%

4.13.2 VERMIAN–CEREBELLAR HYPOPLASIA

includes DANDY–WALKER VARIANTS
vermian or cerebellar hypoplasia without excessive fourth ventricle dilation
usually no hydrocephalus, no torculolambdoid inversion
fourth ventricle communicates with cisterna magna

4.13.3 MEGACISTERNA MAGNA

asymptomatic and essentially a normal variant
by definition, exerts no mass effect and communicates with the subarachnoid space

4.13.4 POSTERIOR FOSSA MASSES

4.13.4.1 Posterior fossa arachnoid cyst

asymptomatic or has mass effect
by definition, does not communicate freely with the subarachnoid space

4.13.4.2 Epidermoid

4.13.4.3 Dermoid

4.13.4.4 Cystic tumor

ASSESSMENT ON IMAGING

COMMUNICATION TO FOURTH VENTRICLE AND CISTERNA MAGNA
AQUEDUCT AND FOURTH VENTRICLE OUTLET PATENCY
HYDROCEPHALUS
TORCULOLAMBDOID INVERSION
VERMIAN AND CEREBELLAR HYPOPLASIA

4.14 STURGE–WEBER SYNDROME

see Ch 11

4.15 TUBEROUS SCLEROSIS

see Ch 11

4.16 VON HIPPEL–LINDAU SYNDROME

see Ch 11

SECTION 5

1. NORMAL

1.1 ABBREVIATIONS

see Ch 14

1.2 LUNG INFLATION IN A NEONATE

correct positioning: anterior rib ends symmetrical and do NOT point upwards
8–9 posterior ribs clear of diaphragms is normal
6–7 is underinflation or FILM IN EXPIRATION
10–11 is overinflation

1.3 AIRWAY

adenoids not visible at birth, 5 mm at 3 months and growing
subglottic shoulders in tracheal air column always normal

1.4 THYMUS

most prominent at 2 years; seen in 2% of 5 year olds

CXR
triangular or quadrilateral
thymic sail sign (enters right horizontal fissure)
thymic wave sign (flowing concave margin from rib to rib)

CT/MR
quadrilateral anterior mediastinal structure isodense to muscle on CT
T1W: higher than muscle, T2W: similar to fat
enlarges till puberty, then slowly involutes

1.5 PULMONARY VASCULARITY

Neonatal physiology
high fetal pulmonary vascular resistance falls once the neonate starts breathing and progressively falls over days
ductus arteriosus constricts with increased blood oxygenation (accelerated by indocid, prevented by prostaglandins)
once LA pressure exceeds RA pressure the physiological R to L shunt across the normal foramen ovale ceases
pulmonary vascular pressure has to fall before L to R shunts can occur

Normal vascularity on CXR
peripheral 1/3 of lung relatively devoid of vascular markings
right descending pulmonary artery where it crosses right upper lobe pulmonary vein is same size as trachea at level of aorta

2. GAMUTS

also see Ch 13 for general lung gamuts

2.1 NEONATE

2.1.1 CYSTIC LUNG MASS

CYSTIC ADENOMATOID MALFORMATION

CONGENITAL LOBAR EMPHYSEMA

ISOLATED PNEUMATOCELE OR CYST

DIFFERENTIAL: CONGENITAL DIAPHRAGMATIC HERNIA

2.1.2 HEART DISEASE PRESENTING EARLY

the classification grid follows heart machine 1

Pink not plethoric

CRITICAL AORTIC STENOSIS/ COARCTATION

Pink plethoric

MASSIVE SYSTEMIC AV SHUNT

PDA IN A PREMATURE NEONATE

Cyanotic oligemic

HYPOPLASTIC LEFT HEART

TRICUSPID ATRESIA, HYPOPLASTIC RIGHT HEART

SEVERE EBSTEIN'S ANOMALY

SEVERE FALLOT'S TETRALOGY

Cyanotic plethoric

D-TRANSPOSITION OF GREAT ARTERIES

TRUNCUS ARTERIOSUS

TOTAL ANOMALOUS PULMONARY VENOUS RETURN
(venous congestion if obstructed)

2.1.3 PLEURAL EFFUSIONS

TRANSIENT TACHYPNEA OF THE NEWBORN

LEFT VENTRICULAR FAILURE

PNEUMONIA

CHYLOTHORAX, HYDROTHORAX
?underlying Turner's syndrome

CYSTIC ADENOMATOID MALFORMATION

2.1.4 PULMONARY HYPOPLASIA

Differential: partial or complete collapse of normal lung

Primary

WHOLE LUNG AGENESIS/HYPOPLASIA

LOBAR AGENESIS/HYPOPLASIA

PULMONARY ARTERY HYPOPLASIA

VENOLOBAR SYNDROMES

Secondary

UNILATERAL
THORACIC MASS

BILATERAL
OLIGOHYDRAMNIOS (Ch 22)
INSUFFICIENT THORACIC SPACE
 HYDROTHORAX, CHYLOTHORAX
 SKELETAL DYSPLASIAS

2.1.5 RESPIRATORY DISTRESS

WET LUNG/TRANSIENT TACHYPNEA OF NEWBORN (TTN)

MECONIUM ASPIRATION
term/post term neonate

HYALINE MEMBRANE DISEASE
preterm neonate

PULMONARY HEMORRHAGE

PNEUMONIA

LOBAR OR LUNG COLLAPSE

VENTILATOR PROBLEMS

PULMONARY INTERSTITIAL EMPHYSEMA

AIR LEAKS: PNEUMOTHORAX, PNEUMOMEDIASTINUM

BRONCHOPULMONARY DYSPLASIA including Wilson–Mikity syndrome

DIFFERENTIAL: CARDIAC CAUSE OF RESPIRATORY DISTRESS

2.1.6 SOLID LUNG MASS

SEQUESTRATION

AVM

BRONCHOGENIC CYST

FLUID FILLED CONGENITAL LOBAR EMPHYSEMA (early)

FLUID FILLED CYSTIC ADENOMATOID MALFORMATION (early)

2.2 CHILD

2.2.1 AIRWAY OBSTRUCTION

FOREIGN BODY

MUCUS PLUG

EPIGLOTTITIS

STRUCTURAL

CHOANAL ATRESIA

AIRWAY STENOSIS

TRACHEOBRONCHOMALACIA

HEMANGIOMA

EXTRINSIC COMPRESSION

PREVERTEBRAL ABSCESS

ESOPHAGEAL MASS

NORMAL BRACHIOCEPHALIC ARTERY

VASCULAR RING

2.2.2 BASE OF TONGUE MASS

LINGUAL THYROID

THYROGLOSSAL DUCT CYST

HEMANGIOMA–LYMPHANGIOMA SPECTRUM

2.2.3 FOCAL HYPERINFLATION

CONGENITAL LOBAR EMPHYSEMA

ACQUIRED AIR TRAPPING

!ALL THESE CAN ALSO PRODUCE COLLAPSE

MUCUS PLUG

FOREIGN BODY

STRICTURE

TUMOR

CARCINOID

PAPILLOMA

EXTERNAL COMPRESSION OF BRONCHUS

2.2.4 GENERALIZED HYPERINFLATION

LEFT VENTRICULAR FAILURE, VENOUS CONGESTION (neonate)

BRONCHIOLITIS

ASTHMA, ABPA

CYSTIC FIBROSIS

2.2.5 LUNG MASS IN A CHILD

Contusion, hematoma

Infection

TUBERCULOUS OR FUNGAL FOCUS

ROUND PNEUMONIA

POST INFLAMMATORY PSEUDOTUMOR

LUNG ABSCESS

HYDATID

SEPTIC EMBOLUS

SARCOIDOSIS

Malformation

PERIPHERAL BRONCHOGENIC CYST

PULMONARY SEQUESTRATION

BRONCHOCELE

Vascular

ARTERIOVENOUS MALFORMATION

Tumor

METASTASIS

OSTEOSARCOMA

EWING'S SARCOMA

RHABDOMYOSARCOMA

NEUROBLASTOMA

NEPHROBLASTOMA

LYMPHOMA, LEUKEMIA

PULMONARY HAMARTOMA

BRONCHIAL ADENOMA

Autoimmune

WEGENER'S GRANULOMATOSIS

Mass not in lung parenchyma

USUALLY LOCULATED PLEURAL EFFUSION

2.2.6 RETROPHARYNGEAL NON TRAUMATIC MASS

LYMPHADENOPATHY

EBV, OTHER VIRAL INFECTION

TB

ABSCESS

TUMOR

HEMANGIOMA–LYMPHANGIOMA SPECTRUM

LYMPHOMA

NEUROBLASTOMA

2.2.7 SUBGLOTTIC SOFT TISSUE MASS

ensure there is no swallowing artifact simulating mass

CROUP EDEMA (symmetrical)

PAPILLOMA

HEMANGIOMA

RETENTION CYST

2.3 HEART MACHINE 1
(abnormalities of cardiac chambers and outflow)

this conventional classification of congenital heart disease is based on the presence or absence of pulmonary arterial plethora (CXR) and the presence or absence of cyanosis

2.3.1 TABLE

	CXR shows no plethora	CXR shows plethora
Child not cyanotic	1. no significant R to L shunt exists 2. no significant L to R shunt exists SIMPLE STENOSES	1. no significant R to L shunt exists 2. L to R shunt causes plethora LEFT TO RIGHT SHUNTS
Child cyanotic	1. significant R to L shunt is present 2. R circulation stenosis or high pressure prevents L to R shunt RIGHT TO LEFT SHUNTS	1. significant R to L shunt is present, or L and R circulations do not mix 2. L to R shunt causes plethora TRANSPOSITIONS OR ADMIXTURES

2.3.2 DEFINITIONS

Cyanosis

desaturated systemic arterial blood

for cyanosis to be clinically visible, 5 g deoxyhemoglobin per 100 ml of systemic arterial blood must be present (i.e. O2 saturation <~85%)

Plethora

engorgement of pulmonary arteries (see HEART MACHINE 2 for signs)

for plethora to be visible on CXR, a L to R shunt has to exceed 2:1

differential: pulmonary venous congestion

Oligemia

underfilling of pulmonary arteries

on CXR, inconspicuity of pulmonary vascular markings in the middle 1/3 of lungs

CONGENITAL HEART DISEASE GAMUT FOR OLIGEMIC LUNGS AND CYANOSIS IS THE SAME AS THE GAMUT FOR NORMAL CXR AND CYANOSIS

2.3.3 OVERALL PREVALENCE OF CONGENITAL HEART DISEASE

bicuspid aortic valve is the single most common abnormality but asymptomatic when isolated and is not included in the conventional classification of congenital heart disease; THEREFORE

VSD is the most common overall (~1/3 of all congenital heart disease)

ASD is the second most common overall

Fallot's tetralogy is the most common cyanotic malformation

D-TGA is the most common cause of a blue cardiac neonate

2.3.4 SIMPLE STENOSES (child not cyanotic, CXR not plethoric)

AORTIC STENOSIS

congenital isolated aortic valve regurgitation is rare

congenital isolated mitral valve stenosis or regurgitation is rare

AORTIC COARCTATION

PULMONARY STENOSIS

congenital isolated pulmonary valve regurgitation is rare

ALSO: ISOLATED L-TGV

L-TGV: double transposition of great vessels (atrioventricular discordance and ventriculoarterial discordance) with correct blood crossover as a result

2.3.5 RIGHT TO LEFT SHUNTS (child cyanotic, CXR not plethoric)

TETRALOGY OF FALLOT AND PSEUDOTRUNCUS

TRICUSPID ATRESIA

EBSTEIN'S ANOMALY

HYPOPLASTIC RIGHT HEART OR VENTRICLE

PERSISTENT FETAL CIRCULATION (pulmonary arterial hypertension)

HYPOPLASTIC LEFT HEART OR VENTRICLE

ALSO: EISENMENGER'S COMPLEX

central pulmonary arterial prominence from a previous L to R shunt; shunt now reversed by pulmonary arterial hypertension

2.3.6 LEFT TO RIGHT SHUNTS (child not cyanotic, CXR plethoric)

shunt needs to be at least 2:1 to see plethora

VSD

ASD

PDA

AVSD

CXR DIFFERENTIAL IS PULMONARY VENOUS HYPERTENSION WITH VENOUS CONGESTION

2.3.7 TRANSPOSITIONS OR ADMIXTURES (child cyanotic, CXR plethoric)

D-TGV (!presents very early)

TAPVR (total anomalous pulmonary venous return)

TRUNCUS ARTERIOSUS

DORV (double outlet right ventricle)/SINGLE VENTRICLE

CXR DIFFERENTIAL IS PULMONARY VENOUS HYPERTENSION WITH VENOUS CONGESTION

2.4 HEART MACHINE 2 (pulmonary venous hypertension)

gamut of conditions causing pulmonary venous congestion

CXR classification is based on whether or not cardiomegaly is present

presence of cyanosis is determined by whether there are any associated R to L shunts or transpositions

2.4.1 PULMONARY ARTERIAL PLETHORA VS VENOUS CONGESTION

the two may coexist

Signs of pulmonary arterial plethora

recruitment of vessels in outer 1/3 of lungs

increase in size of central pulmonary arteries

peripheral lung vessels have a sharp margin

no pulmonary edema

Signs of pulmonary venous congestion

recruitment of vessels in outer 1/3 of lungs
loss of gravitational gradient in vessel size
no increase in size of central pulmonary arteries
peripheral lung vessels have a progressively fuzzy margin
progressive pulmonary edema

2.4.2 NO CARDIOMEGALY

(child or adult)

Obstruction at pulmonary vein level

PRIMARY VENOOCCLUSIVE DISEASE

MEDIASTINAL FIBROSIS

Obstruction at left atrium level

OBSTRUCTED TAPVR (total anomalous pulmonary venous return)
presents early

COR TRIATRIATUM
accessory chamber draining pulmonary veins which empties into the LA via a variably stenosed orifice

LEFT ATRIAL MYXOMA

Non compliant left ventricle

TAMPONADE

CONSTRICTIVE PERICARDITIS

Mitral valve disease (early)

early in the disease no cardiomegaly is present
LA dilation develops in both mitral regurgitation and stenosis
LV dilation develops in mitral regurgitation

2.4.3 CARDIOMEGALY IN A CHILD

Mitral valve disease

most common acquired cause: rheumatic fever

Abnormal left ventricle

MYOCARDIUM

MYOCARDITIS

DILATED CARDIOMYOPATHY

HYPERTROPHIC CARDIOMYOPATHY

HYPOPLASTIC LEFT HEART
presents as a neonate, cyanosis evident

ANOMALOUS CORONARY ARTERY ORIGIN
L coronary artery origin from the pulmonary trunk leads to development of epicardial L to R shunting from the RCA to the LCA and myocardial ischemia secondary to vascular steal
presents as a neonate or infant with myocardial infarcts and ischemic LVF

ENDOCARDIUM

ENDOCARDIAL FIBROELASTOSIS

Obstruction at left ventricle outflow tract

classic 'backwards' left ventricular failure
LV hypertrophy develops first, but LV dilation and cardiomegaly eventually follow

AORTIC STENOSIS

AORTIC COARCTATION

Systemic L to R shunt (LV volume overload)

Fluid overload

RENAL

IATROGENIC

2.4.4 FOR COMPARISON: CARDIOMEGALY IN AN ADULT

ischemic heart disease is numerically overwhelmingly major, with dilated cardiomyopathy and mitral valve disease other statistically important conditions

Acquired mitral valve disease

MITRAL STENOSIS

MITRAL REGURGITATION

Abnormal left ventricle

MYOCARDIUM

ISCHEMIC HEART DISEASE

DILATED CARDIOMYOPATHY

HYPERTROPHIC CARDIOMYOPATHY

SPECIFIC MYOCARDIAL DISEASES

ENDOCARDIUM

ENDOMYOCARDIAL FIBROSIS

Fluid overload

RENAL

IATROGENIC

2.5 SITUS MACHINE

this is a simplified, approximate classification of abnormalities of situs (i.e. sidedness)

TABLE

Chest situs	Abdo situs normal		Abdo situs abnormal or inversus	
Normal	Cardiac levorotation	Cardiac dextrorotation	Cardiac levo or dextrorotation	
	normal state 99.5% normal 0.5% have congenital heart disease	98% have congenital heart disease Commonest are: no cyanosis – L-TGV cyanosis – tricuspid atresia	vast majority have congenital heart disease L to R shunts are common polysplenia and variants are common azygos continuation of IVC is common	
Inversus	Cardiac levo or dextrorotation		Cardiac levorotation	Cardiac dextrorotation
	vast majority have congenital heart disease L to R shunts are common polysplenia and variants are common, azygos continuation of IVC is common		rare 100% have congenital heart disease	95% have normal but mirror image layout (consider Kartagener's syndrome) 5% have congenital heart disease

NOTES

Chest situs

is strictly defined as sidedness based on atrial morphology

sidedness based on bronchial morphology is acceptable (i.e. which is the trilobed lung and which is the bilobed lung)

SITUS NORMAL (OR SOLITUS): trilobed lung on the right, bilobed lung on the left

SITUS INVERSUS: bilobed lung on the right, trilobed lung on the left

SITUS AMBIGUUS: can not tell!

Abdominal situs

determined from liver, spleen and stomach position

SITUS NORMAL (OR SOLITUS): liver on the right, spleen and stomach on the left

SITUS INVERSUS: spleen and stomach on the right, liver on the left

spectrum of variants exists, including bilateral right sidedness (asplenia) and bilateral left sidedness (polysplenia)

Cardiac rotation

apex position determines rotation

LEVOROTATION: cardiac apex points to the left

DEXTROROTATION: cardiac apex points to the right

Side of aorta is not relevant to situs

side of aortic arch is determined by which part of the symmetrical embryonic double aortic arch atrophies, and is not necessarily concordant with atrial or bronchial or abdominal situs

CONDITIONS OF PEDIATRIC THORAX

3. CARDIO-MEDIASTINAL CONDITIONS

3.1 ABSENT PERICARDIUM

CLINICAL

male:female 3:1, L side >> R side

increased incidence of congenital heart disease

IMAGING

CXR (partially absent pericardium)

L auricle herniates through pericardial defect

prominent pulmonary artery (differential: mitral stenosis)

CXR (totally absent pericardium)

heart shifted to the left over the dome of the diaphragm

flattened left heart border

all border forming structures sharply separated

lung herniation around heart

3.2 CARDIOMYOPATHY

see Ch 14

3.3 CONGENITAL HEART DISEASE: CLINICALLY SILENT CONDITIONS

3.3.1 ISOLATED BICUSPID AORTIC VALVE

estimated to be present in 2–5% of population

develops symptomatic aortic stenosis in a minority during adult life

3.3.2 ISOLATED L-TGA

DEFINITION

atrioventricular discordance and ventriculoarterial discordance which 'cancel each other out'

MORPHOLOGY

ascending aorta forms L heart border but arch left sided; ventricular position variable; atrioventricular and ventriculoarterial discordance

any plethora, oligemia or presentation depends on associated anomalies

3.3.3 ISOLATED VENOUS ANOMALIES

Persistent left SVC

drains into coronary sinus

Azygos continuation of IVC

usually asymptomatic in an otherwise normal individual

associated with polysplenia and congenital heart disease

Scimitar or venolobar syndrome

definitions vary from authority to authority

ELEMENTS:

isolated anomalous lower lobe venous drainage (also considered a type of partial anomalous venous return)

lobar hypoplasia

anomalous arterial supply (i.e. sequestration)

IMAGING

CXR

classic appearance is of a curved right inferior pulmonary vein running medially and down towards the diaphragm ('scimitar')

right lower lobe drained by the scimitar is hypoplastic

3.4 CONGENITAL HEART DISEASE: LEFT TO RIGHT SHUNTS

GROUP MORPHOLOGY

variable size communication between homologous chambers leads to shunting down the systemic to pulmonary pressure gradient (i.e. L to R)

only oxygenated blood enters the systemic circulation (hence no cyanosis)

pulmonary circulation has volume or volume and pressure overload (depending on location of shunt) of severity that depends on defect size (need at least 2:1 shunt to see plethora on CXR)

all the chambers with volume overload enlarge; it is easier to identify the chambers that remain relatively normal size because they are excluded from the volume overload; shunt has to be sufficiently large to produce chamber enlargement

CLINICAL: no cyanosis

CXR: plethora

3.4.1 VENTRICULAR SEPTAL DEFECT (VSD)

EPIDEMIOLOGY

incidence 1/1000, female > male
frequently present in other more complex
malformations and may be obligatory
(i.e. required for survival)
most common cardiac abnormality in
trisomies (with or without AVSD)

CLASSIFICATION

MEMBRANOUS/PERIMEMBRANOUS (~80%)
MUSCULAR
CONAL

CLINICAL

size of VSD determines clinical severity
very small VSD is insignificant, but may
have impressive murmurs
COMPLICATIONS: endocarditis, CCF, early
Eisenmenger's syndrome

IMAGING

CXR

left atrium, left ventricle, right ventricle and
pulmonary artery all enlarged
right atrium relatively normal; aorta normal
plethora

3.4.2 ATRIAL SEPTAL DEFECT (ASD)

EPIDEMIOLOGY

incidence 1/2000, often isolated

CLASSIFICATION

Secundum defect (most common)

single defect in the fossa ovalis
associated with Holt–Oram syndrome

Primium defect in isolation (rare)

distal atrial septum defect
an endocardial cushion defect, and usually
part of AVSD

Sinus venosus (5%)

high at the junction of SVC and RA
anomalous right upper lobe pulmonary vein
termination in SVC

Lutembacher syndrome

= ASD and mitral stenosis secondary to
rheumatic fever

CLINICAL

frequently clinically silent, and so not
diagnosed
develops Eisenmenger's syndrome late BUT
Eisenmenger's syndrome may be the first
presentation

IMAGING

CXR

left atrium should be enlarged according to
logic of volume overload, but
decompresses into the right atrium and
only enlarges late if at all
right atrium, right ventricle, pulmonary
artery all enlarged
left ventricle relatively normal; aorta normal
plethora

3.4.3 PATENT DUCTUS ARTERIOSUS (PDA)

CLINICAL

incidence 1/3000, female > male
associated with aortic coarctation
frequent in premature neonates with hyaline
membrane disease – presents as LVF
once pulmonary vascular resistance falls
and a hemodynamically major L to R
shunt develops
eventual Eisenmenger's syndrome if not
closed (indocid, coiling, clipping)
PDA may be essential for survival where
there is RV outflow atresia or stenosis
and no other inflow to the pulmonary
circulation (e.g. pulmonary atresia,
severe Fallot's tetralogy)
PDA may be essential for survival where
there is LV or LVOT atresia and the right
heart provides systemic perfusion

IMAGING

CXR

left atrium, left ventricle, aorta and
pulmonary artery all enlarged
right atrium and ventricle relatively normal
plethora

development of LVF in an otherwise normal
premature neonate is very suggestive of
PDA

3.4.4 ATRIOVENTRICULAR SEPTAL DEFECT (AVSD)

EPIDEMIOLOGY

incidence 1/5000
40% have Down's syndrome (prinicipal
cardiac malformation in Down's)

EMBRYOGENESIS

endocardial cushions divide common
atrioventricular canal into right and left
sides of the heart
if these do not fuse properly, the tricuspid
and mitral valves do not develop
normally and the lower interatrial
septum and upper interventricular
septum are deficient with a large central
defect connecting all four chambers

MORPHOLOGY/TYPES

OSTIUM PRIMIUM ASD
OSTIUM PRIMIUM + CLEFT MITRAL VALVE
LV TO RIGHT ATRIAL (GERRODE) SHUNT
(LOW MITRAL VALVE)
COMPLETE AV CANAL (CLEFT MITRAL AND
TRICUSPID VALVES)
depending on size and location of defects
there are L to R shunts at the atrial level,
ventricular level, LV to RA shunting,
shunting at both atrial and ventricular
levels, or free mixing of blood in all four
chambers

CLINICAL

LVF or massive shunting
early unremitting pulmonary hypertension
and Eisenmenger's syndrome
REPAIR – palliative: PA band; open formal
repair; pacemaker (conduction bundles
usually disrupted in repair)

IMAGING

CXR

everything except aorta enlarged (i.e. gross
cardiomegaly)
plethora

3.5 CONGENITAL HEART DISEASE: RIGHT TO LEFT SHUNTS

GROUP MORPHOLOGY

in all of these there is a significant R to L shunt causing cyanosis; AND there is stenosis, atresia or high pressure of the R circulation preventing a L to R shunt (and, therefore, there is oligemia or no plethora on CXR)
CLINICAL: cyanosis
CXR: no plethora or oligemia

3.5.1 FALLOT'S TETRALOGY
(Fallot's tetrad)

EPIDEMIOLOGY

most common cyanotic heart disease
incidence ~1/2000

CLASSIFICATION

Pentad (with ASD)

Tetrad
see below

Triad (no VSD)

Pseudotruncus
complete RVOT or pulmonary atresia
confluent or non confluent L and R PA
ductus dependent type (PDA provides pulmonary perfusion, usually via morphological PA)
bronchial artery type (absent PA, bronchial arteries supply lungs)

MORPHOLOGY

CLASSIC COMPONENTS
RVOT stenosis or pulmonary artery stenosis or atresia
VSD
overriding aorta
right ventricular hypertrophy (not present at birth, develops gradually)
RVOT stenosis may be multilevel; pulmonary valve may have 1–3 cusps

OTHER FEATURES
30% have a right sided aortic arch
5–10% have an anomalous origin of left anterior descending artery from the right coronary artery

CLINICAL

Shunt type determines clinical presentation

'PINK TET' (L to R shunt)
relatively mild pulmonary obstruction
VSD dominant feature

BALANCED
L/R pressures and flows equal

BLUE (R to L shunt)
severe pulmonary stenosis which is the dominant feature
R to L shunt that develops late in a 'pink tet' as RVOT stenosis progresses (or pulmonary hypertension develops)

Complications
septic embolism, cerebral abscess
polycythemia, thrombosis
right heart failure, systemic venous hypertension
conduit aneurysm following conduit repair

Repairs
PALLIATIVE: routine Blalock–Taussig shunt
DEFINITIVE: 2nd step VSD closure and RVOT patch

IMAGING

CXR
oligemia, concave PA segment
+/– bronchial arterial supply to lungs
heart size normal but there is RV hypertrophy with raised apex ('coeur en sabot')
large aorta, right sided in 30%
pulmonary artery to aortic ratio of <1/3 at the level where the right pulmonary artery crosses behind the ascending aorta generally indicates the need for palliative shunt placement before definitive repair

MR
used to demonstrate atresia vs stenosis of RVOT and origin of pulmonary arteries
demonstrates bronchial collaterals from the aorta that are not accessible to echo
evaluates postoperative status

Angio
aortogram run shows bronchial collaterals

3.5.2 TRICUSPID ATRESIA

MORPHOLOGY

absent tricuspid valve
variably developed rudimentary RV that opens into LV
OBLIGATORY ASD AND VSD
MAY BE PDA DEPENDENT
the only route for blood to reach the pulmonary trunk is through a shunt distal to the tricuspid atresia (i.e. VSD, AVSD, PDA) and the only route for blood to exit the right atrium is through a shunt proximal to the tricuspid atresia (i.e. patent foramen ovale or ASD)

IMAGING

CXR
oligemia
elevated apex, normal size heart, but left ventricular hypertrophy
pulmonary artery segment concave
right sided aorta in 5%

MR (cine)
characteristic 'triangle void' which in the normal is occupied by RV

3.5.3 EBSTEIN'S ANOMALY

EPIDEMIOLOGY

approximately 0.5% of congenital heart disease

MORPHOLOGY

balloon tricuspid valve with displaced posterior +/– septal leaf adherent to right ventricular wall
effective origin of the free portion of the posterior +/– septal leaf some distance from the AV junction
small residual functional right ventricle
large right atrium (includes atrialized RV)
functional right atrial obstruction
ACCOMPANIED BY PATENT FORAMEN OVALE OR ASD (i.e. R TO L SHUNT)

NATURAL HISTORY

may reach adult age depending on right
    heart function

IMAGING

CXR

oligemia
small pulmonary artery, normal aorta
massively enlarged right atrium ('box heart')

Differential diagnosis

Uhl's anomaly (hypoplastic RV)
pulmonary stenosis with ASD

3.5.4 HYPOPLASTIC RIGHT HEART/VENTRICLE

Uhl's anomaly: hypoplastic R ventricle

MORPHOLOGY

complete RVOT obstruction
obligatory R to L shunt and ASD or PFO
PDA dependent with L to R shunt across the
    ductus supplying the lungs

IMAGING

CXR

oligemic lungs, small heart

3.5.5 HYPOPLASTIC LEFT HEART OR VENTRICLE

CLINICAL

a diagnosis usually made on antenatal US
clinically, neonatal circulatory collapse
    occurs with progressive closure of ductus
    arteriosus
rapidly fatal untreated

MORPHOLOGY

hypoplastic left ventricle and aortic valve
    with or without atretic or interrupted
    aortic arch
functional obstruction of left heart flow
obligatory ASD
survival depends on L to R shunt through
    the ASD and R to L shunt through the
    PDA

IMAGING

Antenatal US
see Ch 22

CXR

normal size heart, no plethora
pulmonary edema may be present

3.5.6 PERSISTENT FETAL CIRCULATION

DEFINITION

failure of high fetal pulmonary arterial
    pressure to fall, with persistent R to L
    flow across patent foramen ovale and
    possibly R to L flow via a patent ductus
    arteriosus

TYPES

PRIMARY: no cause identified by definition
SECONDARY: LUNG PATHOLOGY or LUNG
    HYPOPLASIA

MORPHOLOGY

neonatal equivalent of Eisenmenger's
    syndrome: high pressure reduced volume
    pulmonary circulation with blood
    shunted to the systemic circuit

CLINICAL

persistent pulmonary arterial hypertension
indefinite R to L shunt via patent foramen
    ovale
ECMO (extracorporeal membrane
    oxygenation) may lead to pulmonary
    vasodilation

IMAGING

CXR

oligemia or normal

3.5.7 EISENMENGER'S SYNDROME

also see pulmonary hypertension in Ch 13

DEFINITION

reversal of a previous L to R shunt as a
    result of progressive pulmonary arterial
    hypertension (underlying mechanism:
    plexogenic arteriopathy)

MORPHOLOGY

primary L to R shunt
slow onset but progressive pulmonary
    arterial hypertension first matching and
    then exceeding systemic pressures
eventual reversal of shunt and development
    of R to L shunt with progressive cyanosis
may result from any L to R shunt, but is
    usually secondary to undiagnosed ASD
    (other L to R shunts are usually
    symptomatic)
common order of manifestation: (earliest)
    AVSD, VSD, PDA, ASD (latest)

IMAGING

CXR

oligemic periphery
massive proximal pulmonary artery dilation
dilation proportional to duration of disease
calcified pulmonary arteries (pathognomonic
    of pulmonary arterial hypertension)
heart shape has the morphology of old L to
    R shunt

3.6 CONGENITAL HEART DISEASE: SIMPLE STENOSES

GROUP MORPHOLOGY

there is no shunting of mixing of the two
    circulations (and so, no cyanosis and no
    plethora); a stenosis (usually isolated)
    causes pressure overload upstream of the
    stenosis and produces the responsible
    clinical signs
CLINICAL: no cyanosis
CXR: no plethora

3.6.1 AORTIC STENOSIS

CLASSIFICATION

VALVULAR (75%)
SUPRAVALVULAR (WILLIAMS' SYNDROME)

SUBVALVULAR MEMBRANOUS
SUBVALVULAR MUSCULAR

IMAGING

CXR

aortic post stenotic dilation
late left ventriculomegaly (decompensation)

3.6.2 AORTIC COARCTATION

CLASSIFICATION

Localized (juxtaductal)

classic location, just distal to the origin of
the left subclavian artery, with a short
segment involved

Diffuse (preductal)

long segment hypoplasia
50% have congenital heart disease with
PDA; these present early

MORPHOLOGY

severity and location of coarctation
determines the status of collaterals
common collateral pathway is antegrade
flow down internal thoracic arteries and
anterior intercostal arteries and
retrograde flow along posterior
intercostal arteries into the thoracic
aorta
the enlarged intercostal arteries groove the
inferior aspect of their ribs ('rib
notching') – this does not affect ribs 1–3
as their posterior intercostal arteries
arise from the thyrocervical trunks off
the subclavian arteries
if the coarctation is proximal to the left
subclavian artery origin, only right sided
notching is present

CLINICAL

absent, reduced or delayed ('radiofemoral
delay') femoral or pedal pulses
arm (and cerebral) arterial hypertension

IMAGING

CXR

aortic '3' sign (left aortic outline has the
contour of the figure 3)
late left ventricular dilation (once
decompensation develops)

rib notching which first develops between
5 and 10 years
left ventricular decompensation develops
depending on severity of coarctation

CT/MR

axial imaging may miss narrowing
sagittal MR demonstrates narrowing/flap
and change in luminal caliber directly

3.6.3 PULMONARY STENOSIS

EPIDEMIOLOGY

isolated pulmonary stenosis is relatively
common
50% of Noonan syndrome has pulmonary
stenosis (dysplastic valve)

MORPHOLOGY

95% dome shaped mobile valve with pinhole
orifice
5% dysplastic immobile thickened valve
(Noonan syndrome has this type)
secondary right ventricular hypertrophy

IMAGING

CXR

right ventriculomegaly
post stenotic pulmonary trunk or left
pulmonary artery dilation

3.7 CONGENITAL HEART DISEASE: TRANSPOSITIONS AND ADMIXTURES

GROUP MORPHOLOGY

in transpositions (arterial or venous) the
pulmonary and systemic circulations are
separate and in parallel; the blood in
systemic circulation is not oxygenated
(hence cyanosis), and survival depends
on persistent communication between the
two circulations allowing some
bidirectional cross-over (which also
elevates pulmonary circulation pressure
and leads to plethora)
in admixtures the two circulations are
variably fused, so that returning systemic

deoxygenated blood mixes with returning
pulmonary oxygenated blood producing a
more or less homogeneous arterial
outflow (cyanosis is present), while the
pulmonary vasculature is supplied at
systemic pressures resulting in plethora
CLINICAL: cyanosis
CXR: plethora

3.7.1 UNCORRECTED TRANSPOSITION OF GREAT VESSELS (D-TGV)

EPIDEMIOLOGY

incidence 1/3000; male > female
commonest cause of blue cardiac neonate
presents early

MORPHOLOGY

VENTRICULOARTERIAL DISCORDANCE
STRAIGHT NARROW CARDIAC PEDICLE
RVOT empties into the aorta, LVOT empties
into the pulmonary artery
pulmonary artery lies in concavity of aorta,
with two not spiraling but running
straight
survival before intervention is dependent on
an open ductus arteriosus

CLINICAL

Repairs

PALLIATIVE: prostaglandins to keep ductus
open, Rashkind septotomy, Blalock–
Hanlon operative septostomy
DEFINITIVE: arterial switch procedure
(Jatene repair)
REPAIRS DONE IN PAST: Senning repair,
Mustard repair

IMAGING

CXR

'egg on side' heart
plethora (not present initially and develops
gradually; corrective repair may be done
before it develops)
pulmonary venous congestion, LVF

3.7.2 TOTAL ANOMALOUS PULMONARY VENOUS RETURN (TAPVR)

DEFINITION

abnormal insertion of all pulmonary veins into the right atrium

CLASSIFICATION AND MORPHOLOGY

Supracardiac (snowman mediastinum)

vertical common pulmonary vein enters left brachiocephalic vein

Cardiac

common pulmonary vein enters coronary sinus

Infracardiac (usually obstructed)

common pulmonary vein enters portal vein, IVC or hepatic veins via the esophageal hiatus

diaphragm causes extrinsic obstruction and pulmonary venous hypertension and congestion

IMAGING

CXR

if obstructed, congestion, pulmonary venous hypertension, pulmonary edema

if not obstructed – plethora

3.7.3 TRUNCUS ARTERIOSUS

DEFINITION

failure of primitive ventricular outflow (embryonal truncus arteriosus) to divide into an aorta and pulmonary artery, with a single arterial trunk supplying the systemic and pulmonary circulations

CLASSIFICATION AND MORPHOLOGY

truncal valve is incompetent; obligatory VSD is present

multiple classifications exist

Van Praagh classification

I   short pulmonary trunk is present
II pulmonary arteries arise as branches of the truncus
III no pulmonary trunk; pulmonary arteries supplied by PDA
IV atretic aortic arch, truncus supplies the PA; descending aorta is supplied via PDA

Collet and Edwards classification

I   aorta and pulmonary trunk arise from same valve
II pulmonary arteries arise from truncus base
III pulmonary arteries arise from truncus sides
IV pseudotruncus (Fallot's tetralogy, lungs supplied by bronchial collaterals)

CLINICAL

septic embolism, endocarditis
Eisenmenger's syndrome

IMAGING

CXR

global cardiomegaly

plethora

right sided aorta in 40% ('sitting duck heart')

absent RVOT on lateral film

3.7.4 DOUBLE OUTLET RIGHT VENTRICLE (DORV)

DEFINITION

complex intracardiac malformation with abnormal division of ventricular chambers and both aorta and pulmonary trunk arising from the morphological right ventricle

CLASSIFICATION AND MORPHOLOGY

I DORV

morphological RV dominant
VSD to small morphological LV
1.5 valves on RV side
aorta and pulmonary artery are usually transposed

II Taussig–Bing anomaly (rare)

'antiFallot' configuration
incomplete TGV, VSD, overriding PA

IMAGING

CXR

cardiomegaly and plethora

3.7.5 SINGLE VENTRICLE

CLASSIFICATION AND MORPHOLOGY

Without pulmonary stenosis

plethora, cardiomegaly

With pulmonary stenosis

behaves like Fallot's tetralogy

3.8 CONGENITAL HEART DISEASE: IMAGING, SHUNTS AND PROCEDURES

IMAGING

specific detailed imaging of congenital heart disease is beyond the scope of this text

CXR findings for each condition are included in the condition's entry, as these are often the initial findings before any other imaging has been performed

ECHO, MR and ANGIO are all used to image congenital cardiac abnormalities

in general, the findings in these modalities reflect the morphology of the malformation as listed in each entry

where specific issues exist for these modalities, these have been noted within the entry

ECHO allows estimation of pressure gradients and quantitation of stenotic, regurgitant and shunt jets

MR (cine, velocity mapping, etc) allows estimation of pressure gradients and jets; MR also directly demonstrates bronchial artery derived systemic collaterals where pulmonary flow is oligemic

ANGIO measures pressure gradients directly; it is a frequent prelude to either palliative septostomy or definitive patch closure or coil embolization

NUC MED (RBC scan) is used for two major indications in congenital heart disease: to quantitate the size of the left to right shunt (bolus first pass technique) and to monitor LV and RV contraction and ejection fractions with graded exercise

exercise ECHO is in general too technically difficult, and RBC scan provides more reliable functional information

SHUNTS

Blalock–Taussig (BTS): subclavian artery to pulmonary artery; performed for Fallot's tetralogy and related conditions

Waterston–Cooley: ascending aorta to pulmonary trunk; performed for Fallot's tetralogy if a BTS can not be done

Potts: descending aorta to left pulmonary artery; performed for Fallot's tetralogy

Glenn: superior vena cava to right PA (!tends to thrombose); performed for tricuspid atresia, Ebstein's anomaly, occasionally for pulmonary atresia or stenosis

Blalock–Park: left subclavian artery to descending aorta (to bypass coarctation)

PROCEDURES

arterial switch procedure (Jatene repair) for D-TGA

Mustard/Senning repairs (for D-TGA); atrial baffle to cross blood over (!tendency for late right ventricular failure and SVC or pulmonary vein stenoses)

Norwood procedure: hypoplastic L heart conversion to single ventricle and pulmonary artery banding

Rastelli repair: truncus repair

Mueller–Daman pulmonary banding for DORV

potential complications of all procedures: stenosis, residual shunt, aneurysmal dilation

Fontan procedure

a number of different techniques that baffle systemic venous blood to the pulmonary artery when there is only one functioning ventricle; these include:

valved and non valved RA to PA conduit

direct RA to PA anastomosis (e.g. via right auricle)

incorporation of rudimentary ventricle in the baffle

direct cavopulmonary (SVC and IVC) anastomosis

patients tend to develop postoperative systemic venous hypertension and thrombosis; obstruction may lead to congestive cardiac failure

Conduit repairs (general comments)

MATERIALS COMMONLY USED TO CONSTRUCT CONDUITS:

pericardium, Dacron and Goretex

OVER TIME, CONDUIT REPAIRS TEND TO OBSTRUCT:

residual native anastomotic stenosis

prosthetic valve stenosis

diffuse intraluminal narrowing in the conduit (formation of a 'peel')

beware conduit xenograft valves on MR: metallic supporting ring can mimic a flow void where there is none

3.9 KAWASAKI'S DISEASE

see Ch 15

3.10 RHEUMATIC FEVER

see Ch 14

3.11 RIGHT SIDED AORTA AND AORTIC RINGS

GROUP DEFINITION

right sided aorta: aortic arch to right of trachea

aortic ring: either full vascular ring or ring made of part vessels and part atretic vessels that have become cords/ligaments

PATHOGENESIS

CONGENITAL HEART DISEASE – PREFERENTIAL EJECTION INTO RIGHT AORTIC ARCH

NO CHD – ISOLATED ANOMALOUS AORTIC RING INTERRUPTION

EPIDEMIOLOGY

isolated right aortic arch, aberrant left subclavian ~1/1000, probably the most common right sided arch overall

Fallot's tetralogy (~1/2000) with right aortic arch (1/3 of Fallot's tetralogies) and truncus arteriosus are the next most common

3.11.1 ABERRANT RIGHT SUBCLAVIAN ARTERY (SCA)

CLINICAL

incidence ~1/200

usually completely silent

aortic arch is in its normal left sided position with normal origins of right CCA, left CCA and left SCA

proximal R SCA is formed by the descending part of the embryonal right aortic arch

no complete vascular ring exists; anomalous R SCA arises last on the aortic arch and to the right rather than left and ascends behind the esophagus to the thoracic inlet

IMAGING

Fluoro

posterior bump in LAO view on esophagogram

CT/MR

anomalous origin of R subclavian artery as the last great vessel on aortic arch

retroesophageal and often quite vertical course

Angio

see description in clinical

relatively low and wide origin (infundibulum)

3.11.2 RIGHT SIDED AORTIC ARCH, ABERRANT LEFT SUBCLAVIAN ARTERY (SCA)

CLINICAL

incidence ~1/1000

5% have congenital heart disease

MORPHOLOGY

most have no associated congenital heart disease

right sided aortic arch gives origins to L CCA, R CCA and R SCA

descending aorta crosses behind the esophagus from R to L at a variable level

L SCA arises low from a large aortic diverticulum and runs upwards to thoracic inlet

variant: large aortic diverticulum, persistent ligamentum arteriosum; this produces compressive symptoms

variant: isolated L SCA not arising from the descending aorta; this produces subclavian steal

IMAGING

Fluoro

posterior bump in RAO on esophagogram

CT/MR

determines how completely the trachea and esophagus are enclosed by the vascular structures

Angio

see morphology

3.11.3 DOUBLE AORTIC ARCH

MORPHOLOGY

persistence of both embryonic arches
R arch is bigger and lies more superiorly
usually an isolated anomaly with no associated cardiac malformations
L arch may be patent or may be atretic
if L arch is patent, each arch gives origin to its CCA and SCA

CLINICAL

very symptomatic because of a complete tight ring

IMAGING

Fluoro

compression of esophagus by vascular ring

MR

shows morphology of the ring
only modality to directly show the left arch if it is atretic

Angio

see morphology
angio does not show the atretic left arch!

3.11.4 MIRROR IMAGE AORTIC ARCH

CLINICAL

integral part of a total situs inversus (otherwise normal)
excluding above, 98% have congenital heart disease (Fallot's tetralogy is 90% of these)

MORPHOLOGY

R aortic arch with a true mirror image arrangement

left brachiocephalic artery is the first branch, followed by R CCA and then R SCA
left ductus arteriosus runs to left brachiocephalic artery (i.e. anterior to trachea and esophagus) – no vascular ring is present

3.11.5 TRACHEAL COMPRESSION BY NORMAL BRACHIOCEPHALIC ARTERY

CLINICAL

not a vascular ring or malformation
forms a clinical and radiological differential to vascular rings
isolated and common
presents with variably severe compressive symptoms and improves with time

IMAGING

MR

demonstrates degree of compression

3.11.6 LEFT PULMONARY ARTERY SLING

MORPHOLOGY

left PA originates from right PA and runs between trachea and esophagus to L hilum
presents with compressive symptoms

IMAGING

CXR

may have lungs of different vascularity

MR

directly demonstrates origin and course of left PA

3.12 THYMIC HYPERPLASIA

see Ch 14

3.13 THYMIC REBOUND

see Ch 14

4. LUNG CONDITIONS

4.1 ASTHMA

see Ch 13

4.2 BRONCHIOLITIS

DEFINITION

clinical syndrome of respiratory distress, wheeze and lung hyperinflation in infants <18 months

CLINICAL

up to ~18 months
respiratory syncytial virus, others
strong statistical association with subsequent asthma

IMAGING

CXR

normal OR
diffuse hyperinflation
patchy hyperinflation and patchy subsegmental collapse
peribronchial thickening

4.3 BRONCHOCELE

DEFINITION

congenital atretic or acquired stenotic bronchus with buildup of mucus upstream of it and frequent hyperinflation of distal lung

ETIOLOGY

Congenital atresia

Acquired

FOREIGN BODY
POST TRAUMATIC
TUMOR (look for mass central to bronchocele)

IMAGING

CXR/CT

dilated tubular structure in the expected position of a bronchus

may be V shaped if more than one bronchus is involved

thin wall and smooth edges unless superinfected

fluid density content

subtended lung segment normal (sometimes) or hyperinflated, or collapsed, or consolidated, or has fibrotic scarring (or a combination of these)

4.4 BRONCHOGENIC CYST

DEFINITION

mediastinal or pulmonary parenchymal vestigial cyst formed by bronchial epithelium

CLINICAL

filled with mucoid material and lined with columnar epithelium

usually an asymptomatic incidental finding

Central (more common)

mediastinal thin walled cyst, frequently subcarinal but location varies

may be deformed by surrounding structures, may have mass effect

Peripheral (rare)

pulmonary parenchymal peripheral thin walled cyst of variable size

more common on right

NO connection to bronchial tree

may present with compression of bronchus or if superinfected

IMAGING

CXR

mediastinal soft tissue density mass with no specific CXR characteristics; or pulmonary parenchymal soft tissue density rounded well defined mass with sharp edge unless superinfected

?cystic on above criteria

CT/MR

hypodense, water density or hyperdense depending on content

MR signal variable depending on content

no calcification

post contrast, thin enhancing rim with non enhancing center

water density or water signal on MR suggestive

4.5 CHILDHOOD PNEUMONIAS

see main pneumonia entry in Ch 13

ETIOLOGY BY AGE

NEONATAL
see etiology below

1 MONTH TO 5 YEARS OLD
viruses
Pneumococcus
Staphylococcus
Hemophilus
(i.e. particular susceptibility to encapsulated organisms)

OVER 5 YEARS OLD
viruses
Pneumococcus
Mycoplasma
Hemophilus
(i.e. young adult pattern)

TUBERCULOSIS

4.5.1 NEONATAL PNEUMONIA

ETIOLOGY

ascending infection (from birth canal)
ESPECIALLY Group B Streptococcus
OTHER: Streptococcus fecalis, E coli, Staphylococcus, Chlamydia, ureaplasma, Hemophilus

CLINICAL PRESENTATIONS

CLASSICAL CONSOLIDATION
LIKE HYALINE MEMBRANE DISEASE, +/– EFFUSIONS
LIKE MECONIUM ASPIRATION +/– EFFUSIONS

IMAGING

CXR

classical airspace consolidation (relatively uncommon)

granular pattern similar to hyaline membrane disease

patchy overinflation simulating meconium aspiration

may have effusions

4.5.2 ROUND PNEUMONIA

DEFINITION

purely morphological description of spherical airspace consolidation in a child, which mimics a tumor or other mass

ETIOLOGY

pneumococcus, less often other bacterial

occurs <8 years of age; if older child or adult, immune suppression and/or atypical organism likely (e.g. fungus)

PATHOGENESIS

incomplete development of pores of Kohn

containment of consolidation around seeding focus with circumferential growth of consolidated lung rather than lobar 'flooding'

IMAGING

CXR

rounded airspace density usually in lower lobes

edge well defined or soft

may show air bronchograms

radiographic clearing may lag behind clinical cure, resulting in 'post inflammatory pseudotumor'

mimics tumors

4.5.3 TB

see Ch 13 for full discussion

TB

children classically have the pattern of 'immunologically naive' host with peripheral consolidation, central unilateral lymphadenopathy and an effusion

TB is the commonest cause of lung nodule in a child, nodule and lymphadenopathy may calcify

neonates classically develop miliary TB

Fungus

cryptococcus, histoplasma, rarely coccidiomycosis

may have benign laminated or diffuse calcification, hilar lymphadenopathy with/without calcification

4.6 CHILDHOOD UPPER RESPIRATORY INFECTIONS

4.6.1 CROUP (LARYNGO-TRACHEOBRONCHITIS)

CLINICAL

parainfluenza virus, others
barking cough in toddlers

IMAGING

CXR

no findings OR
subglottic mucosal swelling (loss of subglottic shoulders)

4.6.2 DIPHTHERIA

Corynebacterium diphtheriae (immotile club shaped Gram+ rod) producing exotoxin
LOCAL EFFECTS OF TOXIN: sloughed mucosa forms pseudomembrane
SYSTEMIC EFFECTS OF TOXIN: myocarditis, ocular neuropathies

4.6.3 WHOOPING COUGH

caused by Bordetella pertussis (small Gram+ rod) which produces pertussis exotoxins
severe upper bronchitis with focal ulceration progressing to bronchiectasis

IMAGING

CXR

classical description is of a 'shaggy heart'

HRCT

possible subsequent bronchiectasis

4.6.4 BRONCHIOLITIS

see its own entry

4.6.5 EPIGLOTTITIS

CLINICAL

Hemophilus influenzae infection of the epiglottis (also Pneumococcus)
fever, severe dysphagia, drooling, inspiratory stridor
high risk of total airway obstruction: therefore NO INVASIVE EXAMINATIONS

IMAGING

XR

lateral neck film 'as is'
marked thickening and enlargement of epiglottis and aryepiglottic folds

4.7 CONGENITAL DIAPHRAGMATIC HERNIA

DEFINITION

embryonic failure of pleuroperitoneal membranes to completely separate the two cavities with subsequent herniation of abdominal contents into the thorax and lung hypoplasia

CLINICAL

incidence ~1/3000, left >> right, 25% have other malformations
Bochdalek's foramen (posteriorly between diaphragmatic and costal components of diaphragm)
left sided defects usually contain small and large bowel, right sided defects may contain liver or bowel
if sufficiently large to cause significant lung hypoplasia, presents with neonatal respiratory insufficiency and scaphoid abdomen
may develop obstruction, strangulation or infarction of herniated bowel
if small, may present with late bowel obstruction or pneumonia
intraabdominal volvulus is uncommon despite bowel malfixation/malposition

IMAGING

CXR

no normal lung–diaphragmatic interface
at first, intrathoracic lobulated mass with no inferior border (non aerated bowel)
as bowel progressively aerates, intrathoracic bowel develops into a 'cystic mass'
reduced number of air filled bowel loops in abdomen

Fluoro

contrast study diagnostic

CT

generally diagnostic

4.8 CONGENITAL LOBAR EMPHYSEMA

DEFINITION

idiopathic overinflation of one lobe or segment secondary to air trapping by subtending bronchus

CLINICAL

male:female 3:1
15% have cardiac malformations
presents with neonatal soft tissue density lung mass with/without respiratory distress, which progresses to cystic mass as the spaces empty of fluid

IMAGING

CXR/CT

early – soft tissue density lung mass
once fluid resorbs, a cystic hyperinflated hyperlucent lobe with mass effect on rest of lung
LUL > RML > RUL; only 5% occurs in lower lobes
RETAINS PULMONARY VESSELS

Differential

MUST RULE OUT ACQUIRED LOBAR EMPHYSEMA
cystic adenomatoid malformation
simple lung cyst

4.9 CYSTIC ADENOMATOID MALFORMATION

DEFINITION

failure of respiratory endodermal epithelium to induce normal mesenchymal morphogenesis producing a mass of epithelial spaces and mesenchyme

CLASSIFICATION

I   MACROCYSTIC
II MEDIUM SIZE CYSTS (5–10 mm)
III MICROCYSTIC (<5 mm)

CLINICAL

macrocystic CAM has low incidence of other malformations;
type II and III CAMs have high incidence of other malformations

IMAGING

Antenatal US
bright lung mass

CXR/CT
unicystic or polycystic mass with or without respiratory distress
type III CAM is solid on imaging
CONTAINS NO PULMONARY VESSELS

Differential
congenital lobar emphysema
acquired lobar emphysema
simple lung cyst
lung abscess
congenital diaphragmatic hernia (air filled bowel)
unilateral pulmonary interstitial emphysema

4.10 CYSTIC FIBROSIS

see Ch 13

4.11 HISTIOCYTOSIS X
(Langerhans cell histiocytosis)

see Ch 05, Ch 11, Ch 13

4.12 HYALINE MEMBRANE DISEASE (HMD)

DEFINITION

failure of gas exchange and spontaneous ventilation in premature neonates secondary to surfactant deficiency and lung immaturity

EPIDEMIOLOGY

incidence proportional to degree of prematurity
RISK FACTORS: maternal diabetes, Cesarean section
reduced by: steroids, prophylactic surfactant administration

ETIOLOGY

Surfactant deficiency
assess by sphingomyelin:lecithin ratio of amniotic fluid

Distal airspace immaturity
absent alveoli and acini; cuboidal epithelium; thick interstitial mesenchyme

PATHOGENESIS

immature distal airspace with reduced number of alveoli
excessive alveolar/alveolar sac wall tension
patchy poor expansion and patchy atelectasis; markedly increased work of breathing
V/Q mismatch, hypoxia, hypercapnia, respiratory acidosis
focal dense lung ischemia, parenchymal necrosis
fibrinoid and cellular exudate forming dense pink hyaline membranes
heavy beefy red small volume lungs (sink in water)

CLINICAL

Untreated disease
early onset (at birth or within the hour) respiratory distress
progressive central cyanosis and increasing oxygen requirements
inspiratory retraction, tachypnea, expiratory grunting

SEVERE – DEATH
MILD – spontaneous recovery (produces sufficient own surfactant)

With intervention
prenatal steroids to mature lung
adequate ventilation, surfactant administration

ACUTE COMPLICATIONS
air leaks
sepsis
intracranial bleeds
necrotizing enterocolitis

CHRONIC COMPLICATIONS
bronchopulmonary dysplasia, failure to wean
retrolental fibroplasia
short gut syndrome
persistent ductus arteriosus with shunt and left ventricular failure

NB ALSO SEE WILSON–MIKITY SYNDROME

IMAGING

CXR
spectrum from no findings to severe changes
reduced or normal volume lungs (hypoinflation)
reticulogranular diffuse bilateral pattern (visible at ~12 hours)
progressive patchy consolidation with airbronchograms and marked volume loss
eventual lung white out if untreated
normal CXR at 6 hours rules out HMD
see neonatal lung disease – respiratory distress syndrome for appearance of ventilator complications and bronchopulmonary dysplasia
can not rule out Group B Streptococcus as responsible for CXR appearance

4.13 IMMUNE DEFICIENCY IN CHILDREN – ACQUIRED

CLASSIFICATION

AIDS

BONE MARROW REPLACEMENT

LEUKEMIA

METASTASES TO BONE MARROW (e.g. neuroblastoma)

IATROGENIC IMMUNE SUPPRESSION

ORGAN TRANSPLANT

STEROID TREATMENT

CHEMOTHERAPY

IMAGING

CXR
see AIDS overview in Ch 13

MR
assesses extent of bone marrow replacement in leukemia/lymphoma

4.14 IMMUNE DEFICIENCY IN CHILDREN – CONGENITAL

4.14.1 IMMUNE DEFICIENCY OF PREMATURITY

relative and temporary immune deficiency reflecting relative immune immaturity

4.14.2 ANTIBODY DEFICIENCY

all eventually develop lymphoma or leukemia

IgA deficiency (incidence ~1/800)

Ataxia telangiectasia
cerebellar ataxia, skin telangiectasias, recurrent respiratory infections
50% have no thymus or lymphoid tissue
50% have IgA deficiency
INCREASED INCIDENCE OF RADIATION INDUCED MALIGNANCY

Bruton's X-linked agammaglobulinemia
recurrent bronchopneumonias, sinusitis, mastoiditis, skin and urinary tract infections
no lymphadenopathy despite infections
no adenoids – characteristically widened pharyngeal airway

Hyperimmunoglobulinemia E
elevated IgE and depressed cell mediated immunity

Staphylococcal infections with repeated lobar or segmental pneumonias producing pneumatoceles

4.14.3 CELLULAR DEFICIENCY – WHITE CELLS

Chronic granulomatous disease of childhood
neutrophil enzyme deficiencies result in failure of bacterial killing following phagocytosis (hence granulomatous response to bacterial infection)
frequent bacterial and fungal infections

Hereditary neutropenia

4.14.4 CELLULAR DEFICIENCY – LYMPHOCYTES

DiGeorge syndrome
the prototype cell mediated immune deficiency syndrome
abnormal or absent development of lower branchial apparatus, leading to absent thymus and/or parathyroid glands
deficient cell mediated immunity with neonatal hypocalcemia

4.14.5 COMBINED DEFICIENCY

Severe combined immune deficiency
survive beyond 1 year of age only with bone marrow transplantation
develop lymphoma/leukemia

Chronic mucocutaneous candidiasis
= PARTIAL COMBINED IMMUNODEFICIENCY

IMAGING (group)

Imaging features to look for
PNEUMONIA
PRESENCE OF THYMUS
PRESENCE OF LYMPHOID TISSUE
BRONCHIECTASIS
SINONASAL DISEASE
SUPERVENING MALIGNANCY

4.15 INHALED FOREIGN BODY (FB)

CLINICAL

occurs in 1–5 year olds; most common between 1–2 years of age
usually radiolucent solid vegetable matter (e.g. peanut)
LOCATION: RIGHT MAIN BRONCHUS > LEFT MAIN BRONCHUS >> TRACHEA
80% present with an acute episode
if not presenting acutely, child develops persisting cough and/or wheeze
diagnosis delayed in 1/3
GOLDEN RULES: wheeze of new onset (in the absence of known asthma) is FB till proven otherwise; failure of pneumonia to resolve in the usual time course may be a FB

Effect on lung distal to FB
ball valve effect with air trapping
partial collapse
full obstruction with collapse/consolidation
<1% have normal aeration (this classically happens with a tracheal FB)

IMAGING

CXR
DO inspiratory/expiratory CXR pair or FLUORO to unmask air trapping
10% show FB
50% show air trapping
30% show collapse
10% CXR fully normal

CT
problem solving; demonstrates location and shape of foreign body (helical thin section acquisition)

NUC MED (ventilation scan)
shows lobes or segments with non aeration in search for occult FB

4.16 LARYNGOMALACIA, TRACHEOMALACIA

4.16.1 LARYNGOMALACIA

'floppy larynx' (resolves with age)

lax epiglottis and aryepiglottic folds produce an inspiratory stridor at rest that improves with crying or activity

FLUORO: epiglottis/aryepiglottic folds drawn towards larynx with inspiration

4.16.2 TRACHEOMALACIA

'floppy trachea'

abnormally soft tracheal wall that collapses in expiration producing an expiratory stridor

secondary to tracheoesophageal fistula, tracheostomy, extrinsic compression, chronic infection

FLUORO: tracheal collapse with expiration

4.17 MCLEOD/SWYER-JAMES SYNDROME

see Ch 13

4.18 MECONIUM ASPIRATION

CLINICAL

often a term or post term fetus

fetal distress induces a mature fetus to pass meconium

intrauterine or intrapartum hypoxia causes fetal gasping, leading to aspiration of previously passed meconium

IMAGING

hyperinflation, patchy consolidation

interstitial air leaks common (see entry on pulmonary interstitial emphysema)

pneumothorax, pneumomediastinum in about 1/4

often improves by 48 hours but radiological clearing is delayed compared to clinical improvement

beware Group B Streptococcus pneumonia simulating meconium aspiration

4.19 PULMONARY ARTERIOVENOUS MALFORMATION (AVM)

see Ch 15 hereditary hemorrhagic telangiectasia

4.20 PULMONARY SEQUESTRATION

GROUP DEFINITION

segment of lung with abnormal systemic blood supply

4.20.1 EXTRALOBAR SEQUESTRATION

sequestered segment is surrounded by own pleura, lies separate from rest of lung, and has no communication with bronchial tree

lower lobes >> upper lobes, left to right 4:1

variable systemic supply from small aortic branches

systemic venous drainage via IVC, azygos or portal vein to right atrium

high incidence of other malformations

4.20.2 INTRALOBAR SEQUESTRATION

presentation as child or young adult with recurrent infections, hemoptysis or abscess

50% present after 20 years of age

lower >> upper lobes, usually medial left lower lobe

sequestered segment lies within visceral pleura of its lobe and may communicate with the bronchial tree

95% drain to left atrium via pulmonary veins

usually has a single large feeding artery from distal thoracic aorta

IMAGING (group)

CXR

lung mass, usually lower lobe

may present as recurrent segmental or lobar pneumonia in the same location with no complete resolution between episodes

may cavitate or develop an air–fluid level if superinfected

CT

homogenous or heterogeneous lower lobe mass with irregular enhancement

may cavitate if an abscess develops

CT angiography demonstrates systemic arterial supply

Angio

thoracic aortogram diagnostic

4.21 ROUND PNEUMONIA

see the pediatric pneumonia entry

4.22 SARCOIDOSIS (child)

see full entry in Ch 13

CLINICAL

childhood sarcoidosis is unusual, but occurs

100% have bilateral hilar lymphadenopathy

90% have paratracheal lymph nodes

75% show reticulonodular lung pattern

may progress to restrictive lung disease

4.23 VENTILATOR PROBLEMS (and neonatal ICU)

GROUP DEFINITION

pulmonary complications of positive pressure ventilation in premature neonates with hyaline membrane disease

4.23.1 ENDOTRACHEAL TUBE MALPOSITION

endotracheal tube tip is very mobile and
  moves with head rotation and flexion
ideal position is at approximately T1–T2
  (carina is generally opposite T4)
all malpositions produce rapid collapse of
  the non ventilated lung or lobes
RIGHT MAIN BRONCHUS
BRONCHUS INTERMEDIUS
LEFT MAIN BRONCHUS
ESOPHAGEAL

4.23.2 MUCUS PLUGGING
(and lobar collapse)

4.23.3 PULMONARY INTERSTITIAL EMPHYSEMA (PIE)

CLINICAL

dissection by ventilated air into lung
  interstitium and connected spaces
occurs relatively early during mechanical
  ventilation
meconium aspiration is the one condition
  where air leaks are common WITHOUT
  mechanical ventilation

IMAGING

CXR

early: hyperinflated lungs
later: linear air streaks in pulmonary
  interstitium
pneumothoraces (use cross-table dorsal
  decubitus view)
pneumomediastinum
surgical emphysema
pneumopericardium
all abnormal air collections should be
  assumed to be under tension until proven
  otherwise
NOTE: pneumothoraces collect anteriorly
  and at first may only be evident as excess
  expansion or lucency of one hemithorax

4.23.4 BRONCHOPULMONARY DYSPLASIA (BPD)

CLINICAL

disordered development and fibrotic
  dysplastic disorganization of distal
  airspace evolving out of hyaline
  membrane disease in neonates on
  ventilation
related to duration of ventilation and may be
  related to inspired oxygen concentration

MICRO

Early
epithelial loss, hyaline membranes,
  squamous metaplasia, interstitial edema
  with fibroblastic response

Late
cuboidal respiratory epithelial regeneration;
  excess collagen and reticulin with
  thickened walls; mixed lobular
  overdistension and collapse

IMAGING

CXR early ('granular opacities')
evolving features of hyaline membrane
  disease
lack of distal air sacs produces granular
  opacities

CXR late ('cystic bubbles')
coarse cystic pattern with bubbly
  hyperinflation +/– air bronchograms;
  localized bullae, air trapping

NUC MED (V/Q)
V/Q mismatches

4.23.5 WILSON–MIKITY SYNDROME

DEFINITION

defined as bronchopulmonary dysplasia
  occurring without any mechanical
  ventilation

CLINICAL

rare; occurs in premature neonates who are
  not sick enough to be ventilated
postulated response of immature lung to
  inspired oxygen
onset ~2 weeks

4.23.6 UMBILICAL CATHETER MALPOSITION

umbilical artery catheter should dip into the
  pelvis before running upwards along the
  internal iliac artery, with tip ideally
  positioned AWAY from renal artery
  origins (T6–T10 or L3–L4)
catheter in the umbilical vein runs directly
  up and to right of midline (i.e. through
  the ductus venosus) to reach the right
  heart

4.24 WET LUNG/ TRANSIENT TACHYPNEA OF NEWBORN (TTN)

CLINICAL

transient retention of airspace and
  interstitial lung fluid with temporary
  overload of draining lymphatics
commoner in Cesarean section

IMAGING

CXR

hyperinflation, hazy diffuse granular
  pattern, airspace opacities (hyaline
  membrane disease has no hyperinflation)
progresses to interstitial pattern +/–
  effusions
heart size stays normal (in LVF, it enlarges)
resolves in 48 hours

Obstetrics, gynecology, breast

22 Obstetrics

1. NORMAL

all gestational age dates in this chapter are menstrual dates (weeks post LMP)

1.1 ABBREVIATIONS

AC: abdominal circumference
AFI: amniotic fluid index
AFP: alphafetoprotein
beta hCG: beta human chorionic gonadotrophin
BPD: biparietal diameter
BPP: biophysical profile
CRL: crown–rump length
CTG: cardiotocography
EDD: estimated date of delivery
EFW: estimated fetal weight
FIRP: first international reference preparation
FL: femur length (only diaphysis measured)
GA: gestational age (always menstrual, i.e. weeks from LMP)
GS: gestational sac
HC: head circumference
IVF: in vitro fertilization
IUGR: intrauterine growth retardation
LMP: date of last menstrual period
LVOT: left ventricle outflow tract
OFD: occipitofrontal diameter
PID: pelvic inflammatory disease
PROM: premature rupture of membranes
RVOT: right ventricle outflow tract
UA: umbilical artery

FIRST TRIMESTER NORMAL

1.2 FORMULAS

these are approximate, simplified formulas applicable only to the specified gestational interval but with clinically acceptable accuracy within it

GS size vs GA between 5 and 10 weeks of GA (LMP)

LIMITS: 5 TO 11 WEEKS POST LMP OR
8 mm < GS < 55 mm
$GS = (AGE-1)^2/2+5$
$AGE = 1+\sqrt{(2*GS-10)}$

where:
GS size is in mm
AGE is GA in weeks post LMP

CRL vs GA between 5 and 10 weeks of GA (LMP)

LIMITS: 5 TO 10 WEEKS POST LMP OR
1 mm < CRL < 36 mm
$CRL = (AGE-4)^2$
$AGE = 4+\sqrt{(CRL)}$

where:
CRL is in mm
AGE is GA in weeks post LMP

1.3 MEASUREMENTS

Accuracy of measurements done for GA

most accurate measurement at 5 to 6 weeks: mean GS diameter
most accurate measurement at 7 to 12 weeks: CRL (+/– 5 days)
most accurate measurement at 12 to 24 weeks: BPD (+/– 5 days)
over 24 weeks measurements reflect growth and not GA

Corpus luteum cyst (of pregnancy)

<5 cm, resolves by 18 weeks

Heart rate

>90 bpm after 5 weeks
140–150 bpm by 8 weeks

Nuchal lucency

measure at 10–14 weeks (CRL 38–84 mm)
normal is <3 mm
5% of normal have nuchal lucency >3 mm (resolves by 16 weeks)
abnormal nuchal lucency suggests aneuploidy or cardiac malformations
risk increased if lucency is septated (70% aneuploid)
nuchal lucency is used together with maternal age for risk estimation

Yolk sac

largest at 10 weeks at 5 mm

1.4 MILESTONES (LMP)

5 weeks

intradecidual sign, double decidual sign gestational sac, yolk sac, double bleb

6 weeks

heart beat

8 weeks

rhombencephalon (~3 mm cystic vesicle)
midgut herniates into base of cord

9 weeks

early placenta
head and limbs

10 weeks

yolk sac largest at 5 mm
nuchal lucency <3 mm between 10 and 14 weeks

11 weeks

stomach, ossified skull and spine, 4 chamber heart

12 weeks

midgut returns to abdomen
membranes fuse

Intradecidual sign

small gestational sac fully buried in bright decidua

Double decidual sign

larger gestational sac surrounded by a layer of decidua displaces the endometrial cavity line and decidua of the opposite wall over it: there are three layers over the sac: decidua capsularis, endometrial cavity, decidua parietalis of the opposite wall

1.5 PHYSIOLOGICAL BOWEL HERNIATION

elongating bowel herniates into the base of the umbilical cord at 8 weeks and returns by 12 weeks
differentiation between omphalocele and physiological bowel herniation is based on GA and serial scanning
no physiological herniation should be present at CRL >45 mm

1.6 ULTRASOUND CHECKLIST (first trimester)

Number and location of embryos

uterus versus adnexa
(beware pseudogestational sac of ectopic pregnancy)

Is the embryo live?

fetal heart

Measurements and dates

CRL, GS

nuchal translucency (10 to 14 weeks)

Anatomy (when applicable)

HEART: position and rate

HEAD: vesicles, presence of brain, presence of skull

NECK: nuchal translucency

SPINE: is the neural tube closed?

LIMBS: presence

Associated findings

corpus luteum of pregnancy (location, normal vascularity)

implantation bleed (site and size)

fibroids, incidental masses

FIBROID VERSUS CONTRACTION

contraction: deforms inner wall contour, transient

fibroid: frequently deforms both inner and outer wall contours, may contain calcification, fixed

SECOND TRIMESTER NORMAL

1.7 FORMULAS

these are approximate, simplified formulas applicable only to the specified gestational interval but with clinically acceptable accuracy within it

BPD and FL vs GA

LIMITS: 16 to 30 weeks (36 mm < BPD < 78 mm)

BPD = (AGE-4)*3

AGE = BPD/3+4

(accuracy +/– 1 week)

LIMITS: 16 to 26 weeks (21 mm < FL < 51 mm)

FL = (AGE-9)*3

AGE = FL/3+9

(accuracy +/– 1 week)

where:

BPD is in mm

FL is in mm (diaphysis measured only)

AGE is GA (LMP) in weeks

HC from BPD and OFD

HC = (BPD + OFD)*1.62

Formulas that are more accurate

adapted from PM Doubilet, CB Benson, PW Callen in: PW Callen (ed) Ultrasound in Obstetrics and Gynecology; WB Saunders, Philadelphia, 2000

predicted GA (<42 weeks) = exp (2.28 + 0.0151*BPD)

predicted GA (<42 weeks) = exp (2.45+0.0166*FL)

predicted GA (< 42 weeks) = exp (2.39 + 0.0050*BPD +0.0090*FL + 0.0005*AC)

1.8 FETAL TISSUE DIAGNOSIS

Amniocentesis

INDICATIONS

KARYOTYPING

AFP LEVEL

?AMNIONITIS

IMMUNE HYDROPS – BILIRUBIN LEVEL

RISKS

FETAL

ABORTION (~1/300, varies with pregnancy, operator)

INJURY

INFECTION

AMNIOTIC SEPARATION

MATERNAL

HEMORRHAGE

ISOIMMUNIZATION

ADVANTAGES OVER CVS

LOWER ABORTION RATE

LOWER ERROR RATE

Chorionic villus sampling (CVS)

RISKS

FETAL

ABORTION

INFECTION

AMNIOTIC SEPARATION

MATERNAL

HEMORRHAGE

ISOIMMUNIZATION

TECHNICAL PROBLEMS

MOSAICISM (placental genome may differ from fetal genome)

MATERNAL CELL CONTAMINATION

ADVANTAGES OVER AMNIOCENTESIS

EARLIER RESULT

1.9 INDICATIONS FOR ULTRASOUND

First trimester

ACCURATE GA

uterus size disagrees with dates

dates critical to management (e.g. amniocentesis planned, previous IUGR)

adverse past personal history (IUGR, Rhesus disease)

EARLY FETAL ANATOMY OVERVIEW

neural tube for risk of spina bifida or high AFP

nuchal lucency for high risk pregnancy or older maternal age

FAILED EARLY PREGNANCY

threatened abortion

patient with habitual abortion

ABNORMAL PREGNANCY

?ECTOPIC

?MOLAR PREGNANCY

?PREGNANCY AND A MASS

TWIN PREGNANCY OR PATIENT WITH OVULATION INDUCTION

AS PART OF KARYOTYPING

AS PART OF CERVICAL SUTURE

Second trimester

ACCURATE GA AND NUMBER

dates allow planning

discloses twin pregnancies

FETAL ANATOMICAL SURVEY

ultrasound screen for major abnormalities

EXCLUDE LOW LYING PLACENTA

Third trimester

ASYMPTOMATIC HIGH RISK PREGNANCY

MATERNAL RISK FACTORS

diabetes, renal disease, cardiac disease

Rhesus disease

POSITION/PRESENTATION/PLACENTA

low lying placenta in second trimester

malpresentation including breech

ADVERSE PAST HISTORY

IUGR

FETAL DEATH IN UTERO

TWIN PREGNANCY

scans at 28 weeks, 32 weeks routinely done

twin growth, fetal well being

fetal position and presentation

SYMPTOMATIC – FETUS AT RISK

preeclampsia – BPP, UA Doppler
PROM – AFI, BPP
?IUGR
?fetal distress – BPP, UA Doppler
polyhydramnios
documented fetal anomalies – review

SYMPTOMATIC – UTEROPLACENTAL

placenta previa
antepartum bleed
?malpresentation
?retained products

INTERVENTION GUIDANCE

AMNIOCENTESIS
?INFECTION
LUNG MATURITY
ISOIMMUNIZATION DISEASE

CORDOCENTESIS
?KARYOTYPE
ISOIMMUNIZATION DISEASE

FETAL DRAIN INSERTION

1.10 MEASUREMENTS

Abdominal

BOWEL CALIBER IN THIRD TRIMESTER

small bowel caliber <7 mm
large bowel caliber <20 mm

UMBILICAL VEIN DIAMETER

3 mm at 15 weeks
8 mm at 40 weeks

AFI

normal is 7 to 20
highest AFI occurs at 26 weeks

Cervical canal

3 cm < NORMAL LENGTH <5 cm

CNS

BPD

BPD is measured in the transverse plane passing through the thalami and third ventricle (conventionally the plane through the thalami and septum pellucidum); the near and far cranium should be symmetrical shape

CISTERNA MAGNA

2 mm < NORMAL <10 mm

ISOLATED CHOROID CYST

<10 mm

LATERAL VENTRICLE ATRIAL WIDTH

mean 8 mm (>10 mm is definitely abnormal)

separation between choroid plexus and wall <3 mm

NEURAL ARCH OSSIFICATION

L5 ossified at 16 weeks
S2 ossified at 22 weeks

NUCHAL SKIN FOLD THICKNESS

plane of section through septum pellucidum and cerebellum
>6 mm is abnormal

THIRD OR FOURTH VENTRICLES

abnormal if >2 mm

EFW

when based on AC and BPD, has accuracy of +/– 100 g per kg or +/– 10%

Heart rate

120–160 bpm at 20 weeks
110–150 bpm at 36 weeks

Membranes

AMNIOTIC SHELF

fold of amnion (bilayer) projecting into the amniotic cavity and incompletely dividing it
fetus moves freely around the shelf

CHORIOAMNIOTIC SEPARATION

PRIMARY
normal under 15 weeks

SECONDARY
antepartum hemorrhage
amniocentesis

INTERTWIN MEMBRANES

twins are diamniotic dichorionic if membrane >2 mm OR
intertwin peak or intertwin Y signs are present
twins are probably diamniotic monochorionic if membrane <2 mm

Renal

RENAL PELVIS WIDTH IN SECOND TRIMESTER

(continuum of normality and hydronephrosis; no magic cutoff)
in general, normal <5 mm

RENAL PELVIS WIDTH IN THIRD TRIMESTER

(continuum of normality and hydronephrosis; no magic cutoff)
in general, normal is <7 mm

RENAL SIZE

on transverse abdominal scan, renal circumference to abdominal circumference is ~1/3

Thoracic

thoracic circumference:abdominal circumference >80%

1.11 NORMAL HEART

apex points to left, 4 chambers visible, heart fills <50% of thorax
tricuspid valve is closer to apex than mitral valve, both ventricles reach apex (i.e. 'offset cross')
ventricular septum is of same thickness as left ventricle lateral wall, and intact (no color flow across it)
aortic arch has the shape of a walking stick, ductal arch has the shape of a hockey stick, both are similar size; these cross over
septomarginal trabeculae may be visible in right ventricle
echogenic papillary muscle insertions may be visible in left ventricle
normal venous connections are present

1.12 ULTRASOUND CHECKLIST (second trimester)

Fetus

NUMBER, GA, EDD, CORRELATION WITH MENSTRUAL DATES

MEASUREMENTS

BPD, FL, AC, heart rate

HEAD

falx, thalami, cerebellum, cisterna magna, nuchal skin, ventricle and choroid

FACE

orbits, lips, nose

SPINE

skin line, vertebrae

LIMBS

FL, shape, number of digits

THORAX

diaphragm

ABDOMEN

AC, umbilical vein, portal vein, stomach, kidneys, bladder

HEART

(also see normal heart)
heart rate
4 chamber view, LVOT, RVOT, aortic arch, ductal arch

Placenta

POSITION

RELATIONSHIP TO INTERNAL OS
ACCESSORY LOBES
RETROPLACENTAL STRIPE AND COMPLEX

Amniotic fluid

Cervix

THIRD TRIMESTER NORMAL

1.13 FORMULA

Umbilical artery S/D ratio upper limit

this is approximate only and should not be used below 25 weeks' gestation (LMP)

UPPER S/D RATIO LIMIT = 6.5-AGE/10

where:

S/D RATIO: umbilical artery systolic/diastolic velocity ratio

AGE: GA in weeks (LMP)

1.14 AMNIOTIC FLUID INDEX

uterus divided into four quadrants by the midline and umbilicus

deepest pocket of amniotic fluid is measured vertically in each quadrant (cord or limb are allowed to enter the pocket)

AFI is the sum of all quadrants (in cm)

normal AFI is 7 to 20 and varies with GA; highest normal AFI occurs at 26 weeks

polyhydramnios is AFI >24

oligohydramnios is AFI less than 3rd centile

1.15 ASSESSMENT OF FETAL WELL BEING

Indications

HIGH RISK FETUS
DECREASED MOVEMENT
OLIGOHYDRAMNIOS, POLYHYDRAMNIOS
PROM
IUGR
TWINS
POST DATES

HIGH RISK MOTHER
DIABETES, HYPERTENSION, RENAL DISEASE, CARDIAC DISEASE
PREECLAMPSIA
RHESUS DISEASE

AUTOIMMUNE DISEASE
HEMOGLOBINOPATHIES

Biophysical profile (BPP)

COMPONENT 1: CTG: NON STRESS TEST

20 min of fetal heart rate recording, with identification of fetal movement and uterine activity

VALID IF:

28 weeks onwards

beware CNS depressants or fetal quiet sleep simulating abnormal test

beware hyperglycemia, adrenaline, caffeine masking an abnormal test (all these increase fetal reactivity)

REACTIVE NORMAL

normal baseline (120–160 bpm)

2 or more accelerations (of 15 bpm for 15 s) with associated fetal movement

no late decelerations

NON REACTIVE TEST

POOR OUTCOME IN 20%

COMPONENT 2: ULTRASONIC BPP (limited BPP)

ultrasound observation to 30 min (or less if met all normal criteria)

NORMAL BREATHING

more than one period of 60 s or more

NORMAL MOVEMENT

3 or more gross movements

NORMAL TONE

closed fists, flexed spine

one episode of extension or hand opening returns to flexion

NORMAL AFI

relative to normal range for age

BIOPHYSICAL PROFILE SCORING

TOTAL SCORE IS OUT OF 10

EACH PARAMETER SCORED 2 IF NORMAL, 0 IF ABNORMAL

PARAMETERS:

NON STRESS CARDIOTOCOGRAPHY
BREATHING
MOVEMENT
TONE
AFI

PREDICTOR OF OUTCOME BY SCORE

BPP 8–10

normal, low risk of hypoxia

BPP 6

suspicious, repeat in 4 hours

BPP 4

suspicious

probably deliver (if >36 weeks)

BPP 0–2

intrauterine fetal hypoxia

Umbilical artery doppler US

parameters that can be used are S/D ratio, resistive index, pulsatility index (all provide comparable information)

see formula for approximate upper limit of S/D normal for GA; S/D slowly falls with advancing gestation

reversal of umbilical flow highly significant abnormal umbilical cord Doppler analysis predictive of poor fetal outcome

PARAMETERS

S/D RATIO, A/B RATIO: (peak systolic velocity)/(minimal diastolic velocity)

RI (resistive index, Pourcelot index): [peak systolic velocity – minimal diastolic velocity]/(peak systolic velocity)

PULSATILITY INDEX: [peak systolic velocity – minimal diastolic velocity]/(mean velocity)

the simplest of these is the S/D RATIO

ASSOCIATIONS OF ABNORMALLY ELEVATED S/D

with progressively more severe changes, the S/D ratio increases with progressively reducing diastolic flow; diastolic flow becomes totally absent, and may eventually be reversed

FETAL HYPOXIA
IUGR, OLIGOHYDRAMNIOS
FETAL DISTRESS IN UTERO, FETAL DEMISE
PREMATURE DELIVERY
LOW APGAR SCORE

CTG: Contraction stress test (outline)

second line investigation

uses an oxytocin infusion (provocative testing)

aim is 3 uterine contractions <90 s duration per 10 min

NORMAL RESPONSE

no late decelerations

1 week survival is 99%

ABNORMAL RESPONSE

late decelerations (fetal hypoxic bradycardia)

50% have poor outcome

1.16 MEASUREMENTS

Cervical canal

length is measured from the inner os to the outer os

transvaginal US is the gold US standard

transperineal US provides similar measurements

transabdominal US overestimates cervical
length because of compression by the full
bladder

2 cm < NORMAL LENGTH < 4 cm

the population distribution is a Gaussian
curve (mean at ~35 mm in second
trimester)

Heart rate

120–160 bpm at 20 weeks
110–150 bpm at 36 weeks

Myometrium

retroplacental hypoechoic complex consists
of myometrium, decidua and perivillous
vascular space; normal is between 1 and
2 cm

the retroplacental stripe is hypoechoic
between the placenta and myometrium
and corresponds to the placenta/decidual
interface

loss of the retroplacental stripe and thinning
of the retroplacental complex suggests
placenta creta or a variant

focally widened retroplacental complex is
abnormal: see the retroplacental mass
gamut

Placenta

2 cm < NORMAL THICKNESS < 4 cm
retroplacental stripe is normally present

GRADING AND CALCIFICATIONS

GRADE 0 (normal to 30 weeks)
no calcifications
homogeneous echotexture
smooth chorionic plate

GRADE I (normal at >30 weeks)
scattered random punctate calcifications
homogeneous echotexture
minimally undulating chorionic plate

GRADE II (normal at >32 weeks)
linear parallel or comma-like calcifications
irregular chorionic plate

GRADE III (normal at >34 weeks)
confluent calcifications or septal
calcifications
deep chorionic plate indentations

Uterine artery

S/D mean is 2, always <3

1.17 PELVIMETRY

commonest indication is trial of labor in
breech presentation, occasionally others
(e.g. previous pelvic trauma)

Normal diameters

source: Mercy Maternity Hospital Melbourne
1996
INLET TRUE CONJUGATE 11.5 cm
TRANSVERSE 13.5 cm
MID PELVIS AP 12.5 cm
BISPINOUS 10.5 cm
OUTLET AP 11.5 cm
BITUBEROUS 11.5 cm

Method (CT pelvimetry)

low exposure protocol
LATERAL SCOUT: inlet true conjugate, mid
pelvis AP, outlet AP
AP SCOUT: transverse inlet (between iliac
arcuate lines), bituberous (between inner
cortices of ischial tuberosities)
SINGLE THIN SLICE THROUGH FEMORAL
HEAD FOVEAS: bispinous diameter

Method (MR pelvimetry)

SAGITTAL SLICES: inlet true conjugate, mid
pelvis AP, outlet AP
OBLIQUE CORONAL SLICES: transverse
diameters

2. GAMUTS

2.1 FIRST TRIMESTER GAMUTS

2.1.1 EMPTY UTERUS, ADNEXAL MASS

ECTOPIC PREGNANCY

OVARIAN MASS

CORPUS LUTEUM CYST WITH
HEMORRHAGE

TORSION OF OVARIAN CYST OR MASS

TUBAL MASS

TUBOOVARIAN ABSCESS

HYDROSALPINX

PYOSALPINX

ENDOMETRIOMA

UTERINE MASS

FIBROID (may be torted)

BICORNUATE UTERUS, PREGNANCY IN ONE
HORN

BOWEL MASS

APPENDIX ABSCESS

NORMAL BOWEL LOOP SIMULATING MASS

2.1.2 EMPTY UTERUS, POSITIVE beta hCG

ECTOPIC PREGNANCY

EARLY NORMAL PREGNANCY

COMPLETED ABORTION, beta hCG
NOT FALLEN YET

2.1.3 FAILED PREGNANCY CRITERIA

NO GS AT beta hCG >1500 (FIRP)

NO EMBRYO OR YOLK SAC AT GS
> 15 mm

NO FETAL HEART BEAT AT GS
>15 mm

NO FETAL HEART BEAT AT CRL
>5 mm

2.1.4 INTRAUTERINE MIMICS OF GESTATIONAL SAC

HEMORRHAGE

RETAINED PRODUCTS OF
CONCEPTION (incomplete abortion)

ECTOPIC PREGNANCY WITH PSEUDO
GESTATIONAL SAC

ENDOMETRIOSIS

2.1.5 PREDICTORS OF POOR OUTCOME

SUBCHORIONIC BLEED > GS SIZE

beta hCG LOW FOR GS SIZE

FETAL HR <90 BPM AFTER 5 WEEKS
GA

FETAL HR <110 BPM AFTER 6 WEEKS
GA

GS SIZE SMALL FOR CRL (or yolk sac
size)

GS SIZE SMALL FOR ABSOLUTE
DATES (e.g. IVF)

GS LIES LOW IN ENDOMETRIAL
CAVITY

DECIDUAL REACTION IS < 2mm
THICK

2.1.6 PV BLEEDING

ABORTION IN PROGRESS

BLIGHTED OVUM

ECTOPIC PREGNANCY

GESTATIONAL TROPHOBLASTIC
DISEASE

2.1.7 RETAINED PRODUCTS IN FIRST TRIMESTER

Detection

US is specific, but not sensitive

100% if US shows: GS, fetus,
endometrium >5 mm

50% if US shows: endometrium 2–5
mm

10% if US shows: endometrium <2 mm

Differential

RETAINED PRODUCTS (incomplete
abortion)

HEMATOMA

DECIDUAL REACTION, EARLY
INTRAUTERINE PREGNANCY

DECIDUAL REACTION, ECTOPIC
PREGNANCY

2.2 SECOND TRIMESTER GAMUTS

2.2.1 OLIGOHYDRAMNIOS

PROM

IUGR
*see IUGR entry in third trimester conditions
section*

BILATERAL RENAL AGENESIS–
DYSGENESIS

BILATERAL URINARY OBSTRUCTION
(or bladder outflow obstruction)

IMPENDING OR COMPLETE FETAL
DEMISE

2.2.2 POLYHYDRAMNIOS

NO ABNORMALITY FOUND IN 60%

MATERNAL DIABETES

FETAL CNS ABNORMALITY
('will not swallow')

CNS MALFORMATION, ANENCEPHALY

ABNORMAL NEUROLOGY, TRISOMY 18

OBSTRUCTION TO SWALLOWING
('can not swallow')

MOUTH

CLEFT, MICROGNATHIA, MASS

NECK

TERATOMA, HEMANGIOMA, GOITRE

CHEST

MASS IMPEDING SWALLOWING

cystic adenomatoid malformation

sequestration

congenital diaphragmatic hernia

SKELETAL DWARFISM SYNDROMES

BOWEL ATRESIAS OR
OBSTRUCTIONS ('vomiting')

ATRESIAS

ESOPHAGUS

DUODENUM

PROXIMAL SMALL BOWEL

OBSTRUCTION WITHOUT ATRESIA

OMPHALOCELE

HYDROPS

CARDIAC

STRUCTURAL OR ARRHYTHMIA

NON CARDIAC

IMMUNE (Rhesus disease in particular)

PLACENTAL

CHORIOANGIOMA

TWINS

TWIN TRANSFUSION SYNDROME

2.2.3 RAISED MATERNAL SERUM AFP

Beware confounding factors:

NORMAL AFP VARIES WITH GA
INCORRECT GA WILL LEAD TO INCORRECT
AFP ASSESSMENT
AFP IS HIGHER IN blacks and maternal
hepatitis;
AFP IS LOWER IN obesity and diabetes
AMNIOCENTESIS MAY LEAD TO A
TRANSIENT AFP RISE

Twins

CNS

NEURAL TUBE CLOSURE DEFECTS
anencephaly
open spina bifida
amniotic band syndrome
encephalocele

HYDROCEPHALUS

DANDY–WALKER MALFORMATION

Anterior abdominal wall defects
omphalocele
gastroschisis
amniotic band syndrome
bladder extrophy

Renal anomalies
AGENESIS
MULTICYSTIC DYSPLASTIC KIDNEY
HYDRONEPHROSIS

RUPTURED CYSTIC HYGROMA

ESOPHAGEAL OR DUODENAL
ATRESIA

TERATOMA

PLACENTAL HEMATOMA OR
FETOMATERNAL HEMORRHAGE

2.2.4 UMBILICAL CORD MASS OR THICKENING

Focal cord mass

FOCAL ACCUMULATION OF
WHARTON'S JELLY

incidental and not significant

CYSTIC

omphalomesenteric cyst

allantoic cyst

cystic degeneration (mucoid degeneration) of
Wharton's jelly

SOLID

teratoma (solid, cystic or mixed)

hematoma (especially after cordocentesis)

VASCULAR

umbilical vein varix

hemangioma

Diffuse cord thickening

HYDROPS FETALIS

LEAKED URINE

2.2.5 UTERUS LARGE FOR DATES

DATES WRONG

TWINS

MATERNAL DIABETES AND
MACROSOMIA

POLYHYDRAMNIOS

HYDATIDIFORM MOLE

PREGNANCY AND MASS OF OTHER
ORIGIN (e.g. fibroid)

2.2.6 UTERUS SMALL FOR DATES

DATES WRONG

FETAL DEATH IN UTERO

IUGR, OLIGOHYDRAMNIOS

PROM

PSEUDOCYESIS

2.3 THIRD TRIMESTER GAMUTS

2.3.1 LARGE OR THICK PLACENTA

RHESUS DISEASE

MATERNAL DIABETES

MATERNAL ANEMIA

FETAL HYDROPS

FETAL TRIPLOIDY

PARTIAL MOLE

PLACENTAL NEOPLASM

2.3.2 PV BLOOD LOSS

PLACENTA PREVIA

MARGINAL PLACENTAL
SUBCHORIONIC HEMORRHAGE

PLACENTAL ABRUPTION

2.3.3 RETROPLACENTAL MASS

CONTRACTION

FIBROID

RETROPLACENTAL BLEED –
PLACENTAL ABRUPTION

vs SUBMEMBRANOUS BLEED

BEWARE SUCCENTURIATE LOBE
MIMICKING A MASS

2.3.4 SMALL PLACENTA

PREECLAMPSIA, HYPERTENSION,
DIABETES

FETAL ABNORMALITY

CHRONIC INFECTION

POLYHYDRAMNIOS MAY CAUSE A
THIN PLACENTA

2.4 FETAL STRUCTURAL GAMUTS

FETAL ABDOMEN GAMUTS

2.4.1 ABDOMINAL CYSTIC (OR MULTICYSTIC) MASS CLASSIFIED BY LOCATION

RIGHT UPPER QUADRANT

NORMAL GALLBLADDER

CHOLEDOCHAL CYST

BOWEL

NORMAL BOWEL WITH FLUID OR
HYPOECHOIC MECONIUM

DILATED OBSTRUCTED BOWEL

MECONIUM PSEUDOCYST

MESENTERIC CYST

DUPLICATION CYST

OMPHALOMESENTERIC DUCT CYST

RENAL

MULTICYSTIC DYSPLASTIC KIDNEY

HYDRONEPHROSIS

URINOMA

RETROPERITONEAL LYMPHANGIOMA

BLADDER

NORMAL BLADDER

OBSTRUCTION

URACHAL CYST

URETEROCELE

PELVIC

OVARIAN CYST

HYDROMETROCOLPOS

ANTERIOR MENINGOCELE

SACROCOCCYGEAL TERATOMA
variable external and internal components

VASCULAR

UMBILICAL VEIN VARIX

PERSISTENT RIGHT UMBILICAL VEIN

2.4.2 ABDOMINAL SOLID MASS

BOWEL

ABNORMALLY BRIGHT BOWEL
see its own gamut

RENAL

INFANTILE POLYCYSTIC KIDNEY DISEASE

DYSPLASTIC KIDNEY

WILMS' TUMOR

ADRENAL

NORMAL ADRENAL

NEUROBLASTOMA

HEMATOMA

LIVER

HEPATOBLASTOMA

PELVIC

SACROCOCCYGEAL TERATOMA
mixed cystic and solid

2.4.3 ABNORMALLY BRIGHT BOWEL

NORMAL BOWEL AND NORMAL
MECONIUM

SCANNING ARTIFACT

MECONIUM ILEUS

MECONIUM PERITONITIS

DOWN'S SYNDROME

2.4.4 ANTERIOR ABDOMINAL MASS

OMPHALOCELE

OTHER FORMS OF EVISCERATION

TERATOMA

2.4.5 BLADDER NOT SEEN

EMPTY BLADDER (transient by
definition)

RENAL CAUSE

BILATERAL RENAL AGENESIS (Potter's
syndrome)

BILATERAL OBSTRUCTION

BILATERAL MULTICYSTIC DYSPLASTIC
  KIDNEY

INFANTILE POLYCYSTIC KIDNEY DISEASE

BLADDER CAUSE

EXTROPHY

PERSISTENT CLOACA

2.4.6 CALCIFICATION

Must see shadowing to diagnose calcification

PERITONEUM

MECONIUM PERITONITIS

LIVER

TORCHES GROUP INFECTION

HEMANGIOMA

MASS WITH CALCIFICATION

NEUROBLASTOMA

TERATOMA

2.4.7 'DOUBLE BUBBLE'

DUODENAL ATRESIA OR STENOSIS

HIGH JEJUNAL ATRESIA

HIGH SMALL BOWEL OBSTRUCTION
  OF OTHER CAUSE

**STOMACH WITH AN ADJACENT
  FLUID FILLED STRUCTURE**

GALLBLADDER

COLON

DILATED RENAL PELVIS

NON INTESTINAL CYST

2.4.8 ENLARGED FETAL KIDNEYS

UNILATERAL

HYDRONEPHROSIS

MULTICYSTIC DYSPLASTIC KIDNEY

CYSTIC RENAL DYSPLASIA

WILMS' TUMOR

MESOBLASTIC NEPHROMA

BILATERAL

HYDRONEPHROSIS

INFANTILE POLYCYSTIC KIDNEY DISEASE

2.4.9 FREE FLOATING BOWEL

GASTROSCHISIS

RUPTURED OMPHALOCELE

AMNIOTIC BAND DEFECTS

2.4.10 HEPATO-SPLENOMEGALY

HYDROPS FETALIS

TORCHES GROUP INFECTIONS

CARDIAC FAILURE

ANEMIA

?NEUROBLASTOMA

2.4.11 HYDRONEPHROSIS

PELVIURETERIC JUNCTION
  OBSTRUCTION

VESICOURETERIC REFLUX

VESICOURETERIC JUNCTION
  OBSTRUCTION

OBSTRUCTED MOIETY IN A DUPLEX

BLADDER OUTFLOW OBSTRUCTION
  (bilateral hydronephrosis)

2.4.12 KIDNEY ABSENCE
(unilateral)

SHADOW ARTIFACT

HORSESHOE KIDNEY

PELVIC KIDNEY

CROSSED FUSED ECTOPIA

UNILATERAL AGENESIS

2.4.13 SMALL BOWEL OBSTRUCTION

VOLVULUS

ATRESIA

MECONIUM ILEUS (cystic fibrosis)

SECONDARY TO LARGE BOWEL
  OBSTRUCTION

MECONIUM PLUG (cystic fibrosis)

HIRSCHSPRUNG'S DISEASE

2.4.14 STOMACH NOT SEEN

EMPTY STOMACH (by definition,
  transient)

ESOPHAGEAL ATRESIA,
  TRACHEOESOPHAGEAL FISTULA

DIAPHRAGMATIC HERNIA

OLIGOHYDRAMNIOS

FACIAL MALFORMATIONS
  INTERFERING WITH SWALLOWING

FETAL FACE GAMUTS

2.4.15 CATARACTS (bright lenses)

TORCHES GROUP INFECTIONS

METABOLIC DISORDERS

USUALLY ENZYME DEFICIENCIES

IDIOPATHIC

SYNDROMIC

e.g. Alport's syndrome

2.4.16 FACIAL MASS

HEMANGIOMA

TERATOMA

ANTERIOR CEPHALOCELE

PROTRUDING TONGUE

2.4.17 HYPERTELORISM

CEPHALOCELE

MEDIAN FACIAL CLEFT SYNDROME

TRISOMY 13

CRANIAL DYSPLASIAS, SKELETAL
  DYSPLASIAS

2.4.18 HYPOTELORISM

HOLOPROSENCEPHALY

TRISOMY 13

CYCLOPIA

TRISOMY 13

MULTIPLE SYNDROMES

2.4.19 MICROPHTHALMIA

HOLOPROSENCEPHALY SPECTRUM

TRISOMY 13

TORCHES GROUP INFECTIONS

MULTIPLE SYNDROMES

FETAL HEAD GAMUTS

2.4.20 ABNORMAL HEAD SHAPE

PHYSIOLOGICAL COMPRESSION

FETAL DEMISE

ANENCEPHALY

LEMON HEAD

NEURAL TUBE CLOSURE DEFECT
(somewhere along the neuraxis) or

NORMAL VARIANT (i.e. normal fetus)

OSTEOGENESIS IMPERFECTA

CLOVERLEAF SKULL

THANATOPHORIC DYSPLASIA

OTHER SKELETAL DYSPLASIAS

ISOLATED

MICROCEPHALY

CRANIOSYNOSTOSIS

AMNIOTIC BAND DEFECTS

2.4.21 ABNORMAL OR ABSENT SKULL

Brain present

OSTEOGENESIS IMPERFECTA
and other mineralization disorders

ACRANIA

Brain absent

ANENCEPHALY

2.4.22 FOCAL CSF COLLECTION

Midline

DANDY-WALKER CYST AND
VARIANTS

POSTERIOR FOSSA ARACHNOID
CYST

DIFFERENTIAL: VEIN OF GALEN
ANEURYSM (use color doppler)

Lateral

PORENCEPHALY
(focal encephaloclastic defect)

SCHIZENCEPHALY
(focal, usually bilateral dysgenetic clefts)

ARACHNOID CYST
rare compared to the other two
produce mass effect

Unilateral hydrocephalus
rare
most probably due to prior intraventricular
hemorrhage

2.4.23 HYDROCEPHALUS

NEURAL TUBE DEFECT AND CHIARI II

DANDY–WALKER OR VARIANT

AQUEDUCT STENOSIS

VEIN OF GALEN ANEURYSM

INTRAVENTRICULAR BLEED

CONGENITAL INFECTION (TORCHES)

NEOPLASM/ARACHNOID CYST

CRANIAL DYSPLASIAS

ACHONDROPLASIA

THANATOPHORIC DWARFISM

MUCOPOLYSACCHARIDOSES

2.4.24 INCREASED CSF CONTENT

Cortex absent, falx present

HYDRAANENCEPHALY

Cortex present

FALX ABSENT

HOLOPROSENCEPHALY

FALX PRESENT

VENTRICULOMEGALY

HYDROCEPHALUS IS PROVEN WITH SERIAL
SCANNING

see hydrocephalus gamut

Pitfall: pseudohydrocephalus
false identification of fetal brain as CSF on
US (usually where US access is difficult)

FEATURES

Sylvian cistern normal

no dangling choroid

LOOK FOR VENTRICULAR WALLS!

bright specular reflectors which will be
normally positioned

2.4.25 INTRAUTERINE INTRACRANIAL CALCIFICATION

CYTOMEGALOVIRUS

HERPES SIMPLEX VIRUS

TOXOPLASMOSIS

FETAL HEART GAMUTS

2.4.26 ABSENT CRUX

ATRIOVENTRICULAR SEPTAL DEFECT

LARGE VSD

2.4.27 AORTIC ARCH AND PULMONARY ARCH DO NOT CROSS

TRANSPOSITION OF GREAT
ARTERIES

2.4.28 LARGE LEFT VENTRICLE

HEART FAILURE

2.4.29 LARGE LEFT VENTRICULAR OUTFLOW TRACT

TETRALOGY OF FALLOT

TRUNCUS ARTERIOSUS

2.4.30 LARGE RIGHT VENTRICLE

ISOLATED PULMONARY STENOSIS
(no VSD)

AORTIC COARCTATION (preductal)

2.4.31 LARGE RIGHT ATRIUM

EBSTEIN'S ANOMALY

TRICUSPID REGURGITATION

HEART FAILURE

ANOMALOUS PULMONARY VENOUS
RETURN

2.4.32 SMALL LEFT VENTRICLE

HYPOPLASTIC LEFT HEART/VENTRICLE

2.4.33 SMALL LEFT VENTRICULAR OUTFLOW TRACT

HYPOPLASTIC LEFT HEART

AORTIC ATRESIA

AORTIC COARCTATION

2.4.34 SMALL RIGHT VENTRICLE

TRICUSPID ATRESIA

HYPOPLASTIC RIGHT HEART/VENTRICLE

2.4.35 SMALL OR ABSENT RIGHT VENTRICULAR OUTFLOW TRACT

TETRALOGY OF FALLOT

PULMONARY ATRESIA

TRUNCUS ARTERIOSUS

FETAL THORAX GAMUTS

2.4.36 ECHOGENIC OR MIXED CYSTIC/SOLID MASS

DIAPHRAGMATIC HERNIA

CYSTIC ADENOMATOID MALFORMATION

SEQUESTRATION

HEMANGIOMA/LYMPHANGIOMA

TERATOMA

2.4.37 HYPOECHOIC COLLECTION OR CYST

PLEURAL EFFUSION

CHYLOTHORAX

INTRATHORACIC STOMACH

DILATED PROXIMAL ESOPHAGUS, ESOPHAGEAL ATRESIA

BRONCHOGENIC CYST

ENTERIC, NEURENTERIC CYST

2.4.38 PULMONARY HYPOPLASIA

INTRATHORACIC MASS

SKELETAL DYSPLASIA

OLIGOHYDRAMNIOS

HYDROTHORAX/CHYLOTHORAX

ANEUPLOIDY

OBSTETRIC CONDITIONS

3. CONDITIONS OF EARLY PREGNANCY

3.1 ABORTION

DEFINITION

spontaneous evacuation of the pregnant uterus before 20 weeks' gestation, often related to an abnormal embryo

EPIDEMIOLOGY

~20% of all clinically evident pregnancies, ?50% of all pregnancies
~2% of all pregnancies with a detected fetal heart beat
AND ~25% of all pregnancies have first trimester bleeding, of these 1/2 abort

CLINICAL

THREATENED ABORTION
PV bleeding, pain, closed cervix

ABORTION IN PROGRESS
(= inevitable abortion)
PV loss of membranes or embryonic parts, bleeding
variably open cervix

IMAGING (US) IN THREATENED ABORTION

Live intrauterine pregnancy
early pregnancy: it may be too early to see GS, embryonic pole and embryonic heart (see failed pregnancy criteria gamut)

MAY HAVE A SUBCHORIONIC HEMORRHAGE – IMPLANTATION BLEED
anechoic crescentic collection between decidua and GS

PREDICTORS OF POOR OUTCOME
see in gamuts

Failed intrauterine pregnancy

ANEMBRYONIC PREGNANCY (blighted ovum)
GS but no embryo
see failed pregnancy criteria gamut

EMBRYONIC DEMISE (missed abortion)
embryo demonstrable, but no evidence of heart beat or growth (see failed pregnancy criteria gamut)

PRODUCTS OF CONCEPTION (incomplete abortion)
slow fall of beta hCG
endometrial cavity material
see retained products in first trimester gamut
DIFFERENTIAL:
PRODUCTS OF CONCEPTION
HEMATOMA
DECIDUAL REACTION, EARLY INTRAUTERINE PREGNANCY
DECIDUAL REACTION, ECTOPIC PREGNANCY

EMPTY UTERUS (complete abortion)
rapid fall of beta hCG
US is relatively poor at ruling out retained products
see retained products in first trimester gamut

LOW LYING SAC (?inevitable abortion)
GS low in endometrial cavity
GS passing through cervical canal

Ectopic pregnancy
see its own entry

Molar pregnancy
see Ch23

3.2 ECTOPIC PREGNANCY

DEFINITION

implantation and growth of a gestational sac in locations other than the endometrial cavity

EPIDEMIOLOGY

1.5% of all pregnancies, 15% of all maternal deaths, mortality ~1/1000
most significant risk factor is PREVIOUS ECTOPIC PREGNANCY

ETIOLOGY

Abnormal tube

previous PID/salpingitis (40%)
previous surgery, reversal of ligation
endometriosis
other adhesions (e.g. appendicitis)

Abnormal uterus

intrauterine contraceptive device
other structural abnormalities

Abnormal ovulation

particularly in vitro fertilization (IVF) and ovulation induction

PATHOGENESIS

DELAY IN TRANSIT THEORY
LATE LUTEAL FERTILIZATION WITH MENSTRUAL BACKFLUSH THEORY

CLINICAL

asymptomatic OR
pain/bleeding/collapse (and rarely also a palpable adnexal mass)
beta hCG (FIRP) >2000 indicates pregnancy
when beta hCG (FIRP) <2000 diagnosis depends on history and examination
combined intrauterine and ectopic pregnancy rate ~1/10 000 except for IVF, where the rate is high

MACRO

95% ampullary/isthmic (rupture from 6 weeks on)
interstitial in the intramural part of the tube (late rupture)
ovarian or rectovaginal pouch
cervical

ULTRASOUND

Empty uterus and

25% live adnexal embryo (specificity 100%)
50% tubal ring (specificity 95%) (often with extensive ring-like flow on color Doppler)
adnexal mass (with free fluid specificity is >90%)
echogenic/extensive rectouterine pouch fluid
15% ultrasonically normal

Pitfall

PSEUDOGESTATIONAL SAC (decidual reaction of pregnancy, endometrial fluid)
ovoid and central in endometrial cavity
surrounded only by a single layer of decidua
margins ill defined
see entry on double decidual sign in normal

Differential of normal ultrasound

ectopic pregnancy that is not visible
missed abortion/failing intrauterine pregnancy
equivocal beta hCG (e.g. around 2000) with an inconclusive US and clinically stable patient should be monitored with serial beta hCG and serial US

Differential of adnexal mass

see empty uterus with adnexal mass gamut

Interstitial ectopic pregnancy

interstitial ectopic pregnancies rupture late, often with a catastrophic collapse
conventional US criterion is a high fundal pregnancy NOT surrounded by at least 5 mm of myometrium on all sides

3.3 FAILED EARLY PREGNANCY

DEFINITION

failure of normal embryo to form (ANEMBRYONIC PREGNANCY, BLIGHTED OVUM) or death of a formed embryo (FETAL OR EMBRYONIC DEMISE, 'MISSED ABORTION')

ETIOLOGY

Abnormal embryo

ANEUPLOIDY (50% of all spontaneous abortions)
ABNORMAL IMPLANTATION

Other

LUTEAL FAILURE
SMOKING, ALCOHOL
ABNORMAL UTERUS
TORCHES INFECTIONS (?)

CLINICAL

Proceeds to abortion

Missed abortion (evacuated therapeutically)

IMAGING (US)

Anembryonic pregnancy

GS >15 mm with no embryo or yolk sac
if GS is smaller, repeat examination should be done when the normal sac would grow over 15 mm (assume growth rate of 1 mm per day); anembryonic GS grows more slowly

Embryonic demise

embryonic pole with CRL >5 mm and no cardiac activity
if embryo is smaller, repeat examination

Decidual reaction

decidual reaction <2 mm thick or irregular reaction; poorly vascular corpus luteum are associated with a poor outcome

3.4 SUBCHORIONIC (IMPLANTATION) BLEED

CLINICAL

chorion frondosum (embryonic precursor of placenta) is invasive and erosive, and often leads to implantation bleeds (? true incidence, as usually asymptomatic)
if presenting at all, it is with PV blood loss or spotting
more often it is an US finding

IMAGING (US)

hyperechoic crescentic collection between one wall of the sac and the decidua; progresses to hypoechoic over ~2 weeks
predictor of poor outcome if larger than the GS

4. FETAL CONDITIONS

4.1 AMNIOTIC RUPTURE SEQUENCE/AMNIOTIC BAND SYNDROME

DEFINITION

non chromosomal, non recurrent syndrome of non embryologically distributed random fetal defects and malformations

EPIDEMIOLOGY

1 in 5000–15 000 births
amniotic bands demonstrable in 1–2% of malformed neonates

ETIOPATHOGENESIS

Early amniotic rupture sequence (first trimester)

rupture of amnion is followed by fetal adhesion and malformation (?sticky bands)
random deformities, adhesions, bands, slash defects, amputations
fibrous mesodermal bands, restricted motion
does not explain all the abnormalities (in particular, does not explain holoprosencephaly and hydrocephalus)

Late amniotic rupture (second trimester) produces an extraamniotic pregnancy

normal fetus, loose membrane folds

MORPHOLOGY

Head
CLEFTS, CALVARIAL DEFECTS
ENCEPHALOCELE
HYDROCEPHALUS
ANENCEPHALY

Face
'SLASH' DEFECTS
NON EMBRYOLOGICAL CLEFTS

Chest
'SLASH' DEFECTS AND DEFORMITIES

Spine
ANGULATION AND ROTATION DEFORMITIES

AMPUTATIONS

Abdomen
'SLASH' DEFECTS
OMPHALOCELE
GASTROSCHISIS
AMPUTATION OF GENITALIA

Limbs
AMPUTATION
LIMB CONSTRICTION, DISTAL EDEMA
CLUBFOOT
SYNDACTYLY

IMAGING

morphology as above
cardinal imaging finding is of non embryologically distributed random defects IN ASSOCIATION WITH AMNIOTIC BANDS
non embryologically distributed asymmetrical defects are suggestive

4.2 ANEUPLOIDY MARKERS

At 12 weeks

NUCHAL TRANSLUCENCY

At mid trimester anatomical survey

NUCHAL THICKNESS/CYSTIC HYGROMA

SYMMETRIC IUGR

NON IMMUNE HYDROPS

STRUCTURAL
ENDOCARDIAL CUSHIONS
DUODENAL ATRESIA
OMPHALOCELE
HOLOPROSENCEPHALY SPECTRUM
ANY MULTIPLE ABNORMALITIES

SINGLE UMBILICAL ARTERY + ONE OTHER STRUCTURAL ABNORMALITY

4.3 FETAL ABDOMEN

4.3.1 CLOACAL EXTROPHY/BLADDER EXTROPHY

IMAGING

absent normal bladder (even with observation)
variable suprapubic mass or irregularity
associated caudal anomalies (meningomyelocele, anal atresia)
widely separated pubic bones

4.3.2 DUODENAL ATRESIA

EPIDEMIOLOGY

~1/5000, 25% are in trisomy 21 (<5% of Down's syndrome have duodenal atresia)
second most common atresia after ileal atresia
associated with other malformations: anal atresia, esophageal atresia, limb and vertebral malformations; atresia elsewhere in the small bowel

IMAGING (US)

'DOUBLE BUBBLE' SIGN

DIFFERENTIAL
stenosis/web/bands
jejunal atresia/meconium ileus
malrotation

4.3.3 GASTROSCHISIS

CLINICAL

right sided paraumbilical anterior body wall fusion defect with herniation of free floating bowel loops through it (?secondary to vascular accident)
the bowel is non rotated and malfixed, and may be obstructed
non syndromic with normal karyotype; prognosis good

IMAGING

thickened free floating bowel loops in amniotic fluid
possibly polyhydramnios

4.3.4 JEJUNAL OR ILEAL ATRESIA

atresia of small bowel distal to duodenum, postulated secondary to a vascular occlusion agenesis of dorsal mesentery may accompany small bowel atresia; the remaining distal small bowel spirals around the vascular stalk ('Christmas tree' or 'apple peel' deformity)

4.3.5 MECONIUM PERITONITIS

bowel perforation in utero leads to focal or diffuse intraperitoneal free meconium which produces a chemical peritonitis and induces calcification
!cystic fibrosis likely

IMAGING

peritoneal calcifications
meconium from a focal perforation may collect as a MECONIUM PSEUDOCYST
may have dilated loops of bowel
may have bright intraluminal meconium

4.3.6 NORMAL (PHYSIOLOGICAL) BOWEL HERNIATION

see entry in first trimester normal section
should not be present if CRL >45 mm

4.3.7 OMPHALOCELE

CLINICAL

persistent pathological herniation of abdominal contents into the base of the umbilical cord through an anterior abdominal wall defect
unless ruptured, omphalocele is covered by a membrane and the cord inserts into the apex of the membrane
syndromic in ~1/2 and aneuploid in ~1/3 (trisomies 13, 18, 21, monosomy XO)
associations: cardiac defects, neural tube defects, intestinal atresias
overall prognosis depends on underlying syndrome
prognosis of the omphalocele itself depends on size and contents (better prognosis if liver, and if small)

IMAGING (US)

anterior abdominal wall mass containing variable viscera
cord inserts into mass apex

4.3.8 RUPTURED OMPHALOCELE

free floating loops of bowel – a differential diagnosis of gastroschisis

4.4 FETAL CNS

4.4.1 ACRANIA

CLINICAL

rare partial or complete failure of cranial vault development
brain tissue always present: this is not anencephaly

IMAGING

cerebral hemispheres surrounded by a thin membrane

4.4.2 AMNIOTIC BAND DEFECT

asymmetric amputations
other amputations, defects and amniotic bands may be visible

4.4.3 ANENCEPHALY

CLINICAL

~1/1000 (varies), female:male 4:1; risk factors multifactorial, including folate deficiency and previous family history
failure of anterior neuropore closure with secondary non development of brain and cranium

IMAGING

no normal brain or skull above the orbits
echogenic dysmorphic material in place of brain: 'fibrovascular stroma'
polyhydramnios

4.4.4 CHOROID PLEXUS CYST

CLINICAL

up to 1% of normal fetuses (unifocal choroid plexus cyst)

Associations

trisomies 18, 21, monosomy XO
choroid plexus cyst alone – 0.5% risk of trisomy 18
choroid plexus cyst and another malformation – 20% risk of aneuploidy (usually trisomy 18)
50% of trisomy 18 fetuses have choroid plexus cysts

IMAGING

cystic space within the choroid plexus, 3–10 mm
all resolve by 26 weeks
!do anatomical survey

4.4.5 DANDY–WALKER SPECTRUM

see Ch 20

CLINICAL

obstruction of fourth ventricle outlets producing massive cystic dilation, and vermian and cerebellar hypoplasia

IMAGING (US)

posterior fossa cystic mass; hydrocephalus

4.4.6 ENCEPHALOCELE

usually occipital, may contain echogenic brain or cystic CSF
defect in the bony skull or spinal dysraphism differentiates from a soft tissue posterior neck mass such as cystic hygroma

4.4.7 HOLOPROSENCEPHALY SPECTRUM

also see Ch 20

CLINICAL

failure of midline hemispheric cleavage of variable degree with associated orbital and facial malformations; associated with trisomy 13

CLASSIFICATION AND IMAGING

Alobar

thin cortex surrounding a dilated monoventricle
single fused thalamic mass
absent midline structures (falx, corpus callosum, cavum septum pellucidum)
associated agenesis of optic tracts
cyclopia

Semilobar

single ventricle with fused thalami but rudimentary temporal and occipital horns; partly present falx and corpus callosum; hypotelorism

Lobar

well formed ventricle bodies and posterior horns; absent septum pellucidum, box-like anterior horns; falx and corpus callosum present

4.4.8 HYDRAANENCEPHALY

CLINICAL

intrauterine loss of cerebral cortex and other structures (postulated infarction); outlook poor
non syndromic, not associated with aneuploidy or other malformations

IMAGING

absent cortex; occipital cortex may be variably present (posterior circulation territory)
thalami usually absent, choroid plexus may be present
FALX IS PRESENT
usually microcephaly

4.4.9 MICROCEPHALY

common non specific feature of aneuploidy
cranial vault and brain present

4.4.10 NEURAL TUBE CLOSURE DEFECTS

see encephalocele and anencephaly above
see spina bifida in fetal spine entry

4.4.11 POOR CRANIAL MINERALIZATION

most common cause is osteogenesis imperfecta
abnormal calvarium is present, and other bones are also abnormal

4.5 FETAL FACE

4.5.1 ANTERIOR CEPHALOCELE

also see Ch 20
midline herniation of meninges and CSF (meningocele) or meninges, brain and CSF (encephalocele)
associated with hypertelorism and a visible cranial defect

4.5.2 HEMANGIOMA

similar appearance to hemangiomas elsewhere
bright solid mass, may have fine calcifications
may have a capacitive Doppler trace

4.5.3 LACRIMAL DUCT CYST

cystic dilation of the lacrimal duct visible in the third trimester
small cyst inferior to medial canthus
usually resolve spontaneously after birth

4.5.4 LATERAL FACIAL CLEFT

EPIDEMIOLOGY

~1/800 overall, male:female 2:1
only 10% are syndromic (trisomies 13 and 18, triploidy)
more severe clefts tend to be syndromic

CLASSIFICATION

ISOLATED LIP
UNILATERAL LIP AND PALATE
BILATERAL LIP AND PALATE

IMAGING

3D US is likely to become the primary imaging modality

Primary clefting
CLEFT RUNS FROM SURFACE TO LIP AND PREMAXILLA (CLEFT PRIMARY PALATE)

Secondary clefting
DEFECT IN SECONDARY PALATE
often invisible with US

4.5.5 TERATOMA

similar appearance to teratomas elsewhere
solid or complex mixed solid/cystic mass, coarse calcifications

4.6 FETAL HEART

see Ch 21 congenital heart disease

4.6.1 HYPOPLASTIC LEFT VENTRICLE

only single ventricle (right) present, or a rudimentary left ventricle
associated mitral and aortic atresias, hypoplastic aorta

4.6.2 TRANSPOSITION OF GREAT ARTERIES

the cardinal US sign is the failure of right ventricular and left ventricular outflow tracts to cross (normally shown by tilting the off-axially oriented transducer from one to the other showing a criss-cross orientation)

4.7 FETAL KIDNEYS

4.7.1 AGENESIS (Potter's sequence or syndrome)

CLINICAL

incidence 1 in ~3000–4000
bilateral renal agenesis with a predictable sequence of events
obligatory oligohydramnios leads to: pulmonary hypoplasia, low set ears, hypertelorism, limb deformities
neonatal death results from pulmonary hypoplasia

IMAGING

BILATERAL RENAL AGENESIS

adrenals prominent as no kidneys
NO bladder
oligohydramnios from 18 weeks on
pulmonary hypoplasia
cardiac anomalies (15%)

4.7.2 DILATED KIDNEY

Obstruction, bladder normal size

PUJ obstruction (differential: multicystic dysplastic kidney)
VUJ obstruction with ureteric dilation (differential: dilated loop of bowel)

Reflux

Dilated bladder

OBSTRUCTION
POSTERIOR URETHRAL VALVES
URETHRAL ATRESIA
CLOACA

4.7.3 RENAL CYSTIC DISEASE IN UTERO

MULTICYSTIC DYSPLASTIC KIDNEY
CYSTIC RENAL DYSPLASIA
PUJ OBSTRUCTION

4.7.4 RENAL MASS IN UTERO

MULTICYSTIC DYSPLASTIC KIDNEY
INFANTILE POLYCYSTIC KIDNEY DISEASE: BILATERAL
MESOBLASTIC NEPHROMA
NEPHROBLASTOMATOSIS: BILATERAL
NEPHROBLASTOMA

4.8 FETAL NECK

4.8.1 CERVICAL TERATOMA

anterolateral unilateral solid or mixed solid/cystic mass; frequently has calcifications

4.8.2 CYSTIC HYGROMA

all cystic or cystic with septations
posterior and bilateral or posterolateral asymmetrical
most have abnormal karyotype
(BUT if isolated and karyotype is normal, prognosis is good)

LOOK FOR HYDROPS
LOOK FOR OTHER MALFORMATIONS
DO KARYOTYPING

4.8.3 ENCEPHALOCELE

midline posteriorly, spinal dysraphism
LOOK FOR POLYHYDRAMNIOS

4.8.4 GOITRE

anterior bilateral
LOOK FOR MATERNAL THYROID DISEASE

4.8.5 HEMANGIOMA

non specific variable appearance mass, more commonly solid
may have a Doppler trace – capacitive type

4.9 FETAL SKELETON

4.9.1 APPROACH

Dwarfism
characterize
assess thorax
assess mineralization

Terminal reductions
look for other malformations

Amniotic band syndrome

Clubfoot
look for spina bifida

Clenched fists
?trisomy 18

4.9.2 DWARFISM

Osteogenesis imperfecta
MICROMELIA, MULTIPLE FRACTURES
NARROW THORAX
HYPOMINERALIZATION

Thanatophoric dysplasia
NARROW THORAX
CLOVERLEAF SKULL, HYDROCEPHALUS
HYPOPLASTIC SPINE AND LIMBS

Achondrogenesis
HYPOMINERALIZATION
MICROMELIA

Achondroplasia
SHORT LIMBS AFTER 20 WEEKS
LARGE HEAD, HYDROCEPHALUS
POLYHYDRAMNIOS
(HOMOZYGOTE: NARROW THORAX, LETHAL)

4.9.3 HYPOMINERALIZATION

brain in near field not shadowed by near calvarium, starting at 20 weeks
OSTEOGENESIS IMPERFECTA
ACHONDROGENESIS
HYPOPHOSPHATASIA

4.10 FETAL SPINE

4.10.1 CAUDAL REGRESSION SPECTRUM

see Ch 20

CLINICAL

spectrum of sacrococcygeal anomalies: sacrococcygeal atresias, lumbar atresias, neural deficits, anorectal atresias, lower limb abnormalities
strong association with poorly controlled maternal diabetes, also increased incidence in twins
sirenomelia (fused rudimentary lower limb) is probably in the spectrum

IMAGING

ability to demonstrate with US prenatally depends on severity
gross atresias are not a diagnostic problem
cardinal sign of milder forms is absence of lumbar and sacral ossification centers at the time they are normally expected to be visible (see normal)

4.10.2 SPINA BIFIDA

DEFINITION

the entire spectrum of neural tube closure defects (distal to the brain) and secondary associated abnormalities

CLINICAL

most common neural tube defect overall

compatible with survival if the open spina bifida defect is closed, hydrocephalus is shunted and urinary sepsis and obstructive urinary failure avoided

CLASSIFICATION

By level of defect

ANENCEPHALY
see its own entry

CERVICAL, THORACIC (rare)

LUMBAR – HIGH OR LOW

SACRAL

By morphology

SPINA BIFIDA OCCULTA
asymptomatic failure of vertebral neural arch formation; of no clinical significance

COVERED DEFECT
meningocele, rarely myelomeningocele
associated malformations of cord tethering, spinal lipoma, sinuses and fistulas

OPEN DEFECT
myelomeningocele
the most common form is lumbosacral open myelomeningocele

IMAGING (US)

Spinal defect

ASSESS
?COVERED DEFECT
?OPEN DEFECT
?LEVEL OF DEFECT

FINDINGS
abnormally divergent lateral spinal ossification centers (out of series with centers above and/or below)
abnormal angulation of spine
hemivertebrae
defect in skin contour or thin covering membrane only (but 'skin' is present in closed defects)
midline mass covered by a thin sac

Cranial signs

CHIARI II MALFORMATION
banana-shaped cerebellum (as opposed to peanut-shaped cerebellum)

the shape is produced by a combination of cerebellar crowding into a small posterior fossa and compressed cisterna magna and fourth ventricle; the' banana' wraps around the brainstem

LEMON HEAD
present in ~95%
symmetrical flattening or concavity of anterolateral frontal bones

HYDROCEPHALUS/
VENTRICULOMEGALY

4.11 FETAL THORAX

4.11.1 CONGENITAL DIAPHRAGMATIC HERNIA

see Ch 21
congenital herniation of abdominal contents (usually bowel) through a persistent pleuroperitoneal canal; usually left sided

IMAGING (US)

unequivocal intrathoracic viscera (e.g. peristalsing bowel)
multicystic mass behind left ventricle with variable mass effect
hypoplastic lung
right sided hernia: intrathoracic gallbladder
reduced abdominal circumference
diaphragmatic defect (interruption of thin hypoechoic curved diaphragmatic line that separates right lung from liver and left lung from spleen and stomach)

4.11.2 CYSTIC ADENOMATOID MALFORMATION

see Ch 21

Classification

I   macrocystic
II medium (5–10 mm)
III microcystic (<5 mm)

4.11.3 SEQUESTRATION

see Ch 21
segment of lung with abnormal systemic arterial supply, usually left lower lobe
demonstration of arterial feeders from the aorta is diagnostic

4.11.4 BRONCHOGENIC CYST

see Ch 21

4.11.5 ENTERIC OR NEURENTERIC CYST

posterior mediastinal cyst adjacent to the spine
associated vertebral abnormality suggests neurenteric cyst

4.11.6 PENTALOGY OF CANTRELL

cardiac ectopy
omphalocele
intracardiac malformations
anterior diaphragmatic hernia
defects in anterior chest wall

4.11.7 LIMB–BODY WALL COMPLEX

absence of umbilical cord with broad based ventral attachment of fetal thorax and abdomen to membranes/placenta, and associated external viscera

4.12 FETUS OF DIABETIC MOTHER

IMAGING FINDINGS

MACROSOMIA
CARDIAC MALFORMATIONS
NEURAL MALFORMATIONS
CAUDAL REGRESSION SPECTRUM

4.13 SACROCOCCYGEAL TERATOMA

CLINICAL

most common tumor of neonates
arises from pluripotent embryonal cells in sacrococcygeal area
~1/35 000, female > male
most are benign at birth, with increasing rate of malignant degeneration with age
associated with other malformations, polyhydramnios and hydrops

IMAGING

mixed solid and cystic mass arising from fetal pelvis and occupying a variable extent within it, and with a variably large external component

may have areas of calcification (or bone formation)

15% totally cystic

4.14 UMBILICAL CORD ANOMALIES

4.14.1 ABNORMALITIES OF CORD INSERTION

Marginal insertion
cord inserts on the edge of the placenta: Battledore placenta

Velamentous
cord runs between the membranes for a variable distance

Succenturiate lobe
see under placental conditions

4.14.2 ABNORMALITIES OF CORD POSITION

all of these may cause fetal demise, particularly cord prolapse (i.e. cord first presentation)

TRUE KNOT

NUCHAL CORD

CORD PROLAPSE

4.14.3 BASE OF CORD ANOMALIES

Gastroschisis
see its own entry

Omphalocele
see its own entry

Body stalk syndrome
short umbilical cord

pentalogy of Cantrell

Persistent right umbilical vein
look for other anomalies

4.14.4 CORD MASSES OR THICKENING

see under gamuts

4.14.5 SINGLE UMBILICAL ARTERY

<1% incidence

50% risk of other malformation

if another malformation is present, aneuploidy is very likely

4.14.6 UMBILICAL VEIN THROMBOSIS

indicates fetal death

5. FETAL SYNDROMES

5.1 MONOSOMY X
(Turner's syndrome)

EPIDEMIOLOGY

~1/10 000

survives into adult life and may first present with primary infertility

MORPHOLOGY

Head
cystic hygroma (regresses spontaneously, but neck webbing in child and adult thought to be the remnant)

cleft palate

Chest
aortic coarctation

cardiac defects

hypoplastic lungs

Limbs
syndactyly

Placenta
partial mole

5.2 TRIPLOIDY

EPIDEMIOLOGY

1% of pregnancies, most abort

MORPHOLOGY

severe symmetric IUGR

abnormal head shape with hydrocephalus or holoprosencephaly

neural tube defects

cardiac septal defects

multiple other anomalies in no particular pattern

Placenta
PARTIAL MOLE

5.3 TRISOMY 21
(Down's syndrome)

also see Ch 17

EPIDEMIOLOGY

the most common trisomy in liveborn

incidence rises with maternal age: 0.25% at 35 years, 1% at 40 years, 4% at 45 years

OVERALL ~1/660

SCREENING

First trimester nuchal lucency
risk varies with maternal age and width of nuchal lucencies (estimated from nomograms)

allows comparison of risk of Down's syndrome against risk of karyotyping

Karyotyping

MORPHOLOGY

Head

INCREASED NUCHAL LUCENCY (first trimester)

no sharp cutoff, as risk increases with increasing thickness and maternal age

arbitrary conventional 'normal' cutoff is 3 mm

INCREASED NUCHAL SKIN THICKNESS OR CYSTIC HYGROMA (second trimester)

no sharp cutoff (see above)

conventional normal is <6 mm

Chest

atrioventricular septal defect or ventricular septal defect

hydrops fetalis

isolated ascites or pleural effusion

Skeletal

fifth finger middle phalanx hypoplasia

HYDROPS

SECTION 6

Abdomen

duodenal atresia (fetal 'double bubble')
tracheoesophageal fistula
2 VESSEL CORD INCIDENCE NOT
    INCREASED

5.4 TRISOMY 18
(Edwards' syndrome)

EPIDEMIOLOGY

~1/3000, second most common trisomy
lethal in the neonatal period

MORPHOLOGY

Symmetric IUGR

Head

choroid plexus cysts
micrognathia
hydrocephalus

Chest

cardiac defects (all) – usually septal defects,
    complete AV canal or double outlet right
    ventricle

Abdomen

omphalocele

Limbs

clenched fists, overlapping fingers
clubfoot
rocker bottom feet

5.5 TRISOMY 13
(Patau's syndrome)

EPIDEMIOLOGY

~1/5000, lethal

MORPHOLOGY

Symmetrical IUGR

Head

failure of midline neural cleavage
    (holoprosencephaly–monoventricle–
    cyclopia spectrum)
microphthalmia

Chest

cardiac defects (90%): usually septal defects

Abdomen

omphalocele

Limbs

postaxial polydactyly

5.6 VACTERL

composite syndrome of multisystem
    malformations:
V-ERTEBRAL
A-NAL
C-ARDIAC
T-RACHEAL
E-SOPHAGEAL
R-ENAL
L-IMB

5.7 OTHER

5.7.1 WARFARIN EMBRYOPATHY

hydrocephalus, occipital meningocele
microphthalmia, hypertelorism
cardiac malformations
limb reduction anomalies

5.7.2 FETAL ALCOHOL SYNDROME

microcephaly, microphthalmia, micrognathia
cleft lip or palate
cardiac malformations
diaphragmatic hernia
hydronephrosis

5.7.3 MECKEL–GRUBER SYNDROME

autosomal recessive
CNS: posterior encephalocele, microcephaly,
    hydrocephalus
ABDOMEN: cystic renal dysplasia with
    bilaterally enlarged kidneys; secondary
    empty bladder and oligohydramnios
other malformations

6. THIRD TRIMESTER CONDITIONS

6.1 CERVICAL INCOMPETENCE

DEFINITION

preterm dilation of cervix leading to
    pregnancy loss or premature labor

EPIDEMIOLOGY

~1% of all pregnancies

Risk factors

in utero exposure to diethylstilbestrol
previous cervical incompetence and
    pregnancy loss
previous preterm labor
cervical biopsy especially cone biopsy
uterine malformations

CLINICAL

usually presents in second trimester
silent painless cervical dilation
premature rupture of membranes followed
    by premature labor
treated medically (bed rest, tocolytics) in
    third trimester; treated surgically
    (cervical suture cerclage) in second
    trimester

IMAGING (US)

At risk patient monitoring

most patients enter monitoring programs in
    a subsequent pregnancy following an
    initial pregnancy loss

OBSERVATION

progressive cervical canal shortening in
    patients likely to progress to preterm
    delivery

CERVICAL DYNAMIC STRESS
    TESTING

fundal pressure, coughing, standing and
    straining have all been used
shortening of cervix correlates with
    premature delivery
no single cutoff, with 15 mm or 20 mm used
    as criterion for cervical suture

Acute presentation

cervical shortening (e.g. shorter than 15 or 20 mm)

cervical funneling: V shaped upper cervix with progressive dilation of upper cervical canal

spontaneously dilated cervix (can measure diameter as well as length)

membranes bulging through dilated cervix ('hourglass' configuration)

Cervical suture

mid-cervical anterior and posterior point reflector in every transducer craniocaudal plane

6.2 INTRAUTERINE GROWTH RETARDATION (IUGR)

= Intrauterine growth restriction

new term designed to avoid any perceived stigma!

DEFINITION

abnormally low rate of fetal growth relative to that expected for this particular fetus; IUGR is NOT equivalent to SGA

Small for gestational age (SGA)

any fetus that falls below the fifth centile on relevant population growth charts

the usual cause is that this is a normal but small fetus (check parental height!)

IUGR fetuses need to be differentiated from normal SGA

Symmetrical IUGR (~10%)

defined as comparable growth retardation of head and body

Asymmetrical IUGR (~90%)

defined as relative sparing of head (at least early in the course of IUGR) and greater growth retardation of body

EPIDEMIOLOGY

Risk factors

previous pregnancy with IUGR

multiple pregnancy

MATERNAL ILLNESS

diabetes

hypertension, preeclampsia

SLE

renal or cardiac disease

sickle cell disease

MATERNAL SMOKING OR ALCOHOL/DRUG ABUSE

ABNORMAL FETUS

established e.g. by karyotyping or on mid trimester US

6.2.1 SYMMETRICAL IUGR (~10%)

ETIOLOGY

Abnormal fetus

ANEUPLOIDY

SINGLE GENE ABNORMALITIES

NON CHROMOSOMAL MALFORMATIONS

Severe intrauterine insult

INTRAUTERINE INFECTION (TORCHES group)

DRUGS, ALCOHOL, TERATOGENS

SICKLE CELL DISEASE OR MAJOR MATERNAL ILLNESS

Abnormal placenta

EARLY ONSET PLACENTAL FAILURE OR RECURRENT ANTEPARTUM HEMORRHAGE

CLINICAL

classically caused by an abnormal fetus or maternal drug/alcohol use

BPD and HC reduced (or lag) to the same extent as AC and FL

AFI usually normal

may present in first trimester

by definition, fetal measurements must be below 5th centile (this gives a 'small for gestational dates' status); the differential then is of normal SGA versus symmetrical IUGR

the underlying fetal abnormality (e.g. chromosomal abnormality, intrauterine infection) determines the subsequent postnatal course

Postnatal associations of IUGR itself

increased risk of infant death

short stature

learning difficulties, intellectual disability

6.2.2 ASYMMETRICAL IUGR (~90%)

ETIOLOGY

Adverse uterus

HYPERTENSION/PREECLAMPSIA

DIABETES

RENAL DISEASE

CARDIAC DISEASE

OTHER MATERNAL ILLNESS

IDIOPATHIC

Adverse placenta (placental failure)

primary placental failure is a diagnosis of exclusion

Twins and multiple pregnancy

in third trimester twins may be SGA when compared with singleton charts

see 8.2 twins (growth assessment)

CLINICAL

classically caused by an adverse environment in a normal fetus

BPD and HC reduced less (or lag less) than AC and FL

AFI often abnormal

usually presents in third trimester

the 'starved fetus' has reduced reserves to cope with neonatal physiological and pathological stressors

ANTENATALLY, increased incidence of:

fetal death in utero

premature delivery

intrauterine or perinatal hypoxia

POSTNATALLY, increased incidence of:

hypoglycemia, hypothermia

hypocalcemia

polycythemia, thrombocytopenia

necrotizing enterocolitis

pulmonary hemorrhage

IMAGING (symmetrical and asymmetrical IUGR)

Measurement parameters available

DIRECT PARAMETERS
BPD, HC, AC, FL (third trimester error is ~1 week)

DERIVED PARAMETERS
ratios, estimated fetal weight (error 15% or more)

SUPPORTING SIGNS
AFI
umbilical artery Doppler
placental grade
uterine artery Doppler (expected S/D <3)

INTERVAL GROWTH
in the absence of any other information this is the most discriminatory parameter
SGA but normal fetuses grow normally on interval studies (i.e. grow along 'their own' curve)
IUGR fetus growth 'falls off' the centile curves
even if a fetus is not SGA, lack of interval growth is significant and suggests IUGR
interval between examinations has to be SUFFICIENTLY LONG TO EXCLUDE STATISTICAL VARIATION IN MEASUREMENTS
interval growth assessment is valid if the interval is 3 weeks or more (or at least 2 weeks)

Algorithm

GESTATIONAL AGE KNOWN
either precise dates (e.g. IVF) or earlier US

ESTABLISH SMALL FOR GA STATUS
centile tables and 5% cutoff

ESTABLISH SYMMETRICAL FETUS VS ASYMMETRICAL FETUS

ASYMMETRICAL
look for supporting signs
?fetus at risk – consider doing a biophysical profile

SYMMETRICAL
look for supporting signs
look for structural anomalies
antenatal screen
IF ABNORMAL – SYMMETRICAL IUGR
IF NO SUPPORTING SIGNS – INDETERMINATE IUGR VS SMALL BUT NORMAL: do interval measurements

GESTATIONAL AGE NOT KNOWN
ESTABLISH SYMMETRICAL FETUS VS ASYMMETRICAL FETUS

ASYMMETRICAL
look for supporting signs
the diagnosis is probably asymmetrical IUGR

SYMMETRICAL OR INDETERMINATE
look for supporting signs
look for structural anomalies
ASSESS INTERVAL GROWTH AFTER 2 WEEKS

6.3 HYDROPS FETALIS

GROUP DEFINITION

Abnormal fluid in two or more compartments
skin
pleural space
pericardial space
peritoneal space
placenta
polyhydramnios

IMAGING (group)

Early signs
small ascites, pericardial effusion, enlarged right atrium, thick placenta, polyhydramnios

Sequence
polyhydramnios, thickened placenta, hepatomegaly, ascites, hydrops

Additional findings to look for
cardiac arrhythmias
structural fetal abnormality

6.3.1 IMMUNE HYDROPS

EPIDEMIOLOGY

single commonest cause of hydrops, but rapidly dropping with use of rhesus antiD globulin; rarely due to other alloantiboides

ETIOPATHOGENESIS

alloimmunization of rhesus factor (Rh) D negative women from previous Rh D positive blood transfusion or pregnancy
maternal anti RhD causes fetal hemolysis in SUBSEQUENT pregnancy
administration of Rh anti D globulin to Rh D negative women to cover fetomaternal hemorrhage has largely eliminated immune hydrops
alloimmunization for other RBC antigens occurs by an analogous mechanism, but is rare

MACRO AND CLINICAL

anemia, congestive cardiac failure, hydrops fetalis
increased hematopoiesis: hepatosplenomegaly
maternal serum anti Rh D IgG

6.3.2 NON IMMUNE HYDROPS

EPIDEMIOLOGY

as a group, much more prevalent than immune hydrops
~1/2000 to 1/4000
50% of fetal deaths in utero have associated hydrops

ETIOLOGY

PREECLAMPSIA

INFECTIVE
TORCHES GROUP
PARVOVIRUS
RESPIRATORY SYNCYTIAL VIRUS
COXSACKIE VIRUS

TWIN–TWIN TRANSFUSION

ANEUPLOIDY
MONOSOMY XO, TRISOMIES 21, 18, 13; TRIPLOIDY

GENERALIZED CHROMOSOMAL ABNORMALITY

ISOLATED DEFECT OR MALFORMATION

PATHOGENESIS

Cardiogenic

STRUCTURAL CARDIAC MALFORMATION

MYOCARDITIS

ARRHYTHMIAS

DECREASED VENOUS RETURN
COMPRESSION
THORACIC MASS
DIAPHRAGMATIC HERNIA

CYSTIC ADENOMATOID MALFORMATION
SEQUESTRATION

OBSTRUCTION

HIGH OUTPUT FAILURE

AV MALFORMATION

   VEIN OF GALEN AVM

   LIVER HEMANGIOENDOTHELIOMA

   OTHER AVM

TWIN–TWIN TRANSFUSION

Anemia

HEMOGLOBINOPATHY

BONE MARROW FAILURE

INTRAUTERINE NEUROBLASTOMA

INTRAUTERINE LEUKEMIA

Cirrhotic/nephrotic

PLASMA ONCOTIC PROTEIN
INSUFFICIENCY

Lymphedema

LYMPHATIC AGENESIS/APLASIA

CYSTIC HYGROMA

Twin–twin transfusion

6.4 PREECLAMPSIA/ ECLAMPSIA

DEFINITION

PREECLAMPSIA: hypertension, proteinuria,
edema
ECLAMPSIA ('TOXEMIA OF PREGNANCY'):
disseminated intravascular coagulation,
microinfarcts, convulsions

EPIDEMIOLOGY

occurs in the third trimester in ~6% of all
pregnancies; more in primiparas, renal
disease, molar pregnancy

ETIOPATHOGENESIS

postulated shallow placentation leading to
uterine circulation remaining a high
resistance low volume vascular bed
(failure of spiral artery dilation)
secondary global placental ischemia causes
increased placental renin and decreased

prostaglandin secretion (maternal
hypertension via angiotensin), and also
leads to DIC

CLINICAL

Preeclampsia
insidious onset hypertension and proteinuria
with secondary edema
may respond to medical management

Eclampsia
headache, visual disturbances
cerebral edema, pulmonary edema
convulsions, coma
multiorgan failure
necessitates urgent delivery

MACRO

Brain
scattered microinfarcts, microhemorrhages
(including anterior pituitary)
cerebral edema

Heart
micro infarcts, microhemorrhages

Liver
diffusely fatty liver
focal scattered hemorrhagic infarcts

Kidney
petechial hemorrhages
cortical necrosis

Placenta
multiple infarcts
retroplacental hemorrhages

Disseminated intravascular coagulation
arteriolar thrombosis by platelets
distal bland or hemorrhagic microinfarcts
microangiopathic hemolysis
HELLP syndrome: h-emolysis, e-levated
l-iver enzymes, l-ow p-latelet count

IMAGING (US)

uterine artery spectral Doppler analysis and
resistive index have been used with
mixed success to predict development of
preeclampsia; no consensus guidelines as
yet exist

7. PLACENTAL CONDITIONS

7.1 ANTEPARTUM HEMORRHAGE

DEFINITION

passage of cervical blood in the second or
third trimester outside the setting of
established labor

EPIDEMIOLOGY

5% of all pregnancies

ETIOLOGY

(combination of etiology of placental
abruption and placenta previa)
PREECLAMPSIA
HYPERTENSION
COCAINE ABUSE
TRAUMA (especially anterior placenta)
PLACENTA PREVIA
PLACENTA CRETA
ABNORMAL UTERUS
IDIOPATHIC – NO CAUSE FOUND

CLINICAL

MARGINAL HEMORRHAGE
RETROPLACENTAL HEMORRHAGE
PLACENTA PREVIA, HEMORRHAGE

IMAGING (US FINDINGS)

No hematoma found
ALL HEMATOMA HAS EVACUATED
HEMATOMA PRESENT BUT NOT VISIBLE

Placenta previa
see its own entry

Placenta creta
see its own entry

Placental abruption (and retroplacental hematoma)
see its own entry

Fetal death

7.2 PLACENTA CRETA

DEFINITION

abnormally deep invasion by placental villi into or through the myometrium, with failure of postpartum separation often leading to a catastrophic hemorrhage

RISK FACTORS

PRIOR UTERINE SURGERY
PRIOR LOWER UTERINE CESAREAN SECTION, SCAR
PRIOR MANUAL REMOVAL
PLACENTA PREVIA (30%)
MULTIPARITY

CLASSIFICATION

Accreta
chorionic villi reach to myometrium and attach

Increta
chorionic villi invade the myometrium

Percreta
chorionic villi extend through the uterine wall possibly into adjacent organs

CLINICAL

placenta previa (30%)
antepartum hemorrhage
failure of placental separation postpartum
antepartum uterine rupture (especially if percreta)

IMAGING (US)

cardinal sign: absent retroplacental decidual stripe; thinned retroplacental complex
increased number of vascular intraplacental 'lakes' on Doppler US

7.3 PLACENTA PREVIA

DEFINITION

placenta either covering the inner os or sufficiently close to obstruct labor

EPIDEMIOLOGY

~20% of placentas are low lying at 18 weeks and most resolve as the lower uterine segment elongates
0.5% are still low lying at term (risk higher with previous lower uterine segment Cesarean section)
~90% of previas bleed at some point
~10% of antepartum hemorrhage is due to placenta previa

Risk factors
multipara
prior abortion
prior Cesarean section or scarring

CLINICAL

antepartum hemorrhage
premature labor
placental abruption
fetal death in utero

CLASSIFICATION

Complete symmetrical
placenta covers the inner os and is symmetrically attached anteriorly and posteriorly

Complete asymmetrical
placenta completely covers the inner os but is not symmetrical with respect to it

Marginal
placenta on edge of internal os, but does not cross it

Low lying placenta
placental edge is within 2 cm of the inner os

Low lying succenturiate lobe
SUCCENTURIATE LOBE COVERING INNER OS

Vasa previa
VELAMENTOUS INSERTION, CORD RUNS ACROSS INNER OS
SUCCENTURIATE LOBE, LOBAR VESSELS RUN ACROSS INNER OS

IMAGING (US OR MR)

best access for assessment of inner os by US is transvaginal or translabial
previa grading is from placental position relative to internal os

GRADE 1: low lying placenta
GRADE 2: marginal placenta previa
GRADE 3: complete asymmetrical placenta previa
GRADE 4: complete symmetrical placenta previa
BEWARE OF SUCCENTURIATE LOBE
BEWARE OF VASA PREVIA
second trimester low lying placenta should be re-examined in the third trimester in the expectation of 'migration'

Pitfalls

FALSE POSITIVE
overfull bladder compressing LUS, LUS contraction (if the cervix >5 cm, re-scan)

FALSE NEGATIVE (transabdominal US)
lateral previa obscured by fetal head

7.4 PLACENTAL ABRUPTION

DEFINITION

premature separation of placenta from the myometrium by retroplacental hemorrhage (which may not always be visible)

EPIDEMIOLOGY

1% of pregnancies
20% of all perinatal mortality
50% progress onto premature labor
1/3 deliver normally

ETIOLOGY

PREECLAMPSIA
HYPERTENSION
COCAINE ABUSE
TRAUMA (ESPECIALLY IF PLACENTA ANTERIOR)
PLACENTA CRETA
ABNORMAL UTERUS
FETAL DEATH IN UTERO (ORDER OF EVENTS AND CAUSATION THEN UNCLEAR)
IDIOPATHIC

CLINICAL

Marginal hemorrhage
tear of marginal vessels
low pressure hemorrhage

frequent PV blood loss with few symptoms
increased incidence of premature labor
fetal death or distress in utero less likely

Retroplacental hemorrhage

tear of spiral arteries
high pressure hemorrhage between placenta
and decidua, stripping placenta off the
uterine wall
PV bleed may occur or hematoma may be
fully contained behind the placenta
classic 'abruption' presentation: tense
painful uterus
increased incidence of premature labor
fetal hypoxia, distress and demise more
likely

IMAGING (US findings)

sensitivity of US in demonstrating placental
abruption is ~50%
fresh hemorrhage is isoechoic to
myometrium and may be completely
undetected on US
cardinal sign of fresh hematoma between
the placenta/chorion and the
myometrium is thickening of the uterine
wall or the retroplacental hypoechoic
complex (see the differential for
hematoma below)

Hematoma

blood dissects between the membranes and
myometrium and therefore location of
the hematoma is not necessarily the
original location of the hemorrhage

HEMATOMA APPEARANCE AS A FUNCTION OF AGE

HYPERACUTE (1–2 DAYS): hyperechoic to
placenta
ACUTE (3–7 DAYS): isoechoic
EVOLVING (1–2 WEEKS): hypoechoic or
complex mixed (differential is placental
infarct)
LATE (2 WEEKS ON): variably anechoic

MARGINAL HEMORRHAGE

VENOUS LOW PRESSURE HEMORRHAGE
HEMATOMA AT EDGE OF PLACENTA

SUBCHORIONIC HEMORRHAGE

EXTRAMEMBRANOUS VENOUS LOW
PRESSURE HEMORRHAGE
HEMATOMA BETWEEN CHORION AND
MYOMETRIUM

RETROPLACENTAL HEMORRHAGE

ARTERIAL HIGH PRESSURE HEMORRHAGE
HEMATOMA LIFTING PLACENTA
(RETROPLACENTAL MASS ON US)
IF >40% OF PLACENTAL SURFACE IS

DETACHED, THE FETUS IS AT
SIGNIFICANT RISK OF IUGR OR DEATH
DIFFERENTIAL OF RETROPLACENTAL
HEMATOMA
FIBROID
CONTRACTION

7.5 PLACENTAL INCIDENTAL ABNORMALITIES

7.5.1 BATTLEDORE PLACENTA

umbilical cord inserting into side of placenta
instead of the center

7.5.2 CALCIFICATION

see under normal placenta

7.5.3 CIRCUMVALLATE PLACENTA

membranes insert on inner placental
surface and not peripherally
the insertion has a characteristic 'rolled'
edge

7.5.4 FOCAL COLLECTIONS (non tumoral)

on US, fibrin is hypoechoic, hematoma
variable

Subchorionic

HEMORRHAGE, FIBRIN DEPOSITION
focal collection of fibrin or blood on the fetal
aspect of the placenta; fibrin is of no
clinical significance, hemorrhage is
significant only if large

Perivillous and intervillous deposits

FETAL HEMORRHAGE, MATERNAL BLOOD
THROMBOSIS
maternal blood intervillous thrombosis
presents with rounded 1–2 cm thrombi
within the placenta, hypoechoic on US

Decidual septal cyst

decidual tissue penetrating placental
substance and presenting as a cyst in
subchorionic location; of no significance
(hypoechoic on US)

7.5.5 FOCAL INFARCT

wedge shaped area of placental and villous
necrosis, with base on decidua
not seen on US unless hemorrhagic
does not compromise fetal well being unless
extensive (>~40% of placenta)

7.5.6 SUCCENTURIATE LOBE

accessory placental lobe separate from the
main placental mass
connected to main placenta via the placental
vessels
similar risk of placenta previa as main
placenta
increased risk of retained succenturiate lobe
after delivery

7.5.7 VELAMENTOUS INSERTION

cord runs through membranes for a variable
distance before reaching the placenta

7.6 PLACENTAL TUMORS

7.6.1 MOLAR TWIN

hydatidiform molar pregnancy coexisting
with a normal pregnancy

7.6.2 PARTIAL MOLE

CLINICAL

hydropic villi interspersed with normal villi
the placenta is thickened
the placental and fetal karyotype is usually
triploid

IMAGING (US)

enlarged placenta with multiple diffuse
anechoic spaces

7.6.3 CHORIOANGIOMA

CLINICAL

most common non trophoblastic placental
tumor
usually small well defined intraplacental
vascular mass

ASSOCIATIONS (larger tumors only)

polyhydramnios, hydrops fetalis, IUGR
elevated maternal AFP
general placental complications (abruption,
PROM, postpartum hemorrhage, retained
placenta)

IMAGING (US)

well defined solid or mixed echogenicity
mass within the placenta or protruding
from its amniotic surface

7.6.4 TERATOMA

rare solid mass between amnion and chorion
of no clinical significance

8. TWINS

8.1 ACARDIAC TWIN

DEFINITION

failure of cardiac development in one of two
monochorionic twins secondary to
overwhelming placental arteriovenous
anastomoses leading to retrograde
perfusion by the other twin ('pump twin')

EPIDEMIOLOGY

RARE
frequent in exams

PATHOGENESIS

early arteriovenous placental anastomoses
lead to retrograde flow in acardiac twin
normal cardiac development is supressed
and usually head and neck development
is suppressed
there is retrograde flow in the acardiac
twin's umbilical vessels

8.2 TWINS

EPIDEMIOLOGY

Monozygotic
incidence ~1/250, geographically and
ethnically constant
same sex always

1/3 DICHORIONIC DIAMNIOTIC ('DiDi twins')
US FINDINGS
twins same sex always
other findings and risk same as for dizygotic
twins

2/3 MONOCHORIONIC DIAMNIOTIC ('DiMono twins')
US FINDINGS
single placenta
thin intertwin membrane (1 mm or thinner)
vascular shunts may be present
twin transfusion may be present

1% MONOCHORIONIC MONOAMNIOTIC ('MonoMono twins')
US FINDINGS
single placenta
intertwined cords
no separating membrane
twin transfusion may be present

Dizygotic
incidence ~1/80 to ~1/90, VARIABLE
blacks > whites > Asians
increased with family history, personal
history
varies with maternal age, multiparity

US FINDINGS
different sexes or same sex
two gestational sacs in first trimester
placentas separate or fused
twin peak sign or thick separating
membrane

Multizygotic: ovulation induction

COMPLICATIONS

General
singleton perinatal mortality is ~1%

perinatal mortality for DiDi twins is ~9%

FETAL
IUGR (relative to singleton charts) in ~25%
FETAL ANOMALIES (x3)
FETAL DEATH IN UTERO

PLACENTAL
PLACENTA PREVIA
ANTEPARTUM HEMORRHAGE/ABRUPTION
(x3)
PREECLAMPSIA (x3)

DELIVERY PROBLEMS
PROM
PREMATURE LABOR (x12)
CORD ACCIDENTS

OBSTRUCTED LABOR (interlocking twins)
PERINATAL DEATH
POSTPARTUM HEMORRHAGE

DiMono twins (perinatal mortality 25%)
TWIN TRANSFUSION (1/3 of DiMono twins)
TWIN DEMISE – DISSEMINATED
INTRAVASCULAR COAGULATION IN
LIVING TWIN

MonoMono twins (perinatal mortality 50%)
SAME RISKS AS FOR DiMono TWINS
CONJOINT TWINS
ACARDIAC TWIN

ULTRASOUND APPROACH

Determination of type

UNEQUIVOCALLY DIZYGOTIC (always
dichorionic)
different sexes

DICHORIONIC (monozygotic or dizygotic)
two separate GS in first trimester
two separate placentas
two placentas fused (indistinguishable from
single placenta) and:
twin peak sign (triangle of placenta
interposed between two chorionic
membranes)
membrane >2 mm (80% accurate)

MONOCHORIONIC, DIAMNIOTIC
single placenta
thin (<1 mm) intertwin membrane
may require amniography or CT
amniography to prove

MONOCHORIONIC, MONOAMNIOTIC
single placenta
no separating membrane at all
intertwined cords
intermingled fetal parts with no membrane
visible (may require amniography or CT
amniography to prove)
conjoint twins

GROWTH ASSESSMENT

Second trimester
AS FOR SINGLETON
ALL PARAMETERS NORMAL

Third trimester
TWIN GROWTH SLOWS AFTER
30–32 WEEKS RELATIVE TO
SINGLETONS

two followup scans

FL usually stays within normal singleton range

BPD usually slows but stays within normal singleton range

AC is usually reduced relative to singleton growth

BPP is normal

DISCORDANT TWIN GROWTH

discordance is defined as EFW difference of >20%

discordant growth is associated with significantly higher complication rate

may be caused by unequal placentation but also twin transfusion syndrome

NEED TO DETERMINE:

position of twins, placental position

what is the lie of each twin?

which twin is presenting first?

what is the presenting part?

8.3 TWIN DEMISE

First trimester

VANISHING TWIN

the second gestational sac disappears by mid trimester ultrasound, and is presumably completely resorbed

Second trimester

FETUS PAPYRACEUS

flattened residual fetus in an empty gestational sac

usually delivered with the living twin

RISK OF LIVING TWIN DISSEMINATED INTRAVASCULAR COAGULATION AND DEATH IF TWINS MONOCHORIONIC

Third trimester

ECLAMPSIA, MATERNAL DISSEMINATED INTRAVASCULAR COAGULATION

PREMATURE LABOR

OBSTRUCTED DELIVERY

HIGH RISK OF LIVING TWIN DISSEMINATED INTRAVASCULAR COAGULATION IF MONOCHORIONIC

8.4 TWIN TRANSFUSION SYNDROME

DEFINITION

unbalanced transfer of blood from one monochorionic twin to another with complications in both

EPIDEMIOLOGY

1/3 of monochorionic twins have twin–twin transfusion

PATHOGENESIS

abnormal intraplacental arteriovenous connection between arterial pressure sinusoids of one twin and venous pressure sinusoids of the other

COMPLICATIONS

Anemic donor twin

IUGR

oligohydramnios

'stuck twin'

twin demise

Plethoric recipient twin

accelerated growth

congestive cardiac failure

fetal hydrops

polyhydramnios

disseminated intravascular coagulation after demise of donor twin

twin embolization syndrome (embolic material from dead twin entering circulation of live twin)

IMAGING (US)

discordant twin EFW (20% difference or more) and growth rates

discordant amount of amniotic fluid (if sacs separate)

different size umbilical vessels and cords

COMPLICATIONS AS ABOVE

23 Gynecology

1. NORMAL

1.1 ENDOMETRIUM ON US

endometrial thickness is conventionally measured as an anteroposterior DOUBLE LAYER

endometrium appears thinner on MR than on US

'dark' refers to hypoechoic, 'bright' to hyperechoic (relative to adjacent structure)

MENSTRUAL 3 mm
thin echogenic line

PROLIFERATIVE 4–8 mm
early: thin echogenic

late: thick and dark (functional layer) inside a brighter shell (basal layer)

SECRETORY 7–14 mm
bright and uniform (functional and basal layer similar echogenicity)

POSTMENOPAUSAL
conventional upper limit of normal is ~5 mm

HORMONE REPLACEMENT THERAPY
variably increased endometrial thickness

upper limit of normal is ~8 mm

TAMOXIFEN CHANGES
endometrial thickness >5 mm

variable echogenicity, often with cystic spaces

endometrial polyps

association with endometrial carcinoma

1.2 OVARY

INFANT VOLUME: <1 cm3

PREPUBERTAL VOLUME: ~3 cm3 (range ~1 to ~9)

POSTPUBERTAL DIMENSIONS: 2–4 cm x 1.5–2.5 cm x 1–2 cm

size depends on number and size of developing follicles

POSTPUBERTAL VOLUME: ~10 cm3 (range ~3 to ~20)

POSTMENOPAUSAL VOLUME: ~6 cm3 (range ~1 to ~15)

postmenopausal size progressively reduces with age

ARTERIAL TRACE
RESISTIVE INDEX IS USUALLY CLOSE TO 1

LATE FOLLICULAR TO LATE LUTEAL PHASE (ON SIDE OF CORPUS LUTEUM) RESISTIVE INDEX 0.8

FOLLICLES
non dominant follicles measure around 1 cm in diameter

dominant preovulatory follicle size is up to 3 cm in diameter

Corpus luteum (menstruation) normal 1.5–2.5 cm in diameter; upper limit is 4 cm in diameter

1.3 UTERUS, CERVIX, VAGINA

Size

NEONATE 3 X 1 cm

configuration is adult; small amount of endometrial fluid is normal (effect of maternal estrogens)

INFANT 3 X 1 cm (cervix is 1/3 to 2/3)

CHILD 2–4 cm long

NULLIPARA 6–8 X 3-5 X 2–4 cm

MULTIPARA 8–10 X 4–6 X 3–5 cm

POSTMENOPAUSAL 3–7 X 2–4 X 2–3 cm

POSTPARTUM
immediate 20 cm

3 weeks postpartum 10 cm

DETECTION OF RETAINED PRODUCTS OF CONCEPTION
US is specific, but not sensitive

100% if US shows: GS, fetus, endometrium >5 mm

50% if US shows: endometrium 2–5 mm

10% if US shows: endometrium <2 mm

Position and angulation

POSITION RELATIVE TO VAGINA
ANTEVERTED

RETROVERTED

NOTE: CAN BECOME INCARCERATED WHEN PREGNANT

POSITION OF UPPER UTERINE SEGMENT RELATIVE TO LOWER
ANTEFLEXED

RETROFLEXED

US structure
serosa: thin echogenic interface

myometrium: three layers (darker thin outer, arcuate vessels, brighter thick intermediate, darker thin inner)

endometrium: see its own entry

endometrial stripe: thin echogenic interface (formed by two opposed endometrial surfaces) – lost if there is endometrial fluid

MR structure

UTERUS
endometrium is high signal on T2W; has delayed enhancement with Gd

junctional zone of myometrium (the innermost more cellular myometrium) is low signal on T2W, <5 mm thick

myometrium is intermediate signal on T2W; has rapid enhancement with Gd; oral contraceptives cause increased myometrial signal

CERVIX
endocervical glands and mucus have high T2W signal; mucosa enhances with Gd

compact cervical stroma is low signal on T1W and T2W (lower signal than myometrium), and has a thin rim of peripheral intermediate T2W signal similar to myometrium; compact cervical stroma enhances less with Gd than endocervical mucosa or parametrial tissues

VAGINA
fibrous vaginal wall has low T1W and T2W signal

vaginal mucosa and secretions are high on T2W sequences (and are often not visible postmenopause)

2. GAMUTS

2.1 GENERIC (all modalities)

2.1.1 ACUTE OVARY

FOLLICULAR RUPTURE

CORPUS LUTEUM BLEED

ACUTE TORSION

TUBOOVARIAN ABSCESS

RUPTURED ECTOPIC

2.1.2 ADNEXAL MASS

ECTOPIC PREGNANCY

OVARIAN

CORPUS LUTEUM WITH BLEED

OVARIAN CYST WITH BLEED

ENDOMETRIOMA

OVARIAN TUMOR

  ADENOMA/CYSTADENOMA

  CARCINOMA/CYSTADENOCARCINOMA

  TERATOMA

TUBAL

HYDRO/PYOSALPINX/TUBOOVARIAN
  ABSCESS

UTERINE

BICORNUATE UTERUS AND GESTATION IN
  ONE HORN

PEDUNCULATED FIBROID

LOOP OF BOWEL OR CECUM

APPENDIX ABSCESS/DIVERTICULAR
  ABSCESS/CROHN'S ABSCESS

2.1.3 OVARIAN MASS OR CYST

Simple cyst

PHYSIOLOGICAL (always <4 cm)
reexamine in 6 weeks or 2 menstrual
  periods' time

INCLUSION CYST

BENIGN CYSTADENOMA

MALIGNANT
  CYSTADENOCARCINOMA

NON OVARIAN CYSTIC SPACE
  (e.g. bladder diverticulum)

Complex mass

PHYSIOLOGICAL CYST WITH BLEED

ECTOPIC PREGNANCY

ENDOMETRIOMA

TERATOMA

CARCINOMA

TUBOOVARIAN ABSCESS

OVARIAN TORSION

NON OVARIAN (e.g. hydrosalpinx)

Markers of malignancy

SIZE >10 cm
COMPLEX STRUCTURE, THICK WALLS,
  NODULES, NECROSIS
DOPPLER: RI <0.4

FIXITY
ASCITES, PERITONEAL DEPOSITS, NODAL
  METASTASES
AGE

2.1.4 THICKENED ENDOMETRIUM

Pregnancy associated

DECIDUAL REACTION
see Ch 22

EARLY INTRAUTERINE PREGNANCY

ECTOPIC PREGNANCY

RETAINED PRODUCTS OF
CONCEPTION

Gestational trophoblastic disease

MOLAR PREGNANCY

Endometrial polyp

Endometrial carcinoma

postmenopausal endometrium >5 mm off
  hormone replacement therapy is
  suspicious

Hormonal stimulation

ANOVULATORY CYCLES

HORMONE REPLACEMENT THERAPY

TAMOXIFEN THERAPY

IUCD WITH PROGESTERONE

Mimics of thickened endometrium

ADENOMYOSIS

HEMATOMETRA OR PYOMETRA

2.1.5 UTERINE CAVITY FILLING DEFECT

POLYP

CLOT

ADHESIONS

SUBMUCOSAL FIBROID

TB ENDOMETRITIS

RETAINED PRODUCTS

HYDATIDIFORM MOLE

PREGNANCY

2.1.6 UTERINE MASS
(non pregnancy)

FIBROID

ADENOMYOSIS

ENDOMETRIAL POLYP

ENDOMETRIAL MALIGNANCY

SARCOMA

CHORIOCARCINOMA

GYNECOLOGICAL CONDITIONS

3. GENERAL CONDITIONS

3.1 ADENOMYOSIS

DEFINITION

abnormal presence of foci of normal basal
  endometrium deep within the
  myometrium

PATHOLOGY

no association with endometriosis
focal or diffuse distribution of ectopic
  endometrium with marked surrounding
  smooth muscle hyperplasia (small blood
  filled cystic structures with white cuffing
  or coarse trabeculated appearance)

IMAGING

US

DIFFUSE
diffuse thickening of the myometrium
global uterine enlargement with no change
  in echotexture

FOCAL
more circumscribed thickening with possible
  ill defined changes in echotexture
  ('adenomyoma')

CT

non specific uterine enlargement

MR

DIFFUSE
diffuse uterine enlargement

diffusely or segmentally thickened junctional zone (>12 mm)

may contain foci of cystic change or hemorrhage

FOCAL

irregularly expanded uterine wall with an ill defined margin containing foci of high T2W signal surrounded by low T2W signal

differential is a leiomyoma with degeneration

3.2 CERVICAL CARCINOMA

DEFINITION

carcinoma of the ectocervix (squamous, more common) or the endocervix (adeno, less common) related to human papilloma virus infection

EPIDEMIOLOGY

second most common female carcinoma after breast

Risk factors

SQUAMOUS

age at first intercourse

number of sexual partners

HPV 16/18 infection

smoking

ADENOSQUAMOUS

in addition to above:

nulliparity with fertility problems

in utero exposure to diethylstilbestrol

ETIOPATHOGENESIS

cervix growth at puberty everts the endocervical columnar mucosa onto the ectocervix; the everted mucosa undergoes metaplasia to squamous epithelium, forming the TRANSITION ZONE

transition zone epithelium infection by oncogenic human papilloma virus (HPV 16, 18) leads to viral DNA incorporation and cervical intraepithelial neoplasia (CIN)

other promoting factors (?smoking) are required for progression to malignancy, which arises almost always in the transition zone

CIN shows orderly progression to carcinoma in situ, microinvasive carcinoma and invasive carcinoma

with postmenopausal atrophy the transition zone is pulled back into the endocervical canal

CLINICAL

Presentation

FROM SCREENING PROGRAM

WITH LOCAL SYMPTOMS

post coital hemorrhage, infection, pelvic pain

ureteric obstruction, renal failure if high grade and bilateral

Spread

uterus, bladder, rectum; ureters

laterally into broad ligament and parametrium

down along the vaginal fornices

posterolaterally along sacrouterine ligaments

PERINEURAL/PERIVASCULAR INVASION

LYMPHATIC

Staging (TNM and FIGO identical)

stage is the main predictor of 5 year survival

T STAGING

Tis carcinoma in situ

T1a microscopically invasive carcinoma

T1b1 confined to cervix, <4 cm

T1b2 confined to cervix, >4 cm

T2a outside cervix but not to parametrium or lower third of vagina

T2b outside cervix with parametrial invasion but not to lower third of vagina

T3a lower third of vagina, but not pelvic side wall

T3b to pelvic sidewall or ureteric obstruction

T4 invades bladder or rectal mucosa or extends beyond pelvis

N STAGING

N1 pelvic side wall nodes, internal, external and common iliac nodes, presacral and lateral sacral nodes

M STAGING

M1 distant metastasis

STAGE GROUPING (Federation Internationale de Gynecologie et d'Obstetrique)

0 Tis N0 M0

IA T1a N0 M0

IB1 T1b1 N0 M0

IB2 T1b2 N0 M0

IIA T2a N0 M0

IIB T2b N0 M0

IIIA T3a N0 M0

IIIB T3b any N M0 or up to T3a N1 M0

IVA T4 any N M0

IVB any T any N M1

MACRO

FUNGATING: exophytic, ulcerating mass (more commonly SCC)

BARREL TUMOR: endocervical tumor (more commonly adenocarcinoma, more commonly postmenopausal)

MICRO

CERVICAL INTRAEPITHELIAL NEOPLASIA (I–III)

(70%) SQUAMOUS CELL (well, moderately, poorly differentiated)

(30%) ADENOCARCINOMA

IMAGING

CT

used for distant M and N stage (lungs, liver, paraaortic and pelvic side wall lymphadenopathy)

unhelpful in T staging below at least T2b – use MR

MR

principal staging modality (multiplanar thin section T2W sequences)

on T2W: cervical carcinoma is high signal compared to compact cervical stroma and to myometrium

Gd T1W sequences can differentiate live tumor and areas of necrosis or hematoma (no enhancement)

stage T1 tumor has an intact rim of low signal cervix around it

loss of clear low signal rim in all planes and a 'fuzzy' cervix to parametrium interface is a sign of likely tumor spread outside the cervix

nodular or massive invasion is unequivocal T2b disease

tumor extension along vagina produces expansion of the vaginal wall (differential is exophytic tumor immediately next to a normal thin vaginal wall)

signs of likely pelvic side wall invasion: high T2W signal in pelvic side wall muscle; vascular encasement; direct nodular extension is unequivocal abnormal nodes are detected on size criteria alone (signal intensity not helpful)

there often are small presacral nodes of uncertain significance

RADIATION FIBROSIS VS RECURRENCE

after 6 months radiation fibrosis is usually low signal on T2W sequences, while tumor recurrence is high

PET (FDG)

primary cervical carcinoma is FDG avid, but is next to FDG-filled bladder (differentiation often requires catheterization)

PET is probably the most sensitive modality for N staging

local recurrence is a firm indication for PET

3.3 ECTOPIC PREGNANCY

see Ch 22

3.4 ENDOMETRIAL CARCINOMA

DEFINITION

malignant Mullerian endometrial tumor with carcinomatous differentiation

CLINICAL

commonest invasive gynecological carcinoma

most patients are postmenopausal

Risk factors

HYPERESTRONISM

HYPERPLASIA WITH ATYPIA

ENDOMETRIAL ATROPHY

Staging (TNM and FIGO identical)

T STAGING

Tis   carcinoma in situ

T1a   confined to endometrium

T1b   invades inner half of myometrium

T1c   invades outer half of myometrium

T2a   invades endocervical glands but confined to uterus

T2b   invades cervical stroma but confined to uterus

T3a   invasion of serosa or adnexa or carcinomatous cells in peritoneal fluid or washings

T3b   invasion of vagina

T4   invasion of bladder mucosa or bowel mucosa

N STAGING

N1   regional lymph nodal metastases

note: regional nodes are only pelvic side wall and paraaortic nodes; other nodes are M1

M STAGING

M1   distant metastases

STAGE GROUPING (Federation Internationale de Gynecologie et d'Obstetrique)

0	Tis N0 M0
IA	T1a N0 M0
IB	T1b N0 M0
IC	T1c N0 M0
IIA	T2a N0 M0
IIB	T2b N0 M0
IIIA	T3a N0 M0
IIIB	T3b N0 M0
IIIC	any T below T4, N1 M0
IVA	T4 any N M0
IVB	any T any N M1

MICRO

(85%) ENDOMETRIOID TYPE

irregular neoplastic glands

MULLERIAN TUMOR RANGE

ADENOCARCINOMA

ENDOMETRIAL STROMAL SARCOMA
see separate entry

MIXED MALIGNANT MULLERIAN TUMOR
see separate entry

(5%) SQUAMOUS/ADENOSQUAMOUS

aggressive tumors with poor prognosis

IMAGING

US

diffuse endometrial thickening

focal endometrial thickening or irregularity

area of focally altered echotexture

in general, rarely present with uniform endometrial thickness <5 mm (no cutoff exists; the risk of endometrial carcinoma increases with endometrial thickness)

pitfall: endometrial carcinoma within non expanded endometrium

Hysterosonography

clarifies position, origin and size of any endometrial mass

allows sonographically guided suction biopsy

CT

uterine enlargement with hypodense eccentric central mass

not helpful in T staging unless there is unequivocal transgression of the myometrium

useful in M and N staging

MR

the principal locoregional staging investigation

on T2W: endometrial carcinoma is similar signal intensity to endometrium or lower; it is higher signal intensity than junctional zone

on Gd enhanced images: it enhances later and often less than myometrium

edge between myometrium and carcinoma determines local tumor stage: T1a is where no transgression of the junctional zone has occurred; T1b and T1c show invasion through the junctional zone and into the myometrium

loss of sharp serosal to parametrial fat interface adjacent to tumor is a sign of likely tumor infiltration into parametrium; nodular or massive extension is unequivocal invasion

regional node MR signal is unhelpful in determining malignant vs benign status; node involvement is on size criteria alone (conventionally, >1 cm transverse dimension)

3.5 ENDOMETRIAL HYPERPLASIA

DEFINITION

totally benign or benign but premalignant excessive endometrial proliferation

ETIOLOGY

HIGH LEVELS OF ESTROGEN, UNOPPOSED ESTROGEN

anovulatory cycles (particularly perimenarchial or perimenopausal)

polycystic ovary syndrome

unopposed hormone replacement therapy

tamoxifen
estrogenic tumors (usually ovarian)

CLINICAL

DYSFUNCTIONAL UTERINE BLEEDING
'BREAKTHROUGH' ON HRT OR
POSTMENOPAUSAL BLEEDING

MICRO

Non premalignant

regresses with administration of
progesterone or removal of estrogen drive

SIMPLE
hyperplasia of both glands and stroma
gland to stroma ratio preserved and gland
density normal

COMPLEX
hyperplasia of glands only, gland branching,
increased gland density

With atypia (premalignant)

focal or multifocal
'back to back' glands
cytological atypia, abnormal mitoses, loss of
normal cellular polarity, complex
multilayering
25% progress to carcinoma

IMAGING

US

thickened echogenic endometrium
does not cycle normally (if patient
premenopausal)

Hysterosonogram

uniformly thickened echogenic endometrium
allows US guided suction biopsy

3.6 ENDOMETRIAL POLYP

DEFINITION

focal non neoplastic polypoid proliferation of
endometrium

CLINICAL

focal endometrial failure to shed with
menstruation; progressive growth with
each hormonal cycle
incidental finding or presents with abnormal
perimenopausal or postmenopausal
bleeding

single or multiple, up to 2 cm in size,
pedunculated or sessile nodular; may
have hyperplasia, cystic gland dilation,
squamous metaplasia
not premalignant, but tends to recur

IMAGING

US

focal thickening of endometrial echo
does not change texture and does not cycle
(if patient premenopausal)
may contain a small cyst or cysts

Hysterosonography

rounded pedunculated or sessile
endometrial mass projecting into fluid
filled lumen
allows US guided suction biopsy

Fluoro (hysterosalpingography)

filling defect: rounded if pedunculated,
broad based if sessile

MR

well shown on heavily T2W weighted
sequences: moderately high T2W signal,
higher than that of submucosal fibroid
but often lower than that of the
endometrium

3.7 ENDOMETRIAL STROMAL AND MIXED TUMORS

DEFINITION

Mullerian endometrial tumor with stromal
or mixed carcinomatous and stromal
differentiation

CLASSIFICATION

see Mullerian tumor range entry

3.7.1 LOW GRADE STROMAL SARCOMA

3.7.2 MIXED MULLERIAN TUMOR

bulky aggressive high grade tumor of older
patients with tendency to hematogenous
metastases

3.8 ENDOMETRIOSIS

DEFINITION

ectopic endometrial glands and stroma
outside of the uterus

ETIOLOGY

retrograde menstruation with implantation
theory
metastatic type spread

CLINICAL

asymptomatic endometriosis much more
common than symptomatic, true
incidence hard to determine
pelvic pain/dyspareunia (rectal symptoms if
in rectovaginal pouch)
infertility (?mechanism; ~1/4 of women with
endometriosis)
small bowel/ureteric symptoms
ECTOPIC PREGNANCY

MACRO

early endometriotic nodules are small
blue-gray serosal nodules
repeated hemorrhage produces a
cystic/multicystic core containing brown
blood products ('chocolate cyst') with
surrounding reactive inflammation and
fibrosis

OVARIAN

PELVIC
tubal/broad ligament/rectovaginal pouch
on or in bladder/rectum/vagina/small
bowel/ureter
may obstruct Fallopian tubes

DISTAL
surgical scars (implantation endometriosis)
liver, lungs, etc (hematogenous spread)

MICRO

Simple

cyclical epithelium, glands, stroma

Complex

blood products/granulation/fibrosis
endometrium may be unrecognizable

IMAGING

US

endometriomas have variable US appearance, depending on contents, recent hemorrhage and degree of fibrosis

simple fluid filled cyst or echogenic complex cyst or mixed cystic–solid mass or solid-appearing mass

may have echogenic reflective foci; some of these shadow (calcification)

classically multiple, with thick walls; do not regress with followup

MR

ENDOMETRIAL IMPLANTS

peritoneal or extraperitoneal nodules with signal initially paralleling that of normal endometrium

as the implants hemorrhage, signal changes to that of blood products

ENDOMETRIOMA

complex solid–cystic mass containing blood products at various stages of evolution

variable T1W signal but predominantly high (and does not saturate with fat suppression)

variable T2W signal but with at least some areas of high signal

low T1W low T2W hemosiderin rings and rims

blood product layering

3.9 GESTATIONAL TROPHOBLASTIC DISEASE

3.9.1 CHORIOCARCINOMA

DEFINITION

very aggressive gestational neoplasm of cytotrophoblast and syncytiotrophoblast with tendency to hemorrhagic hematogenous metastases

EPIDEMIOLOGY AND ETIOLOGY

incidence ~1/45 000, geographic variation

follows a molar pregnancy (50%), spontaneous abortion (30%), or normal pregnancy (20%)

delay of months to years between initiating pregnancy and overt gestational trophoblastic disease; it is very rare during the initial pregnancy

CLINICAL

presents with bloodstained PV discharge

beta hCG is usually elevated (> levels of hydatidiform mole)

highly aggressive and lethal without treatment but very responsive to chemotherapy

even in presence of distal metastases (except brain) survival is ~80%

Spread

predominantly hematogenous (and often present at diagnosis)

lungs, brain, liver, kidneys

MICRO

bilaminar architecture of central cytotrophoblast surrounded by syncytiotrophoblast

AVASCULAR but angioinvasive (hence behavior)

NO VILLI (villi rules choriocarcinoma out)

IMAGING

MR/CT

hemorrhagic cerebral metastases with surrounding edema

rounded 'cannon ball' lung metastases

variable appearance and size uterine mass with differing degree of invasion; hemorrhagic and cystic change

3.9.2 HYDATIDIFORM MOLE

DEFINITION

abnormal benign proliferation of aneuploid trophoblast with characteristic hydropic degeneration (producing a grape-like mass)

ETIOPATHOGENESIS

Complete mole

empty ovum fertilized by one or two spermatozoa

MONOSPERMIC 46XX (incidence 85%)

one 23X sperm with duplication

low invasive potential

DISPERMIC 46XY (INCIDENCE 15%) OR 46XX (rare)

higher invasive potential

Partial mole (usually triploid 69XXX karyotype)

MATERNAL GENOME DUPLICATION

triploid embryo, morphologically normal placenta

PATERNAL DUPLICATION/DOUBLE SPERM

triploid embryo, partial mole

CLINICAL

incidence ~1/1500, geographic variation, tends to occur at extremes of age

Presentation

uterus enlarged for dates

threatened abortion, molar abortion

abnormally high beta hCG levels, hyperemesis gravidarum, theca-lutein cysts, preeclampsia

MORPHOLOGY

Complete mole

ABNORMAL CONCEPTUS WITHOUT AN EMBRYO

large intrauterine mass of grape-like vesicles with no placenta or embryo

hydropic degeneration of all villi (distension with central fluid filled cavities)

Partial mole

ABNORMAL CONCEPTUS WITH AN EMBRYO

the embryo usually dies early

placenta with intermixed normal and hydropic villi

'Norwegian fjord' histology

NATURAL HISTORY

TREATMENT: complete evacuation of molar pregnancy

10% develop persistent trophoblastic disease

Persistent trophoblastic disease

persistence of molar tissue after evacuation

indicated by persistence of beta hCG

usually treated by chemotherapy without tissue confirmation

INVASIVE MOLE

penetration of myometrium and myometrial blood vessels by molar villi (complete mole or partial mole)

MOLAR EMBOLISM TO LUNGS

embolism of invasive molar tissue to lungs with survival and growth; emboli have hydropic villi (rules out choriocarcinoma)

CHORIOCARCINOMA

IMAGING

US

COMPLETE MOLE

distended uterus filled with rounded cystic masses within a homogeneous mass
'snowstorm' appearance on early US reports
no fetal parts, no placenta
theca-lutein cysts

MOLAR TWIN

normal pregnancy in one gestational sac and a complete mole in the other

PARTIAL MOLE

embryo or fetus usually present (and frequently has IUGR or may be dead)
placentomegaly, thickness >4 cm
'Swiss cheese' placenta with cystic vacuolations

INVASIVE MOLE

focal intramyometrial cystic–solid masses or focal areas of increased echogenicity
increased surrounding color Doppler flow (intramyometrial shunts and neovascularity)
reduced uterine artery resistive index

3.9.3 PLACENTAL SITE TROPHOBLASTIC TUMOR

rare; follows normal pregnancy, presents with enlarged uterus, amenorrhea and often elevated beta hCG
cords, sheets, nodules of cytotrophoblast, no bilaminar architecture
moderately angioinvasive; treated with surgery (poor response to chemotherapy)

IMAGING

solid or mixed solid–cystic focal mass or multifocal masses within the myometrium

3.10 HEMATOCOLPOS/ HEMATOMETRA/ PYOMETRA

CLINICAL

dilation of uterus or uterus and vagina secondary to outflow obstruction
HEMATOCOLPOS: vagina distended with blood (imperforate hymen)
HEMATOMETRA: uterus distended with blood (cervical stenosis, imperforate hymen); may have obstruction of one horn (see Mullerian duct developmental anomalies)
HEMATOMETROCOLPOS: combination of the above
PYOMETRA: usually secondary to superinfected malignant or benign cervical stenosis or following incomplete abortion, retained placenta or instrumentation; uterus distended with pus

IMAGING

US/CT/MR

vagina and or uterus distended with complex fluid
clot and debris may layer in posterior vagina
gas in body of uterus indicates pyometra

3.11 LEIOMYOMA

DEFINITION

(= 'fibroid')
common, benign, hormonally dependent tumor of uterine smooth muscle

EPIDEMIOLOGY

25% of women >35 years old; frequently multiple; regress after the menopause

MORPHOLOGY

rounded expansile mass surrounded by a pseudocapsule of compressed normal myometrium, whorled cut surface
benign smooth muscle cells in bundles/whorls, intermixed fibrovascular stroma

most undergo some kind of ischemic degeneration (particularly in pregnancy: hemorrhagic (red) degeneration)

Rare invasive forms

benign metastasizing leiomyomatosis (metastatic lung deposits with typical 'benign' histology)
disseminated peritoneal leiomyomatosis (?in situ transformation)

IMAGING

XR

a massive fibroid uterus is a soft tissue density midline pelvic mass displacing bowel gas upwards (differential is bladder)
calcified fibroids have a 'popcorn' or 'stippled' pattern

US

variable appearance depending on composition, position and number of leiomyomas
diffuse or nodular uterine enlargement
nodular uterine contour (subserosal fibroids)
displaced or distorted endometrial echo (submucosal fibroids)
pedunculated leiomyomas may mimic an adnexal mass

'YOUNG' MUSCULAR LEIOMYOMA

rounded hypoechoic regular mass with moderate sound attenuation

PROGRESSIVE DEGENERATION

increasing sound through transmission
increasing diffuse or patchy echogenicity possibly with smaller cystic areas

CENTRAL CYSTIC DEGENERATION

irregular hypoechoic area with posterior acoustic enhancement

CALCIFICATION

stippled or linear shadowing reflectors

Hysterosonography

clarifies position of the submucosal fibroid

CT

isodense myometrial masses, or may have low density core with significant cystic degeneration
calcification is quite specific if present

MR

variable T1W signal, often isointense to myometrium

variable T2W signal, but usually low relative to myometrium and endometrium

position can be intramyometrial; submucosal (darker than endometrial polyps); or subserosal (the fibroid usually has a 'claw' of myometrium stretched around it)

degeneration produces patchily variable areas better visible on T2W as patchy areas of high signal; infarction is higher than myometrium on both T1W and T2W

3.12 LEIOMYOSARCOMA

rare uterine smooth muscle cell sarcoma

large fleshy grossly invasive mass with areas of hemorrhage and necrosis

tendency to hematogenous spread, particularly to lungs

3.13 MULLERIAN DUCT DEVELOPMENTAL ABNORMALITIES

EPIDEMIOLOGY

as a group, common (?0.5%)

frequently silent and do not impair normal fertility and pregnancy

more severe malformations associated with primary infertility, recurrent abortion, premature labor and uterine rupture

CLASSIFICATION/MACRO

Agenesis

UTERUS UNICORNIS UNICOLLIS

agenesis of one uterine horn and tube

rarely, an isolated rudimentary horn is present

unilateral renal agenesis may be associated

Total/partial non fusion

UTERUS BICORNIS (bicornuate uterus)

partial division of uterus

two clearly separate horns, one cervix, one vagina

UTERUS BICOLLIS

duplication of uterus and cervix

two uterine horns, two cervices, one vagina

UTERUS DIDELPHYS

complete duplication

two uterine horns, two cervices, two vaginas

SEPTATE UTERUS

complete or partial non resorption of the midline septum

Incomplete development

INFANTILE UTERUS

small body and cavity compared with cervix

increased incidence of infertility

HYPOPLASTIC UTERUS

T SHAPED UTERUS

mildest and usually asymptomatic form

Mullerian (paramesonephric) duct remnant

'HYDATID OF MORGAGNI'

simple paramesonephric duct residual cyst in the broad ligament

identifiable as a separate cystic structure only if spatially separate from the ovary

Wolffian (mesonephric) duct remnants

not an abnormality of Mullerian duct development, but associated

GARTNER'S DUCT CYST

static asymptomatic simple cyst in the broad ligament

Gartner's duct: adult remnant of the fetal mesonephric duct

PARAOOPHORON

adult remnant of the mesonephric duct system

collection of small ducts in the broad ligament adjacent to the ovary

usually asymptomatic but may generate cysts

IMAGING

Fluoro (hysterosalpingography)

may occasionally be required to demonstrate the presence of a septum or the presence and patency of a Fallopian tube in a partly fused or a totally duplex system

US/MR

US may have difficulty in demonstrating the degree of myometrial (as opposed to endometrial) fusion

MR has better demonstration of the cervices and septa, and allows definitive classification of the abnormality

imaging manifestations are direct equivalents of the macroscopic findings above

3.14 MULLERIAN TUMOR RANGE

theoretically, any of these differentiations can occur in any Mullerian derived epithelium

in practice only some types are sufficiently common in particular locations

Epithelial differentiation

see Mullerian epithelial tumor classification in ovarian neoplasms entry

Sarcomatous and mixed differentiation

ENDOMETRIAL STROMAL SARCOMA

MIXED MULLERIAN TUMOR

both stroma and parenchyma of Mullerian origin

ADENOFIBROMA (rare, benign)

ADENOSARCOMA (malignant, low grade)

CARCINOSARCOMA (malignant, high grade)

3.15 NABOTHIAN CYSTS

simple cervical cysts that result when glandular epithelium is overgrown by squamous metaplasia in the transition zone

IMAGING

simple unilocular cysts immediately deep to the endocervical canal and external os

3.16 OVARIAN NEOPLASMS

3.16.1 GERM CELL TUMORS

3.16.1.1 DYSGERMINOMA

CLINICAL

uncommon; equivalent of seminoma in males

10–30 year olds

mass with gray-white cut surface and few foci of hemorrhage

polygonal cells in cords, lymphocytic reactive infiltrate

radiosensitive with good prognosis

IMAGING

US

multilobulated solid ovarian mass with vascularized septa

3.16.1.2 CHORIOCARCINOMA

rare; the principal differential is metastasis from gestational choriocarcinoma

3.16.1.3 YOLK SAC TUMOR

4–20 year olds

large hemorrhagic necrotic mass

endodermal sinus histology (glomerulus like)

3.16.1.4 EMBRYONAL CELL CARCINOMA

rare

3.16.1.5 IMMATURE TERATOMA

rare; 1–20 year olds, solid mass

3.16.1.6 MATURE TERATOMA

(97% of germ cell tumors)

see its own entry

3.16.2 LYMPHOMA

solid hypoechoic ovarian mass, often bilateral

3.16.3 METASTASES TO OVARY

Hematogenous

breast, endometrium, melanoma

Lymphatic

endometrium, ?gastrointestinal

Transcelomic

stomach and colon

less frequently pancreas

'Krukenberg tumor' is an adenocarcinoma metastasis to the ovary, presumably transcelomic

IMAGING

bilateral ovarian SOLID masses (bilateral ovarian primary epithelial tumors usually have a significant cystic component)

3.16.4 MULLERIAN EPITHELIUM TUMORS

DEFINITION

neoplasms arising from ovarian surface Mullerian epithelium

EPIDEMIOLOGY

90% of all ovarian malignancies; 45–60 year olds

Risk factors

nulliparity

early menarche, late menopause

family history

hereditary non polyposis colorectal cancer syndrome (Lynch type II)

risk is REDUCED with oral contraceptives

CLINICAL AND STAGING

present late (often with abdominal distension)

BILATERALITY COMMON

CA125 is elevated

Pseudomyxoma peritonei

seeding of peritoneal serous surfaces with malignant cell nests, particularly mucinous adenocarcinoma

malignant mucoid ascites and loculated collections

Spread

transcelomic

lymphatic

hematogenous late

Staging (TNM and FIGO identical)

T STAGE

T1a   one ovary, capsule intact, no malignant cells in peritoneal washings or on ovarian surface

T1b   as above, but both ovaries

T1c   either of above with tumor breaching ovarian surface or present in ascites/peritoneal washings

T2a   tumor on tubes and uterus; peritoneal washings clear

T2b   tumor on other pelvic structures; peritoneal washings clear

T2c   T2a or T2b but with tumor cells in peritoneal washings

T3a   microscopic peritoneal deposits beyond pelvis

T3b   macroscopic peritoneal deposits beyond pelvis, <2 cm

T3c   macroscopic peritoneal deposits beyond pelvis, >2 cm

N STAGE

N1   regional nodal metastases (pelvic and paraaortic nodes)

M STAGE

M1   distant metastases

STAGE GROUPING (federation internationale de gynecologie et d'obstetrique)

IA   T1a N0 M0

IB   T1b N0 M0

IC   T1c N0 M0

IIA   T2a N0 M0

IIB   T2b N0 M0

IIC   T2c N0 M0

IIIA   T3a N0 M0

IIIB   T3b N0 M0

IIIC   T3c N0 M0 or any T N1 M0

IV   any T any N M1

CLASSIFICATION AND MORPHOLOGY

Serous (40%)

spectrum from simple cyst (benign end) to multiloculated cysts with papillary projections to solid tumor with hemorrhage or necrosis (malignant end)

3.16.4.1 SEROUS CYSTADENOMA

3.16.4.2 SEROUS PAPILLARY CYSTADENOMA

3.16.4.3 SEROUS CYSTADENOCARCINOMA

Mucinous (10%)

usually larger than serous tumors (grow to up to 30 cm in diameter)

spectrum from large cysts filled with clear mucus to mixed solid/cystic masses with areas of necrosis and hemorrhage

3.16.4.4 MUCINOUS CYSTADENOMA

3.16.4.5 MUCINOUS CYSTADENOCARCINOMA

Endometrioid (20%)

mixed cystic/solid with nodules, hemorrhage and necrosis

ENDOMETRIOID ADENOMA (rare)

ENDOMETRIOID ADENOFIBROMA (rare)

3.16.4.6 ENDOMETRIOID ADENOCARCINOMA

3.16.4.7 ENDOMETRIAL STROMAL SARCOMA

3.16.4.8 MIXED MALIGNANT MULLERIAN TUMOR

Abnormal vagina-like (5%)

CLEAR CELL ADENOFIBROMA (rare)

3.16.4.9 CLEAR CELL ADENOCARCINOMA

Wolffian urothelium-like

BENIGN BRENNER TUMOR

MALIGNANT BRENNER TUMOR

TRANSITIONAL CELL CARCINOMA

Undifferentiated carcinoma (10%)

IMAGING (US, CT AND MR)

large multicystic low density mass filling the pelvis may simulate complex loculated ascites and makes lateralization difficult; bilateral similar abutting masses may be indistinguishable from a unilateral mass

Serous cystadenoma

large simple unilocular cyst
occasional internal septum or papillary projection may be present
occasionally bilateral
sometimes has calcification

Serous cystadenocarcinoma

large, often >10 cm
multiloculated, thick septa, numerous papillary projections
echogenic material in loculations

Mucinous cystadenoma

prominent septation
echogenic material in septa (mucin)
internal debris or mucin may mimic solid, but are mobile
rupture can produce pseudomyxoma peritonei

Mucinous cystadenocarcinoma

bilateral in ~25%
features form a spectrum with mucinous cystadenoma and serous cystadenocarcinoma
papillary projections less common than with serous cystadenocarcinoma
peritoneal metastases produce pseudomyxoma peritonei
high protein content may lead to hyperintense T1W signal

Endometrioid carcinoma

frequently bilateral
variable appearance; cystic, solid, mixed cystic and solid mass

Clear cell adenocarcinoma

variable cystic or solid or mixed mass

Brenner tumor

predominantly small solid masses
may show calcification

Undifferentiated carcinoma

solid or solid with central necrosis

Pseudomyxoma peritonei

free abdominal and pelvic fluid (ascites)
multiple loculated peritoneal fluid collections with variably echogenic contents
lentiform capsular collections on abdominal solid viscera (classically liver and spleen)
peritoneal and visceral implants (enhance with Gd)

Recurrence after pelvic exenteration

recurrent mass or nodules on CT or MR compared to baseline; often FDG avid; cystic when sufficiently large; may diffusely involve the peritoneum

3.16.5 SEX CORD STROMAL TUMORS

DEFINITION

endocrine tumors of the ovarian parenchyma and stroma (deep to the surface epithelium); both are formed from embryonal sex cords

CLINICAL

benign or malignant
present with hyperestrogenism (abnormal bleeding, precocious puberty, etc) or mass/metastases

Endocrine

GRANULOSA TUMOR, FIBROTHECOMA, SERTOLI TUMOR, LEYDIG TUMOR

Fibroblastic (non endocrine)

FIBROMA (associated with Meigs' syndrome: ovarian fibromas, ascites, pleural effusions)
FIBROSARCOMA

IMAGING

US

usually solid hypoechoic or whirled (like a uterine leiomyoma)
may be bilateral

3.17 OVARIAN NON TUMORAL MASSES

3.17.1 ABSCESS

see salpingitis

3.17.2 ECTOPIC PREGNANCY

see Ch 22

3.17.3 ENDOMETRIOMA

see endometriosis

3.17.4 LUTEOMA OF PREGNANCY/THECA LUTEIN CYSTS

see entry under ovarian physiological and benign cysts

3.17.5 MASSIVE OVARIAN EDEMA

intermittent torsion with secondary engorgement and swelling

3.17.6 OVARIAN TORSION

see its own entry

3.18 OVARIAN PHYSIOLOGICAL AND BENIGN CYSTS

3.18.1 CYSTIC CORPUS LUTEUM/LUTEAL CYST

DEFINITION

cystic corpus luteum is <3 cm
luteal cyst is >3 cm

IMAGING

thick walled unilocular cyst, usually with echogenic content (blood and blood clot); may be partly collapsed and so more solid

surrounding vascular ring, often with capacitive flow

recent hematoma may mimic a solid mass (but is avascular)

by definition resolves spontaneously or on followup (usually within 2 months)

3.18.2 CYSTIC FOLLICLE/ FOLLICULAR CYST

DEFINITION

cystic follicle is <3 cm
follicular cyst is >3 cm

IMAGING

thin walled, unilocular cyst

contents may be totally fluid or mixed echogenicity (hemorrhage)

by definition resolves spontaneously or on followup (usually within 2 months)

3.18.3 EPITHELIAL INCLUSION CYST/TUMOR

DEFINITION

static cyst lined by non neoplastic tubal type epithelium

'tumor' if >3 cm

IMAGING

thin walled unilocular simple cyst, usually small, but may be up to 10 cm in size

3.18.4 PERITONEAL INCLUSION CYST

CLINICAL

mesothelial lined peritoneal cysts next to the ovary

present as an incidental finding or with mass

postulated etiology is a mixture of post infective, post surgical, post traumatic or endometriotic causes

IMAGING

loculated fluid collections with intervening septa, and including the ovary

3.18.5 THECA-LUTEIN CYSTS

DEFINITION

bilateral cystic ovarian enlargement resulting from supraphysiologic beta hCG drive

CLINICAL

bilateral multiple follicular cysts and luteinization

increased risk of torsion

Increased beta HCG:

TWINS
MOLAR PREGNANCY
CHORIOCARCINOMA
OVULATION INDUCTION

IMAGING

US

bilateral thick walled enlarged (up to 10 cm) ovaries containing multiple cystic spaces with regular but thick septa

bilateral 'soap-bubble' enlarged ovaries

may have ascites

tend to regress in a period of weeks to months with cessation of stimulus

3.19 OVARIAN TERATOMA
(ovarian mature teratoma)

97% of ovarian germ cell tumors

DEFINITION

mature differentiated tumor of pluripotent ovarian germ cells

'ovarian dermoid' is a misnomer; a true 'dermoid' is a complex ectodermal inclusion cyst and not a tumor

CLINICAL

10% bilateral

tumor of young adults, but also the commonest ovarian tumor in children

usually presents with pelvic mass, rarely with acute torsion

1% transformation of ectodermal epithelium into squamous cell carcinoma

MORPHOLOGY

round cystic unilocular

Rokitansky mural tubercle (internal 'bump' in the cyst, containing the different layer elements)

ectodermal element usually dominant: sebum, hair, teeth (30%); neural tissue

endodermal epithelium

mesodermal epithelium (not kidney, pancreas or spleen): bone, fat, cartilage

MONOPHYLETIC TERATOMA

mature teratoma differentiating along one pathway only

THYROID TISSUE (STRUMA OVARII)
INTESTINAL TISSUE
CARCINOID TISSUE

IMAGING

US

diffusely echogenic with focal echogenic areas

'dots and dashes' (ultrasonic appearance of matted hair)

may contain shadowing reflectors

may have a shifting sebum–fluid level

may have internal mobile structures

occasionally cystic

PITFALL: can be confused with a loop of bowel with echogenic contents!

CT

mixed density well circumscribed mass with frequent calcification and fat–fluid levels

recognizable teeth and fat are pathognomonic

MR

well circumscribed heterogeneous mass

some fat signal usually present (and true fat suppresses with fat suppression)

fat–fluid levels, fluid–fluid levels

septa and solid components enhance with Gd

3.20 OVARIAN TORSION

CLINICAL

torsion of an ovary on its vascular pedicle

venous and lymphatic obstruction precedes arterial occlusion with resultant venous engorgement and venous infarction

may mimic appendicitis or present as 'left sided appendicitis'

frequently caused by ovarian masses (particularly teratomas and theca-lutein cysts) but also by large ovarian or paraovarian cysts

recurrent torsion manifests as massive ovarian edema

IMAGING

US

complex mixed multicystic or complex solid adnexal or pelvic mass

may be recognizable as an enlarged ovary if contains follicles

absent color or spectral Doppler flow (pathognomonic if this is present in a recognizable ovary)

arterial Doppler traces may be present early in the clinical course

free pelvic fluid or blood

twisted pedicle may show as a round echogenic structure with concentric hypoechoic layers or coiled vessels on color Doppler

cause of the torsion may dominate the findings, with absent vascularity not prominent

3.21 OVARIAN VENOUS INCOMPETENCE AND HYPERTENSION

CLINICAL

classically presents with pelvic dragging pain worse after prolonged standing or may have dyspareunia

may have vulval or perineal varices or recurrent upper leg varicose veins

IMAGING

CT

usually an incidental finding of a markedly dilated left gonadal vein running from the left renal vein towards the ovarian fossa (along a normal ureter)

differential is of a dilated contrast filled ureter (wrong contrast phase)

Angio (ovarian venogram)

dilated left (more commonly than right) ovarian vein

left gonadal vein competent if not locatable on a left renal venogram with Valsalva, or if retrograde flow stops at a venous valve (with Valsalva)

gonadal vein injection with retrograde flow to pelvis indicates incompetence

causation of varices proven if outlined with contrast

right ovarian vein enters the IVC and may need to be looked for with a 'rim' catheter

3.22 POLYCYSTIC OVARY SYNDROME

DEFINITION

syndrome of enlarged ovaries with multiple follicular cysts, elevated luteinizing hormone (LH), infertility and endocrine abnormalities

CLINICAL

Infertility only

Stein–Leventhal syndrome

polycystic ovaries and infertility

endometrial hyperplasia, oligomenorrhea

hirsutism, obesity

MORPHOLOGY (ovary)

luteinization, hyperplasia, enlargement

cortical fibrosis (ovary encased in a fibrous shell), anovulatory cycles

multiple peripheral primary follicles

IMAGING

US

multiple small cystic follicles arranged either at ovarian periphery or scattered through the parenchyma

increased parenchymal echogenicity

may have echogenic ovarian margin

~2/3 of patients have ovarian enlargement

US CRITERIA (TA US): at least 10 follicles between 2 and 18 mm in diameter in a single plane

US CRITERIA (TV US): at least 15 follicles between 2 and 10 mm in diameter peripheral to an echogenic stroma

3.23 SALPINGITIS AND PELVIC INFLAMMATORY DISEASE (PID)

DEFINITION

acute or subacute inflammation of the Fallopian tubes with or without extension to the pelvic peritoneum

ETIOPATHOGENESIS

Ascending mucosal infection

SEXUALLY TRANSMITTED DISEASE (gonococcus, chlamydia)

SUPERINFECTION OF IUCD (polymicrobial, beware actinomyces infection)

POST INSTRUMENTATION

POST PARTUM (anaerobic gangrenous infection)

Tuberculous salpingitis

hematogenous spread from a focus elsewhere

50% have tuberculous endometritis

Spread from pelvic abscess

appendix or Crohn's abscess

CLINICAL/MACRO

Acute salpingitis and PID

acute salpingitis in isolation

pyosalpinx

tuboovarian abscess

peritonitis

Chronic salpingitis

FOLLICULAR SALPINGITIS

tubal epithelial fold adhesions and scarring

meshwork of adherent folds and cystic spaces

SALPINGITIS ISTHMICA NODOSA

formation of isthmic mucosal diverticula

HYDROSALPINX

LUMINAL FIBROSIS AND
 OBLITERATION

Complications

TUBAL ECTOPIC PREGNANCY

TUBAL INFERTILITY
incidence ~10% after one episode of PID
incidence ~25% after two episodes of PID

Tuberculous salpingitis
smooth fibrotic tube (patent)
multiple strictures (beading)
tuboovarian calcification
cavities, sinus tracts
ragged uterine cavity
the usual outcome is sterility

IMAGING

US

SALPINGITIS/PID
may have no findings at all (particularly in
 early uncomplicated salpingitis)
free pelvic fluid (clear or complex) – totally
 non specific finding
visible Fallopian tube with thickened wall
 (>5 mm)
non specifically increased vascularity of
 uterus, ovaries, adnexa
'cogwheel' Fallopian tube (cogwheel shaped
 transverse section of Fallopian tube with
 central hypoechoic area)
dilated tortuous fluid filled adnexal structure
 (hydro or pyosalpinx) with mucosal folds
 forming incomplete septa
'tuboovarian complex': matted ovary and
 tube (with Fallopian tube recognizable as
 such) but before tuboovarian abscess is
 visible
focal cystic space with an irregular wall and
 increased peripheral vascularity
 (tuboovarian abscess)
differentiation from ovarian or tubal
 neoplasm may be impossible on imaging
 findings in isolation (and requires
 appropriate history and tenderness/pain
 on direct probe pressure)

ENDOMETRITIS
endometrial cavity fluid or debris or
 complex fluid (pyometra)
free pelvic fluid (clear or complex)
gangrenous endometritis: shadowing
 reflectors in the uterine cavity that move
 (differential: post instrumentation air)

CT
free pelvic fluid, edema and stranding of
 pelvic fat
edematous Fallopian tubes and ovaries
hydrosalpinx, pyosalpinx
complex enhancing adnexal mass with
 possible central necrosis and liquefaction
 and peripheral contrast enhancement
gas within abscess specific

Hysterosonography
contraindicated in acute infection
role in documenting endometrial adhesions
 following curettage (Asherman's
 syndrome) or endometritis

Fluoro (hysterosalpingography)
contraindicated in acute infection

TUBAL PATENCY
free spill of uterine contrast through one or
 both tubes outlining serosal bowel
 surface is proof of patency
contrast outlining a fixed space may be
 within an abscess or hydrosalpinx

ENDOMETRIAL CAVITY
filling defects (TB endometritis)
adhesions (post curettage – Asherman's
 syndrome or post endometritis)

SALPINGITIS ISTHMICA NODOSA
pathognomonic nodular or mushroom
 shaped contrast filled diverticula arising
 from the isthmic portion of a tube

3.24 VAGINAL NEOPLASIA
(overview)

3.24.1 VAGINAL CLEAR CELL ADENOCARCINOMA

average age of presentation ~20 years old
2/3 of cases have been exposed to
 diethylstilbestrol in utero
develops from vaginal adenosis
nodular/sessile/papillary mass, hobnail cells
 (glycogen, large nuclei)

3.24.2 VAGINAL INTRAEPITHELIAL NEOPLASIA

analogous to cervical intraepithelial
 neoplasia
association with prior cervical intraepithelial
 neoplasia or cervical carcinoma

3.24.3 VAGINAL RHABDOMYOSARCOMA

see rhabdomyosarcoma entry in soft tissue
 tumors
rare invasive rhabdomyosarcoma of children
most occur before 2 years of age
fleshy soft grape-like conglomerate arising
 from anterior vaginal wall (sarcoma
 botryoides)
myxoid stroma with round or elongated
 malignant cells and a dense subsurface
 tumor cell layer (cambium layer)
aggressive and invasive; tends to recur
 locally

3.24.4 VAGINAL SQUAMOUS CELL CARCINOMA

3.25 VULVAR CARCINOMA

human papilloma virus, chronic infection,
 smoking (carcinogens in urine)
60 years and older
squamous cell carcinoma of vulvar skin
 (firm indurated ulcer or more aggressive
 verrucous)
mass, itch, bleeding or discharge

Staging (TNM and FIGO identical)

T STAGE
T1a vulva/perineum only, <2 cm, invasion
 <1 mm
T1b vulva/perineum only, <2 cm, invasion
 >1 mm
T2 vulva/perineum only, >2 cm
T3 invades lower urethra, vagina, anus
T4 invades bladder mucosa, rectal
 mucosa, upper urethra or fixed to bone

N STAGE
N1 unilateral femoral or inguinal nodes
N2 bilateral femoral or inguinal nodes

M STAGE
M1 distant metastasis (including pelvic
 lymph nodes)

FIGO STAGE GROUPING
IA T1a N0 M0
IB T1b N0 M0
II T2 N0 M0
III up to T3, N1 M0 or T3 N0 M0
IVA any T N2 M0 or T4 any N M0
IVB any T any N M1

1. NORMAL AND APPROACH

1.1 ARTIFACTS

Mammo unit
grid lines

Patient
talc powder or deodorant (simulates malignant microcalcifications)
hair, jewelry, tattoos, other body parts!

Cassette
dirt
moisture
fingerprints, scratches

Processor
static
fog
roller marks
water spots, drying patterns

1.2 LOCALIZATION AND TRIANGULATION

Triangulation CC – MLO – lateral
CC and LAT correctly locate the position of an abnormality in orthogonal planes
CC and MLO triangulate:
upper outer quadrant projects highest on MLO
inner lower quadrant projects lowest on MLO
lower outer quadrant, central breast and upper inner quadrant all superimpose in mid-MLO close to the level of the nipple
a lesion in high MLO is in the upper outer quadrant/axillary tail
a lesion in low MLO is in the inner lower quadrant
MID-MLO LESION LOCALIZATION:
lateral on CC = lower outer quadrant; mid-CC = central breast; medial on CC = upper inner quadrant
IF IN DOUBT, DO A TRUE LATERAL
ONE OR TWO LESIONS?
any one lesion is the same distance back from the nipple (along the line perpendicular to edge of pectoralis major) in CC, MLO and LAT views (corollary: if this distance varies significantly between two views, there are two different lesions)

Confirmation that a lesion is the same on US and mammo
if can not confirm by correlation of features and location, inject a tiny amount of contrast or air under US and repeat mammography

1.3 MAMMOGRAPHY REPORTING CHECKLIST

Quality and exposure
symmetrical films that are sufficiently dark
sufficient breast tissue on film, uniform breast density (i.e. sufficient compression), no overlapping folds, no artifacts
IF ASYMMETRY
has there been previous surgery?
is one breast edematous or infiltrated?
is there a non breast reason for insufficient reach on one side (e.g. chest wall abnormality, painful frozen shoulder, etc)

Previous mammograms
the most recent previous films and the most remote previous films
anything between those two that may be of help

Checklist
overall breast parenchyma density and distribution (?symmetry)
breast plate contour and shape (?symmetry)
breast plate examined in smaller 'chunks': masses, architectural distortion, non specific densities, calcifications
retromammary fat
mammary cone apex, axilla (MLO view)
subareolar area
magnifier review: microcalcifications
if there is one finding, do not stop: WHAT ELSE IS THERE?

1.4 NORMAL APPEARANCE

Mammo
breast density depends on age and hormonal status
normal varies very widely despite above, from largely fat replaced to dense
both sides are reasonably symmetrical
breast parenchyma distributed similarly on both sides, with more parenchyma in central breast, upper outer breast and axillary tail

with involution, breast parenchyma persists longest in central and upper outer areas
parenchyma consists of intersecting rounded curved shadows ('trabeculae', 'ligaments of Cooper') and softer rounded or fluffy densities (glandular tissue) dispersed among breast fat
large tubular ducts course under nipple
intramammary arteries commonly calcify
retromammary fat is a regular low density stripe
axilla contains lymph nodes, or may contain axillary tail of breast (i.e. breast parenchyma)

US
breast fat is hypoechoic to glandular tissue
amount of glandular tissue depends on age and hormonal status
breast fat lobules regular, ovoid or lens shaped, change shape and appearance as transducer is rotated
breast parenchyma and trabeculae: curved hyperechoic concave structures that change shape with changing transducer orientation
nipple normally shadows; under nipple are major subareolar ducts
pectoralis regular hypoechoic; ribs rounded shadowing reflectors (in cross section)

1.5 NORMAL HISTOLOGY

Ducts
two cell epithelium (columnar, myofibroblasts)
basement membrane, collagen/elastin/fibroblast cuff

TDLUs (terminal ductal lobular unit)
<1 mm in reproductive resting state
terminal duct: two cell epithelium, no stromal cuff
looser myxomatous intralobular stroma
firmer denser collagenous extralobular stroma

1.6 POSITIONING AND ROUTINE PROJECTIONS

Standard mammography projections
MEDIOLATERAL OBLIQUE ('MLO')
cassette along angle of pectoralis major (therefore different from patient to patient but the same for any one patient)

(elevate breast up, do not compress down)
need to see pectoralis major to level of
nipple
need to see retromammary fat (stripe free of
glandular tissue)
nipple in profile, no drooping breast,
inframammary fold opened

CRANIOCAUDAL ('CC')
horizontal cassette
(elevate breast up, do not compress down)
should reach back at least within 1 cm of as
far as the MLO view (along line through
the nipple perpendicular to pectoralis
edge)
may see a little pectoralis on CC view
even with optimal positioning (including
elevation of inframammary fold) the
lateral breast is routinely not on the film

Additional projections
EXTENDED CC (to image lateral breast)
patient rotated so that lateral breast is
included on film
TRUE LATERAL (vertical cassette)
CLEAVAGE (both medial breasts on film)
TANGENTIAL
for a cutaneous or subcutaneous palpable or
otherwise localizable mass
ROTATIONAL (to confirm presence of an
abnormality)
breast rolled 10 to 20 degrees off baseline
view
LATEROMEDIAL ('true lateral')
REVERSE OBLIQUE

Coned compression magnification
done in view of concern
for calcium characterization should be done
true lateral rather than MLO (looking for
layering)

1.7 SCREENING MAMMOGRAPHY RECOMMENDATIONS

American Cancer Society
baseline between 35 and 40
annual or biannual between 40 and 50 years
annual over 50 year old
if high risk, screening starts at 30 years

Breastscreen Australia
BIANNUAL
>50 years old with no risk factors
will accept self referred 40–50 year old

ANNUAL
personal history of carcinoma
strong family history of carcinoma (2x 1st
degree relatives)
atypical hyperplasia
lobular carcinoma in situ

1.8 WORKUP OF PALPABLE ABNORMALITY

double check that patient, referrer and
technologist are all dealing with one and
the same palpable abnormality
size, position and shape (for larger masses)
should be concordant on physical
examination, mammography and
ultrasound

Mammography
technologist should place a marker on each
of the two standard views while the
breast is positioned for that exposure

Sonography
if it is palpable, it should be ultrasonically
visible
if it is ultrasonically visible, it should be
accessible to US guided biopsy

'Lumpy breast'
prominent breast tissue ('lumpy breast')
should have normal mammographic and
ultrasound findings, and no suspicious
findings on physical examination (i.e.
absence of mammo or US findings should
not preclude from further management
on suspicious clinical grounds)

2. GAMUTS
2.1 MAMMOGRAPHY

2.1.1 ABNORMALITY SEEN IN ONE MAMMOGRAPHIC VIEW ONLY

Microcalcification on one view only
poor technique, position, motion artifact or
exclusion on one view

Density ('DIS' or 'NON') or architectural distortion
exclusion on one view – try extended CC
view to include lateral breast on film

summation shadow – try rotational or
compression views to resolve overlying
structures

2.1.2 DEALING WITH ARCHITECTURAL DISTORTION ('ARC') AND NON SPECIFIC DENSITY ('NON')

CONVERT TO 'DIS', 'STEL', OR
SUMMATION SHADOW WITH FURTHER
WORKUP
USE: HISTORY
KEY IN DIAGNOSES OF SCAR, FAT
NECROSIS, ABSCESS
USE: PHYSICAL EXAM/US
MAY CONVERT LESION TO A MASS ('DIS')
USE: COMPRESSION MAGNIFICATION
VIEW IN PROJECTION WHICH
DEMONSTRATED THE LESION
CONVERTS LESION TO A SUMMATION
SHADOW (disappears with compression
magnification) OR PERSISTING DENSITY
(does not disappear with compression
magnification)

2.1.3 DESCRIPTIVE TERMS FOR MAMMOGRAPHIC/US ABNORMALITIES

Discrete mass ('DIS')
also called circumscribed mass ('CIRC')
DENSITY OR ECHOGENICITY
EDGE OR CAPSULE
SIZE AND CALCIFICATION
SHAPE AND ORIENTATION
POSITION AND NUMBER
patient age is relevant to incidence of
malignancy

Stellate lesion ('STEL')
CORE OF LESION: SIZE AND DENSITY
STRANDS: LENGTH AND REGULARITY

Calcification ('CAL')
SIZE AND FORM
DENSITY AND UNIFORMITY
DISTRIBUTION
MICROCALCIFICATION
LOBULAR
DUCTAL (IMPLIES MALIGNANCY/DCIS)
MACROCALCIFICATION
DUCTAL
PERIDUCTAL
VASCULAR
FOCAL
EGGSHELL

Architectural distortion ('ARC')

distorted pattern of breast ligaments, breast parenchyma, or breast plate shape or density but not a STEL

Non specific density ('NON')

not characterizable mammographically as one of the above

2.1.4 DISCRETE MASS ('DIS') CLASSIFIED BY MAMMOGRAPHIC DENSITY

Low density

lower density than breast parenchyma: descriptor is 'hypodense'

LIPOMA

OIL CYST, GALACTOCELE

Mixed low and high density

LYMPH NODE

classically has a fatty hilum

FIBROADENOLIPOMA (hamartoma)

HEMATOMA, FAT NECROSIS, GALACTOCELE

Isodense to breast parenchyma

CYST

ABSCESS

FIBROADENOMA, PHYLLODES TUMOR

HEMATOMA, SCAR

PAPILLOMA, HEMANGIOMA

PAPILLARY CARCINOMA, MUCINOUS CARCINOMA, MEDULLARY CARCINOMA

High density

higher density than breast parenchyma: descriptor is 'dense' or 'hyperdense'

CYST

ABSCESS

HEMATOMA, SCAR

PHYLLODES TUMOR

CARCINOMA

SARCOMA, METASTASIS

SILICONE INJECTION

2.1.5 DISCRETE MASS ('DIS') CLASSIFIED BY QUALITY OF ITS EDGE

often requires focal compression to move away overlying tissue

Benign mass

HALO SIGN

thin regular rim of lucent fat around the mass

OR SHARP EDGE

Suspicious mass

SPICULATION OF EDGE

COMET TAILS

elongated streak of density running from the mass in one direction

FUZZY MARGIN

ARCHITECTURAL DISTORTION/ SPICULATION (SEE STELLATE LESION)

2.1.6 INCREASED BREAST DENSITY OR SKIN THICKENING ON MAMMOGRAM

PREVIOUS RADIOTHERAPY

MASTITIS

LYMPHATIC DRAINAGE OBSTRUCTION

(axillary clearance, replacement by tumor)

VENOUS OBSTRUCTION

(e.g. SVC obstruction)

INFILTRATING CARCINOMA

INFLAMMATORY CARCINOMA

POST SURGICAL OR POST PROCEDURAL

AS PART OF GENERALIZED SKIN EDEMA

(e.g. nephrotic syndrome)

2.1.7 LESIONS OF NO PATHOLOGIC INTEREST PRODUCING MAMMOGRAPHIC FINDINGS

Skin

NIPPLE NOT IN PROFILE

PAPILLOMA

SEBACEOUS CYST/SEBACEOUS CALCIFICATION

SCAR

Fat

HEMATOMA

FAT NECROSIS

LIPOMA

Glands

GALACTOCELE

Blood vessels

HEMANGIOMA

Lymph nodes

NORMAL INTRAMAMMARY NODES

LYMPHADENOPATHY

lymphoma

systemic disease with reactive lymphadenopathy

Hormone replacement therapy (HRT) changes

Breast implants/capsule after implant removal

2.1.8 MACROCALCIFICATION BY PATHOLOGY OF ORIGIN

Periductal mastitis/plasma cell mastitis

dense uniform calcification

follows major ducts

periductal calcification: rings, cigar shapes

intraductal calcification: linear

Arterial

elongated tortuous 'tram track' calcification following the course of arteries

Fat necrosis/hematoma/scar

small rings/blebs with central low density or isodense

liponecrosis microcystica calcificans

calcified oil cyst (liponecrosis macrocystica calcificans)

eggshell calcification (thin calcification in wall of cyst or oil cyst)

Skin

dystrophic in scar, burns or keloid

Papilloma

irregular dense calcification in papilloma morphology

Fibroadenoma

coarse dense clumped irregular (popcorn) calcification

flecked calcification

eggshell calcification

Hemangioma

same as hemangioma elsewhere

punctate bizarre

Sutural

calcium deposition on surgical sutures

in scar

often outlines the suture knot

Implant capsule calcification

coarse linear calcification in fibrous periimplant capsule

2.1.9 MICROCALCIFICATION BY PATHOLOGY

Ductal (malignant)

follows small ducts, and takes on their shape

casting small (linear)

branching calcifications imply ductal
calcification
granular small (needle tip)
variable, irregular density (pleomorphic
calcifications)
clustered, focal, few or numerous
may be sectorial or converge on nipple

Lobular (benign)

sharply outlined hemispherical small
soft edge hemispherical small
homogenous, regular, uniform density
scattered numerous bilateral
clustered (single or multiple rounded
clusters)
'cups and saucers': rounded in craniocaudal
view, hemispherical convex downwards
in true lateral view (layering milk of
calcium in dilated terminal lobular units)

Skin calcifications

fine rings of calcification at mouths of skin
ducts
bilateral multifocal scattered

2.1.10 POOR CONTRAST MAMMOGRAM

POOR COMPRESSION
kVp too high
UNIFORM BREAST DENSITY
UNDERDEVELOPED FILM

2.1.11 STELLATE LESION ('STEL')

HEMATOMA, SCAR, FAT NECROSIS
DEALING WITH SCAR
baseline and magnification compression
views at 6 months post op (radioopaque
scar markers on skin)
bilateral mammography at 12 months
scar usually biggest at 6 months and does
not enlarge from 12 months on
DOCUMENTED KNOWN STABLE SCAR CAN BE
LEFT ALONE
CARCINOMA
'white star' (central density with radiating
spicules)
possibly retraction or tenting of breast plate
similar in all projections
SCLEROSING ADENOSIS
RADIAL SCAR/COMPLEX SCLEROSING
LESION
'black star' or 'sheaf of wheat' (absent
central density, parallel spicules)
no retraction or tenting
may vary between projections

2.1.12 WHITE MAMMOGRAM

Unilateral

UNILATERAL INADEQUATE
COMPRESSION
UNILATERAL INCREASED BREAST
DENSITY (see gamut)

Bilateral

UNDEREXPOSED FILMS
DENSITY SETTING TOO LOW
REACHED mAs LIMIT
PHOTOCELL OVER FAT OR AIR
UNDERDEVELOPED FILMS
DROP IN DEVELOPER TEMPERATURE
INSUFFICIENT DEVELOPER DWELL TIME
FIXER CONTAMINATION OF DEVELOPER

2.2 GENERIC (all modalities)

2.2.1 LOCATION OF ORIGIN FOR VARIOUS CONDITIONS

Nipple

PAGET'S DISEASE OF THE NIPPLE
ADENOMA

Main ducts

DUCT ECTASIA
INFLAMMATORY FIBROCYSTIC CHANGE
periductal mastitis
plasma cell mastitis
obliterative mastitis
GALACTOCELE
PAPILLOMA

Terminal ducts

FIBROCYSTIC CHANGE (FCC)
simple FCC
FCC with fibrosis
cysts
DUCTAL HYPERPLASIA
DCIS (ductal carcinoma in situ)
DUCTAL CARCINOMA – INVASIVE

Lobules

FIBROCYSTIC CHANGE
simple adenosis
sclerosing adenosis
effects of hormone replacement therapy
FIBROADENOMA/PHYLLODES TUMOR
LOBULAR HYPERPLASIA
LCIS (lobular carcinoma in situ)
LOBULAR CARCINOMA – INVASIVE

2.3 ULTRASOUND

2.3.1 ULTRASOUND SIGNS OF BENIGN VS MALIGNANT MASSES

After Thomas Stavros

Malignant

sonographic spiculation or rind (PPV 92%)
angular margins (PPV 70%)
microlobulation (PPV 75%)
branching or nodular extensions
depth:width >1 (PPV 82%)
posterior shadowing
markedly hypoechoic (PPV 70%)
microcalcification

Benign

uniform hyperechoic (NPV 100%)
depth:width <1 (NPV 99%)
macrolobulations (3 or fewer)
bright pseudocapsule
(must have at least two benign features for a
benign diagnosis)

Unhelpful

size
internal homogeneity
mildly hypoechoic or isoechoic
normal or increased through transmission

BREAST CONDITIONS
3. GENERAL
3.1 BREAST CARCINOMA

GROUP DEFINITION

heterogeneous group, numerically
dominated by invasive ductal carcinoma
NOS

GROUP EPIDEMIOLOGY

incidence increases with age
commonest female carcinoma
Australia: lifetime risk 1/15 and slowly
increasing
United States: lifetime risk 1/8

Classification

INVASIVE CARCINOMA (= 100%)
lobular 10%
ductal NOS 75% (55% pure, 20% mixed)
medullary 5%

mucinous 5%

tubular ? (infrequent)

papillary ? (infrequent)

adenoid cystic (rare)

special presentations: Paget's disease of the nipple, inflammatory carcinoma

CARCINOMA IN SITU

DUCTAL

20–40% of carcinoma found at screening

comedo DCIS is ~5% of palpable carcinoma

non comedo DCIS

LOBULAR

??incidence

Risk factors

PRIOR CARCINOMA (marker of field change)

CARCINOMA IN SITU (precursor and/or marker of field change)

GENETIC

FAMILY HISTORY

1 first degree relative (relative risk x2)

2 first degree relatives (relative risk x6)

p53: Li–Fraumeni syndrome

17q21 BRCA-1 locus (codes C-erb oncogene); BRCA-2 gene

HORMONAL

UNOPPOSED ESTROGENS

early menarche and late menopause

nulliparity, obesity

unopposed estrogen hormone replacement therapy

polycystic ovary syndrome

estrogen secreting tumor

FIBROCYSTIC DISEASE WITH INCREASED RELATIVE RISK

sclerosing adenosis (x2)

moderate–severe epithelial hyperplasia without atypia (x2)

epithelial hyperplasia with atypia (x5)

ENVIRONMENTAL

migrants assume incidence of new location

increased in exposure to high dose radiation

GROUP PATHOGENESIS

hyperplasia with atypia may progress to carcinoma in situ

DCIS progresses to invasive carcinoma

LCIS is a marker of field change

breast carcinoma is localized for a variable period before spreading (carcinoma size is a prognostic factor)

Spread theories: centrifugal spread (lymph nodal stage is a prognostic factor) vs early systemic micrometastases (supported by improved patient survival in adjuvant chemotherapy trials)

GROUP CLINICAL PRESENTATION, STAGING AND SPREAD

Presentation

BREAST LUMP

UNRELATED BREAST SYMPTOMS, INCIDENTAL FINDING

FOUND AT SCREENING

METASTASES PRESENTING FIRST

Spread

INTRAMAMMARY

intraductal within own segment

diffuse involvement of breast lymphatics

multifocal incidence may be impossible to distinguish from intramammary satellite spread

LYMPHATIC

relatively early

in general, orderly (see lymphoscintigraphy)

if primary lymphatic drainage is blocked (e.g. by tumor), drainage to collateral node basins may occur

DRAINAGE PATTERNS

central and lateral breast (and nipple) drain to axillary nodes, then supraclavicular nodes

medial breast may drain to internal thoracic nodes

cross-breast drainage may occur

HEMATOGENOUS

exact timing of spread subject of controversy and probably varies with tumor aggressivity and type

lungs, bones, liver, brain, other locations

Staging

TNM

T STAGE

T1mic	<0.1cm of invasive tumor (microinvasion)
T1a	0.1 cm < size < 0.5 cm
T1b	0.5 cm < size < 1 cm
T1c	1 cm < size < 2 cm
T2	2 cm < size < 5 cm
T3	size > 5cm
T4	any size, with direct extension to chest wall or skin
T4a	extension to chest wall
T4b	skin edema, ulceration, or nodules
T4c	both
T4d	inflammatory carcinoma

NOTES

Paget's disease of the nipple is staged on its associated mass

chest wall does not include pectoralis major muscle

N STAGE

N1 mobile ipsilateral axillary nodes

pN1a micrometastases only (< 0.2 cm)

pN1b i 1–3 nodes, 0.2 cm < met size < 2cm

pN1b ii >3 nodes, 0.2 cm < met size < 2 cm

pN1b iii transcapsular spread, met size < 2 cm

pN1b iv met size > 2 cm

N2 matted or fixed ipsilateral axillary nodes

N3 ipsilateral internal thoracic nodes

STAGE GROUPING

STAGE 0	Tis N0 M0
STAGE I	T1 N0 M0
STAGE IIA	up to T1 N1 M0, or T2 N0 M0
STAGE IIB	T2 N0 M0 or T3 N0 M0
STAGE IIIA	up to T3 N2 M0 or T3 N1 M0
STAGE IIIB	T4 any N M0
STAGE IV	any T any N M1

GROUP PROGNOSTIC FACTORS

Local recurrence

completeness of excision and adequacy of surgical margins

presence of field change, i.e. multifocal tumor, carcinoma in situ (lobular, ductal) elsewhere or DCIS to margin of resection

Systemic recurrence

NODAL STAGE (correlates with primary size)

PATIENT AGE (in general, tumor more aggressive in younger patients)

HISTOLOGIC TYPE (DCIS has best prognosis, pure special types have good prognosis)

GRADE

Other factors

presence and degree of expression of estrogen (and progesterone) receptors (predicts treatment response)

neovascularization (increased tumor neoangiogenesis is a predictor of systemic metastases)

DNA flow cytometry (indicates degree of aneuploidy), oncogene expression (predicts tumor dedifferentiation and hence aggressivity)

3.1.1 DUCTAL CARCINOMA IN SITU (DCIS)

CLINICAL

usually asymptomatic; up to 5% of all palpable carcinomas, 20%–40% of screen detected carcinomas

may present with Paget's disease of the nipple

non comedo DCIS carries risk of invasion of ?1% per year
comedo DCIS frequently invades
overall absolute risk of invasive carcinoma is ~25% in 10 years

PATHOLOGY

Subtypes

COMEDO CARCINOMA

only palpable DCIS; high grade by description
small ducts distended with neoplastic ductal epithelium and central necrosis (can be squeezed out: hence 'comedo')

SOLID

CRIBRIFORM

MICROPAPILLARY

Grading

WELL DIFFERENTIATED

POORLY DIFFERENTIATED

IMAGING

Mammo

cardinal finding: clusters of malignant microcalcifications
pleomorphic, granular; angular microcalcifications
angular clusters; 'broken needles'; 'crushed rock'
branching microcalcifications (implying ductal casts)
no benign features (i.e. no layering)
may have associated ill defined or lobulated discrete mass or non specific density
INVASIVE NON DCIS COMPONENT may evoke reactive architectural distortion or spiculation

US

may have no findings
microcalcifications may be visible as dot reflectors
mass may or may not be present

Biopsy

if microcalcifications were the presenting findings, biopsy specimen must contain multiple typical calcifications
fine needle aspiration not appropriate
US guided biopsy often not possible as there is no associated mass
stereotactic core biopsy or vacuum assisted biopsy possible (do specimen X-ray); if there is discordance between specimen

histology grade and mammographic microcalcification grade, consider lumpectomy
hook needle localization and excisional biopsy may be therapeutic if histologic margins clear and all microcalcifications removed with specimen

3.1.2 LOBULAR CARCINOMA IN SITU (LCIS)

('lobular neoplasia')

CLINICAL

has no symptoms or signs, an incidental histological finding
true incidence not well established
marker of subsequent invasive disease (both breasts)
frequently bilateral and multifocal
overall absolute risk of carcinoma is ~25% in 10 years (anywhere in either breast)

PATHOLOGY

lobular neoplastic cells distending and distorting acini

IMAGING

no imaging findings – at all
therefore, if an imaging abnormality was biopsied, at least one other pathologic diagnosis should be made

3.1.3 DUCTAL CARCINOMA NOT OTHERWISE SPECIFIED (NOS)

CLINICAL

~75% of all breast cancer
no special histologic or clinical features

PATHOLOGY

usually scirrhous carcinoma: very hard white mass with retraction of surrounding tissue
pure ductal NOS 2/3, mixed with other types 1/3
epithelial neoplastic cells in cords, nests, glands, lumps or tubules
invasive component by definition (direct, vascular, perineural)
variable amount of reactive desmoplasia

IMAGING

Mammo

CLASSIC FINDINGS

stellate mass ('STEL')
central isodense or hyperdense opacity
extensive radiating spiculation, relatively uniform in all views
retraction and distortion of breast plate, skin retraction
may have malignant type microcalcifications (associated DCIS: important if extensive as it implies field change)

OTHER FINDINGS

mass in isolation ('DIS' or 'CIRC'); usually has ill defined or lobulated or spiculated edge; density usually iso or high to breast parenchyma; rarely, a well rounded mass
architectural distortion ('ARC') in isolation (with mass difficult to appreciate)
malignant microcalcifications in association with above

US

US FEATURES OF MALIGNANCY

hypoechoic solid mass with posterior shadowing
taller than wider
sonographic spiculation or rind or microlobulations, disrupts tissue planes
angular margins, extension into ducts
may have microcalcifications

ALTERNATIVE US FINDINGS

mass without specific features

NUC MED (lymphoscintigraphy)

CONCEPT OF SENTINEL LYMPH NODE

lymphatic drainage of tissue is to its particular dedicated nodes and nodal basins (unless obstructed), and is reproducible
nodal metastases will form in the first node draining a particular volume of tissue ('sentinel node')
sentinel node status predicts the status of the entire nodal basin with a high degree of accuracy (well documented for breast carcinoma and melanoma)
sentinel node can be identified by peritumoral radiocolloid injection and subsequent imaging/radioguided surgery with a gamma probe

COLLOIDS AVAILABLE

unfiltered Tc-sulfur colloid (large slowly moving particles that enter lymphatics relatively poorly)
filtered Tc-sulfur colloid

Tc-antimony colloid (colloid of choice, not yet approved by FDA)

(non radioactive) patent blue dye (used intraoperatively)

FINDINGS

'flare' around tumor with peritumoral injection (may be lead screened)

dynamic images may show lymphatic channels running to nodal basins

series of static images identify first order nodes (sentinel nodes) and higher echelon nodes

BEWARE of sentinel nodes in unexpected locations (e.g. internal thoracic nodes)

PET (FDG)

not commonly used for diagnosis of primary staging and problem solving tool

metastatic breast carcinoma is reasonably FDG avid

demonstrates axillary nodes and distal metastases (subject to partial volume and low metabolism limitations)

Staging investigations

variable combinations of MDP bone scan, chest X-ray or CT, brain CT or MR, whole body CT or even whole body PET

3.1.4 INVASIVE LOBULAR CARCINOMA

CLINICAL

10% of all breast cancer

20% bilateral, frequently multicentric

rubbery ill defined mass, focal thickening, focal tenderness

PATHOLOGY

pure or mixed with other types (e.g. tubulolobular)

small regular cells invading surrounding tissue single file

may have associated lobular carcinoma in situ

IMAGING

Mammo

variable appearance, including all of stellate density, discrete mass, non specific opacity and architectural distortion

occasionally diffuse breast changes

microcalcifications rare

US

no specific features (see US signs of malignancy)

3.1.5 MEDULLARY CARCINOMA

CLINICAL

5% of breast carcinoma

commoner in younger women

presents as a rapidly growing mass

relatively aggressive clinical behavior but pure medullary carcinoma has better prognosis than ductal carcinoma NOS

PATHOLOGY

soft relatively well defined mass, may have areas of hemorrhage or necrosis

highly cellular tumor with syncytial-like sheets and masses of anaplastic cells and frequent mitoses

prominent lymphocytic infiltrate between neoplastic cells

no reactive desmoplasia

IMAGING

Mammo

discrete mass with variably defined margins

US

hypoechoic, homogenous rounded mass

3.1.6 MUCINOUS CARCINOMA

CLINICAL

2% of all breast cancer

older patients, slowly growing tumor

better prognosis for pure mucinous carcinoma than for ductal carcinoma NOS

PATHOLOGY

soft, mucinous mass

mucinous 'lakes' which dissect through tissue planes

small islands, clumps and glands of neoplastic cells of which some are vacuolated (intracytoplasmic mucin)

IMAGING

Mammo

discrete mass with variable edge

US

hypoechoic mass, may have increased through transmission

3.1.7 TUBULAR CARCINOMA

CLINICAL

rare

prognosis of pure tubular carcinoma very good

often multicentric

PATHOLOGY

neoplastic single cell layer tubules, with no myoepithelial cells

prominent stromal elastosis (mimics radial scar)

calcifications in about 50%

cribriform type DCIS common, LCIS may occur

IMAGING

Mammo

spiculated mass, may mimic radial scar

satellite/multicentric foci

may have malignant microcalcifications

3.1.8 PAPILLARY CARCINOMA

CLINICAL

uncommon (1–2%), older patient

slowly growing central mass, often with nipple discharge

PATHOLOGY

soft mass often inside a dilated duct or cyst

neoplastic epithelium forming papillary processes, no myoepithelial cells

IMAGING

Mammo

large well circumscribed subareolar mass

variable microcalcifications – malignant or may appear benign

US

complex cystic/solid mass, often a cyst with a solid intracystic component
may be entirely solid

3.1.9 CRIBRIFORM CARCINOMA

CLINICAL

uncommon (2–3%) but with excellent prognosis

PATHOLOGY

associated with well differentiated cribriform DCIS
stromal invasion recapitulates cribriform arrangement

IMAGING

no distinguishing features

3.1.10 ADENOID CYSTIC CARCINOMA

CLINICAL

rare, excellent prognosis

PATHOLOGY

histologically, same as adenoid cystic carcinoma of salivary glands (Ch 12)

IMAGING

no distinguishing features

3.1.11 INFLAMMATORY CARCINOMA (a special presentation)

CLINICAL

1% of breast carcinoma
presentation mimics mastitis
enlarged breast with erythema, skin edema (peau d'orange), skin thickening and increased warmth
usually no discrete mass
aggressive disease with very poor prognosis

PATHOLOGY

poorly differentiated invasive ductal carcinoma diffusely involving the breast
tumor cells in breast lymphatics and dermal breast lymphatics
reactive dermal inflammatory response
(not all inflammatory carcinoma has dermal lymphatic involvement, and dermal lymphatic involvement can occur without an 'inflammatory' presentation)

IMAGING

Mammo

cardinal sign is increased breast density and skin thickening in the absence of an explanatory history
often there is no mammographic (or palpable) mass
thickened breast trabeculae
may have scattered malignant type microcalcifications

3.1.12 PAGET'S DISEASE OF THE NIPPLE (a special presentation)

CLINICAL

uncommon presentation of carcinoma, with intraepithelial neoplastic extension to involve the nipple by large pale 'Paget's cells' with large nuclei
invariably, underlying DCIS (often comedo) with or without an invasive component; only half of patients have a palpable mass
red itchy 'eczematous' nipple with eventual nipple destruction

IMAGING

Mammo

often no abnormality
nipple and areolar thickening or microcalcification
may have an associated subareolar mass

3.2 BREAST RECONSTRUCTION (autologous)

variable amount of fat and soft tissue density (muscle) with possible fluid collections, clips and surgical scar

3.3 DUCT PAPILLOMA

benign solitary epithelial papilloma arising within a major duct and presenting with single duct discharge
two cell histology (epithelial and myoepithelial cells) around a fibrovascular core

IMAGING

Mammo

usually no findings
occasional mass or subareolar calcifications

US

dilated duct with homogenous intraductal mass

Ductography

duct obstruction by intraluminal mass (acute angles around mass)
intraductal mass without obstruction, duct dilation

3.4 DUCT PAPILLOMA MIMICKERS

3.4.1 PAPILLOMATOSIS

peripheral multiple intraductal papillomas
cellular atypia, tend to recur

3.4.2 INTRADUCTAL PAPILLARY HYPERPLASIA

epithelial hyperplasia, cellular atypia
papillary pattern

3.4.3 INTRADUCTAL PAPILLARY CARCINOMA

see its own entry
no fibrovascular core or myoepithelial cells

3.5 FAT NECROSIS

CLINICAL

post operative, post traumatic; resolution of hematoma by fat necrosis
acutely, often a mass with induration or bruising
slow transformation of mass/collection to retractile scar

PATHOLOGY

necrosis, oil cysts, dystrophic calcification, lipid laden macrophages, fibroblasts with fibrotic reaction

IMAGING

Mammo

EARLY

collection: discrete mass, isodense or denser than parenchyma with variable margins

more diffuse hemorrhage/necrosis: ill defined but focal increase in density

LATE

stellate mass with variable central density (fat density, lucent, isodense, denser than parenchyma)

variable amount of architectural distortion

may develop coarse macrocalcifications

OIL CYST: low density rounded mass; may have eggshell calcification

MAJOR DIFFERENTIALS are CARCINOMA (because of the mass and stellate fibrotic response) and SURGICAL SCAR (effectively, controlled trauma with some fat necrosis and prominent fibrotic reaction)

US

EARLY

collection of variable appearance: cystic, complex, hyperechoic

area of induration or altered echotexture without a collection

LATE

variable appearance hypoechoic mass with variable amount of tissue plane distortion and shadowing

oil cyst: cystic anechoic structure with posterior enhancement; occasionally internal echoes

3.6 FIBROADENOMA

DEFINITION

benign breast stromal neoplasm usually presenting as an isolated mass

CLINICAL

commonest benign breast mass (overall incidence up to 10% of breast masses)

younger patient (20–40 years old) but occurs at any age

small painless mass (1–4 cm), commonly multiple, occasionally painful or hormonally responsive

involutes with perimenopausal changes, and commonly calcifies ('popcorn' macrocalcification)

PATHOLOGY

intralobular stroma supplies clonal component; epithelial component is hormonally dependent; compressed surrounding breast tissue forms capsule

risk of malignancy increased by x2 for simple fibroadenomas, x4 for complex fibroadenomas with proliferative fibrocystic disease

Pericanalicular type (commonest)

intact glandular spaces, normal two cell epithelium

Intracanalicular type

glandular component compressed into cords by the stromal component

IMAGING

Mammo

discrete isodense or dense mass ('DIS') usually with a benign edge

may have gentle lobulation

coarse 'popcorn' macrocalcification (stromal calcification in involuting hyalinized fibroadenoma)

punctate microcalcification (epithelial calcification)

US

CLASSIC APPEARANCE

ovoid elongated mass, depth:width ratio <1

bright pseudocapsule or few gentle lobulations

distorts and displaces surrounding breast parenchyma, but does not disrupt or invade tissue planes

homogeneous hyperechoic, no posterior shadowing

VARIANTS

calcification with shadowing

cystic spaces

variable echogenicity, may be hypoechoic

complex internal structure (complex fibroadenoma)

3.7 FIBROCYSTIC CHANGE

GROUP DEFINITION

benign extremely common hormonally responsive proliferative/involutive heterogeneous change of breast parenchyma

GROUP EPIDEMIOLOGY

occurs in 30–50 year olds, most prominent in premenopausal 10 years

prominent histologic feature of breast parenchyma in 30% of population, minor feature in another 30%

single commonest cause of breast symptoms and breast 'lump' or 'lumpiness'

GROUP ETIOPATHOGENESIS

inappropriate patterns of growth and involution

more prevalent in high estrogen states, and hormonally responsive (?abnormal endorgan response)

less common with oral contraceptive use (?balanced estrogen and progesterone)

Components of fibrocystic change are:

GLANDULAR

involution

proliferation (non hyperplastic or hyperplastic)

STROMAL

fibroblast proliferation

myofibroblast proliferation

INFLAMMATORY

inflammatory cell infiltration, inflammation

MECHANICAL

obstruction

cyst formation

CLASSIFICATION/PATHOLOGY

With symptoms or signs or imaging findings

SIMPLE (no added risk of carcinoma)

FIBROSIS

stromal proliferation

ADENOSIS

glandular proliferation

glands back to back

CYSTIC CHANGE

mechanical obstruction of terminal ductal lobular unit (TDLU)

TDLUs unfolding into cysts

flat/cuboid/columnar epithelium lining cysts

apocrine metaplasia, papillary nodules

benign cells

INFLAMMATORY (no added risk of carcinoma)

DUCT ECTASIA

inspissated cheesy secretions

patchy focal wall destruction

patchy squamous metaplasia

PERIDUCTAL MASTITIS

leakage of secretions beyond ducts

lymphocytic, macrophage, fibroblastic and granulomatous response

PLASMA CELL MASTITIS

leakage of secretions beyond ducts

lymphocytic, macrophage, plasmacyte response

OBLITERATIVE MASTITIS

duct destruction, periductal fibrosis

SCLEROSING (x2 risk of developing carcinoma)

SCLEROSING ADENOSIS

stromal FIBROBLASTIC proliferation

adenosis with benign back to back glands

process lobulocentric

RADIAL SCAR

stromal MYOFIBROBLASTIC proliferation

elastin deposition (as in wound healing)

contraction, retraction, fibrosis

benign adenosis

COMPLEX SCLEROSING LESION

defined as radial scar of >1 cm in size

Without symptoms or signs; microcalcification only imaging finding

LOBULAR MICROCALCIFICATIONS

milk of calcium layering in dilated TDLUs

HYPERPLASIA (from no added risk to x5 risk of developing carcinoma)

INCREASED NUMBER OF CELLS ABOVE BASEMENT MEMBRANE

MAY BE DUCTAL OR LOBULAR

HYPERPLASIA WITHOUT ATYPIA (no added risk to x2 risk)

MILD

3–4 cells thick, no atypia

~70% of all hyperplasia, no added risk

MODERATE–SEVERE

cells fill ducts, bridge, swirl

~20% of all hyperplasia, carcinoma risk x2 (marker of increased risk, not a precursor)

HYPERPLASIA WITH ATYPIA (x5 relative risk of developing carcinoma, 10% of all hyperplasia)

absolute risk of developing carcinoma ? 10% in 15 years

DUCTAL HYPERPLASIA WITH ATYPIA

incomplete filling of ducts and no necrosis

spectrum with DCIS

lead time to carcinoma approx 8 years

LOBULAR HYPERPLASIA WITH ATYPIA

less than 50% fill-out of TDLU

spectrum with LCIS

lead time to carcinoma approx 12 years

3.7.1 CYSTS, CYSTIC CHANGE

Mammo

solitary mass or more commonly multiple masses

isodense, benign sharp margin unless overlapped or obscured by breast parenchyma

classically has 'halo' sign

cyst wall may calcify ('eggshell' calcification)

US

CLASSIC

anechoic rounded purely cystic structure with pencil thin margins and posterior acoustic enhancement

multiple

VARIANT

intracystic debris

thin septa (adjacent cysts squeezed together)

US ASPIRATION

if to dryness, no residual and no suspicious features, no fluid cytology

CYTOLOGY OR BIOPSY IF

atypical US or mammographic appearance

residual solid after aspiration

bloodstained fluid

3.7.2 LOBULAR MICROCALCIFICATIONS

Mammo ('benign lobular type microcalcifications')

homogeneous regular uniform rounded sharp edge or soft edge microcalcifications

classically, rounded in CC view and hemispheric (convex down) in true lateral view ('cups and saucers' sign)

scattered throughout breast parenchyma, frequently bilateral

may be clustered or solitary

NO malignant calcification features

3.7.3 ADENOSIS

Mammo

generalized patchy increase in breast parenchymal density without focal masses or architectural distortion has been called 'adenosis'

3.7.4 FIBROSIS

Mammo

mass of variable appearance (from discrete well circumscribed to stellate to non specific density)

may have coarse calcifications

US

hypoechoic mass

3.7.5 DUCT ECTASIA, PERIDUCTAL MASTITIS, PLASMA CELL MASTITIS, OBLITERATIVE MASTITIS

Mammo

tortuous subareolar ducts

ductal macrocalcification

intraductal macrocalcification: coarse elongated dense 'cigar' calcification following large subareolar ducts

periductal macrocalcification: coarse 'ring' en face, elongated 'cigar' in profile

usually bilateral and symmetrical

may branch (but MACROcalcification)

3.7.6 SCLEROSING ADENOSIS

Mammo

cluster of discrete pleomorphic microcalcifications

diffuse microcalcifications (but not 'cups and saucers' of lobular milk of calcium)

infrequently, an associated mass

3.7.7 RADIAL SCAR, COMPLEX SCLEROSING LESION

NOT a scar; usually impalpable

Mammo

DEFINITION: radial scar is <1 cm, complex sclerosing lesion is >1 cm

stellate abnormality with low density central area and long radiating spicules ('black star')

appearance varies between views, may only show well in one view (flat abnormality)

can not be differentiated from carcinoma on mammography alone

usually requires a full excisional biopsy for definitive histological diagnosis

3.7.8 DUCTAL HYPERPLASIA

Mammo

only finding (present in minority of ductal hyperplasia) is microcalcifications

microcalcifications similar to DCIS microcalcifications and form a spectrum linear, pleomorphic, clustered, irregular, angular, branching (casting)

3.8 GALACTOCELE

CLINICAL

collection of retained milk or related secretions, either in dilated lobule or secondary to extravasation during pregnancy or lactation; may only be intermittently present; often multiple

IMAGING

Mammo

variable density well circumscribed discrete mass(es)

true lateral view may show a fat–fluid level

US

well defined fluid collection

cardinal sign is a fluid–fluid level that shifts with shift in patient position (milk–fluid level), echogenic half above, hypoechoic or anechoic half below

aspiration returns milky fluid

3.9 GYNECOMASTIA

DEFINITION

physiological or pathological benign over-prominence of otherwise normal male breast glandular tissue and fat

CLINICAL

Physiological

very common in adolescence, and frequently bilateral but asymmetrical

presents with soft painless mass under nipple, mass is occasionally tender

proliferation of ducts, parenchyma and stroma

Pathological

HYPERESTROGENIC STATES

cirrhosis, liver failure (most commonly alcoholic)

estrogen therapy of prostate cancer

estrogen secreting tumors (e.g. testicular, adrenal)

anabolic steroids

HYPOANDROGENIC STATES

Klinefelter's syndrome

testicular failure

antiandrogenic therapy

IMAGING

particularly in adolescence gynecomastia is frequently asymmetrical

Mammo

prominent breast or breast 'mass' is composed of normal breast parenchyma and fat

US

normal but prominent breast tissue (same echotexture as in a female breast)

prominent subareolar ducts may be present

3.10 HORMONE REPLACEMENT THERAPY (HRT) EFFECTS

CLINICAL

HRT most commonly given postmenopausally for osteoporosis prevention

occasional other indications (post gonadal failure, pituitary failure, other)

IMAGING

Mammo

diffusely bilaterally increased breast density developing over months

no dominant mass or architectural distortion

asymmetrical densities may occur

cysts may develop

3.11 IMPLANTS

CLINICAL

two major indications: breast reconstruction post mastectomy and cosmetic augmentation

LOCATION: subpectoral (especially in reconstruction) or subglandular

eventually develop a surrounding host fibrous capsule (which may calcify)

Saline implants

silicone shell filled with saline

Silicone

single wall (silicone shell, silicone gel)

double wall (silicone shell, saline jacket, silicone shell, silicone gel)

single wall implants often develop small silicone gel 'bleeds' around them even when grossly intact, and may develop small silicone granulomas

free silicone lies outside the implant if ruptured:

INTRACAPSULAR RUPTURE

rupture of implant shell but host capsule intact

EXTRACAPSULAR RUPTURE

rupture of implant shell with no capsule or rupture of both implant shell and the capsule

free intramammary silicone, eventual silicone uptake in regional lymph nodes

Free silicone injections

blebs of silicone injected into breast tissue

usually leads to an inflammatory response with eventual fibrosis

IMAGING

Mammo

SCREENING VIEWS

disclaimer: cosmetic prostheses reduce sensitivity of screening mammography by obscuring breast parenchyma

compression is limited compared to normal breast

implant is a homogeneous rounded dense mass (if double wall, the outer saline jacket is lower density)

implant wall often has 'wrinkles'

host capsule may have eggshell calcification

intracapsular rupture: no findings

extracapsular rupture: silicone outside of capsule

free silicone looks like multiple rounded dense masses obscuring breast parenchyma, with or without calcification

implant cavity post implant removal is an irregular area of architectural distortion and calcification where the host capsule has collapsed

EKLUND VIEWS

'milking' breast parenchyma forwards over the prosthesis

allows more glandular tissue to be imaged separately

US

prosthesis appears as an anechoic space, may have reverberation

old silicone has internal echoes

capsular fibrosis is bright

leakage of silicone appears as a cystic space

silicone granuloma forms a variable mass

free silicone injection – 'snowstorm'

intracapsular rupture: folded wall floating within silicone gel usually inside host capsule (ultrasound 'linguine' sign)

MR

saline has fluid signal

silicone gel is bright on T1W and T2W sequences

at 1.5T silicon is 70 Hz off resonance from fat

silicone gel bleed (with intact implant shell) fills in the 'wrinkles' ('keyhole' sign)

intracapsular rupture: ruptured implant wall appears as folded or crumpled line inside the gel (MR 'linguine' sign)

3.12 LACTATION EFFECTS

IMAGING

Mammo

'active breast'

diffusely bilaterally massively increased breast density

expansion of parenchymal component, obscuration of fat

dilated subareolar ducts

galactoceles, small oil cysts

3.13 LIPOMA, HAMARTOMA

3.13.1 LIPOMA

CLINICAL

focal benign fatty mass composed of mature adipocytes

IMAGING

Mammo

well circumscribed fat density mass

US

may not be visible separately from breast fat

fat echogenicity well circumscribed mass

3.13.2 HAMARTOMA
(fibroadenolipoma)

CLINICAL

benign hamartomatous focal mass composed of normal breast elements; variable amount of encapsulation on histology

may present as a palpable mass

MAMMO

well encapsulated area of normal glandular parenchyma and normal fat, separate from the rest of the breast

US

usually indistinguishable from normal breast tissue

3.14 MALE BREAST CANCER

CLINICAL

uncommon, often over 60 years old

tends to present early with a mass

most are invasive ductal carcinoma NOS

early lymphatic and systemic spread, with early skin and pectoralis involvement

IMAGING

Mammo

discrete mass or stellate mass

malignant microcalcifications

same mammographic findings as in a female

US

same malignant characteristics as in a female

3.15 MAMMARY LYMPH NODES

CLINICAL

totally normal finding; axillary or intramammary nodes (more common in upper outer breast)

enlarged for the same reasons as anywhere else in the body (malignancy, inflammation)

may mimic mass or cyst

IMAGING

Mammo

normal: soft tissue density kidney shaped discrete mass with a fatty hilum

pathological: enlarged, rounded, with loss of hilum

US

normal: well circumscribed hypoechoic mass with a fatty hilum

pathological: more hypoechoic, enlarged, rounded with loss of hilum and perhaps hypervascular on color Doppler

3.16 MASTITIS/BREAST ABSCESS

CLINICAL

focal pyogenic infection of breast, usually ascending along a duct, eventually leading to abscess formation

common in breast feeding

pain, redness, swelling, discharge

IMAGING

Mammo

may have no findings

pain usually limits compression

diffuse edema, thickened parenchyma

variably well defined mass (depending on degree of fibrosis)

US

normal

diffusely altered echotexture

focal complex cystic/solid mass of variable appearance

abscess: focal fluid collection with posterior acoustic enhancement and with variable amount of echogenic debris

3.17 PHYLLODES TUMOR

DEFINITION

stromal tumor of low malignant potential usually presenting as a large rapidly growing mass

CLINICAL

older patient than for fibroadenoma (usually 40–50 years old), but clinically indistinguishable

~15% have aggressive behavior: local recurrence, hematogenous metastases (lymphatic spread rare)

PATHOLOGY

intralobular stroma supplies clonal component

gray-yellow mass with areas of cystic or occasionally necrotic change

leaf like pattern with nodules protruding into cystic spaces

low grade tumor microscopically similar to fibroadenoma, high grade tumor merges into undifferentiated soft tissue sarcoma

IMAGING

Mammo
discrete mass

US
hypoechoic well marginated mass
may have cystic spaces

3.18 RADIOTHERAPY CHANGE

CLINICAL

usually given following partial mastectomy, and so superimposed on surgical change

occasionally given alone or as neoadjuvant therapy

edema, swelling, thickening of skin, tenderness, redness

changes worst at 6 months, and slowly subsiding over 18 months to 2 years

IMAGING

Mammo
skin thickening
diffusely increased breast density
thickened breast trabeculae

3.19 SURGICAL CHANGE

3.19.1 BREAST REDUCTION SURGERY

CLINICAL

classically, a T incision (below the breast with the stem of the T extending to nipple)

variable amount of breast tissue removed

IMAGING

Mammo
bilateral variably symmetrical change
reduced amount of breast parenchyma in non anatomical locations
long surgical scars often extending to nipple area
dystrophic calcifications, oil cysts

3.19.2 SURGICAL SCAR

CLINICAL

usual seen on screening or diagnostic mammo following excisional biopsy of a mass

other circumstances are following abscess drainage or other general surgical intervention

compression is usually limited by pain in the first weeks or months

RECOMMENDATIONS FOR IMAGING FOLLOWUP

early baseline at 6 months: screening mammograms, two compression magnification views with markers on skin scar (compression as tolerated) to establish baseline

may have a baseline US

surgical changes usually most marked around 6 months and slowly subside, retract or involute after that; scars do not enlarge after 12 months

return to screening as appropriate for benign or malignant nature of excisional biopsy or partial mastectomy specimen

IMAGING

Mammo
in many cases, no findings

hematoma/seroma/fat necrosis/oil cyst at surgery site

hematoma and seroma: discrete soft tissue mass that slowly resorbs over weeks to months and develops surrounding fibrosis

fat necrosis and oil cyst: fat density containing mass that slowly shrinks and may turn into a pure oil cyst (often with eggshell calcification)

reduced breast volume

architectural distortion centered on scar (breast tissue scar, not skin scar)

developing stellate mass or stellate shape without appreciable mass (should retract and shrink from ~6 months on, not grow)

collections/hematomas slowly shrink and are replaced by scarring over 6 to 12 months

sutural calcifications

macroscopic dystrophic calcifications (may be eggshell in oil cyst wall)

pleomorphic microcalcification generally viewed with suspicion, especially if a DCIS component was present pre-excision

US
in many cases, no findings

interstitial fluid or mixed fluid–solid collection in surgical bed, slowly evolving and shrinking

established scar has architectural distortion and may shadow without appreciable mass

General pathology, PET and nuclear medicine, exam techniques

POSITRON EMISSION TOMOGRAPHY

1. PET BASIC CHEMISTRY AND TRACER BIOLOGY

1.1 F-18 CHEMISTRY

F-18 is cyclotron produced, with half life of 110 min (target contains O-18 water)
Transportation of either FDG or F- is feasible within a 2 hour travel time radius

F-18 based tracers

FLUORIDE (F-)
see below

FLUORODEOXYGLUCOSE (FDG)
see below

FLUOROMETHYLTYROSINE (FMT) AND FLUOROETHYLTYROSINE (FET)
related metabolism markers likely to be the next oncological imaging tracer
distribution is similar to FDG, but there is only low grade brain and myocardial uptake
tumor avidity similar to FDG, with marginally lower sensitivity but much better specificity

FLUOROMISONIDAZOLE (FMISO)
hypoxia marker currently used in clinical trials

1.2 F-18 FLUORIDE KINETICS

F- has analogous kinetics and distribution to MDP but allows higher resolution tomographic skeletal imaging
if a small amount of F- is administered with FDG, the skeleton can be used for anatomical localization or co-registration (but may make bone marrow metastases invisible)

1.3 F-18 FLUORO-DEOXYGLUCOSE (FDG) KINETICS AND DISTRIBUTION

FDG biological behavior

FDG is an imperfect glucose analog
taken up by glucose transporters (Glut 1 to Glut 5)
trapped in the cytoplasm after hexokinase or glucokinase phosphorylation

Glucose transporters
Glut 1 insulin independent: tumor
Glut 3 insulin independent: brain
Glut 4 insulin dependent: muscle and myocardium
FDG uptake is competitively inhibited by glucose (hence poor images in hyperglycemia)
FDG is excreted in urine as a result of glomerular filtration followed by incomplete proximal convoluted tubular resorption
tissues with low levels of glucose 6 phosphatase (myocardium, brain; some tumors) accumulate FDG in proportion to their rate of glycolysis
tissues with high levels of glucose 6 phosphatase (liver, kidney, intestine, muscle) have lower FDG activity with increasing time after administration due to tissue clearance

Mechanism of increased tumoral FDG uptake

older theory: inefficient metabolism with greater uptake of glucose compared to utilization; possibly increased anaerobic metabolism compared to aerobic metabolism
newer theory: upregulation of insulin independent glucose receptors (particularly Glut 1); this may be linked to hypoxia and be mediated through oncogene expression

Normal F-18 FDG distribution

BRAIN (gray matter > white matter)
cerebral cortex, basal ganglia, thalami, cerebellar cortex and deep gray nuclei; less so brainstem; less so white matter
spinal cord

NORMAL HEAD AND NECK UPTAKE IN:
extraocular muscles
oral and nasal mucosa
airway maintenance by genioglossus and pharyngeal muscles

larynx if patient has been speaking
accessory muscles of respiration (muscle relaxant should be used to minimize this)

MYOCARDIUM (variably, depending on glucose and insulin levels and metabolic status)
left ventricle uptake variable
right ventricle uptake usually faintly visible

BLOOD POOL (low grade)
if blood is aspirated back into the FDG syringe and allowed to incubate, RBC may become selectively labeled with FDG resulting in increased blood pool activity

BOWEL
(stomach; gastroesophageal junction; cecum, colon and rectum – all low grade linear, may have a lumen)

LIVER
low to moderate grade uniform

SPLEEN
low grade uniform
(less than liver)

MUSCLE AND SOFT TISSUE
low grade (at rest; it is increased post exertion or if the patient is active during the uptake period)

URINARY
renal pelves, bladder (unless washed out with diuretic)

TESTES

CHILDREN
normal lymphoid tissue (e.g. adenoids) – low grade; metaphyseal growth plates – regular and low grade

LACTATING BREAST AND POSTPARTUM UTERUS

Methods of regulating FDG uptake

increased myocardial FDG uptake can be achieved by insulin administration (and concurrent glucose administration to prevent hypoglycemia: 'hyperinsulinemic euglycemic clamp')
cerebral uptake is decreased by sedatives
skeletal muscle uptake is decreased by muscle relaxants (e.g. diazepam)
fasting ensures no hyperglycemia is present and competitive inhibition by glucose is minimal
diuretic (usually with a catheter) decreases urinary FDG activity
in general, insulin administration to decrease glucose levels increases glucose

and FDG uptake in skeletal muscle, fat and soft tissue and may lead to less uptake in tumor (and hence lower tumor conspicuity)

Difference between attenuation corrected and non attenuation corrected images

NON ATTENUATION CORRECTED IMAGES

marked attenuation of deep structures (more than intuitively expected) because both photons need to be registered for an event to be recorded

diffuse very low grade lung activity visible; better accuracy of detection of very small or low grade lung uptake

skin shows linear low grade activity, and two layers of skin (e.g. axillary fold) may simulate a mass

ATTENUATION CORRECTED IMAGES

lungs show low activity (relative to mediastinum)

uniform soft tissue uptake with depth

skin edge invisible

movement between transmission and emission maps may manifest as abnormally hot edge on one side of the image and abnormally cold edge on the opposite side

SUV calculation

SUV: STANDARDIZED UPTAKE VALUE

a semiquantitative measure of regional FDG uptake normalized for injected dose and patient size

SUV = RC/(given dose/patient weight)

where RC is regional FDG concentration (in activity per unit volume, such as Bq/ml) corrected for decay

patient weight is used as a close approximation of total body distribution volume

SUV is most commonly corrected for weight, but may be corrected for body surface area or lean body mass

whole body SUV is 1 by definition

SUV of resting muscle and soft tissue is ~0.8

SUV of blood pool is 1–2

SUV of liver is 2–3

malignant SUV is usually taken to be greater than 2–3

2. FLUORODEOXYGLUCOSE GAMUTS

2.1 GENERIC

2.1.1 ABNORMAL DIFFUSELY INCREASED UPTAKE OF FDG

Diffuse tumor infiltration

Diffuse inflammation

e.g. PERITONITIS, PNEUMONIA, RETROPERITONEAL FIBROSIS

Post radiation change

CHARACTERISTIC PLEURALLY BASED LINEAR UPTAKE AND/OR ESOPHAGEAL LINEAR UPTAKE

Post chemotherapy or bone marrow transplant bone marrow activation

DIFFUSELY INCREASED UPTAKE IN RED MARROW AREAS OR BONE MARROW EXPANSION PATTERN

Large postoperative area

e.g. FLAP OR SKIN GRAFT SITE

Paget's disease

DIFFUSE UPTAKE IN THE AREA OF INVOLVEMENT

2.1.2 ABNORMAL FOCAL UPTAKE OF FDG WHICH IS NOT A TUMOR

Focal muscular activity

most severe if the muscle is exercised during the FDG uptake period, but elevated uptake persists for some hours after exercise

EXTRAOCULAR MUSCLES: NORMAL

LARYNX: TALKING

PARASPINAL MUSCLES, NECK MUSCLES: TENSION

ACCESSORY MUSCLES OF RESPIRATION AND DIAPHRAGMATIC CRURA: COAD/COPD

GLUTEI/QUADRICEPS FEMORIS: WALKED AFTER FDG INJECTION

DELTOIDS, PECTORALS: CARRYING A LOAD, ETC

Granulomatous inflammation

SARCOIDOSIS

Other inflammation

ACUTE PANCREATITIS

ACTIVE ARTHRITIS

RESORBING HEMATOMA

Infection

PNEUMONIA

ABSCESS

GRANULOMATOUS INFECTION

TB, MAC

FUNGAL INFECTION (esp histoplasmosis)

Urinary

PROMINENT CALYX

DIVERTICULUM (calyceal or bladder)

URINARY CONTAMINATION

REFLUX INTO VAGINA

URINARY DIVERSION SURGERY

e.g. ILEAL CONDUIT

Surgical

HEALING SURGICAL WOUND

HEALING FRACTURE

COLOSTOMY, ILEOSTOMY

permanent, mildly elevated uptake

Hyperplasia or metabolically active tissue

GRAVES' DISEASE

LACTATING BREAST

2.1.3 FALSE NEGATIVE PET SCAN

Small volume tumor

count recovery is incomplete below ~2 full width half maximums of the camera

small volume tumor becomes averaged with counts from surrounding normal tissue

this is most prominent in lung; for lung masses, negative FDG scan with size <1–1.5 cm should be treated with caution

Relatively low glucose avidity tumor

prostate

carcinoid
well differentiated malignancy

FDG avid tumor hidden by urine

transitional cell carcinoma
renal cell carcinoma
cervical carcinoma (bladder)

Moderately FDG avid tumor in FDG avid normal tissue

low grade glioma
moderately differentiated hepatocellular carcinoma

Treated tumor

metabolic true negative!

2.1.4 POOR FDG INTENSITY CONTRAST ('poor quality scan')

Patient related

OBESITY
HYPERGLYCEMIA
INSUFFICIENT UPTAKE TIME
OVERDELAYED SCAN

Scanner related

INCORRECT ENERGY WINDOWS
INCORRECT TRANSMISSION SCAN
MISREGISTRATION PROBLEMS

Injection related

TISSUED DOSE

SINGLE PHOTON NUCLEAR MEDICINE

3. NUCLEAR MEDICINE BASIC PHYSICS

3.1 ABBREVIATIONS

A: atomic mass (number of protons and neutrons)
Gy: Gray (mGy: milliGray)
mCi: milliCurie
MBq: MegaBecquerel
Sv: Sievert (mSv: milliSievert)
T 1/2: half-life (in units of time)
Z: atomic number (number of protons)

3.2 RADIOACTIVE DECAY FORMULAS

THE ONLY FORMULA THAT EVER NEEDS TO BE REMEMBERED

$A(t) = A(0)*e^{[(-0.693/\text{half-life})*t]}$
where: A(0) is initial activity, A(t) is activity at time t later, e is 2.71828 (Euler's number), and half-life is expressed in the same time units as time t

3.3 CONVERSIONS

CURIE/BECQUEREL

1 milliCurie (mCi) = 3.7×10^7 disintegrations per second

1 MegaBecquerel (MBq) = 1×10^6 disintegrations per second
1 mCi = 37 MBq
1 MBq = 0.027 mCi

RAD/REM/GRAY/SIEVERT

1 Gray (Gy) = 100 rad
1 rad = 10 milliGray (mGy)
1 Sievert (Sv) = 100 rem
1 rem = 10 milliSievert (mSv)
NOTE: 1 Sievert (Sv) is numerically equal to 1 Gray, but used in description of equivalent dose (i.e. measure of overall radiation burden to the entire organism); 1 rem (Roentgen equivalent man) is numerically equal to 1 rad, but used in the description of equivalent dose

3.4 NUCLIDES IN COMMON MEDICAL USE

Nuclide	T 1/2	Decay	Photon keV (RELATIVE ABUNDANCE %)	Produced in
Diagnostic				
Tc-99m	6 hr	isomeric	140 (89%)	Generator (Mo-99)
I-123	13.2 hr	electron capture	159 (83%)	Accelerator
Ga-67	78.3 hr	electron capture	93 (37%), 185 (20%), 300 (17%)	Accelerator
Tl-201	73.1 hr	electron capture	X-rays of 69-83 keV; 135 (2.5%), 167 (10%)	Accelerator
In-111	2.8 days	electron capture	171 (90%), 245 (94%)	Accelerator
Xe-127	36 days	electron capture	172 (26%), 203 (7%), 375 (17%)	Accelerator
Cr-51	28 days	electron capture	320 (9%)	Accelerator
Se-75	120 days	electron capture	121 (17%), 136 (59%), 265 (59%), 280 (25%)	Accelerator
I-131	8 days	beta minus	364 (81%)	Reactor
Therapeutic				
I-131	8 days	beta minus	364 (81%); therapeutic beta 0.606 meV	Reactor
Sr-89	51 days	beta minus	no gammas; therapeutic beta 1.463 meV	Reactor
Sm-153	46.7 hr	beta minus	103 (29%); therapeutic beta 640, 710, 810 keV	Reactor
Y-90	64.1 hr	beta minus	no gammas; therapeutic beta up to 2.3 meV	Reactor

3.5 DECAY MODES
(overview)

ISOMERIC TRANSITION

high energy of nucleus is released as a characteristic photon with nucleus reaching a stable configuration without a change in A or Z

Example: Tc-99m
half-life 6.01 hours

generated by saline elution of a Mo-99 column which beta minus decays with half-life of 66 hours to Tc-99m

time from elution to next maximum yield is 23 hours (result of the combination of parent and daughter decays)

decay: isomeric transition to Tc-99 (half life 2 x 10^5 years) with characteristic gamma photon of 140.5 keV 89% of the time (remainder is internal conversion)

no particulate emissions from the nucleus (internal conversion produces low energy electrons)

low radiation burden: gamma photon and low relative abundance of ejected electrons

ELECTRON CAPTURE

heavy (high Z, protons in excess) nuclei 'engulf' a low energy orbital electron, with one proton converted to one neutron (Z:A to Z-1:A) and overall mass number unchanged

excess nuclear energy released as characteristic gamma photons; as orbital electrons fill the empty shell, excess energy is released as X-rays (orbital photons) or Auger electrons (ejected orbital low energy electrons)

Example: Tl-201
half-life 73.1 hours

decays by electron capture to Hg-201 (stable)

low relative abundance gamma photons not sufficient for imaging

characteristic orbital electron X-rays ('mercury X-rays') in the 69–83 keV are used for imaging, but undergo significant attenuation

moderately high radiation burden: Auger electrons ejected

BETA MINUS DECAY

heavy (high Z, neutrons in excess) nuclei convert one neutron to one proton, with a high energy electron ejected from the nucleus (beta minus particle) and excess energy released as characteristic gamma photons; other emissions may also occur (i.e. Auger electrons, X-rays)

Example: I-131
half-life 8 days

decays by beta minus decay to Xe-131 (stable); characteristic gamma photon of 364 keV (relative abundance 81%) is higher than optimal for single photon imaging

the nuclear electron is energetic, and deposits considerable energy as it slows down

high radiation burden, primarily from the electron; used in therapy with I-123 preferred diagnostic nuclide based on radiation dosimetry

POSITRON ('BETA PLUS') DECAY

light (low Z, protons in excess) nuclei convert one proton to a neutron, with a high energy positron ejected from the nucleus

the positron travels a variable distance before slowing down (average travel radius depends on characteristic energy of the positron)

once sufficiently slow to interact with other particles, it annihilates with any electron releasing two 511 keV photons at (nearly) 180 degrees

Example: F-18
half-life 110 min

decays by positron decay to O-18 (stable) with a 0.635 meV positron, which has a maximal range in soft tissue of 2.4 mm

3.6 NUCLEAR MEDICINE STUDIES IN PREGNANCY AND BREAST FEEDING

PREGNANCY

only study performed with reasonable frequency is V/Q scanning (there should be no known intracardiac or intrapulmonary shunt in the mother)

dose to fetus is less than 1 mSv at half doses of ventilation and perfusion agents (Technegas and MAA)

all other studies should only be performed after dose to the fetus is estimated and the potential risk to fetus against benefit to fetus and mother is assessed

as a general rule, no nuclear medicine studies (other than V/Q scanning) are performed in pregnancy

I-131 IN PREGNANCY IS AN ABSOLUTE CONTRAINDICATION

even small doses of I-131 can result in ablative doses to the fetal thyroid

pregnancy test for all females of reproductive age who are to have I-131 scanning is recommended

BREAST FEEDING

Stop for 4 hours
Cr-51 EDTA; Tc-99m IDA and derivatives; Tc-99m DMSA, DTPA, HMPAO, sestamibi, phosphonates; In-111 white cells; F-18 FDG

Stop for 12 hours
Tc-99m MAA, red cells, white cells, MAG3, Technegas

Stop for 24 hours
Tc-99m pertechnetate (thyroid dose), I-123 iodide or MIBG, Tl-201

Stop completely
I-131, I-131 MIBG, Ga-67

26 General pathology

1. CELL INJURY AND DEATH

1.1 CELL INJURY AND DEATH

MORPHOLOGY OF CELL INJURY

Cellular edema

POTENTIALLY REVERSIBLE CHANGE

dropping ATP levels, anerobic glycolysis, dropping pH, Na/K pump failure, cellular edema, dispersal of ribosomes

IRREVERSIBLE CHANGE

mitochondrial swelling and membrane disruption

nuclear chromatin autolysis, cytoskeletal destruction

reperfusion injury: free oxygen radicals and intracellular calcium flux

total loss of cell membrane integrity, extracellular flux of enzymes

Fatty change

liver, less commonly kidney, heart

failure of fatty acid oxidation and metabolism but preserved fatty acid uptake

accumulation of intracellular triglycerides

MORPHOLOGY OF CELL DEATH

morphology of cell death depends on the time elapsed since irreversible cellular damage

in biopsy specimens morphological changes continue until histological fixation

Autolysis

autodigestion by enzymes contained within the dead cell

nuclear pyknosis and fragmentation, cytoplasmic eosinophilia

Apoptosis (programmed cell death)

programmed active cell death as part of normal tissue remodelling and cell population turnover; also may occur with viral infections; postulated failure occurs in neoplasia

compared to cell death from injury, apoptosis is very fast (1–2 hours) and does not produce secondary inflammation

1.2 TISSUE NECROSIS PATTERNS

COAGULATIVE NECROSIS

result of ischemic hypoxia (except CNS)

cell death with preservation of structural proteins; 'ghost' cells in preserved tissue architecture

the macroscopic equivalent is the bland (non hemorrhagic) infarct

LIQUEFACTIVE NECROSIS

cell death followed by autolysis and tissue digestion by lysosomal enzymes

bland CNS infarcts, superinfected necrotic tissue; semiliquid featureless material

CASEOUS NECROSIS

typically occurs in tuberculous infection ('crumbly white cheese')

coagulative necrosis with complete loss of identifiable cell and tissue outlines

FAT NECROSIS

fatty acids released from dead adipocytes (trauma, pancreatitis) precipitate as hard white calcium soaps

FIBRINOID NECROSIS

occurs in autoimmune vasculitides/immune complex disease

eosinophilic necrosis of blood vessel wall with immunoglobulin, fibrin and complement precipitation

1.3 EFFECTS OF RADIATION

DETERMINISTIC EFFECTS OF RADIATION

Definition

severity of effect increases with dose and is predictable; reflects cell death in actively dividing cell populations

Whole body effective dose

1 Sievert

sublethal dose

transient bone marrow suppression and lymphopenia

transient nausea and vomiting

temporary sterility

5 Sievert

usually a lethal dose

bone marrow death

radiation enteritis

permanent sterility

lens cataracts

10 Sievert

lethal dose

bone marrow death, pancytopenia

extensive loss of bowel epithelium

acute radiation pneumonitis

dry skin desquamation

death of bone marrow failure and electrolyte disturbances within 2 weeks

100 Sievert

acutely lethal dose

acute cerebral edema and death

STOCHASTIC EFFECTS OF RADIATION

Definition

severity of effect is independent of dose; **probability** increases with dose; reflects sublethal DNA damage with effects on cell growth and replication

Recognized stochastic effects

CARCINOGENESIS

HERITABLE GENETIC DEFECTS

EMBRYONAL TERATOGENESIS

ICRP 60 ORGAN WEIGHTING FOR DETERMINING EFFECTIVE DOSE

represents relative contribution of different organs to the overall lifetime risk of stochastic effects

the effective dose from selective irradiation of specific organs is the absorbed dose multiplied by the weighting; the integral of uniform dose to all body organs is 1 by definition

because the ICRP carcinogenesis model is multiplicative, organ weighting factors reflect the current prevalence of common malignancies

Organ or tissue	Weighting factor
gonads	0.20
red bone marrow, stomach, lung, colon	0.12
bladder, breast, liver, esophagus, thyroid, 'tissue not otherwise specified'	0.05
bone surface (i.e. periosteum), skin	0.01

PRINCIPLES OF PROTECTION FOR DIAGNOSTIC USE OF RADIATION (ICRP 60)

Non diagnostic background radiation levels are 2–3 mSv per year, and greater at high altitudes

EXAMPLES OF DOSES

Examination	Effective dose (mSv): this has wide variation!
CXR	0.01
PELVIS XR or ABDO XR or LUMBAR SPINE SERIES	0.4–1
CHEST CT or ABDO CT or PELVIS CT (very factor dependent)	6–10
HEAD CT	2
MAMMOGRAPHY	0.1, but breast dose is 1–2 mSv
TI MYOCARDIAL PERFUSION SCAN, Tc MYOCARDIAL PERFUSION SCAN	20–25 (Tl); 8 (Tc)
Tc BONE SCAN	8
Ga SCAN (dose varies)	10–20
I-131 THYROID SCAN	360
F-18 FDG SCAN (dose varies)	2–10

Medical exposure guidelines

no dose limits prescribed; each episode judged on its own merits to yield net benefit

Occupational exposure guidelines

RECOMMENDED LIMIT
'barely tolerable' limit: 20 mSv per year effective dose, averaged over 5 years, and no greater than 50 mSv in any one year

SPECIFIC TISSUE LIMITS ARE:
ocular lens 150 mSv per year (threshold for cataracts is 2 Sv)
hands 500 mSv per year
for a pregnant radiation worker, same limits apply to fetus as to any member of public: 2 mSv per year; principal requirement is minimization of the risk of accidental large exposure

Exposure in emergencies
aim: to prevent deterministic effects
limits: effective dose 0.5 Sv, skin equivalent dose 5 Sv

EFFECTS OF RADIATION ON EMBRYO AND FETUS

Gestational age (LMP)	Embryonal stage	Effect	Spontaneous rate in the non irradiated
0–4 weeks	preimplantation	either cell death or no effect at all	
4–10 weeks	early organogenesis	malformations (100 mSv)	~5%
10–17 weeks	late organogenesis	loss of 30 IQ points per Sv	IQ <70 (2 SD) occurs in 1%
17–27 weeks	late organogenesis	lower risk of mental deficit	

POSSIBLE GROWTH RETARDATION WITH DOSE >200 mSv
INCIDENCE OF CHILDHOOD MALIGNANCY (ESPECIALLY LEUKEMIA) ~0.03–0.1 per Sv

NOTE that no effects are expected in the preimplantation period other than subclinical death of any fertilized zygote, not different in character from spontaneous death of a fertilized zygote
THEREFORE no basis exists for different treatment of reproductive age females provided no menstrual periods have been missed
EXCEPTION is I-131, where the risk of severe fetal detriment in the event of accidentally or deliberately misleading patient history is sufficient to recommend confirmation of non pregnant status using beta hCG level

2. NEOPLASIA

2.1 GROWTH PATTERNS

PHYSIOLOGICAL OR PATHOLOGICAL GROWTH PATTERNS

Change in cell size
ATROPHY

HYPERTROPHY

Change in cell number
INVOLUTION, APOPTOSIS

HYPERPLASIA

Change in differentiation lineage
METAPLASIA

PATHOLOGICAL ONLY GROWTH PATTERNS

Dysplasia
abnormal proliferation beyond physiological needs

ultrastructural and cytological premalignant features

not neoplastic by definition, may be reversible

merges into carcinoma in situ

Neoplasia
abnormal proliferation in absence of stimulus or after cessation of stimulus

ultrastructural and cytological premalignant or malignant features

limited or absent response to external control

BENIGN (no capacity to invade, expansile growth)

MALIGNANT (capacity to invade, infiltrative growth)

2.2 TUMOR CHARACTERISTICS

ULTRASTRUCTURAL

altered genome (losses, incorporation)
oncogene expression and amplification
aneuploidy
abnormal tumor products
loss of differentiated organelles

CYTOLOGICAL

nuclear pleomorphism and atypia
increased nuclear–cytoplasmic ratio and hyperchromasia
mitoses and atypical mitoses
cellular pleomorphism and atypia
dedifferentiation of cell appearance

HISTOLOGICAL

cellular pleomorphism
loss of cell polarity and orientation
loss of cell adhesion and stratification
invasion and spread
tumor angiogenesis

3. INFLAMMATION

3.1 ACUTE INFLAMMATION

DEFINITION

first line circulatory and phagocytic response to tissue injury

CLINICAL MANIFESTATIONS

tumor et rubor cum
color et dolor
(and loss of function)

VASCULAR RESPONSE

vasodilation and increased vascular permeability (either controlled endothelial response or endothelial loss)
passage of plasma proteins (including immunoglobulins, complement, etc) into the interstitial compartment
increased interstitial oncotic pressure with water accumulation

PHAGOCYTIC RESPONSE

margination, extravasation and chemotactic migration of white blood cells (first line – neutrophils; second line – macrophages)
recognition of 'foreign' or 'injurious' entity, phagocytosis
bacterial killing by lysosomal enzymes and peroxide ('respiratory burst')
extracellular release of inflammatory mediators, lytic enzymes, peroxide

BYSTANDER INJURY

release of neutrophil or macrophage enzymes and free radicals
cell damage by inflammatory mediators
immune complex deposition
thrombosis

OUTCOMES OF ACUTE INFLAMMATION

Resolution
complete restoration of normal tissue architecture and function

Regeneration
preservation of stromal 'scaffolding'
clearance of inflammatory exudate and dead cells
parenchymal repopulation by cell division

Healing by organization and scarring
failure of clearance of inflammatory exudate or necrotic tissue
vascular ingrowth, then fibrovascular granulation tissue, then fibrous organization, finally collagenous scar

Conversion to chronic inflammation

3.2 CHRONIC INFLAMMATION

DEFINITION

inflammation of prolonged duration with coexistent processes of tissue destruction, inflammatory response and healing; by definition, granulomatous inflammation is chronic (see its own entry)

INITIATION

Conversion from acute
persistence of abnormal stimulus (e.g. foreign body, TB)
abnormal host (e.g. immune suppression, congenital neutrophil deficits)

privileged location (e.g. around a prosthesis, ischemic tissue)

abnormal autoimmune response

Chronic ab initio

stimulus incites lymphocytic not neutrophil response

lymphocytic autoimmune response

INFLAMMATORY CELLS

Macrophages

bacterial kill, or bacterial kill following immune activation (e.g. TB)

immune role: antigen presenting cell, secretes cytokines and inflammatory mediators

Lymphocytes, plasma cells

Fibroblasts

local tissue fibroblasts activated by macrophage cytokines

reparatory and granulation response

OUTCOMES OF CHRONIC INFLAMMATION

Clearance of stimulus and healing by scar

Autoimmune chronic inflammation – persistence

Balance between host and stimulus – persistence

3.3 GRANULOMATOUS INFLAMMATION

DEFINITION

a granuloma is a focal collection of mononuclear cells

GRANULOMA CLASSIFICATION

Non immune granulomas

non activated macrophages, foreign body giant cells, fibroblasts, minimal lymphocytes and plasma cells

NON TOXIC FOREIGN MATERIAL

plastic particles, carbon particles, sutures, silicone

Fe, Al

NON TOXIC ENDOGENOUS MATERIAL

necrotic bone, urate tophi, keratin

TOXIC FOREIGN MATERIAL (leads to macrophage death)

silica, asbestos fibers, talc powder

Immune granulomas

activated and non activated macrophages, immune activated giant cells, lymphocytes, plasma cells, fibroblasts

require intact cell mediated immunity (i.e. do not occur in advanced immune deficiency)

require induction of the immune response (i.e. do not occur with first exposure of naive host)

INFECTIVE IMMUNE GRANULOMAS

INTRACELLULAR ORGANISMS

tuberculosis/non tuberculous mycobacteria (MAC)

leprosy

syphilis

sarcoidosis (?virus?)

FUNGI

cryptococcus

histoplasmosis

aspergillosis

PARASITES (with eosinophilia)

schistosomiasis

leishmaniasis

cutaneous candidiasis

HYPERIMMUNE GRANULOMAS

HAPTENS

Zr, Be

Nickel (skin)

ORGANIC ALLERGENS

hypersensitivity pneumonitis

allergic sinonasal aspergillosis

AUTOIMMUNE

Wegener's granulomatosis

Crohn's disease

sarcoidosis

rheumatoid arthritis

3.4 HYPERSENSITIVITY REACTIONS

TYPE I

ATOPIC/ANAPHYLACTOID/ANAPHYLACTIC REACTIONS

excessive IgE secretion directed at a foreign antigen (usually incidental and harmless)

binding of presynthesized IgE to tissue mast cells

mast cell degranulation following exposure to the antigen, with secretion of leukotrienes and prostaglandins

LOCAL TYPE I HYPERSENSITIVITY: ATOPIC REACTIONS

SYSTEMIC TYPE I HYPERSENSITIVITY: ANAPHYLACTOID OR ANAPHYLACTIC REACTIONS

TYPE II

DIRECT CYTOTOXIC REACTIONS

autoantibody mediated, often with involvement of cell mediated immunity

lead to death of the involved cells

EXAMPLES: immune hemolysis; some drug mediated autoimmunity

TYPE III

IMMUNE COMPLEX DISEASE

in conditions where there is antigen excess antigen–antibody complexes are soluble and circulate freely

depending on size, immune complexes become deposited on vascular and glomerular basement membranes or in synovium

vasculitis caused by immune complex deposition typically shows fibrinoid necrosis

where antibody is in excess to local antigen, complexes precipitate at the site of the antigen (e.g. hypersensitivity pneumonitis)

TYPE IV

DELAYED TYPE HYPERSENSITIVITY (DTH)

autoimmune reaction with activation of cell mediated immune mechanisms

cell mediated immunity itself is not DTH, even with bystander injury

DTH is clearly manifest when a cell mediated response occurs to a harmless antigen (e.g. Mantoux reaction)

in granulomatous infections contributions of cell mediated immunity and DTH are hard to separate (e.g. TB)

STIMULATORY (TYPE V)

antibodies against a hormonal receptor result in abnormal target tissue activation

the only clinically significant example is Graves' disease

4. AIDS

ACQUIRED IMMUNE DEFICIENCY SYNDROME

DEFINITION

constellation of clinical manifestations of immune suppression resulting from infection with the human immunodeficiency virus (HIV)

ETIOLOGY

HIV-1 (most cases of AIDS)

HIV-2 (Africa)

HIV is an RNA retrovirus targeting CD4 positive T lymphocytes ('helper T cells')

Modes of transmission

sexual intercourse: heterosexual in Africa; predominantly male homosexual in developed countries

intravenous drug abuse (with cross contamination)

transfusion of blood or blood products

vertical transmission

PATHOGENESIS

HIV selectively binds and enters CD4+ T lymphocytes, and viral RNA is copied to DNA by viral reverse transcriptase

viral DNA may become incorporated into host cell DNA as a provirus with no virus replication (latency); clinical equivalent is the asymptomatic carrier state

alternatively, viral DNA leads to synthesis and release of new virions by the host cell (productive infection); latency may be converted to productive infection when infected CD4+ cells become activated

an immune response to the HIV virus develops leading to anti HIV antibodies and lymph node hyperplasia, but the virus is not eradicated because of the extreme variability of its glycoprotein coat

the HIV virus causes death of CD4+ cells (?mechanism)

cell mediated immunity deteriorates in a predictable way as the CD4 cell count drops, and a predictable sequence of secondary infections and eventually tumors occurs

the non immune defense mechanisms (neutrophil based defenses, complement cascade, etc) are comparatively unaffected

CLINICAL

HIV conversion illness

HIV viremia with fever, myalgia, arthralgia occurs in ~1/2 of infections

Asymptomatic carrier state

virions present in blood stream

seroconversion, anti HIV component antibodies

generalized lymphadenopathy may be present

AIDS related complex (CD4+ <400)

prolonged fever, night sweats

weight loss and diarrhea

anemia

superficial mucosal fungal infections

AIDS (CD4+ <200)

SPECIFIC INFECTIONS

THORAX (Ch 13 3.1, 3.46.6)

pneumocystis carinii pneumonia

cytomegalovirus pneumonia

tuberculosis (initially immune form, then non immune form)

non tuberculous mycobacterial infections

ABDOMEN (Ch 06 8.1–8.9, Ch 07 3.20)

deep fungal infections (Candida, Histoplasma, Cryptococcus, Coccidioides)

Cryptosporidium parvum diarrhea

Isospora belli enteritis

HIV cholangitis

CNS

CNS toxoplasmosis or cryptococcosis

cytomegalovirus retinitis, enteritis

herpes simplex and zoster infections

progressive multifocal leukoencephalopathy (papova virus infection)

SPECIFIC TUMORS

Kaposi's sarcoma (Ch 13 3.32, Ch 05 5.7)

primary CNS lymphoma

OTHER TUMORS

AIDS lymphoma

SCC of the anus, cervix

HIV ENCEPHALOPATHY (Ch 11 7.2.2)

LATE BACTERIAL INFECTIONS

27 Exam techniques

SECTION 7

1. HOW TO READ FILMS: GENERAL TOPICS

FILM READING MACHINE: AN ALGORITHM

film reading for any anatomically based imaging modality is essentially the same orderly progression through set logical steps which (if followed) will ensure that the final diagnosis or differential diagnosis is made on the basis of the findings present on the film and is clinically and academically defensible

the steps are: DETECTION, LOCALIZATION, CHARACTERIZATION, VALIDATION, CROSS REFERENCE, DIAGNOSIS OR DIFFERENTIAL DIAGNOSIS, and SIGNIFICANCE

DETECTION

see ABNORMALITY DETECTION PROCESSES

LOCALIZATION

in all anatomically based imaging modalities ANATOMICAL LOCATION OF THE ABNORMAL FINDING is the property of the finding that most rapidly and time-effectively narrows the differential diagnosis to a manageable number of possibilities

therefore 'WHERE IS IT?' comes before 'WHAT IS IT?'

LOCALIZATION should be expressed in specific anatomical terms at the best level of confidence possible, but not beyond that

for projectional modalities (plain film, angio, fluoro, mammo) a view at right angles or from a different angle is often required for unequivocal localization

for cross sectional modalities localization may require out-of-plane tracing of multiple structures to confirm their correct shape and identity (e.g. bowel loops)

CHARACTERIZATION

CHARACTERIZATION is the description of the abnormality's imaging appearance and qualities, and allows the differential diagnosis to be reduced further based on appearance and likely tissue composition of the abnormality

therefore 'WHAT DOES IT LOOK LIKE, AND WHAT IS IT MADE OF?' comes before 'WHAT IS IT?'

characteristics of an abnormality or a finding can be either MODALITY DEPENDENT or MODALITY INDEPENDENT

CHARACTERIZATION should use descriptors at the most specific level of confidence possible (whether modality dependent or modality independent) but not beyond that

for cross sectional modalities in particular the SHAPE of the abnormality or structure has to be determined from several contiguous slices, and will fall into one of three broad categories: LUMP, TUBE, and SHEET (see MODALITY INDEPENDENT DESCRIPTORS)

for plain film in particular, only four physiological densities (as well as metal) exist: air, fat, fluid/muscle/blood/soft tissue and bone (see MODALITY DEPENDENT DESCRIPTORS)

VALIDATION

VALIDATION is confirmation that a finding is real, and not a pitfall such as a superposition shadow, a motion artifact, a normal variant, flow artifact, etc

therefore, 'IS IT REAL?' comes before 'WHAT IS IT?'

VALIDATION is best done by relating the finding to other findings on the study, but may need a further imaging study to clarify

CROSS REFERENCE

CROSS REFERENCE is the conscious correlation of all imaging findings made in a study and an attempt to fit them into one or more than one meaningful pattern (it is the imaging equivalent of Occam's razor)

BEWARE: oral exam films have unrelated multiple abnormalities far more commonly than occurs in real life

therefore, 'CAN THESE FINDINGS BE RELATED?' comes before 'WHAT ARE THESE?'

DIAGNOSIS OR DIFFERENTIAL DIAGNOSIS

at this point, there should be one definite diagnosis ('Aunt Minnie'), a reasonably certain single diagnosis or a very short list of differential diagnoses (say, 3 or 4), all made at the best possible level of confidence ('WHAT IS IT?')

it is possible (especially in an oral exam) that there are one, two or three concurrent unrelated diagnoses or differential diagnoses

always ask: 'WHAT ELSE CAN IT BE?'; this is the lowest your index of suspicion is allowed to fall!

in sorting the residual differential, previous films ('THE ANSWER IS IN THE BAG') and key details of the patient's history ('THE PATIENT HAS THE ANSWER') should be used first before asking for additional investigations

SIGNIFICANCE

once the diagnosis or diagnoses are made, is it significant in this particular patient, and does it answer the referrer's question ('DOES IT MATTER?')

this is particularly relevant where there is more than one diagnosis, and only one of them is important (or perhaps none answer the clinical question)

in an oral exam, if the diagnoses made on the film do not appear to be relevant, look again!

ABNORMALITY DETECTION PROCESSES

THE ABNORMALITY DETECTION PROCESS

DETECTION is the first step in the film reading algorithm

before an abnormality can be further worked up or diagnosed, it has to be found

detection is a deliberate, active search process and not passive film contemplation

DETECTION is a binary classification into 'normal' and 'abnormal'

before an abnormality can be recognized as an abnormality the reader requires a competent knowledge of the normal and the full range of normal

an abnormality can be classified as 'possibly abnormal' but requires further action to clarify its status (see 'CAN'T TELL' in TRAPS and GAMBITS)

DETECTION consists of three non mutually exclusive processes: pattern recognition (gestalt), mechanical search (systematic review) and goal directed search

PATTERN RECOGNITION
(GESTALT)

as used here, gestalt is the process of using pattern recognition to reach a diagnosis

gestalt is the fastest way to read a film; it is also highly dangerous!

pattern recognition relies on a memory bank of characteristic appearances and semiconscious matching of the film to one appearance

an 'Aunt Minnie' diagnosis is the classic example of pattern recognition

day to day 'stack reading' at a low index of suspicion and high throughput speed consists predominantly of gestalt

safe efficient pattern recognition requires sufficient experience and adequate levels of alertness and concentration

pattern recognition is very prone to errors, particularly errors of omission

Errors of GESTALT

subtle findings are missed

more than one finding–extra findings are usually missed

'mimic' pattern: sufficient features of one condition simulated by another condition lead to false recognition

the non characteristic pattern gets misclassified

an unfamiliar pattern is not recognized

Strengths of pattern recognition

fast

with a sufficient memory bank of images the 'first impression' is often the correct diagnosis when it functions as a semiconscious feature integrator

MECHANICAL SEARCH
(SYSTEMATIC REVIEW)

systematic review is an ordered review of all components of an imaging study, in a specific but meaningful order and without omissions (i.e. the imaging equivalent of Descartes' principle of 'reduction to the manageable')

as used here, mechanical search is the physical process of carrying out a systematic review

mechanical search is most effective when the review pattern is the same every time for a particular type of examination (see SAMPLE CHECKLISTS)

systematic review requires the knowledge of normal to the same extent as do pattern recognition and goal directed search: it concentrates the normal–abnormal classification on one feature at a time

mechanical search is the usual method used by beginners to a particular examination or a particular modality (e.g. MR) before a sufficiently large memory bank is built up

as commonly used in abbreviated form in 'good manners' stack reading, it is a last minute look through areas known to be weaker or in danger of omission when read by gestalt ('CHECK AREAS')

many oral exam films are designed to catch the candidate who uses gestalt exclusively, and has poor mechanical search patterns!

Weaknesses of systematic review

long, effort intensive, and boring

a finding or constellation of findings that lie outside the standard mechanical search are missed

when findings in different areas are not related to each other, an underlying pattern may not be recognized

Strengths of systematic review

most inclusive of all the three strategies

least likely to make errors of omission

most 'stand alone' strategy: does not require any clinical question as input, and does not require an extensive memory bank of abnormal appearances

mechanical search is the safest method if reading films when fatigued: although it slows the reading even further, it in part compensates for reduced concentration levels

GOAL DIRECTED SEARCH

goal directed search is active problem solving using the film as evidence

it requires initial input information which poses one or several questions (i.e. hypotheses); the search consists of answering these questions (i.e. hypothesis testing using the available evidence)

goal directed search requires an excellent knowledge of pathology and patterns of disease; it also requires perspective and an ability to estimate likelihoods of various competing conditions in a patient of a particular age and gender

goal directed search requires a working knowledge of the expected imaging manifestations of any one particular condition under consideration, on the particular modality that is being read

this is the usual mode of film reading in clinicoradiological correlation sessions, particularly if the case is unfamiliar and the study is too large to be read either with gestalt or mechanically

in film reading orals, misleading or ambiguous clinical information is a frequent gambit to test the robustness of the candidate's goal directed search and clinical logic!

Weaknesses of goal directed search

impossible in the absence of input information (can not formulate the hypothesis to be tested)

highly susceptible to 'GARBAGE IN GARBAGE OUT' failures: with a misleading initial question, the film reading will be wrong (in particular, the significance of findings will be misinterpreted)

will miss the incidental unrelated abnormality or second pathology unless noted in passing

can misclassify the unexpected and the atypical manifestations of a condition

can be very time consuming if the hypothesis net is cast wide

Strengths of goal directed search

intellectually the most satisfying mode

will answer the sensibly put clinical
question – every time
provides greatest possible yield of significant
findings in least possible time (where
gestalt is not suitable or not used)
medicolegally it is probably the safest,
provided a search is made for incidental
unrelated conditions

PITFALLS IN ABNORMALITY DETECTION

these are the commoner causes of detection
failure in film reading, and the list is by
no means exhaustive

Between gestalt and systematic review

no abnormality or pattern seen on gestalt
failure to activate or complete systematic
review
result: missed findings

Between gestalt and goal directed search

no abnormality or pattern seen on gestalt
inadequate clinical information or
misleading initial questions: failure to
pick up unrelated abnormalities or
failure to identify abnormalities as
significant on goal directed search
result: missed unrelated findings; findings
found but significance misinterpreted

At goal directed search

misleading or inappropriate clinical
information and questions directly
causing misinterpretation of
abnormalities

At systematic review

tired, distracted or called away
fail to check part of the mechanical list or
picked up the list at a different point
from where it was left off
result: missed findings (you 'CAN'T FIND
WHAT YOU DON'T LOOK FOR')

Organization, communication failure

too many findings with failure to remember
or communicate them all

'GOOD MANNERS' WORKPLACE FILM READING

the balance in clinical film reading is
between throughput speed, reader
fatigue, and rate of misreading (either

misses – errors of detection, or mis-calls
– errors of interpretation)
mode of reading or the combination of
modes will depend on the nature of the
stack, levels of clinical suspicion, and
patient population specific to the location
(e.g. suburban practice draining family
physician referrals versus practice in a
cancer hospital)
the safest way overall is to use a
combination of all the three detection
modes in a complementary pattern that
is responsive to the time available ('good
manners' film reading)
'GOOD MANNERS' film reading will
minimize the misses in abnormality
detection, and use of the FILM READING
MACHINE algorithm (or any other non
random logical approach) will minimize
the errors of interpretation
this varies from person to person and stack
to stack; what follows below is not at all
prescriptive but an example of a starting
point

Suggested 'good manners' film reading

do not look at the request initially
put up the entire current study (if there are
clearly separate unrelated studies on the
same patient, deal with them separately)
note the patient's age and gender: age,
gender and study being done (and its
source) are already a powerful predictor
of the pathology to be expected
gestalt the entire study, looking for a pattern
to emerge
DO NOT STOP AT ONE PATTERN
read the request: what is the question being
asked? (if it is a stupid irrelevant
question, use the demographic
information to double guess the real
reason the patient has had the study)
shortlist 2 or 3 conditions that most likely
underlie the presentation and are being
asked about
pull out relevant PREVIOUS FILMS, and put
them up at this point (previous report is
a poor second)
use goal directed search for manifestations
of these conditions
DO NOT STOP IF A PATTERN STARTS
EMERGING
apply a short, sharp, concentrated
mechanical search (particularly to
complex cross sectional studies with
multiple images)
save time by bypassing areas already
carefully looked at in goal directed
search – or double check them if so
inclined

in particular, beware of WHAT IS NOT ON
THE FILM (e.g. the missing spleen)
DO NOT STOP UNTIL THE SEARCH HAS
FINISHED
apply the remainder of the FILM READING
MACHINE ALGORITHM: localize,
characterize, validate and cross
reference each finding (this usually
happens very quickly and subconsciously
in simpler cases; and will need to be
done explicitly in the difficult cases)
draw up a diagnosis or differential diagnosis
ask the following:
WHAT ELSE CAN IT BE?
WHAT AM I MISSING?
DOES MY DIAGNOSIS MATTER?

SAMPLE CHECKLISTS FOR SYSTEMATIC REVIEW

PLAIN FILM

CXR
MEDIASTINUM AND VESSELS
LUNGS AND VASCULARITY
BONES AND SOFT TISSUES
ABDOMEN AND DIAPHRAGM
SECOND REVIEW: PNEUMOTHORAX, LUNG
COLLAPSE, TRACHEAL POSITION, RIB
NOTCHING, CARDIAC VALVE
CALCIFICATION

Abdomen XR
BOWEL GAS AND FREE GAS
SOLID ORGANS AND RETROPERITONEUM
PELVIS
BONES
LUNG BASES
SECOND REVIEW: BILIARY/PORTAL VEIN
GAS, PRESACRAL AREAS/SACRUM,
PARACOLIC GUTTERS

Pelvis XR
ALIGNMENT, RINGS AND COLUMNS
SI JOINTS AND SACRUM
SIDE WALL SOFT TISSUES
VISCERA
SECOND REVIEW: SACRAL ARCS,
PRESACRAL AREAS, HERNIAS

Joint XR
ALIGNMENT
CORTICAL SURFACES
EFFUSIONS
CARTILAGE LOSS, CHONDROCALCINOSIS
EROSIONS, CYSTS, SCLEROSIS

OSTEOPHYTES, PERIOSTEAL BONE, POROSIS
SOFT TISSUES, CALCIFICATION
SECOND REVIEW: GROWTH PLATES, LOOSE BODIES

Hands
SYMMETRY AND DISTRIBUTION
BONE DENSITY
CARTILAGE LOSS, CHONDROCALCINOSIS
JOINT ANKYLOSIS
EROSIONS, CYSTS, SCLEROSIS
OSTEOPHYTES, PERIOSTEAL BONE, POROSIS
ENTHESOPATHY
SOFT TISSUES, CALCIFICATION
DEFORMITIES

Skull
PITUITARY FOSSA
VAULT + SUTURES
ORBITS, GREATER WING OF SPHENOID, LESSER WING OF SPHENOID
PETROUS TEMPORAL BONES
SINUSES

Spine
ALIGNMENT
VERTEBRAL BODIES + DISKS
PEDICLES + NEURAL ARCHES
PARASPINAL SOFT TISSUES
SECOND REVIEW: BOWEL, RIBS, SI JOINTS, PELVIS

Mammo
SYMMETRY
TECHNICAL ADEQUACY
BREAST PLATE CONTENTS
BREAST PLATE SHAPE
RETROMAMMARY SPACE
SKIN AND CHEST WALL
PREVIOUS MAMMO

CONTRAST STUDIES

Barium studies (short checklist)
BARIUM SURFACE: EN FACE AND IN PROFILE
LUMINAL SHAPE AND SIZE
WALL THICKNESS
BOWEL POSITION AND MOTILITY
LOOK OUTSIDE THE BARIUM COLUMN

IVU/IVP
PRELIMINARY FILM
KIDNEY NUMBER + POSITION
PARENCHYMA WIDTH + CONTOUR
FOCAL MASSES + FOCAL DISTORTION

MUCOSAL SURFACE + PAPILLAE
CONTRAST COLUMN FILLING DEFECTS OR TRANSITION ZONES
SYMMETRY
LOOK OUTSIDE THE CONTRAST COLUMN

CROSS SECTIONAL

CT or MR head
GRAY MATTER + WHITE MATTER
VENTRICLES + CISTERNS
SINUSES + ARTERIES
SKULL + EXTRAAXIAL TISSUES
ORBITS + TEMPORAL BONES
SPHENOID + PITUITARY
SECOND REVIEW: CT POSTERIOR FOSSA BLOOD, GRAY-WHITE JUNCTION, LACUNAR INFARCTS; MR: EARLY DEMYELINATION, LACUNAR INFARCTS

CT abdo
SCOUT VIEW/TOPOGRAM
SOLID ORGANS: LIVER, SPLEEN, KIDNEYS, ADRENALS, PANCREAS
PORTOBILIARY: SMA, PV, CBD, GALLBLADDER, DUODENUM
VESSELS + RETROPERITONEUM: URETERS, NODES, GREAT VESSELS
PELVIS: BLADDER, PROSTATE, SEMINAL VESICLES, UTERUS, OVARIES, RECTUM; SIDE WALLS
BONES + SUBCUTANEOUS TISSUE
BOWEL: STOMACH, DUODENUM, SMALL BOWEL (upper left clump, mid abdominal clump, right iliac fossa clump); CECUM, APPENDIX, COLON, SIGMOID, RECTUM

CT chest
SCOUT VIEW/TOPOGRAM
MEDIASTINUM + MASSES: ARTERIES, VEINS, HEART; LYMPH NODES AND VASCULAR HILA; ESOPHAGUS; PLEURAL AND PERICARDIAL SPACES
LUNGS + ENDOBRONCHIAL: LUNGS, HILA, BRONCHIAL PATENCY
AXILLAE + CHEST WALL: AXILLAE, SUBCUTANEOUS TISSUES, BREASTS, RIBS
LIVER + ADRENALS
KIDNEYS, SPLEEN, PANCREAS

CT or MR lumbar spine
CT SCOUT VIEW/TOPOGRAM
VERTEBRAE + NEURAL ARCHES
DISKS + FAR LATERAL BULGES
DURAL SAC + NEURAL EXIT FORAMINA
CORD + NERVE ROOTS

SAMPLE ETIOLOGICAL SIEVE

MNEMONIC: TIM VIN TAM
T-RAUMA
I-NFECTION
M-ALFORMATION
V-ASCULAR
I-ATROGENIC
N-EUROPATHIC
T-UMOUR
A-UTOIMMUNE
M-ETABOLIC

MODALITY INDEPENDENT DESCRIPTORS

SHAPE

Lump (i.e. mass)
cardinal finding: one can see the upper and lower border of the lump on cross sectional imaging as well as its in-plane borders (i.e. can 'get above and below')
a tube in cross section and a lump look the same

Tube
cardinal findings:
in-plane tube is elongated, but one can see its upper and lower border on cross sectional imaging
tube in cross section is a stack of coins: it has no close upper or lower border on cross sectional imaging
a sheet in cross section and a tube that lies in the imaging plane look the same

Sheet
(example: abdominal oblique muscles; horizontal fissure; carcinoma infiltrated omentum, thin pleural effusion)
cardinal findings:
a sheet in cross section is always elongated in the plane, and no close upper or lower border is present
a sheet parallel to the plane of section is not easily visible: it presents as a gradual change in characteristics of adjacent structures and another imaging sequence in cross section (or appropriate reconstruction) may be required

INTERNAL STRUCTURE

CAVITY, INTRACAVITARY SOLID
FLUID–FLUID LEVEL
AIR–FLUID LEVEL
COMPLEX (CONTAINS VESSELS, SPACES, etc)

EDGE

SHARP OR ILL DEFINED
ROUNDED, ANGULATED, LOBULATED, SPICULATED
BRANCHING

MASS EFFECT

MASS EFFECT
VOLUME LOSS ('negative mass effect' is an unfortunate example of indiscriminate application of short hand terminology!)

MODALITY DEPENDENT DESCRIPTORS

PLAIN FILM

Density
AIR
FAT
SOFT TISSUE/BLOOD/FLUID
BONE
METAL

Specific internal structure
AIR BRONCHOGRAMS
BONY TRABECULATION
COARSE CALCIFICATION
TUBULAR CALCIFICATION
RECOGNIZABLE BODY PARTS (FETUS, TEETH, etc)

LOSS OF INTERFACE
(silhouette sign)
FOR AN INTERFACE TO BE VISIBLE ON XR, TWO STRUCTURES OF DIFFERENT DENSITY HAVE TO BE APPOSED ALONG AN EDGE PARALLEL TO THE XRAY BEAM

BARIUM

see descriptors entry in gastrointestinal chapter

US

ECHOGENICITY (relative to something): FLUID (i.e. SONOLUCENT), HYPOECHOIC, ISOECHOIC, HYPERECHOIC (ECHOGENIC)
SHADOWING AND ITS EDGE
THROUGH TRANSMISSION (POSTERIOR ACOUSTIC ENHANCEMENT)
INTERNAL CONTENTS, DEBRIS
COLOR DOPPLER FLOW
SPECTRAL DOPPLER WAVEFORM
MOTION AND ITS PATTERN

CT

Absolute density
RELATED TO NORMAL STRUCTURE OF WELL DOCUMENTED STABLE DENSITY e.g.
CSF
FAT
BLOOD
MUSCLE
LIVER
BONE

Relative density
HYPODENSE
ISODENSE
HYPERDENSE

Contrast enhancement characteristics
NON ENHANCING
BLOTCHY, PERIPHERAL, CENTRAL, DIFFUSE
PHASES OF ENHANCEMENT: ARTERIAL, PORTAL VENOUS, NEPHROGRAPHIC, DELAYED

LOSS OF INTERFACE
(silhouette sign)
FOR AN INTERFACE TO BE VISIBLE ON CT, TWO STRUCTURES OF DIFFERENT DENSITY HAVE TO BE APPOSED ALONG A PLANE NOT PARALLEL THE PLANE OF CROSS SECTIONAL IMAGING

MR

T1 weighted, T2 weighted, proton density sequences
ABSOLUTE SIGNAL: HIGH, INTERMEDIATE, LOW
RELATIVE SIGNAL: HYPERINTENSE, ISOINTENSE, HYPOINTENSE
ABSENT SIGNAL: SIGNAL VOID, AIR VOID, BONE VOID, FLOW VOID; METAL ARTIFACT

Diffusion weighted sequence
ABSOLUTE SIGNAL: AREA OF DIFFUSION RESTRICTION
(beware of T2W shine-through)

FLAIR, STIR sequences
ABSOLUTE SIGNAL: HIGH, LOW, etc

Contrast enhancement characteristics
AS FOR CT

NUC MED

TRACER UPTAKE

INCREASED
DIFFUSELY INCREASED
FOCALLY INCREASED
LINEAR/ELONGATED
ROUNDED
ARTICULAR
IN THE SHAPE OF...

DECREASED (photopenia)
FOCAL PHOTOPENIA
DIFFUSE PHOTOPENIA

'HOT SPOT' and 'COLD SPOT'
'hot spot' and 'cold spot' are too colloquial to appear favorably in formal reports or in exams!

Phases of any study with intravenous injection
RIGHT HEART FIRST PASS TRANSIT, PULMONARY TRANSIT
LEFT HEART FIRST PASS TRANSIT
PERFUSION PHASE (i.e. systemic perfusion, 'radioangiogram')
BLOOD POOL PHASE (= INTERSTITIAL SOFT TISSUE PHASE): reflects distribution of tracer both in the intravascular compartment and in the interstitial compartment, depending on tracer
FOR SPECIFIC LATER PHASES, see nuc med entries in the normal part of the systemic chapters

MAMMO

see specific descriptors in Ch 24

2. SURVIVING THE FRANZCR PART II EXAMS

INTRODUCTION

AIMS OF STUDY BEFORE THE AUSTRALIAN PART II EXAM

PASSING THE FRANZCR PART II EXAM
(EQUIVALENT TO US BOARDS)
SAFE INDEPENDENT PRACTICE

PART II EXAM AS IT STANDS AT END OF 2001

Both the pathology and radiology
components are to be sat together

MCQ

Radiology: 80 five part MCQ over 2 hours,
non penal marking system
Pathology: MCQ will be introduced from
2002 to replace short answers

Radiology report writing

8 stations of 14 minutes each; one, two,
three cases per station

Oral examinations

Pathology: 25 minutes, pot session
(pots may be replaced by specimen
photographs)

Radiology: 6 x 25 minutes each, film
reading sessions
Musculoskeletal
CNS/head and neck
Chest/cardiovascular
Abdominal
Pediatrics
Obstetrics, gynecology and mammography

WHAT YOU NEED TO DEVELOP TO PASS THE PART II EXAM

Knowledge base

Performance

Exam technique

THE KNOWLEDGE BASE

COMPONENTS OF THE KNOWLEDGE BASE

Normal

knowledge of normal anatomy and limited
knowledge of normal physiology as they
appear on all the relevant modalities
used for radiology exams more than for
pathology exams; constantly used in
radiology day to day work

Gamuts

lists of differential possibilities for a
particular finding
used for radiology exams and is basic
radiology working knowledge

Condition descriptions

uniform knowledge of a circumscribed
subject sufficient to allow safe practice
used for pathology and radiology MCQ; and
for radiology report writing exams

RESOURCES USED TO BUILD UP THE KNOWLEDGE BASE

READING (pathology, radiology)
FILM LIBRARIES

HOW TO ORGANIZE YOUR KNOWLEDGE BASE

By organ system, pathology and radiology together

knowledge of the pathology of a condition is
frequently sufficient to work out the
radiological appearance on first
principles
the pathology and radiology exams are sat
together, and so there is no point covering
the same ground in two isolated passes

By modality

gamuts should be organized by modality,
because that is how you will need to
recall them
modality based organization is used in film
library preparation for the orals and the
report writing

TIMING OF ACQUISITION OF YOUR KNOWLEDGE BASE

you must plan your study ahead, or risk
running out of time!

Three pass technique

First pass: primary acquisition
Second pass: first revision
Third pass: second revision

Timing of primary acquisition

these are suggested times in weeks,
assuming a 5 day working week; the
order is not important

SECTION I MUSCULOSKELETAL

1. Musculoskeletal normal and gamuts
2. General musculoskeletal conditions and
   syndromes
3. Joint conditions
4. Trauma and degenerative musculoskeletal
   conditions
5. Musculoskeletal tumors
this section should take approximately
8 weeks, with least time spent on
musculoskeletal tumors

SECTION II ABDOMINAL

6. Gastrointestinal system (4)
7. Hepatopancreatobiliary system (4)
8. Adrenal, renal and urinary tract (4)
9. Male reproductive system (2)

SECTION III CNS

10. CNS normal and gamuts
11. Conditions of the CNS
12. Head and neck (4)
chapters 10 and 11 combined should take
approximately 8 weeks

SECTION IV THORAX

13. Lungs (4)
14. Heart and mediastinum
15. Vascular conditions
16. Hematology (3)
chapters 14 and 15 combined should take
approximately 4 weeks

SECTION V PEDIATRICS

17. Pediatric musculoskeletal
18. Pediatric gastrointestinal
19. Pediatric urogenital
20. Pediatric CNS
21. Pediatric thorax
this section should take approximately
8–9 weeks and should ideally be done
during your pediatric rotation

SECTION VI OBSTETRICS, GYNECOLOGY, BREAST

22. Obstetrics (4–5)
23. Gynecology (4)
24. Breast (2)

SECTION VII GENERAL

25. PET and nuclear medicine (2)
26. General pathology (2)
27. Exam techniques (you are reading this
    chapter now!!)

AIDS as a separate topic should take about 1 week (because of the radiology)

COMMENTS

this makes a total of approximately 60 to 70 weeks of primary acquisition

where to get extra time: use holidays (counts as double time)

KEEPING TO TIME IS CRUCIAL, CRITICAL AND LIFESAVING

Timing of first revision

1 WEEK PER CHAPTER EXCEPT:

scale shorter topics in proportion

reduce pediatrics to 1–2 weeks

total first revision should fit into approximately 14 weeks

where to get extra time: use holidays (counts as double time)

order of first revision should follow the order of acquisition

KEEPING TO TIME IS VITAL

Timing of second revision

total of 2 weeks

approximately 2 days per chapter

RESOURCES AND READING FOR THE KNOWLEDGE BASE

you should have a generalist pathology textbook and a generalist radiology textbook

in-depth reading of the radiology primary acquisition phase should be done from specialist radiology texts, using this book as an overview and a guide

first and second revisions should be made using your notes, this book, and the generalist text

PERFORMANCE

Definition

Ability to competently carry on the function of a radiologist

Components

INTERPRETATION OF IMAGING STUDIES

WRITTEN COMMUNICATION SKILLS

ORAL COMMUNICATION SKILLS

(PRACTICAL PROCEDURE SKILLS)

	Knowledge base	Performance skills	Exam technique
radiology MCQ	gamuts, conditions		practice MCQ books
pathology MCQ	condition descriptions		practice MCQ books
report writing exam	condition descriptions first, gamuts second	interpretation of imaging studies written communication skills	timed report practice
pathology oral	condition descriptions	oral communication skills	path museum pots
radiology orals	gamuts first, condition descriptions second	interpretation of imaging studies oral communication skills	solo film library work paired film library work tutorials gamesmanship

EXAM TECHNIQUE

REPORT WRITING TECHNIQUE

History provided for each case will be truthful, but very limited; both gestalt and goal directed search will miss findings

READING THE FILMS

1. Apply your mechanical search pattern
2. List findings at best possible level of confidence
3. (internally) Verbalize findings
4. Stop early and consider diagnosis
5. Re-read the presentation history: do the findings fit?

WRITING THE REPORT

HEADING

  AGE, GENDER, INVESTIGATION

FINDINGS

point form at best possible level of confidence

CONCLUSION

one diagnosis (or, if several conditions present, one diagnosis per condition)

OR VERY SHORT DIFFERENTIAL

two or three most likely conditions

FURTHER TESTS IF RELEVANT

justify why you want to do further tests

IF YOU ARE SHORT OF TIME, WRITE DOWN THE CONCLUSION FIRST!

ORAL EXAM TECHNIQUE

see surviving oral exams

3. SURVIVING ORAL EXAMS

THREE PREREQUISITES FOR SUCCESSFULLY PASSING THE ORALS

Interpretation of imaging studies

see the section on how to read films: general topics

Oral communication skills

not something that can be learnt from a core review of imaging book

Gamesmanship

the subject of this section

THE THREE T'S OF SUCCESSFULLY HANDLING THE ORALS

these are listed in order of importance, and time should be spent on each accordingly

T-echnique

this is good film reading technique that does not falter under extreme pressure: see section 1

T-iming (see below) and

T-raps (see below)

if you fail to prepare these three areas, you will instead reach a fourth T: T-error!

THE SECOND T: TIMING AND PROGRESSION THROUGH CASES

Flow control

your goal in an oral is to correctly get through a sufficient number of cases to allow your examiner to pass you

accept that you will not diagnose ALL the cases correctly

expect that you will need to diagnose (or approach) MOST cases correctly in order to pass

expect that if you make a gross clinically catastrophic error, you will automatically fail no matter how good the rest of your performance is

it is in your interests to say only what is necessary, or what will keep up your end of the exchange; it is equally in your interests to say as much of what is necessary as possible, say it as coherently as possible, and in the least disjointed manner

Why am I showing you this film?

every case has an underlying reason for it being selected as a case; it has nothing to do with the condition demonstrated in the case, and only 50% to do with the final diagnosis

if you can work out this reason, you have passed and dispatched the case

this is a game; but you are not allowed to declare it a game! Therefore, DO NOT open your final 'kill' delivery with 'Well, you are showing me this film because ...'

Your examiners are human

they are subject to the same petty annoyances as you are: tiredness, boredom, irritation, hunger, the full bladder, broken night of sleep, etc

the candidate who allows for these human factors is more likely to pass than the candidate who is self-absorbed in his or her terror, even if the two say exactly the same things in an oral: make it easy for your examiners to pass you!

Timing of a case
(suggested sequence)

When the film goes up:

1. LOOK AT THE LABEL, and ensure you are seen to have looked at the label. This will give you name, age, gender of the patient (and, if you are lucky) the likely ethnicity and the hospital of origin

2. INTRODUCE THE FILM. Give a short, sharp description of the study, the sequences, and the age and gender of the patient

3. STOP TALKING and resist the overpowering urge to fill the silence with blabbing

4. this is your 20 SECONDS OF GOLDEN SILENCE. Concentrate on applying the FILM READING MACHINE and in particular on ABNORMALITY DETECTION. You should NEVER start talking until you have finished at least a rudimentary mechanical search

in preparation for the orals you should use a timer to give yourself a full 20 seconds for film reading before you start speaking. Inevitably, the time you will take in the oral will be shorter because of the adrenalin rush

5. ONE SHOT PRESENTATION: once you start presenting the case, you should do so in one, logical, flowing sequential exposition, and not stop until you have reached the end of it. Do not lose your time and your examiners' attention!

6. THE PAUSE. This is a natural break, and an opportunity for the examiner to move you on to the next case. After what you think is a very long pause, one of three things will happen: i) the film will come down; ii) you will be asked a question; iii) nothing at all will happen. In case of iii) you have to ask yourself: 'WHAT AM I MISSING?'

see 'why is this film not coming down?'

Presenting a case in an oral

WHEN THERE IS ONE DOMINANT FINDING

DESCRIPTION

modality independent descriptors first

modality dependent descriptors second

at the best possible level of confidence, but not beyond that!

LOCATION

in as precise anatomical terms as possible!

PERTINENT NEGATIVES

each one of these should only be mentioned for a good reason; DO NOT state the diagnosis yet: this is a game!

DIAGNOSIS OR DIFFERENTIAL

STANDARD STEM:

In this (patient age, gender – obtained from label) presenting with (potted history – proves you listened to the examiner) ...

ENDING DEPENDS ON YOUR CONFIDENCE LEVEL:

the findings are characteristic of ...

the most likely diagnosis is ...

the differential diagnosis is A, B or C ...

possible conditions underlying this finding could be X, Y or less likely Z ...

SIGNIFICANCE AND WRAP-UP

if you end up with a poor level of confidence, you need to either suggest a way out (e.g. look at previous films, do another test) or concisely explain why you can not be any more specific (this has to be defensible)

DO NOT SUGGEST FURTHER INVESTIGATIONS THAT ARE NOT WARRANTED

WHEN THERE ARE MULTIPLE FINDINGS

this can work well with a set formula:

'this study demonstrates several findings ...'

then go through the description and location of each finding starting with the most important one

CROSS REFERENCE

'... the findings fit an underlying pattern of ...'

'... the findings could all be produced by one process ...'

'... it is difficult to bring all the findings into one pattern ...'

'... there most likely are two different underlying pathological processes ...'

DIAGNOSIS OR DIAGNOSES

STANDARD STEM:

In this (patient age, gender) presenting with (potted history), the (study) demonstrates (one, two, several, related, unrelated) findings which...

ENDING DEPENDS ON YOUR CONFIDENCE LEVEL:

'are all different manifestations of ...'

'are compatible with condition X but coexistent condition Y could produce finding...'

'probably reflect two different underlying conditions:...'

SIGNIFICANCE

a comment (if not already made) on what you think the order of significance of these conditions is to this patient

WHEN THE FILM CARRIES A WIDE DIFFERENTIAL AND YOU NEED MORE INFORMATION

this works well with a set formula:

PERTINENT NEGATIVES

these are very important here. You need to convey that you have attempted to narrow down your differential

'I can not identify any features that would help me (diagnose the cause for the finding; narrow down the differential) ...'

DIFFERENTIAL DIAGNOSIS

once again, a set formula:

'without any additional information (pregnant pause: a cue for the examiner to intervene) this finding has a wide differential diagnosis. In this (age, gender) patient presenting with (cardinal symptom), conditions that enter the differential are ...'

THE VOICE OF THE CASE: ACTIVE OR PASSIVE

I strongly recommend that you use the active voice in your presentation, but keep it third person as much as is possible

when you make positive findings, put them in third person active voice: 'this film shows'; 'a fracture runs', 'the study demonstrates', 'the T12 vertebral body contains'

when you make strong negative findings, put them in third person active voice: 'this CXR shows no pneumothorax', 'the mass contains no high T1 signal'

when you make tentative negative findings, it is good practice to put them in first person active voice: 'I am unable to identify the cause for the demonstrated hydrocephalus...' (this implies: I am looking! I do not have much time! I am still suspicious! If the examiner wants to help you and you are missing the finding you are looking for, your attention will be gently directed)

What the examiner says
(and does not)

listen, listen, listen to the examiner's opening of the case! This will not be actively misleading, but WILL contain omissions. What the story does not contain is as important as what it does.

THE HELPFUL OPENING

this gives you a clinical history which is not self evident from the film

USE THE CLINICAL QUESTION YOU HAVE DEDUCED FROM THE EXAMINER'S OPENING TO CONDUCT A GOAL DIRECTED SEARCH immediately after you gestalt the film

answer this deduced question in the 'significance' part of your presentation

THE 'YOU ARE ON YOUR OWN' OPENING

While NOT MISLEADING, this history is sufficiently non specific and does not allow a goal directed search

'this woman presented with cough'
'abdominal pain'
'preoperative chest Xray'
'this man had a CT for headache'

here it is fair game for you to construct your gamuts based on age and gender, and you need to rely heavily on your systematic review

if you can not make a diagnosis, ask yourself: 'WHAT AM I MISSING?'

if after another review you still can not answer this question, you are probably looking at a TRAP FILM or a NORMAL/NEAR NORMAL FILM

THE OMISSION: ANOTHER CONDITION

it is routine for oral cases to contain more than one unrelated condition

it is almost as routine for examiners to give you a perfectly helpful history which will lead you to discover only one of the conditions

sometimes a critical item of information will be omitted from the clinical history, and be conspicuous by its omission

you are expected to win this information by sensibly asking for it (see the entry on how to ask questions!)

EXAMPLE: brain CT for trauma that also shows an orbital tumor (you get a good history of trauma!)

THE APPARENTLY GENERAL QUESTION

in many cases the candidate who is struggling with detection of findings may be offered a veiled hint

this consists of a question on general anatomy, pathology or radiology invariably concerning the structure the examiner wants you to look at more closely

How to use your hands and the pointer

bring your own pointer with a rounded, non scratchy end

DO NOT

wave the pointer vaguely at the film

point to every structure you are currently looking at

substitute pointing for proper description

point with your sweaty sticky finger

DO

hold one end of the pointer in each hand when not using it. This will also stop you from poking your fingers into the film or covering your mouth with your hand

point (short, sharp and deliberate) when describing an abnormality where there may be any doubt that you have detected it correctly or localized it correctly

Use of the bright light and magnifier

expect that if you do not use the bright light when you should, you will seriously jeopardize your chances of passing the oral

the first time you need to pull a film down to bright light it, ASK

NO EXAMINER should refuse you the right to examine the films as you see fit

THIS DOES NOT MEAN you can cook the films with the bright light

there will always be a magnifier in the mammo oral (and also, you may have to hang the films up correctly yourself)

use the magnifier, or miss calcifications at your own peril

How to hang yourself

CRITICIZING FILMS

beauty is in the eye of the beholder!

the old, cruddy, scratched, oversolarized piece of celluloid hanging in front of you was probably lovingly collated by your examiner many years ago and used ever since!

FAILING TO STOP (verbal diarrohea)

this is probably the biggest candidate killer. All the examiner has to do is sit back and listen as you hang yourself with more and more implausible scenarios. Listen to what you are saying. Stop talking when you are beginning to surprise yourself!

SAYING THE UNREASONABLE

this is a postgraduate examination, and you do not have to be right; you just have to be reasonable

by corollary, the unreasonable, the heretical and particularly the plain dangerous will fail your oral for you

leave the heresies to the abstract submission form for the annual scientific meeting

THE RABBIT IN THE HEADLIGHTS SYNDROME

the candidate who freezes in the steely glare of the light box

this condition is terminal till next year's oral exams

ARGUING WITH THE EXAMINER

you either have to produce irrefutable scientific evidence to back you up – on the spot; OR come back with the evidence next year

THE THIRD T: TRAPS AND GAMBITS

How to ask questions when you need more information

the cardinal rule is: DO NOT ASK QUESTIONS; MAKE STATEMENTS

if you ask a question of your examiner, this interrupts the flow of your presentation and forces you to wait until the examiner responds

it also lets the examiner waste your time (if so inclined)

you should put the examiner in a position where the examiner has to respond; give him or her an opportunity to respond; and treat any non utterance as a response

therefore, convert your question into a conditional statement; give the examiner an opportunity to respond (pregnant pause), and then proceed with the most likely answer to your conditional statement

WEAK QUESTION: '... it would be important to know if this is a chronic or acute appearance.' ('Yes, I agree. How could you do that?' – this leads to a fruitless discussion about clinical history, previous films, etc etc)

STRONG STATEMENT: '... the differential diagnosis in this case depends on whether this appearance is acute or chronic. (pregnant pause) Because interstitial patterns are more commonly chronic, and in the absence of anything on the film to help me decide, I will assume this pattern is chronic.'

What to do when the film is normal (or near normal)

this is NOT A TRAP but a test of your logical thinking and confidence

these situations occur in real life as well – all the time!

WHAT TO DO

this best fits a set pattern:

1. ask yourself 'WHAT AM I MISSING?' and do a repeat mechanical search; stay silent!

2. gambit: use the history. 'I am looking for evidence of conditions X, Y and Z which are common indications for this test with this presentation in a (gender, age); but I do not see anything that I can confidently diagnose as significant. (pregnant pause)'. You just may get mercy. If not...

3. the normality gambit: 'There are a number of important conditions which present with (cardinal symptom) in a (gender) patient of this age, and have a normal (examination type). I could perform (second examination, previous film, history, etc) to rule these out'.

IMPORTANT CONDITIONS WHICH PRESENT WITH NORMAL EXAMINATIONS

CXR
- PULMONARY EMBOLISM
- ASTHMA
- ASPIRATED FOREIGN BODY IN A CHILD

ABDOMEN
- BOWEL INFARCTION (EARLY)

PELVIS
- INSUFFICIENCY FRACTURE

JOINT XR
- AVASCULAR NECROSIS (EARLY)
- SEPTIC ARTHRITIS (EARLY)
- OSTEOMYELITIS (EARLY)

BRAIN MR
- SUBARACHNOID HEMORRHAGE

MAMMO
- ANYTHING AT ALL, AND ESPECIALLY CANCER

'This is what I would do'

expect that at least once in the oral exam you will be given a case where cavalier inaction on your part will kill the patient and fail the oral for you

once you have decided on a course of action, it is not in your interests to present this lifesaving information as a weak afterthought: '... pneumothorax chest drainage could be suggested ...' Say what you will really do – plainly and directly!

do not overuse this; it is as easy to irritate the examiner as it is to irritate the referring clinician

'I do not know' and how not to say it

DO NOT START YOUR DIFFERENTIAL WITH WHAT THE DIAGNOSIS IS NOT

when the terror stricken candidate gets to that all-important diagnosis or differential diagnosis part of the presentation, the usual overwhelming urge is to call out the memorized gamut verbatim, no matter how unlikely some of it is

even worse, the candidate with mental block on what the differential diagnosis really is, starts listing any and all conditions known to cause some or all of the imaging findings on the film. This is usually accompanied by many guttural sounds signifying uncertainty and unhappiness!

DO have sufficient self discipline to verbalize all this agony internally. When you get to the differential diagnosis, state what is most likely, and also what is important even if less likely, and demonstrate perspective and ability to trim your gamuts to each individual case!

'TELL ME WHAT IT COULD BE, NOT WHAT IT COULD NOT BE'

'YES, NO, AND CAN'T TELL'

there are three possible answers to any 'yes or no' question: 'YES, NO and CAN'T TELL'

do not use 'I don't know ...' in presenting a case where you mean 'I can't tell ...'.

'CAN'T TELL'

an 'I can't tell...' is when you are unable to proceed in your diagnostic algorithm, and there is nothing helpful on the film

most candidates know a sufficient amount by the time of the oral – but they do not extrapolate their knowledge to unfamiliar or stressful situations. The 'can't tell' may be the very reason why you are being shown the film

DEFENSE: you need a good reason for why you can't tell, which should ideally be apparent on the film or evident from the absence of information

'DON'T KNOW'

when you are asked a closed question of your knowledge base ('what is the prevalence of dizygotic twinning in Outer Mongolia in 18 to 22 year old primigravidas?') and you do not know the answer, this is an 'I don't know'

if you think you are being asked something beyond what you can be expected to know, then a straight 'I do not know that, but I know where and how to get the answer' may suffice [www.ncbi.nlm.nih.gov – the pubmed site]

if this is something you should have known, a political 'I don't know' defense may just get you out of trouble: 'I am not certain about the exact prevalence of Outer Mongolia primigravida dizygotic twinning, but in European countries it is in the order of 1 in 80 or 90, and I know that it is less frequent in Asians; therefore ...'

How to win that extra film

this is a very common game in oral exams, and a frequent task you will face

inevitably, the extra film that is being withheld contains the reason why you are being shown the case

if you at all can, keep at least some attention on the stack of films in the examiner's hands (examiners are trying to avoid this from happening on the grounds that it constitutes 'cheating')

as a cardinal rule, you need a VALID REASON for requesting (and receiving) an extra examination, or even a previous film

if you at all can, DO NOT ASK for the film directly; convert your request to a statement so that if no film is forthcoming, you can recover immediately and continue with your presentation

GETTING THE OLD FILM

e.g. DIFFUSE LUNG DISEASE: ACUTE vs CHRONIC

'... the differential diagnosis for this appearance is wide, and depends on whether this change is acute or chronic (pregnant pause), which is easiest to determine from an old film (second pregnant pause); in its absence ...'

THE POST TREATMENT FILM

this is a free ride: if there are surgical or especially radiation therapy changes on the study you are looking at, you can ask for the pretreatment examination

Why is this film not coming down?

this is the hardest thing to handle in oral exams

it often indicates you are missing a finding, or have not reached an adequate stage in your reasoning ('WHY AM I SHOWING YOU THIS FILM?')

occasionally it is there just to see whether you can be provoked into verbal diarrhea!

1. repeat your mechanical search (stay silent!)

2. think back to the opening of the case: what was the clinical question implicit in the history? Have you answered it? What was NOT said in the history? Have you addressed it?

3. construct several hypotheses based on the history and the findings visible to you (different hypotheses from what you have used already). THESE HAVE TO BE PLAUSIBLE. Do a repeat goal directed search – here it is good to state your negative findings as pertinent negatives. DO NOT look for findings of unreasonable or exotic or outlandish conditions

4. should you take some further clinical action? Your diagnosis or differential may well be right, but the examiner is waiting for you to demonstrate practical common sense. If so, the action required of you is a rather obvious one

5. if at this point you get no further leads, it is probably worthwhile trying to salvage the oral by moving on to the next case. A straight approach just might win you mercy: 'I am unable to take this case any further with this history and the findings evident to me'

SOME TRAPS

THE BIG HAPPY DISTRACTOR

this is the most common trap, and is quite legitimate

it consists of an obvious but irrelevant finding, and a small important finding that is the reason for showing you the film!

if the answer is too simple, or the film seems too easy, you are probably looking at the big happy distractor

e.g. CXR with gross pleural plaques – and a missing pedicle

THE CORNER FINDING

this is a legitimate trap

it consists of a finding in an infrequently checked area

EXAMPLE
CXR with rheumatoid shoulders

THE TOO BLACK AND THE TOO WHITE

these two extremes of density can conveniently hide abnormalities, particularly in CXR and MAMMO

my personal favorite is the bilateral pneumothoraces in an overexposed, too black film!

THE MISSING FILM (contrast, pre contrast, another view)

this is a time honored and legitimate trap (IT IS NOT WHAT I SHOW YOU, IT IS WHAT I DO NOT SHOW YOU THAT MATTERS!)

especially when an examination conventionally consists of a number of runs, sequences or acquisitions, the absence of one should make you question what it is that is on it and not being shown (see the entry on how to earn that extra film)

e.g. post contrast only CT head; cervicothoracic junction not shown on XR, 10 minute IVP/IVU film with no preliminary

THE NAME, TIME, AND SIDE MARKER

if I want to hang you with a film of dextrocardia, I will give you the film to put up yourself, and you will put it up the wrong way around if you do not check the side marker

if you do not read the label, you will assume the two films I have put up for you are from the same date

to make matters worse, I can use the top panel of the X-ray box to hide the label

THE TOO MANY FINDINGS (INFORMATION OVERLOAD)

this is usually applied if you are already doing well, to see how you handle multiple or conflicting findings

SYMPTOMS: that sinking feeling as your short term memory overloads

DEFENSE: '... this is quite an abnormal study that contains many findings, including... I will examine it as quickly as I can, but I will take some time as I need to be thorough ...'

with some luck, you will be directed to specific parts of the examination!

FINDINGS DO NOT MATCH HISTORY

the examiner's history always takes precedence over the film findings; either you have not found something ('WHAT AM I MISSING?'), or you are misinterpreting it ('WHAT ELSE CAN IT BE?') or ... you are correct!

If your findings are confident ones, you need to verbalize the discrepancy: '... findings A and B are unusual in patients presenting with (cardinal symptom), and do not explain it' (pregnant pause)

THE LOGICAL REASONING CASE

this is not a trap film in the usual sense. Detection of findings here is usually not a problem, and they may even be pointed out for you with measurements or arrows. Characterization is also usually straightforward. It is just that the case is a constellation of findings for which you do not know a differential, nor do you recall ever having seen an 'Aunt Minnie' picture.

Such cases are both uncommon and elegant. Take a deep breath: you will need to use reasoning to get through this!

Suggested reading and reference texts

GAMUTS AND LISTS

Bisset RAL, Khan AN and Thomas NB. Differential Diagnosis in Obstetric and Gynecologic Ultrasound. 2nd ed. Saunders, London, 2002.

Chapman S and Nakielny R. Aids to Radiological Differential Diagnosis. 3rd ed. WB Saunders, London, 1995.

Chhem RK and Cardinal E (eds). Guidelines and Gamuts in Musculoskeletal Ultrasound. Wiley-Liss, New York, 1999.

Datz FL. Gamuts in Nuclear Medicine. 3rd ed. Mosby, St Louis, 1995.

HANDBOOKS

Harnsberger HR. Head and Neck Imaging. 2nd ed. Mosby, St Louis, 1995.

Manaster BJ. Handbook of Skeletal Radiology. 2nd ed. Mosby, St Louis, 1997.

Osborn AG and Tong KA. Handbook of Neuroradiology: Brain and Skull. 2nd ed. Mosby, St Louis, 1996.

PATHOLOGY

Basic:
Cotran RS, Kumar V and Robbins T. Robbins' Pathologic Basis of Disease. 6th ed. WB Saunders, Philadelphia, 1998.

Woolf N. Pathology: Basic and Systemic. WB Saunders, London, 1998.

Advanced:
Jaffe ES, Harris NL, Stein H, Vardiman JW (eds). WHO Classification of Tumors: Pathology & Genetics, Tumors of Hematopoietic and Lymphoid Tissues. IARC Press, Lyon, 2001.

Kleihues P and Cavenee WK (eds). WHO Classification of Tumours. Pathology and Genetics. Tumours of the Nervous System. IARC Press, Lyon, 2000.

McGee JO'D, Isaacson PG and Wright NA (eds). Oxford Textbook of Pathology. Oxford University Press, Oxford, 1992.

GENERAL RADIOLOGY AND NUCLEAR MEDICINE TEXTS

Basic:
Brandt WE and Helms CA. Fundamentals of Diagnostic Radiology. 2nd ed. Williams and Wilkins, 2000.

Thrall JH and Zeissman HA. Nuclear Medicine: The Requisites. 2nd ed. Mosby, St Louis, 2001.

Wegener OH. Whole Body Computed Tomography. 2nd ed. Blackwell, Boston, 1992.

Advanced:
Edelman RR, Zlatkin MB and Hesselink JR. Clinical Magnetic Resonance Imaging. 2nd ed. WB Saunders, Philadelphia, 1996.

Grainger RG, Allison DJ, Adam A and Dixon AK. Grainger and Allison's Diagnostic Radiology. 4th ed. Churchill Livingstone, Edinburgh, 2001.

Henkin RE, Boles MA, Dillehay GL, Halama JR, Karesh SM, Wagner RH, Zimmer AM. Nuclear Medicine: Priciples and Practice. Mosby, St Louis, 1996.

Taybi H and Lachman RS. Radiology of Syndromes, Metabolic Disorders and Skeletal Dysplasias. 4th ed. Mosby, St Louis, 1996.

NEURORADIOLOGY

Basic:
Castillo M. Neuroradiology Companion. JB Lippincott, Philadelphia, 1995.

Advanced:
Atlas SW. MRI of the Brain and Spine. 3rd ed. Lippincott-Raven, Philadelphia, 2002.

Kleihues P and Cavenee WK (eds). WHO Classification of Tumours. Pathology and Genetics. Tumours of the Nervous System. IARC Press, Lyon, 2000.

THORACIC RADIOLOGY

Goodman LR. Felson's Principles of Chest Roentgenology. 2nd ed WB Saunders, Philadelphia, 1999.

Webb WR, Muller NL, Naidich DP. High Resolution CT of the Lung. 2nd ed. Lippincott-Raven, Philadelphia, 1996.

GENITOURINARY RADIOLOGY

Barbaric ZL. Principles of Genitourinary Radiology. 2nd ed. Thieme, New York, 1994.

MUSCULOSKELETAL RADIOLOGY

Anderson J, Read JW and Steinweg J. Atlas of Imaging in Sports Medicine. McGraw-Hill, Sydney, 1998.

Harris JH and Harris WH. The Radiology of Emergency Medicine. 4th ed. Williams and Wilkins, Baltimore, 2000.

Martire JR and Levinson EM. Imaging of Athletic Injuries. McGraw Hill, New York, 1992.

Resnick D. Diagnosis of Bone and Joint Disorders. 4th ed. Saunders, Philadelphia, 2002.

PEDIATRIC RADIOLOGY

Graf R. Guide to Sonography of the Infant Hip. Thieme, Stuttgart, 1987.

Kirks DR, Thorne N and Griscom MD. Practical Pediatric Imaging. 3rd ed. Lipincott Williams & Wilkins, 1998.

Meerstadt PWD and Gyll C. Manual of Neonatal Emergency X-Ray Interpretation. WB Saunders, London, 1994.

NUCLEAR CARDIOLOGY

Zaret BL and Beller GA. Nuclear Cardiology: State of the Art and Future Directions. 2nd ed. Mosby, St Louis, 1999.

BREAST RADIOLOGY

Cardenosa G. Breast Imaging Companion. 2nd ed. Lippincott-Raven, Philadelphia, 2000.

Tabar L and Dean PB. Teaching Atlas of Mammography. 3rd ed. Thieme Verlag, Stuttgart, 2000.

OBSTETRIC AND GYNECOLOGIC IMAGING

Basic:
McGahan JP and Porto M. Diagnostic Obstetrical Ultrasound. JB Lippincott, Philadelphia, 1994.

Advanced:
Callen PW. Ultrasonography in Obstetrics and Gynecology. 4th ed. WB Saunders, Philadelphia, 2000.